Laparo-Endoscopic
Surgery

To my family

Laparo-Endoscopic Surgery

Edited by Iris B. Brune

Chirurgische Klinik und Poliklinik der TU-München

Klinikum Rechts der Isar

Munich, Germany

Second edition
revised and extended

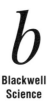

**Blackwell
Science**

© 1996 by
Blackwell Science Ltd
Editorial Offices:
Osney Mead, Oxford OX2 0EL
25 John Street, London WC1N 2BL
23 Ainslie Place, Edinburgh EH3 6AJ
238 Main Street, Cambridge
    Massachusetts 02142, USA
54 University Street, Carlton
    Victoria 3053, Australia

Other Editorial Offices:
Arnette Blackwell SA
    224, Boulevard Saint Germain
    75007 Paris, France

Blackwell Wissenschafts-Verlag GmbH
    Kurfürstendamm 57
    10707 Berlin, Germany

    Zehetnergasse 6
    1140 Vienna
    Austria

First published 1993
Title: *Laparo-Endoskopische Chirurgie*,
edited by Iris B. Brune & K. Schönleben
Publisher: Hans Marseille Verlag GmbH
Munich, Germany
Second edition 1996

Set by Layout und Grafik 1000 GmbH, Munich, Germany
Printed by Druckhaus Darmstadt, Germany
Bound by Fikentscher, Darmstadt, Germany

The Blackwell Science logo is a
trade mark of Blackwell Science Ltd,
registered at the United Kingdom
Trade Marks Registry

DISTRIBUTORS

Marston Book Services Ltd
PO Box 269
Abingdon
Oxon OX14 4YN
(*Orders*:   Tel: 01235 465500
                   Fax: 01235 465555)

USA
Blackwell Science, Inc.
238 Main Street
Cambridge, MA 02142
(*Orders*:   Tel: 800 215-1000
                         617 876-7000
                   Fax: 617 492-5263)

Canada
Copp Clark, Ltd
2775 Matheson Blvd East
Mississauga, Ontario
Canada, L4W 4P7
(*Orders*:   Tel: 800 263-4374
                   Fax: 905 238-6074)

Australia
Blackwell Science Pty Ltd
54 University Street
Carlton, Victoria 3053
(*Orders*:   Tel: 3 9347 0300
                   Fax: 3 9347 5001)

A catalogue record for this title
is available from the British Library

ISBN 0-86542-900-6

Preface, Introduction, the Critical Comments
by J.R. Siewert as well as Chapters 3, 27 and 33
were translated by Suzyon O'Neal Wandrey, Berlin, Germany
Graphics: Rolf Ochs, Karlsruhe and
Dr. med. Katja Dalkowski, Munich, Germany

The figures in Chapter 16 were published by
courtesy of Professor Dr. med. Klaus Schönleben,
Ludwigshafen, Germany

Cover illustrations:
Several methods are available for securing the mesh
to Waldeyer's fascia: the use of the hernia stapler
or intra or extra-abdominally knotted single sutures.

Table of Contents

List of Principal Contributors

Prof. Dr. J.-L. Alain
Service de Chirurgie Pédiatrique
Hôpital Universitaire Dupuytren
2, avenue Martin-Luther-King
87042 Limoges Cedex
France

R. W. Bailey MD
Greater Baltimore Medical Center
6569 N. Charles Street, Suite 708
Baltimore, Maryland 21204
USA

D. H. Birkett MD
Department of Gastrointestinal Surgery and Surgical
Endoscopy
Boston University Medical Center Hospital
88 East Newton Street
Boston, Massachusetts 02118-2393
USA

Prof. M. A. Bruhat
13, boulevard Charles-De-Gaulle
6300 Clermont-Ferrand Cedex 1
France

Dr. I. B. Brune
Chirurgische Klinik und Poliklinik der TU München
Klinikum Rechts der Isar
Ismaninger Straße 22
81675 Munich
Germany

John A. Coller MD
Lahey Clinic
41 Mall Road, Box 541
Burlington, Massachusetts 01805
USA

J. F. Donovan Jr. MD
Department of Urology
University of Iowa
200 Hawkins Drive
Iowa City, Iowa 52242
USA

Dr. J.-L. Dulucq
Maison de Santé Protestante
de Bordeaux Bagatelle
203, route de Toulouse
33401 Talence Cédex
France

Priv. Doz. Dr. H. Feussner
Chirurgische Klinik und Poliklinik der TU München
Klinikum Rechts der Isar
Ismaninger Straße 22
81675 Munich – Germany

M. Gagner MD
Department of General Surgery
Cleveland Clinic Foundation
9500 Euclid Avenue
Cleveland, Ohio 44195
USA

R. J. Ginsberg MD
Department of Thoracic Surgery
Memorial Sloan Kettering Cancer Center
1275 York Avenue, Suite C 881
New York, New York 10021
USA

P. Goh MD
Minimally Invasive Surgical Centre
National University Hospital
5 Lower Kent Ridge Road
Singapore 0511

Prof. Dr. K. T. Hell-Türler
Chirurgische Abteilung
Medizinische Fakultät
Universität Basel
Dammerkirchstraße 32
4056 Bâle
Switzerland

J. G. Hunter MD
Department of Surgery
Emory University School of Medicine
1364 Clifton Road, N.E.
Atlanta, Georgia 30322
USA

G. H. Jordan MD
400 West Brambleton Avenue,
Suite 100
Norfolk, Virginia 23510
USA

Prof. Dr. F. Köckerling
Chirurgische Klinik und Poliklinik
der Universität Erlangen-Nürnberg
Maximiliansplatz 1
91054 Erlangen – Germany

M. Mack MD
Cardiothoracic Surgery – Associates of North Texas, P. A.
7777 Forest Lane C 202
Dallas, Texas 75230
USA

C. K. McSherry MD
525 East, 86th Street
New York, New York 10028
USA

Dr. A. L. de Paula
Department of Surgery – Hospital Samaritano
Pça. Walter Santos no. 1
Setor Coimbra
CEP 74535-270 Goiânia – GO
Brasil

Prof. Dr. J. Périssat
Service de chirurgie digestive
Centre de chirurgie Laparoscopique
Maison du Haut l'Evêque
Avenue de Magellan
33604 Pessac Cedex
France

Dr. J. Rassweiler
Urologische Abteilung – Städtisches Krankenhaus Heilbronn
Jägerhausstraße 26
74074 Heilbronn
Germany

R. J. Rosenthal MD
Division of Endoscopic Surgery
Cedars-Sinai Medical Center
Los Angeles, California 90048
USA

S. Rubin MD
Department of Pediatric Surgery
Children's Hospital of Ontario
401 Smyth
Ottawa, Ontario K1H 8L1
Canada

A. A. Ryberg MD
Department of Surgery
Creighton University School of Medicine
601 North 30th Street
Omaha, Nebraska 68131
USA

Prof. Dr. Dr. h. c. mult. Kurt Semm
Perlacherstraße 24
82031 Munich
Germany

Prof. Dr. J. R. Siewert
Chirurgische Klinik und Poliklinik der TU München
Klinikum Rechts der Isar
Ismaninger Straße 22
81675 Munich
Germany

A. D. Smith MD
Department of Urology – Long Island Jewish Medical Center
270-05 76th Avenue
New Hyde Park, New York 10040
USA

L. E. Smith MD
Department of Surgery
George Washington University
2150 Pennsylvania Avenue
Washington, D.C. 20087
USA

Prof. Dr. R. Stoppa
Clinique chircurgicale de L'Université Amiens
Hôpital Nord
Place Victor Pauchet
80054 Amiens Cedex 1
France

Prof. Dr. M. Trede
Chirurgische Klinik
Klinikum Mannheim
Universität Heidelberg
Theodor-Kutzer-Ufer 1-3
68167 Mannheim
Germany

Dr. A. Ungeheuer
Chirurgische Klinik und Poliklinik der TU München
Klinikum Rechts der Isar
Ismaninger Straße 22
81675 Munich
Germany

Prof. Dr. J. Waldschmidt
Abteilung für Kinderchirurgie
Freie Universität Berlin
Universitätsklinikum Benjamin Franklin
Hindenburgdamm 30
12200 Berlin
Germany

Dr. J. M. Weerts
Department of Surgery
Clinique St.-Joseph
75, rue de Hesbaye
4000 Liège
Belgium

S. D. Wexner MD
Department of Colorectal Surgery
Cleveland Clinic Florida
3000 West Cyprus Creek Road
Fort Lauderdale, Florida 33309
USA

K. A. Zucker MD
Department of Surgery
Presbyterian Hospital
718 Encino Place
Albuquerque, New Mexico 87131
USA

Preface

Laparoscopic surgery started in 1989 and spread throughout the surgical world within an incredibly short time due to the success of laparoscopic cholecystectomy. Meanwhile, we can look back on 7 years of experience and a considerable number of patients in basic techniques such as appendectomy and cholecystectomy. The operative techniques as well as the equipment have much improved during this time.

Development is still progressing, but at a much slower pace than in the beginning and in certain fields, a steady state seems to be close. For this reason, the time has come to evaluate the place of laparoscopy among the different therapeutic options. In which indications is laparoscopic surgery considered the treatment of first choice, where is it a valuable alternative to conventional surgery, and where is it still in the clinical experimental stages? Which procedures are suitable for widespread use (provided the surgeon has adequate training and experience in open surgery as well as in laparoscopy) and which operations should – at least for the moment – be performed only in specialized centers within clinical trials?

To answer these questions, this book includes critical comments from leading "conventional surgeons" and gives their opinion on the role of laparoscopy today as compared to other therapeutic alternatives, particularly with respect to conventional open surgery. Another question that has been resolved and warrants critical discussion is the use of laparoscopy for malignant disease. While the patient obviously seems to benefit from the minimally invasive access in palliative procedures, laparoscopy for cure of a malignancy is still far from being considered oncologically safe. This becomes evident when one considers that only a few of the 30–40 % of surgeons who would consider approaching colonic cancer by laparoscopy in their patients would choose the laparoscopic option if they had a colonic carcinoma themselves.

The precursor of this book was published in 1993. In the last 3 years, further developments have been made, but maybe not always in the predicted ways. Laparoscopic cholecystectomy has become the treatment of choice for symptomatic gallstones, just as everybody expected it to. Laparoscopic colon surgery, on the other hand, is evolving very slowly, probably due to the higher degree of technical difficulty and the justified hesitance against laparoscopic surgery for malignant disease. Therefore, contrary to the general expectations, laparoscopic colon surgery cannot be considered a routine technique in every situation.

This book is still far from defining the place of laparoscopy once and for all: its goal is to present the surgeon with the spectrum of operations performed via a minimally invasive access today without laying claim to completeness. Each operative technique has been extensively described and illustrated. This work will hopefully contribute to the knowledge and information of the surgeon, but it can never replace practical experience. Therefore this book should be considered to be an additional aid to practical hands-on courses and operations under the assistance of an experienced laparoscopist.

Dr. Iris B. Brune

General Considerations

1. Introduction

J. R. SIEWERT

Introductory passages should define the path of a book and accompany it throughout the years. This book is dedicated to minimally invasive surgery. It is very difficult, if not impossible, to point it in "the right direction". However, this book appears to be on the right track. The authors have described all currently tried and tested and, for the most part, standardized minimally invasive operative techniques. However, their primary goal was not to weigh these techniques, but simply to comment on them. The result is a virtual kaleidoscope of the current technical possibilities – it is a true reference book of minimally invasive techniques, and: "He who searches will find".

The preface to a book should also accompany it throughout the years. This raises the question: "Which of the facts presented here are of lasting value?". Minor access surgery will stand its ground in any area where the effects of creating an access for open surgery are out of proportion with the expected benefits of the operation. You do not have to be a prophet to foresee this. Partial incision of the abdominal wall is weighted differently in different cases, e.g., depending on whether one simply plans to remove the gallbladder or perform a complex operation in accordance with established oncological principles. The case of thoracotomy is similar, and the neurosurgical situation is the most convincing. The challenge of operating through a trocar has led to the development of new surgical procedures, the modification of proven techniques of open surgery, and the revival of previously discarded surgical procedures. However, one should be careful to avoid a re-make of the previous mistakes of conventional surgery. Minimally invasive techniques should not be developed so as to avoid or be contrary to the established principles of open surgery, but rather, they should be designed as a continuation of classical surgery with new and different methods. With mutual promotion and assistance, minimally invasive surgery will find its niche and become firmly established there. Otherwise, two techniques that differ only in their access will drift apart – a situation which no surgeon should wish for. The goal should be to avoid having two indications and two different measures of operative success.

In this respect, this book is a contemporary document that describes the current possibilities in minimally invasive surgery. It is an indispensable almanac for any surgeon who already practices minimally invasive surgery or wishes to do so. It is valid today: by the time the next edition is published (which I hope will be the case), many of the described procedures will still be around and various new procedures will have been introduced. However, future possibilities should still be discussed when compiling a state-of-the-art report. The editors must be commended in enlisting truly competent authors, which has allowed the book to achieve the highest standards.

May minimally invasive surgery find maximally invasive and wide-spread success!

Munich, April 1996

2. Historical Development of Laparoscopic Surgery

I. B. BRUNE

An Arabic doctor named Abdul Qasim, living in Cordoba during the 10th century (936-1013), is believed to have performed the first endoscopy in the human body [36]: He inspected the cervix uteri using a speculum. The light was provided by reflection in a glass mirror.

However, the first laparoscopic report dates from the beginning of the 20th century. On September 23, 1901, Georg Kelling, a surgeon from Dresden, Germany, presented a report in Hamburg entitled "The Inspection of the Oesophagus and the Stomach with Flexible Instruments". That same year he published an article on "Oesophagoscopy, Gastroscopy and Coelioscopy" in the *Münchner Medizinische Wochenschrift* [20]. He performed the laparoscopy, or as he termed it, coelioscopy, using an angled cystoscope developed by Max Nitze in 1877 (Fig. 1). After creating a pneumoperitoneum with the insufflation of air that was filtered through sterile cotton, he inspected the abdominal cavity in dogs. With the help of a "Fiedler Trocar" organs were palpated and the liver was lifted up.

Also, in 1901 D. O. Ott, a gynaecologist from Petrograd, Russia, reported on "Ventroscopic Illumination of the Abdominal Cavity During Pregnancy" using culdoscopy. The light was provided by a mirror fixed on his forehead [23].

Hans-Christian Jacobaeus from Sweden wrote about "The Possibility of Using Cystoscopy for Examination of Serous Cavities" in 1901 [15] and reported on 69 patients in whom he had performed 109 laparoscopies. He inspected the intra-abdominal organs and watched the peristaltic activity of the small bowel. Already at this time he had pointed out the danger of intestinal injury causing peritonitis from blind puncturing of the abdominal cavity.

Bertram M. Bernheim from the United States published a paper entitled "Organoscopy: Cystoscopy of the Abdominal Cavity" [3]. He performed a diagnostic laparoscopy with the help of a proctoscope. C. Fervers used oxygen to produce a pneumoperitoneum [8], but while coagulating adhesions caused an intra-abdominal explosion that fortunately caused no injury. Carbon dioxide was first used in 1924 by R. Zollikofer from Switzerland to create a pneumoperitoneum [40]. It was the introduction of carbon dioxide that made the use of electrocoagulation possible in laparoscopic surgery.

In 1929 H. Kalk from Germany published "Experience with Laparoscopy Together with the Description of a New Instrument" [18]. The new instrument was a laparoscope with a 135° angled view that he used for diagnostic laparoscopy to inspect the liver and peritoneum. One of his major indications for diagnostic laparoscopy was carcinoma of the gallbladder. He also performed biopsies of spleen and liver. In 1935 Kalk reported on 300 laparoscopies with only one complication, which was a colonic perforation [19].

In 1934 J. C. Ruddock, an American internist, developed a new lens system with an integrated biopsy forceps, which he used during "Peritoneoscopy" for taking liver biopsies [29]. Janos Veress from Hungary presented his "New Instrument for Puncture of the Thoracic or Abdominal Cavity and Pneumothorax Therapy" in 1938. Presently, the Veress needle is still the most commonly used device for the creation of a pneumoperitoneum.

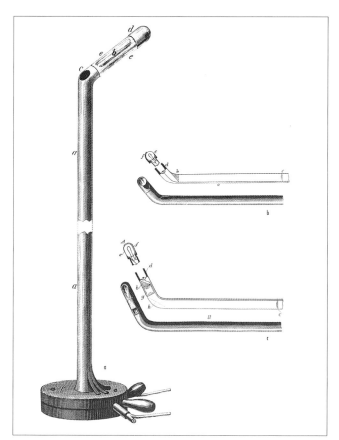

Fig. 1. Cystoscope developed by Max Nitze in 1877. The instrument had a diameter of 21 Charrière and was provided at the end with a platinum wire (b) that was covered by a glass tube (e). The endoscope was cooled by an irrigation system

M. Royer in Argentina and W.Y. Lee in the United States independently in 1941 performed laparoscopic cholecystographies by instilling contrast medium. In 1955 L. Wannagat pursued laparoscopic radiological diagnostic studies, and developed laparoscopic splenoportography and transhepatic cholangiography.

The first report on intraoperative monitoring of the intra-abdominal pressure was by Raoul Palmer from France in 1947 in "Techniques and Instrumentation in gynecological Coelioscopy" [24]. Initially, Palmer performed culdoscopy with the patient in the kneeling position, but because of poor results he gradually changed to laparoscopy with the patient in the Trendelenburg position and with a pneumoperitoneum [25].

The importance of a constant intra-abdominal pressure was recognized in the 1960s [7]. Great progress was achieved by the gynaecologist Kurt Semm from Germany when he developed an automatic pressure-regulated insufflator that kept the intra-abdominal pressure at a constant preset level throughout the operation.

Initially, the main purpose of laparoscopy was that of diagnosis with biopsy capability. The first therapeutic procedure was lysis of adhesions [8]. Therapeutic laparoscopy was championed by Kurt Semm in the field of gynaecology for some time prior to its extension into gastrointestinal surgery [32]. Publications by Frangenheim in 1965 [9], Steptoe in 1967 [35] and Hulka in 1976 [14] illustrated the progress made over these years. However, throughout the 1960s and 1970s there were only a few publications on gastrointestinal laparoscopy [10, 11].

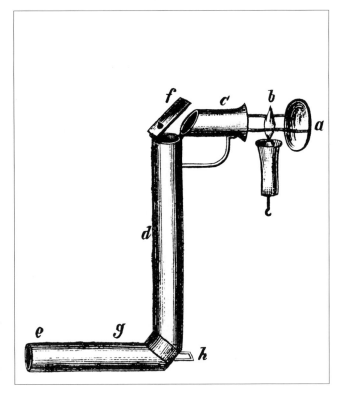

Fig. 2. Angled cystoscope created by John D. Fisher in 1827. The light of a candle (b) is reflected by a convex lens (a) on a mirror, (f) and another convex lens is placed in the horizontal part of the instrument

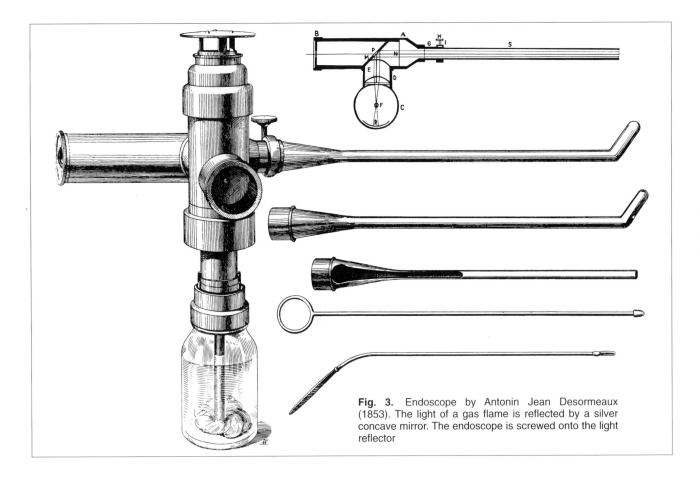

Fig. 3. Endoscope by Antonin Jean Desormeaux (1853). The light of a gas flame is reflected by a silver concave mirror. The endoscope is screwed onto the light reflector

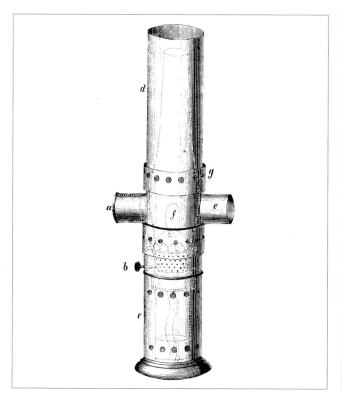

Fig. 4. Ernst Fürstenheim modified the Desormeaux endoscope and placed an oil lamp in a metal sheath

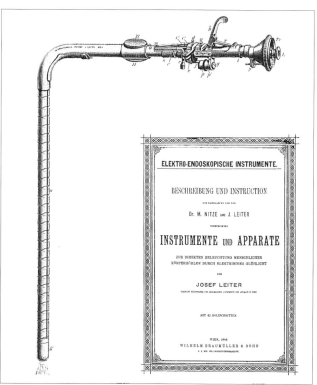

Fig. 5. Oesophagoscope designed by Max Nitze and produced by Josef Leitner in 1880. Later the "Lobster-tail" construction was covered with a rubber tube to avoid lesion of the mucosa

To reduce injury to the bowel from the blind placement of the first trocar using the method originally described by Jacobaeus in 1910, Hasson developed the technique of open access to the peritoneal cavity in 1974 [13].

With the improvement of non-invasive diagnostic modalities, such as ultrasonography, CT scanning and MRI, as well as CT scan or ultrasound-guided puncture techniques, the importance of laparoscopy for diagnostic purposes became less. In the 1970s and 1980s laparoscopy was mainly considered an alternative to peritoneal lavage or exploratory laparotomy in abdominal emergencies or for patients with abdominal pain in whom non-invasive diagnostic procedures did not provide the diagnosis [2].

Laparoscopic therapeutic procedures were well established in gynaecology [14] when in 1978 the first tentative gastrointestinal therapeutic procedures were performed. Cholecystotomy and later cholecystectomy were first performed in the animal model [6, 26, 27]. Progress in the early 1980s was slow with the first laparoscopic appendectomies in patients being performed by Semm [31] in Germany and Mouret in France in 1983.

In 1988 French authors Jaques Périssat [27], Francois Dubois [6] and Philippe Mouret reported the first laparoscopic cholecystectomies in patients. Périssat developed the technique of percutaneous cholecystostomy with lithotripsy in 1989 [27]. In that same year Reddick and Olsen in the United States described the use of laser dissection during laparoscopic cholecystectomy [28].

After this slow and tedious evolution, which took nearly one century, laparoscopic surgery developed in an explosive manner following the first laparoscopic cholecystectomy. This rev-

olution in the surgical world became significantly patient driven once they realized the obvious benefits of laparoscopy compared with the large incision of an open operation. On the other hand, industry made rapid technical progress possible by adapting to surgical demand and supplying the "high-tech" equipment that became more necessary for laparoscopy than for an open operation.

Between 1990 and 1991, laparoscopic cholecystectomy changed from being an experimental procedure to the method of choice for treatment of uncomplicated gallbladder stones. As surgeons became more experienced with laparoscopy, the number of procedures performed laparoscopically grew. However, the use of laparoscopy as the method of access for a significant number of procedures, such as intestinal resection, splenectomy or nephrectomy, cannot yet be considered to be routine or the first method of choice. The results of these operations need to be critically evaluated in controlled studies particularly for the treatment of a potentially curable malignancy.

Development of Laparoscopic Instruments

One of the first endoscopes was the angled instrument designed by John D. Fisher in 1827 [12], which used a candle and reflecting mirrors for illumination (Fig. 2). Antonin Jean Desormeaux [5] equipped his endoscope with a gas lamp (Fig. 3). In 1863 Ernst Fürstenheim [12] modified and simplified this device (Fig. 4). At the end of the nineteenth century, a gastroscope was produced by Josef Leitner [21] with the advice of Max Nitze in 1880 (Fig. 5) and Johann von Mikulicz in 1881 (Figs. 6 and 7).

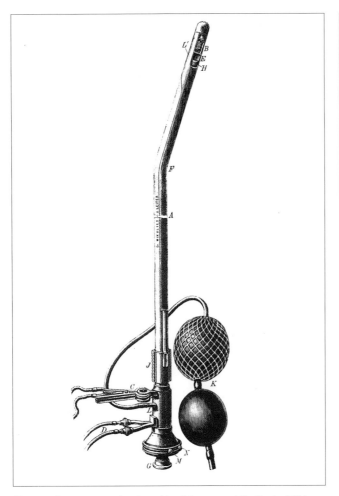

Fig. 6. Gastroscope developed by Johann von Mikulicz in 1881

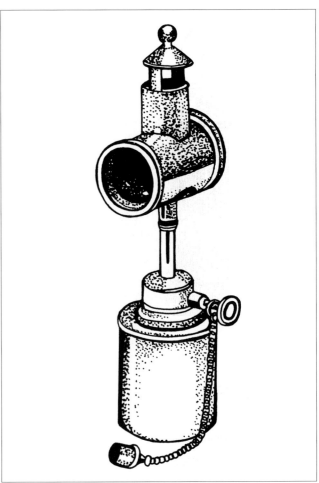

Fig. 8. Extracorporeal endoscopic light source: The light of a candle was reflected by a silver-plated mirror

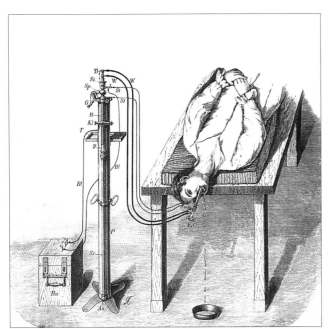

Fig. 7. Gastroscopy with a rigid endoscope in 1883. The procedure was quite painful and often compared with "swallowing a sword"

The instrument available to Kelling in 1901 for his first "Coelioscopy" was a cystoscope with an angled view, which was developed by Max Nitze (Fig. 1) in 1872 [22]. The instrument was designed and produced by Josef Leitner (1830-1892) in Vienna, Austria [21]. The first laparoscope with a 0° forward view was introduced by W. Kremer in 1927. H. Kalk developed a prograde optical system with an angle of 135° [18]. The solid-rod lens system developed by Hopkins in 1959 remains the current standard, and is the heart of the excellent laparoscopes available from the Karl Storz Company.

The first extracorporeal light source was developed by R.P. Arnaud (1651-1723), a French surgeon and gynaecologist [1, 30]: It was made of a candle in a silver-plated box that reflected the light with the help of a convex lens in one beam (Fig. 8). The first intracorporeal light sources were provided by an incandescent platinum wire attached to the tip of the laparoscope, which was inserted into the abdominal cavity. Gustave Trouvé [37, 38] presented his "polyscope" with a platinum wire at the tip in 1873 in Vienna (Figs. 9 and 10). Max Nitze and Josef Leitner developed their "Electro-endoscopic instruments" in 1883 (Fig. 11). In 1886 small Edison-Mignon lamps were fixed on the endoscope.

Only in 1964 was the first cold light developed, in which light was generated by an extracorporeal light source and transmitted through flexible glass fibres (Fig. 12).

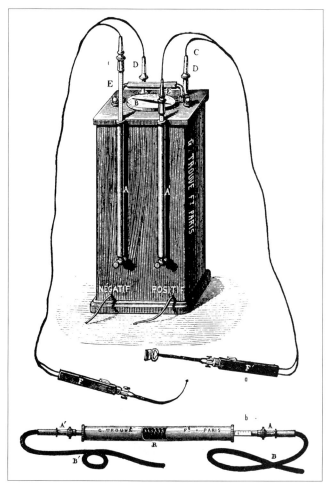

Fig. 9. Polyscope invented by Gustave Trouvé in 1873: The intensity of the electric current and therefore the brightness of the incandescent platinum wire was regulated by a "rheostat"

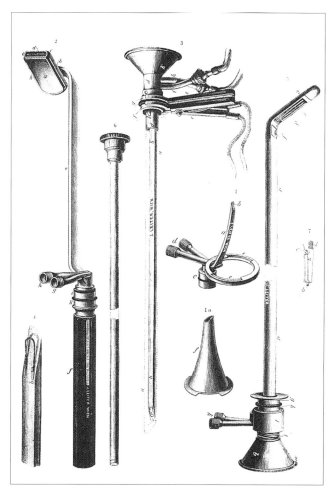

Fig. 11. The "electro-endoscopic" instruments of Max Nitze and Josef Leitner (1883). From left to right: light source of the enteroscope, laryngoscope, cystoscope (180°), urethroscope, otoscope, cystoscope (90°) and an exchange platinum wire

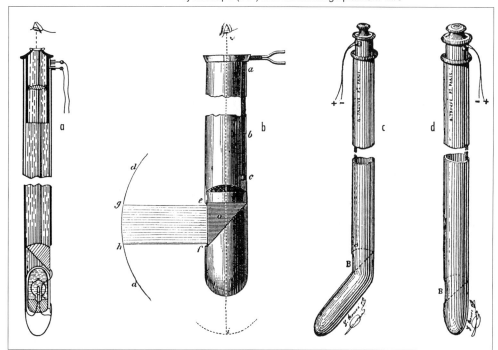

Fig. 10. The "polyscope" was designed for gastroscopy and cystoscopy. The incandescent platinum wire at the tip provided a bright illumination, but produced so much heat that the examination had to be limited to 20 s

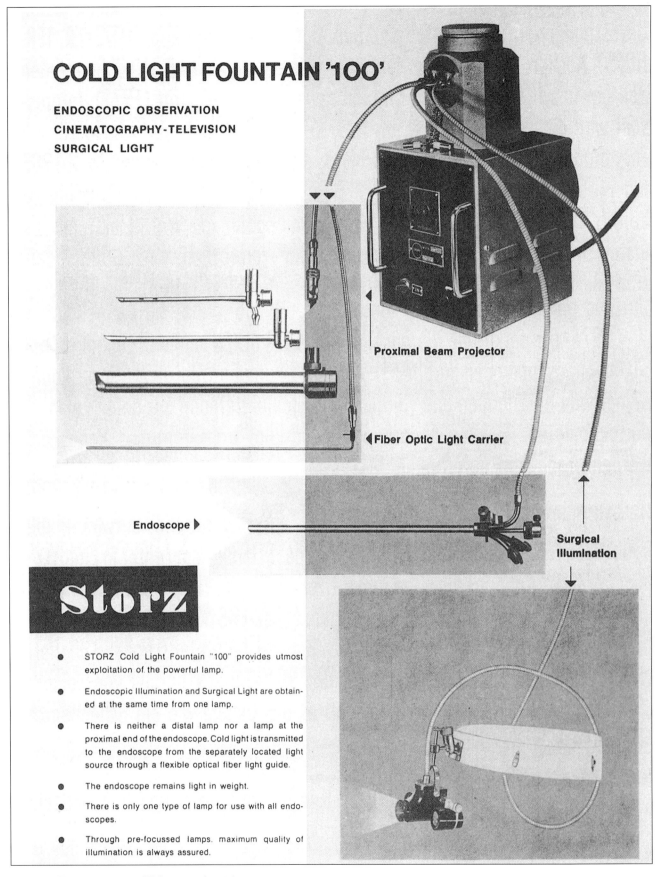

COLD LIGHT FOUNTAIN '100'

ENDOSCOPIC OBSERVATION
CINEMATOGRAPHY-TELEVISION
SURGICAL LIGHT

Proximal Beam Projector

◀ **Fiber Optic Light Carrier**

Endoscope ▶

Surgical Illumination

Storz

- STORZ Cold Light Fountain "100" provides utmost exploitation of the powerful lamp.

- Endoscopic Illumination and Surgical Light are obtained at the same time from one lamp.

- There is neither a distal lamp nor a lamp at the proximal end of the endoscope. Cold light is transmitted to the endoscope from the separately located light source through a flexible optical fiber light guide.

- The endoscope remains light in weight.

- There is only one type of lamp for use with all endoscopes.

- Through pre-focussed lamps, maximum quality of illumination is always assured.

Fig. 12.   First extracorporeal light source fountain

Imaging and Documentation

The problem surrounding the documentation of endoscopic procedures was recognized early in the development of endoscopy. Early endoscopic photographs of his own larynx were taken by Johann Nepomuk Czermak in 1858 (Fig. 13) [4].

In 1874 Theodor S. Stein [33, 34] was taking photographs of pathological conditions found at cystoscopy with a camera that he modified for the purpose (Figs. 14 and 15). Jacobaeus in 1912 included eight black-and-white and five colour laparoscopic drawings in his monograph, whereas Korbsch illustrated his "Lehrbuch und Atlas der Laparo- und Thorakoskopie" in 1927 with 17 aquarels of laparoscopic pictures.

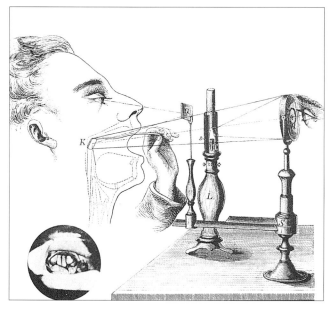

Fig. 13. In 1858, Johann Nepomuk Czermak performed laryngoscopy on himself and took a photograph of his own larynx

In 1931 Hennings developed a camera that could be mounted on a gastroscope. He also used this camera for laparoscopic photography. The first laparoscopic black-and-white photographs were published by Kalk in 1942, followed shortly by coloured pictures. To obtain ideal light conditions, Caroli and Foures first used an intracorporeal electronic flash in 1955.

After initial trials of black-and-white television transmission (Stoichita and Steclaci), early laparoscopic operations were projected onto a color TV screen in 1968 by Kalk and Lindner in Hamburg. Presently, excellent image quality can be produced in RGB or Betacam format with the only drawback being the cost of equipment.

References

1. ARNAUD GA: Mémoires de chirurgie, avec quelques remarques historiques sur l´état de la médecine et de la chirurgie en France et en Angleterre. London, Paris (1768).
2. BERCI G: Endoscopy. Appleton-Century-Crofts, New York (1976).
3. BERNHEIM BM: Organoscopy: cystoscopy of the abdominal cavity. Ann Surg 53 (1911) 764-767.
4. CZERMAK JN: Gesammelte Schriften, Leipzig (1879).

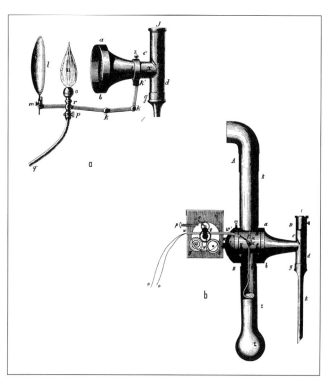

Fig. 14. The "photoendoscope" designed by Theodor S. Stein in 1874. The light was provided by a gas flame

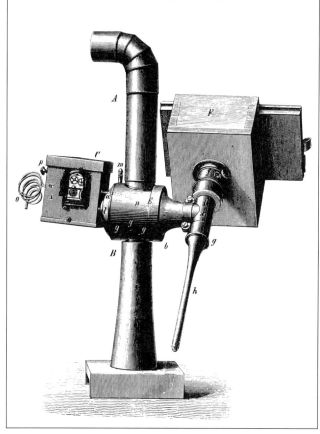

Fig. 15. The endo-camera by Stein called "Heliopiktor" with a magnesium flashlight for endo-photography

5. DESORMEAUX AJ: De l´endoscope et de ses applications au diagnostic et au traitement des affections de l´urèthre et de la vessie. Paris (1865).
6. DUBOIS F, BERTHELOT G, LEVARD H: Cholécystectomie par coelioscopie. Nouv.Presse Méd.18 (1989) 980-982.
7. EISENBURG J: Über eine Apparatur zur schonenden und kontrollierten Gasfüllung der Bauchhöhle für die Laparoskopie. KlinWochenschr 44 (1966) 593.
8. FERVERS C: Die Laparoskopie mit dem Cystoskop. Med Klin 31 (1933) 1042-1045.
9. FRANGENHEIM H: Die Coelioskopie in der Unterbauchchirurgie. Dtsch Med Wochenschr 43 (1965) 1909-1911.
10. GOMEL V: Laparoscopy. Can Med Assoc J 111 (1974) 167-169.
11. GOMEL V: Laparoscopy in general surgery. Am J Surg 131 (1976) 319-323.
12. GRÜNFELD J: Zur Geschichte der Endoskopie und der endoskopischen Apparate Mediz Jahrb, Wien (1879) 237-291.
13. HASSON HM: Open laparoscopy: a report of 150 cases. J Reprod Med 12 (1974) 234-238.
14. HULKA JF et al.: Spring clip sterilization: one year follow-up of 1079 cases. Am J Obstet Gynecol 125 (1976) 1039-1043.
15. JACOBAEUS HC: Über die Möglichkeit die Zystoskopie bei Untersuchung seröser Höhlungen anzuwenden. Münch Med.Wochenschr 57 (1910) 2090-2092.
16. JACOBAEUS HC: Kurze Übersicht über meine Erfahrungen mit der Laparo-Thorakoskopie. Münch Med Wochenschr 58 (1911) 2017-2019.
17. JACOBAEUS HC: Über Laparo- und Thorakoskopie. In: Brauer (ed.): Beiträge zur Klinik der Tuberkulose und spezifischen Tuberkuloseforschung. Kabitzsch, Würzburg (1912).
18. KALK H: Erfahrungen mit der Laparoskopie (zugleich mit der Beschreibung eines neuen Instrumentes). Z Klin Med 111 (1929) 303-348.
19. KALK H: Indikationsstellung und Gefahrenmomente bei der Laparoskopie. Dtsch Med Wochenschr 46 (1935) 1831-1833.
20. KELLING G: Über Oesophagoskopie, Gastroskopie und Koelioskopie. Münch Med Wochenschr 49 (1901) 21-24.
21. LEITNER J: Elektroendoskopische Instrumente. Wien (1880).
22. NITZE M: Eine neue Beobachtungs- und Untersuchungsmethode für Harnröhre, Harnblase und Rektum. Wiener Med Wochenschr 24 (1879) 649-652.
23. OTT DO: Ventroscopic illumination of the abdominal cavity in pregnancy. Z Akush Zhenskikh Boleznei 15 (1901) 7-8.
24. PALMER R: Technique et instrumentation de la coelioscopie gynécologique. Gynecol Obstet 46 (1947) 420.
25. PALMER R: La stérilité involontaire en France et dans le monde. Masson, Paris (1950).
26. PÉRISSAT J et al.: Laparoscopic treatment for gallbladder stones and the place of intracorporeal lithotripsy. Surg Endosc 4 (1990) 135-136.
27. PÉRISSAT J et al.: Laparoscopic cholecystectomy: gateway to the future. Am J Surg 161 (1991) 408.
28. REDDICK EJ et al.: Laparoscopic laser cholecystectomy. Laser Med Surg News Adv (1989) 38-40.
29. RUDDOCK JC: Peritoneoscopy. West J Surg 42 (1934) 392-405.
30. SEGAL A: La longue histoire de l´endoscopie. Tribune Médicale, April 20-27.
31. SEMM K: Endoscopic appendicectomy. Endoscopy 15 (1983) 59-64.
32. SEMM K: Operative pelviscopy. Br Med Bull 42 (1986) 284-295.
33. STEIN ST: Der Heliopiktor, automatisch-photographischer Apparat zur Darstellung von mikroskopischen, anatomischen und chirurgischen Abbildungen. Berl Klin Wochenschr 46 (1873) 551-552.
34. STEIN ST: Das Photo-Endoskop. Berl Klin Wochenschr 47 (1874) 31-33.
35. STEPTOE PC: Laparoscopy in gynecology. Livingstone, Edinburgh (1967).
36. TOELLNER R: Illustrierte Geschichte der Medizin. Salzburg (1986).
37. TROUVÉ G: Polyscope électrique et lampe de sureté pour poudrières et mines. Les Mondes 44 (1877) 611-615.
38. TROUVÉ G: Manuel d´électrologie médicale. Paris (1893).
39. VERESS J: Neues Instrument zur Ausführung von Brust- oder Bauchpunktionen und Pneumothoraxbehandlung. Dtsch. Med. Wochenschr 64 (1938) 1480-1481.
40. ZOLLIKOFER R: Zur Laparoskopie. Schweiz Med Wochenschr 5 (1924) 264-265.

3. | The Pneumoperitoneum – Errors and Risks

K. SEMM

Introduction

An operated abdomen was considered a contraindication to routine laparoscopic liver diagnosis as developed by Kalk in 1926. Massive intestinal and omental adhesions due to blunt abdominal trauma may also be present in the nonoperated abdomen. Since adhesions often remain undetected, blind puncture of the abdomen is always very risky, regardless of whether one is inserting a Veress insufflation needle or a 5 mm examining trocar (O.D.).

Trocars with an outside diameter of 10 mm should never be inserted primarily.

Preconditions

Nowadays, techniques are available which permit the insertion of puncture instruments into the abdomen under visual control in virtually any patient. If careful attention is paid to the techniques as well as to the safety measures and security tests described below, pneumoperitoneum can be induced in over 99 % of all patients without creating any particular risk for the patient.

Mistakes in the induction of pneumoperitoneum

The induction of pneumoperitoneum has been tried and tested millions of times. However, serious injuries resulting in the death of the patient or lawsuits occur again and again. These injuries can be prevented.

Selection of an unsuitable puncture site for the Veress needle

The caudal region of the umbilical fossa is the ideal needle insertion site in over 95 % of all patients. Because hardly any fat accumulates underneath the umbilical fossa, the abdominal wall is thinnest there (Fig. 1).

If attempts to create a pneumoperitoneum in the umbilical region are unsuccessful, an alternative site must be found. The insufflation needle may, for example, be inserted in the posterior vaginal fornix (Fig. 2) or in any site in the abdomen up to the costal arch. The *Quadro-Test* can help the surgeon to find an adhesion-free area under "physiological vision" in 99 % of all patients.

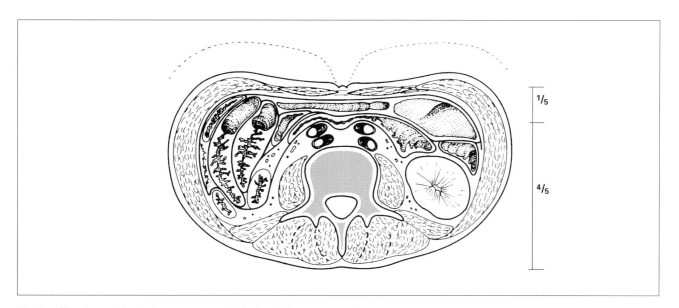

Fig. 1. Slice through the body at approximately the level of the umbilicus (see also Fig. 9). Hardly any fat is located underneath the umbilicus. The broken line indicates the potential locations of fatty deposits

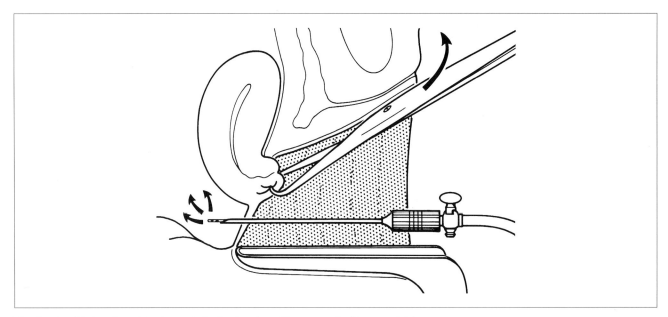

Fig. 2. Insufflation of gas into the posterior fornix using a Veress needle *(frozen pelvis)*

Failure to observe safety measures

Nine safety measures have been developed. They allow the laparoscopic surgeon to safely induce pneumoperitoneum in up to 99 % of all patients without creating any particular risk of vascular or intestinal injury. This high success rate can even be achieved in operated abdomens with massive adhesions, *e.g.,* in patients with a history of peritonitis.

Note: The nine safety measures described below are sometimes modified or omitted by the individual surgeon. However, Laparoscopy/Pelviscopy was discredited prior to the introduction of these safety measures.

Equipment test (Fig. 3)

A proper insufflator must be able to gauge the four physical parameters included in the Quadro-Test (Fig. 4).
1. **Insufflation pressure**, which is the pressure required to transport the gas to the tip of the Veress needle
2. **Gas flow per minute**, which is the amount of gas entering the abdominal cavity per minute
3. **Intra-abdominal pressure**, which is the current pressure, *i.e.*, static pressure, in the induced intra-abdominal bubble
4. **Gas volume used**, which is 1) the size of the intra-abdominal gas bubble and 2) the total amount of gas instilled into the abdominal cavity

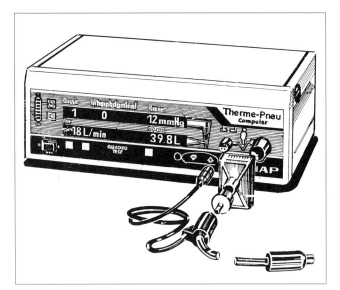

Fig. 3. The gauges on the insufflator measure the following four physical measurement parameters: insufflation pressure in mmHg, intra-abdominal pressure in mmHg, the current gas flow rate in liters per minute, and the total gas volume used in liters

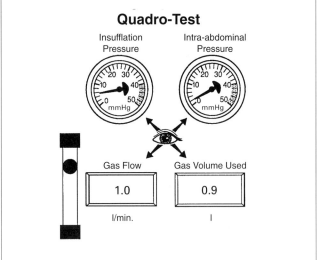

Fig. 4. Quadro-Test: The abdomen is filled "under physiological vision" by simultaneously gauging the four physical measurement parameters. The insufflation pressure indicates the position of the tip of the needle.

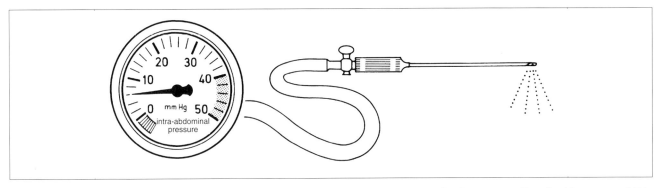

Fig. 5. Needle test to determine the inherent resistance of the tube and the Veress needle. Pressure reading should not exceed 5 to 7 mmHg at a gas flow rate of 1 L/min

Needle test (Fig. 5)

Before starting the procedure, the insufflation needle and its spring-loaded stylet must be checked to ensure that they are functioning properly. That is that they spring back into position properly. At a gas flow rate of 1 L/min, including the insufflation tube, the insufflation pressure reading should never be in excess of 5 to 7 mmHg of the free atmospheric pressure. An unclean needle or water in the gas-carrying tube are two reasons for higher resistance.

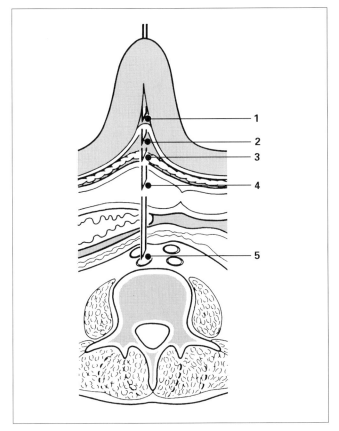

Fig. 6. The tip of the needle can be positioned in the following locations: 1. Preperitoneal → preperitoneal emphysema. 2. Subperitoneal → pneumoperitoneum. 3. Greater omentum → omental emphysema. 4. Intestine → intestinal or gastric flatulence. 5. Retroperitoneal → vessel puncture with gas embolism or → mediastinal emphysema

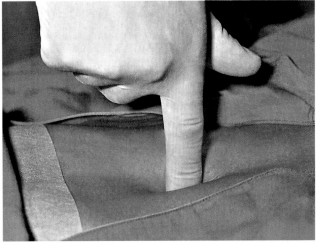

Fig. 7. Palpation of the aorta, *i.e.*, of its bifurcation site, through the umbilicus and against the spine

Correction techniques: Turn the switch to maximum gas flow for a few seconds, then repeat the test at a gas flow rate of 1L/min. If the insufflation pressure still exceeds 8 mmHg, change the needle or the gas-carrying tube.

Explanation: The flow resistance should be equal to the atmospheric pressure when the needle is located between the parietal peritoneum and visceral peritoneum, *i.e.*, in the free abdominal cavity. The pressure gauge registers increased insufflation pressure when the tip of the needle is lodged against any structure.

The increased pressure reading tells the surgeon that the tip of the needle is not in the free peritoneal cavity, but in a confined area, *e.g.*, the omentum, the preperitoneum, or a loop of the bowel (Fig. 6).

The insufflation pressure reading provides the operating surgeon the most important information in the initial phase of pneumoperitoneum induction. Without this reading, the operator would be unable to recognize obstruction of insufflation.

Aorta palpation test (Fig. 7)

Injury to the greater trunk vessels (aorta, vena cava, common iliac arteries and veins) is the greatest danger in abdominal

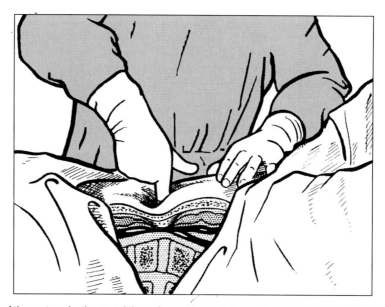

Fig. 8. Schematic diagram of the aorta palpation test. It is performed by applying moderate pressure with the tip of the index finger

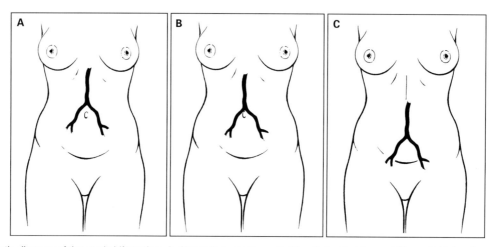

Fig. 9. Schematic diagram of the aortic bifurcation. **A.** Above the umbilicus. **B.** Directly behind the umbilicus. **C.** Below the umbilicus

endoscopy. Therefore, the location of these vessels and of the aortic bifurcation site must first be determined by palpating them through the umbilicus (Fig. 8). The bifurcation site may be above, behind or below the umbilicus (Fig. 9).

Note: Once the greater vessels have been palpated, one generally will no longer be at risk to puncture them.

Spring test (Fig. 10)

When the Veress needle is inserted perpendicular to the abdominal wall, three spring movements are seen as it passes through the skin, the fascia, and the peritoneum (Fig. 10). The click that occurs as the needle passes through the peritoneum sometimes is not audible.

Insertion technique: One hand raises the abdominal wall in order to stabilize the insertion site. This lifts the abdominal wall only and causes hardly any elevation of the peritoneum (Fig. 12).

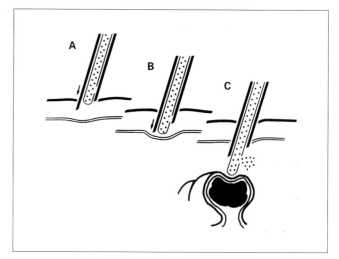

Fig. 10. How the Veress needle works. **A.** Perforation of skin. **B.** Fascia. **C.** Parietal peritoneum

The other hand holds the Veress needle (the stopcock should be open, as in Fig. 11) in a three-finger grasp. The little finger of this hand should be firmly propped against the abdominal wall to prevent sudden advances into the abdominal cavity.

Hiss test (vacuum phenomenon) (Fig. 13)

When one believes the needle is correctly situated in the abdominal cavity (stopcock still open), the abdominal wall should again be lifted with the one hand. A clearly audible hiss of air is heard as air rushes in through the needle if the needle is in the correct position. If this is not the case, the needle should be rotated. If still no hissing noise is heard, one should proceed with great caution to the next insufflation steps.

In patients with massive adhesions, a water aspiration test can be performed instead of the hissing test (Fig. 14). The water should flow in rapidly as the abdominal wall is lifted. Placing a drop of water on the opening of the Veress needle instead of injecting 10 ml of water does not suffice.

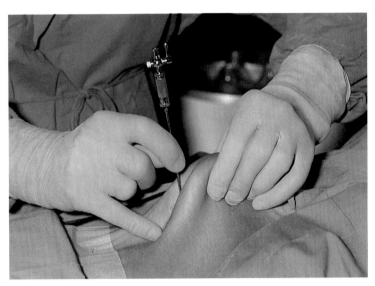

Fig. 11. Lifting of the caudal abdominal wall and perpendicular insertion of the Veress needle ensures perforation of the thinnest site in the abdominal space. Note how the little finger is propped against the abdomen

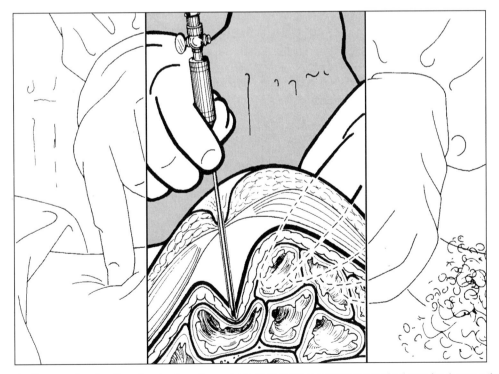

Fig. 12. Schematic diagram of perforation showing how the parietal peritoneum is sometimes pushed very far down as the needle passes through the skin and umbilical fascia

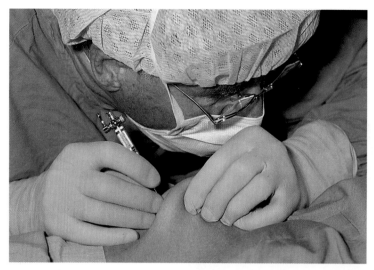

Fig. 13. If the needle is situated between the parietal peritoneum and the visceral peritoneum, a slight hissing noise can be heard as the abdominal wall is lifted

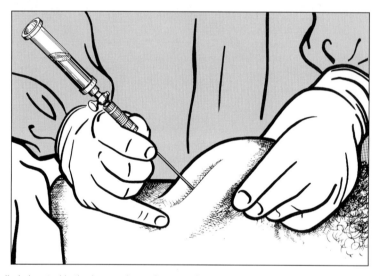

Fig. 14. If the tip of the needle is located in the interperitoneal space, the physiological NaCl solution will slowly flow in when the abdominal wall is lifted

Aspiration test (Fig. 15)

The tip of the needle may still be located in the stomach, the transverse colon, or in a distended loop of bowel, even though these safety tests indicate a correct needle position.

We therefore recommend that one instills 5 ml of physiological saline solution (Fig. 15A). The instilled liquid cannot be aspirated when the needle is correctly located in the free peritoneum (Fig. 15B). If bowel contents or blood is aspirated, the needle position must be changed (Fig. 15C).

Insufflation of gas: Quadro-manometer test (Fig. 4)

Negative pressure test using a manometer (Fig. 16): The hissing phenomenon described above can be reproduced using a manometer to measure intra-abdominal pressure. If the abdominal wall is lifted when the tip of the needle lies within the free abdominal cavity, the manometer will indicate a negative pressure of −5 to −9 mmHg. This is shown either on the digital readout or by the fact that the needle of the manometer migrates to the negative range (Fig. 16).

Quadro-Test 1 = insufflation pressure measurement. This test starts with a raised abdominal wall. After the gas inflow stopcock has been opened and adjusted to 1 L/min, the pressure reading should equal the reading obtained in the needle test compared with free atmospheric pressure.

If the gas flow resistance compared with free atmospheric pressure is higher than the initial value, the needle is not situated in the free abdominal cavity. Instead, the opening of the Veress needle is obstructed by an adhesion, preperitoneal fat, omentum, a loop of bowel, or an adhesion. After raising the abdominal wall several times while rotating but not lifting the needle, the manometer pressure reading compared with the free atmospheric pressure should now correspond to the original measurement.

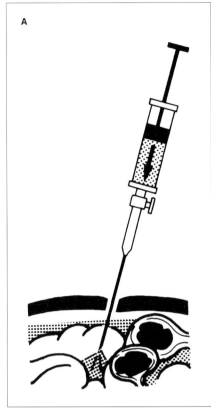 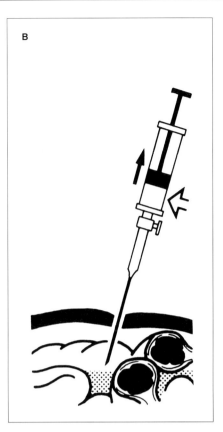 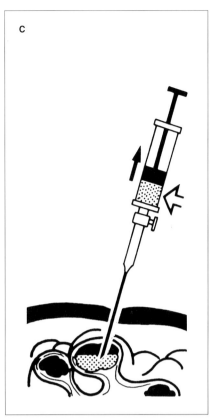

Fig. 15. Aspiration test. **A.** Injection of 5 ml saline solution. **B.** If the solution was injected in the space between the visceral peritoneum and the parietal peritoneum, the solution can no longer be aspirated. **C.** If the solution was injected into a loop of bowel or into the omentum, etc., the solution can be aspirated

If this is not the case even after repeatedly raising the abdominal wall and after gently dislodging the tip of the needle, the needle opening does not lie within the free abdominal cavity. In this case, the needle must be withdrawn. After cleaning the needle, one can begin again with the needle test. If insufflation still is not possible under the described conditions after 2 to 3 attempts at insufflation, other insertion sites must be explored.

If the tests indicate that the hole of the needle is probably located between the visceral peritoneum and the parietal peritoneum, one may proceed with gas insufflation.

Quadro-Test 2 = gas flow test. Gas flow should remain constant at 1 L/min. Flow resistance can reduce the gas flow. After one liter of gas has been insufflated, the gas inflow is switched to "high flow". At an insufflation pressure of

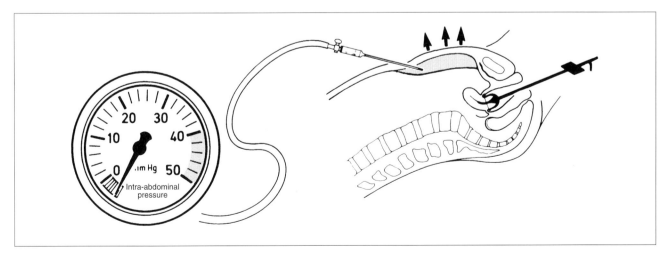

Fig. 16. Negative pressure test: The needle of the manometer migrates to the negative pressure range after the abdominal wall is lifted if the test was positive (Fig. 13)

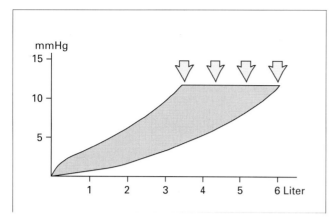

Fig. 17. The intra-abdominal pressure rises in proportion with the size of the gas bubble. If the pressure reading lies outside the curve, the needle is not positioned in the free abdomen

40 mmHg (= maximum value), 2 to 3 L/min of gas flow through the Veress needle and, later, up to 12 L/min flow through the trocar.

Quadro-Test 3 = intra-abdominal pressure test. The intra-abdominal pressure, which increases in proportion with the size of the gas bubble (Fig. 17), should never exceed 12 mmHg. Higher pressure should be discussed with the anesthesiologist.

Quadro-Test 4 = volume test. Volume control: The size of the normal pneumoperitoneum is determined by the age, height, depth of anesthesia, and obesity of the patient. The graph in Figure 17 shows the pressure versus volume ratio. One should proceed very cautiously if the measured values lie outside this range.

Example: The intra-abdominal pressure increases rapidly although only a small volume of gas has been used. This means that the gas is being insufflated into a small cavity in-

stead of into the free abdomen. This is normal in patients with multiple previous abdominal surgeries, but one should take particular care to ensure that the needle really does not lie in a loop of bowel, the stomach, the omentum, or the preperitoneal region before proceeding. The gas volume used is primarily proportional to the size of the intra-abdominal gas bubble. Tests 3 and 4 must correspond.

Note: The amount of CO_2 insufflated is limited by static pressure, *i.e.*, intra-abdominal pressure, not by volume.

The insufflator can be switched to "high flow" once 1 liter of gas has been insufflated and a static pressure reading of 1 to 3 mmHg has been obtained. Two to 3.5 liters of gas then flow into the abdomen at the insufflator's inherent maximum pressure of 40 mmHg.

A filling pressure of over 150 mmHg would be required to achieve a higher inflow volume through the Veress needle. However, this would be an irresponsible violation of physiological safety precautions.

Upon reaching the preselected static pressure (normally not over 12 mmHg), the insufflator automatically terminates gas inflow. Using manometer control permits optimal filling of the abdomen under "physiological vision".

Once the pneumoperitoneum is completed, a sounding test is generally performed. Using a 150 mm long, 0.8 mm gauge needle, the abdominal wall is punctured approximately 3 cm below the umbilicus. The needle is attached to a 10 ml Luer-Lok filled with ca. 2 ml of water. A continuous flow of gas bubbles should occur as one pulls up on the plunger of the syringe while slowly pushing down on the needle. Interruption of bubbling signalizes needle obstruction, *i.e.*, the tip of the needle lies in contact with adhesions or the intestine. Sounding is performed centrally and diagonally right and left, until an adhesion-free area is found. Then and only then is the 5 mm examining trocar guided under direct vision in Z-puncture fashion to the presumably adhesion free gas bubble (Fig. 24).

Pitfalls in the creation of a pneumoperitoneum

If the surgeon fails to pay careful attention to the above-mentioned safety measures, e.g. Quadro-Test etc. and the preconditions for the technical equipment, life-threatening consequences for the patient frequently occur.

Incorrect insufflation pressure and volume

As was already stated, the primary insufflation pressure should not exceed the initial resistance pressure for the connecting tube and the Veress needle. Otherwise, the needle does not lie between the visceral and parietal peritoneum, *i.e.*, in the free peritoneum. Primary filling of the abdomen with up to one liter of carbon dioxide gas can prevent negative effects on the anesthesia (shock).

Physiological limitation of the insufflation volume: The intra-abdominal pressure of 12 ± 1 mmHg is limited by the following physiological factors:
1. Pressure in the vena cava reaches a maximum of 15 mmHg. Intra-abdominal pressure in excess of 12 mmHg would obstruct the return of blood from the lower extremities, which would result in substantial circulation disturbances (Fig. 18).

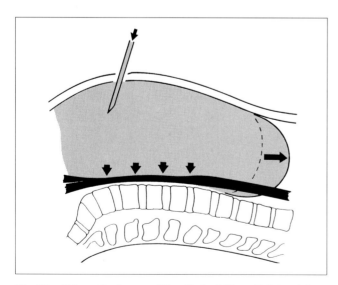

Fig. 18. Schematic diagram of the effects of 12 mmHg intra-abdominal pressure on the vena cava and the diaphragm

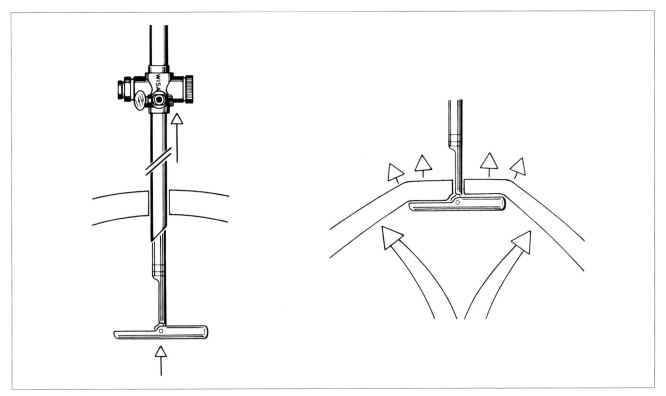

Fig. 19. Abdominal Cavity Expander (ACE) according to Semm, a mechanical abdominal wall elevator used to enhance the expanding capacity of the pneumoperitoneum. Available in sizes 5 and 10 mm

2. The increase in intra-abdominal pressure reduces diaphragm excursion and therefore the respiratory volume (Fig. 18).

In patients of normal height, 12 mmHg of pressure raises the abdominal wall with 12 to 15 kg and the diaphragm with ca. 8 kg. This significantly reduces the respiratory volume, which the anesthesiologist can only partially compensate for with manual ventilation techniques.

Once the abdomen has been inflated up to 12 mmHg – never higher! – the insufflator automatically takes over to ensure that the gas volume is maintained constant at the preselected pressure level. Gas lost while changing instruments or due to a leaky trocar is automatically refilled at a rate of up to 10 L/min, whereby the insufflation pressure *must not* exceed 40 mmHg.

Sometimes adequate abdominal wall elevation cannot be achieved. The ACE device (**A**bdominal **C**avity **E**xpander) can be very helpful in these cases (Fig. 19).

Gas bubble induced at the wrong site

If one does not pay careful attention to the safety tests for pneumoperitoneum induction and to the Quadro-Test, in particular, preperitoneal gas bubbles, omental emphysema

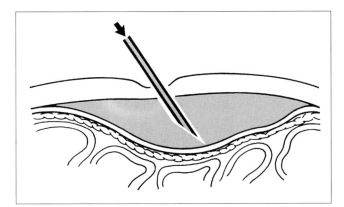

Fig. 20. Preperitoneal emphysema induced due to lack of attention paid to insufflation pressure

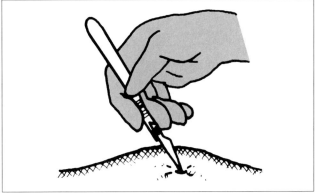

Fig. 21. Scalpel held at wrong angle when making the incision in the lower umbilical fossa. Consequences: Injury to the aorta and/or the common pelvic arteries and veins

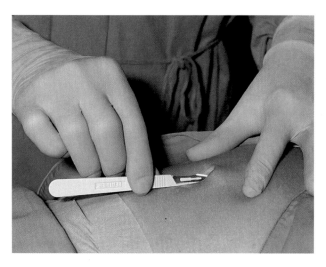

Fig. 22. Ideal scalpel position for avoiding injury to the greater trunk vessels while making the abdominal skin incision

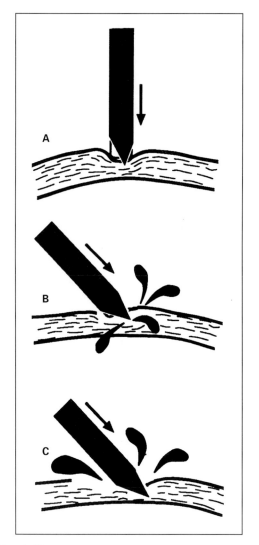

Fig. 23. A. The needle causes hardly any damage when it collides perpendicular to the vessel. The Veress needle acts as a scalpel in situations **B** and **C**

(Fig. 20), or filling of the bowel with carbon dioxide gas can occur. Generally, it is not possible to remove gas from artificially created cavities. In this case, the most sensible thing to do is to terminate the pelviscopy or laparoscopy in order to avoid further complications.

Note: Serious risks usually do not arise from the primary complication, but from the complications of the complication.

Vessel injury caused by the scalpel

In some hospitals, a routine subumbilical or intraumbilical incision is made using a scalpel. Known complications of this technique are severing of the iliac vessels and cutting of the aorta. Therefore, the use of this technique should be restricted. We recommend performing primary puncture with the Veress needle alone.
   The risk of cutting the aorta remains, even when the abdomen is properly filled. This injury may result in the death of the patient. Therefore, when cutting the cutis, the scalpel should never be held perpendicular to the abdominal wall, but parallel to it (Figs. 21 and 22).

Vessel injury caused by the Veress needle

The risk of injury to the greater trunk vessels is extremely low when the Veress needle collides perpendicular to the vessel. However, if the Veress needle is guided in at a certain angle to the vessel, it automatically becomes a scalpel (Fig. 23). The slitting of a greater trunk vessel – occasionally with a tragic outcome – has been reported. Therefore, the Veress needle should always be introduced perpendicular to the abdominal wall [11, 12].

Vessel injury caused by the trocar

Vascular and intestinal injuries caused by the trocar were the primary reasons that the technique came into disrepute. Therefore, we always perforate the abdominal wall under visual control via a trocar. Figure 24 illustrates the procedure, and the captions describe the individual steps.
   Figures 25 to 27 show typical images that can be seen when perforating the layers of the abdominal wall by rotating the elliptical trocar sleeve. These images are clearly visible through an endoscope or on a video monitor. Performing this procedure under direct vision using the 5 mm examining trocar excludes the risk of injury to the vessels or intestines in over 99 % of all cases.
   In some cases, the intestines are perforated due to radical attempts to somehow find a portal to the abdomen. If this problem is recognized immediately, the damage can be corrected by performing a mini laparotomy though the already inserted trocar. At any rate, wide laparotomy is no longer performed.

Injury to the bowel

The causes of injury to the bowel are the same as those for the vessels. Perforation of the bowel with the Veress needle does not require further surgical recourse. However, lacerations with the scalpel or the trocar must, in some cases, be corrected endoscopically or via laparotomy.
   The risk of abdominal injury is minimal when pneumoperitoneum is induced under Quadro-Test control and with trocar

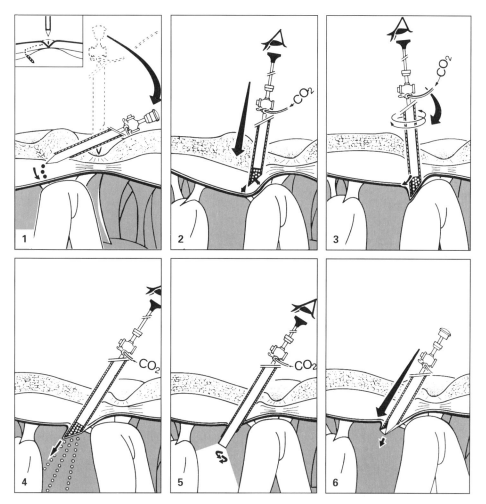

Fig. 24. Peritoneal perforation under direct vision using a 5 mm examining trocar. **1.** The elliptically tipped sleeve of a 5 mm trocar carrying a conical point trocar is guided down the muscle following the Z-puncture pattern. **2.** The conical point trocar is then replaced with a 5 mm pelviscope. Advancement of the trocar sleeve through the abdominal muscles to the peritoneum is achieved under direct vision with drilling-pressing action. **3.** If adhesions (intestinal or omental) are located below the trocar, the surface appears white due to total light reflection. **4.** By laterally shifting the elliptical trocar sleeve to the rectal fascia and the peritoneum, one reaches the translucent peritoneum, where the vessels can be identified. **5.** The parietal peritoneum is perforated by applying blunt pressure under direct vision. One then has an unobstructed view into the abdomen with massive adhesions. **6.** In case step 5 is unsuccessful (*e.g.*, because the fasciae are too thick), peritoneal perforation under visual control is continued in the classical manner after removing the examining trocar and inserting the conical point trocar

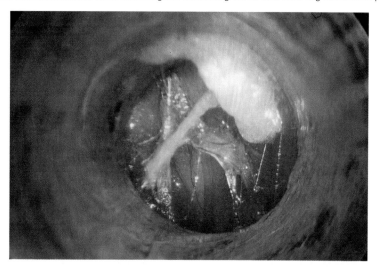

Fig. 25. After removing the conical point trocar (Fig. 24/2) and inserting the 5 mm examining trocar, the red muscles can be identified. The elliptical tip of the trocar is slowly advanced through the muscles

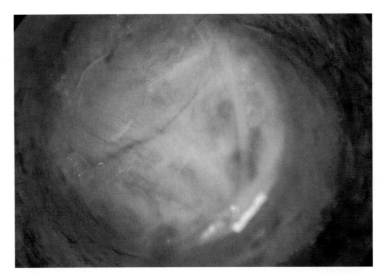

Fig. 26. The trocar sleeve has passed through the muscles and comes in contact with the fasciae and, perhaps, with underlying adhesions. The elliptical tip is advanced until ...

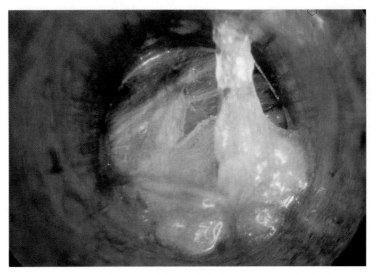

Fig. 27. ...the translucent, vascularized peritoneum becomes visible and the instruments can be freely maneuvered

insertion under direct vision. As soon as the examining trocar has been inserted, a 360 ° inspection is made (Fig. 28) to ensure that the omentum has not been perforated, because massive adhesions may develop on the anterior wall of the omentum after laparotomy (Fig. 29). If the omentum has been perforated, as in Figure 29A, the endoscope should be retracted millimeter by millimeter back to the muscle layer. The pierced tissue should then be inspected to be absolutely sure that no intestinal injury has occurred.

Abdominal wall hernia

In the beginning, gynecological laparoscopists pierced the linea alba just inferior to the umbilicus in order to avoid hemorrhage. Intestinal and omental strangulation (Fig. 30) and, in some cases, total omental prolapse (Fig. 31) were common complications. By making a Z-puncture into the layers of the abdominal wall (Fig. 24/1), primary intestinal prolapse or the later development of hernias can be prevented.

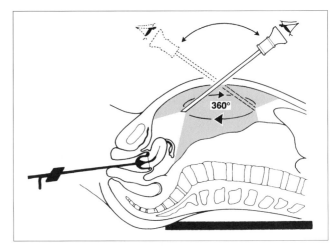

Fig. 28. Once the perforation of the parietal peritoneum has been achieved, one should make a 360 ° inspection to ensure that the abdominal cavity is free of adhesions

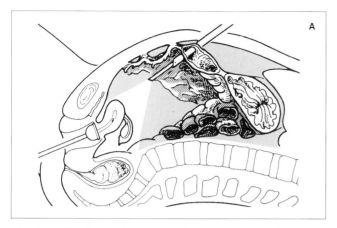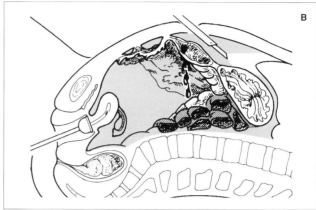

Figs. 29A, B.   Omental perforation. **A.** demonstrates perforation of the omentum or, in this case, of the transverse colon due to failure to introduce the examining trocar under visual control. One has an unobstructed view into the minor pelvis. **B.** The injury to the omentum or transverse colon can be identified as soon as one tests the 360° panorama view (Fig. 28)

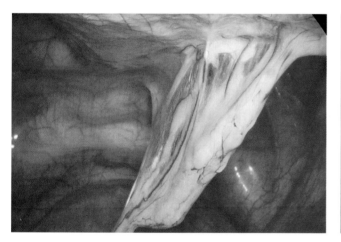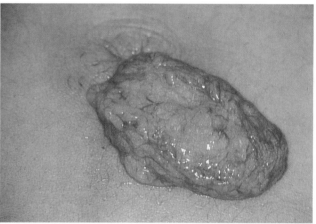

Fig. 30.   Omentum or intestine has become attached to the fissure made by piercing the linea alba with the trocar

Fig. 31.   Here omental prolapse occurred within a few hours of laparoscopy, because a linear puncture was made through the umbilicus, *i.e.*, the linea alba. Serious complications including intestinal strangulation can occur in partial prolapse

Peritoneal hypothermia

In the early days of diagnostic laparoscopy, the abdominal cavity was filled with a maximum of only 5 liters of gas, whereas up to a few hundred liters of carbon dioxide may be insufflated into the abdominal cavity in laparoscopic operations today. However, the designers of this state-of-the-art equipment completely forgot one thing: Due to the size of the peritoneal surface, hypothermia of the abdominal cavity occurs when gas that is not warmed to body temperature is used.

Carbon dioxide gas is bottled in liquid form at a pressure of around 49 bar (temperature-dependent). Sudden vaporization of the gas produces carbon dioxide snow (-96 °C). The insufflator and the connecting tube compensate for this, to a certain extent, and warm the gas to just below room temperature (±20 °C).

Measurements show that temperatures in the abdominal cavity can fall below 32 °C during pelviscopy. Furthermore, the rectal temperature may be reduced by as much as 1 to 3 °C, depending on the length of surgery and the volume of gas used.

Peritoneal contact with the carbon dioxide gas leads primarily to clearly observable hypothermia. The uncontrolled insufflation of cold carbon dioxide gas into the abdominal cavity causes an unspecific peritoneal low-temperature stimulus due to hypothermia. This decreases the well-being of the pelviscopied or laparoscoped patient and gives rise to multiple complaints. Without a doubt, hypothermia of the abdomen (Fig. 32) is frequently the cause. This problem could be largely avoided by using prewarmed gas (Fig. 33).

The Women's Clinic of the University of Kiel performed 3-year studies on the use of gas preoperatively warmed to body temperature. The use of prewarmed gas significantly reduced the intake of postoperative pain-killers by 31%, and shoulder pain was reduced by 47%. Furthermore, tachycardia was observed in only 11% of the patients, which substantially facilitated the task of the anesthesiologist.

The carbon dioxide gas was warmed using a *WISAP Flow Therme* (Fig. 34). Its warming tube can be connected to any insufflator. The Flow Therme has been tried and proven in several months of clinical use, and the tube can be steam sterilized.

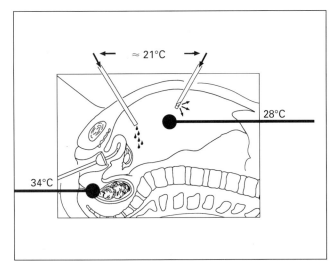

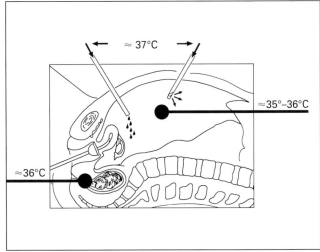

Fig. 32. Schematic diagram of hypothermia observed in Kiel, Germany after a 3-hour pelviscopy session (sterility operation)

Fig. 33. The intra-abdominal temperature is kept constant by using a heated CO_2 gas insufflator (isothermia)

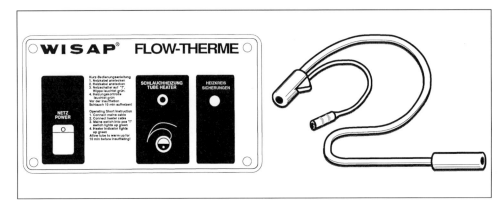

Fig. 34. WISAP Flow Therme and heating tube – can be attached to any CO_2 or N_2O gas insufflator

In view of the fact that uncritical insufflation of cold carbon dioxide gas until now, we would also like to point out the fact that the physiological solutions used for rinsing purposes in endoscopy are cooling mediums which can drastically reduce the body temperature. The warmers, which have been standardized to 37 °C until now, should absolutely be adjusted to 40 to 41 °C (requires little technically effort). This would ensure that rinsing water at least approximates the body temperature of 37 °C.

Conclusions

Initial technical difficulties in the induction of pneumoperitoneum first brought the technique of Laparoscopy into disrepute. Modern CO_2 insufflators should gauge four measurement parameters: the insufflation pressure, the amount of gas insufflated per minute, the current intra-abdominal pressure, and the total gas volume used. The operated abdomen can thus be filled with CO_2 "under vision" using the Quadro-Test. Insertion of the trocar under endoscopic vision almost completely excludes the risk of intestinal and vascular injuries. The insufflation of cold CO_2 gas causes abdominal hypother-

mia and pain or tachycardia, associated with it. This can be prevented by using gas that has been prewarmed to body temperature. The risks and errors that were associated with the creation of pneumoperitoneum in the past are now outdated.

References

1. ANSARI AH: Vaginal induction of pneumoperitoneum for laparoscopy. Obstet. Gynec 48 (1976) 251–252.
2. BUECHNER HA: Pneumopericardium following laparoscopy. Chest 77 (1980) 811–812.
3. CORSON SE: Routine Pneumoperitoneum. Obstet. Gynec 47 (1976) 638.
4. GOETZ O: Die Röntgendiagnostik bei gasgefüllter Bauchhöhle: eine neue Methode. Münch Med Wschr 65 (1918) 1275.
5. HASSON HM: Modified instrument and method for laparoscopy. Am J Obstet. Gynec 11 (1971) 886–887.
6. HASSON HM: Safe Pneumoperitoneum in Laparoscopy. In: Phillips J, Keith ML (eds.): Principles and Techniques. New York, Med Book Corp Stratton Intercont (1974) 265–267.
7. LEMAY M ET AL.: Post-laparoscopy pneumoperitoneum. Clin Invest Med 1 (1978) 211–212.

8. Morgan HR: Laparoscopy: induction of pneumoperitoneum via transfundal puncture. Obstet. Gynec 54 (1979) 260–261.
9. Neely MR et al.: Laparoscopy: routine pneumoperitoneum via the posterior fornix. Obstet. Gynec 45 (1975) 459–460.
10. Nicholson RD et al.: Pneumopericardium following laparoscopy. Chest 76 (1979) 605–607.
11. Sander RR et al.: Pneumopericardium following laparoscopy. Chest 76 (1979) 605–607.
12. Semm K: Pneumoperitoneum mit CO_2-Visum 6 (1967) 139–141.
13. Semm K: Die Laparoskopie in der Gynäkologie. Geburtsh Frauenheilk 27 (1976) 1029–1042.
14. Semm K: Weitere Entwicklungen in der gynäkologischen Laparoskopie – Gynäkologische Pelviskopie. In: Schwalm H, Döderlein G (eds): Klinik der Frauenheilkunde und Geburtshilfe. Erg 5. Urban & Schwarzenberg, München (1971) 326/1–32639.
15. Semm K: Gynecologic pelviscopy. Obstet. Gynec Digest 14 (1972) 21–25.
16. Semm K: Die moderne Endoskopie in der Frauenheilkunde. Frauenarzt 13 (1972) 300–307.
17. Semm K: Pelviskopie und Hysteroskopie: Farbatlas und Lehrbuch. Schattauer, Stuttgart New York Toronto (1976). Übersetzt in Englisch, Französisch, Italienisch, Portugiesisch, Spanisch.
18. Semm K: Die Automatisierung des Pneumoperitoneums für die endoskopische Abdominalchirurgie. Arch Gynaek 232 (1980) 738–739.
19. Semm K: Die operative Pelviskopie. In: Döderlein G, Wulf KH (eds): Klinik der Frauenheilkunde und Geburtshilfe. Vol. 3, Erg 3. Urban & Schwarzenberg, München Wien Baltimore (1983) 351–424/20.
20. Semm K: Operationslehre für endoskopische Abdominal-Chirurgie Pelviskopie – Laparoskopie (mit kompletter Literaturübersicht 1975 – 1983). Schattauer, Stuttgart-New York, 485 p. 1984 (Übersetzungen: Japanisch: Central Foreign Books Ltd., Tokyo, 2 Volumes 1986; Englisch: Year Book Medical Publishers Inc., Chicago-London 1987; Italienisch: Publicazioni Mediche, Neapel 1987; Chinesisch: Shanghai Scientific and Technical Publ., Shanghai 1988).
21. Semm K: Sichtkontrollierte Peritoneumperforation zur operativen Pelviskopie. Geburtsh Frauenheilk 48 (1988) 436–439.

4. | Laparoscopic Surgical Instruments

I. B. BRUNE

Introduction

Equipment and instrumentation have a much greater impact and importance in laparoscopic surgery than in open surgery. This is caused by the fact that in laparoscopy, direct contact with the intra-abdominal situs is not possible. Visualisation as well as tactile exploration of the operative field are always only indirectly achieved through optical systems and instruments.

Imaging Systems

The imaging system includes the laparoscope, light source and light cable, camera and monitor.

Laparoscopes

The safety and speed of a laparoscopic operation essentially depend on the quality of the video image because, an impaired view may lead to complications during dissection and hinder control of a haemorrhage. A frequently used optical system is based on the Hopkins rod lens system: It provides excellent light transmission and a large angle of view that leads to a full-format video image. They may be sterilised by steam autoclave at 134 °C or 273 °F.

The laparoscopes are available with diameters of 5, 7 and 10 mm as well as a view angled at 0, 12, 30, 45, 70, 90 or 120 ° (Fig. 1). The smallest diameter available is 1.9 mm: It allows diagnostic laparoscopy in local anesthesia through the incision of the Veress needle.

Light Cables

Light transmission can be achieved by fluid- or fibre cables. In a fibre cable the light is transmitted by glass fibres. They are very light and reinforced with a metal spiral which makes them more rigid and resistant to deformation than fluid cables. They can be steam sterilised at 134 °C (273 °F). The fibre light cables are available with fibre bundles measuring 1.6, 2.5, 3.5 or 4.5 mm in diameter and having a length of 1.8, 2.3, 3.0 or 3.6 m. The diameter of the fibre bundle should always be chosen to be slightly larger than the lens system. The fibre bundles should not be too large, otherwise too much light intensity would be lost.

Fluid light cables transmit through liquid permitting a more even transmission of light across the spectrum. For this reason they are often used for videotaping and laparoscopic photography. A disadvantage is a loss of brightness of 20–30 % compared with fibre cables, reducing the light intensity. Fluid light cables are available in a length of 1.8 m and with a diameter of 3, 4 or 5 mm.

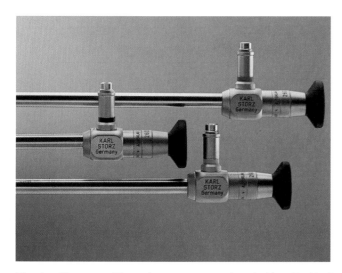

Fig. 1. Shown are 10-mm laparoscopes equipped with a Hopkins' rod lens system (K. Storz GmH, Tuttlingen, Germany)

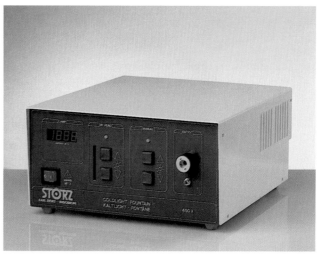

Fig. 2. Cold light fountain with manual or automatic regulation of light intensity (K. Storz GmbH, Tuttlingen, Germany)

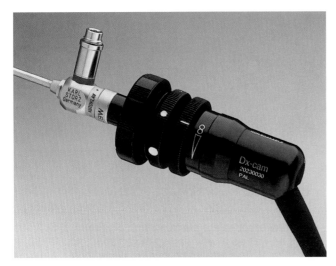

Fig. 3. Camera connected with the laparoscope (K. Storz GmbH, Tuttlingen, Germany)

Cold Light Source

Light sources of 250, 300 or 400 watt may be used. The light intensity can be regulated manually or automatically (Fig. 2). Automatic modification may be integral (the complete video signal is used for regulation) or with a "spot-modus". (Only the signal in a window in the centre of the image is used.)

Camera

Development of cameras in the past decade has been aimed at obtaining cameras that are small, lightweight and easy to use, while producing a picture with optimal sharpness, high resolution and excellent colour reproduction (Fig. 3). The camera should be insulated against high-frequency (HF) disturbance from coagulation and have a high light sensitivity. Whenever sterile camera covers are not available, the camera head and the cable should be soakable.

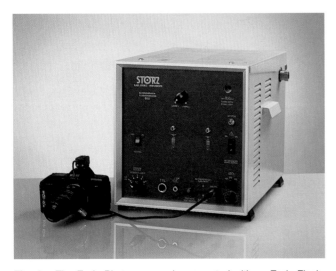

Fig. 4. The Endo-Photo camera is connected with an Endo-Flash, providing an automatically regulated light intensity for the exposure

For high-quality video documentation, the Digivideo (K. Storz GmbH, Tuttlingen, Germany) digitally enhances the contrast achieved by the camera.

The new "Reverse Video" (K. Storz GmbH, Tuttlingen, Germany) is a digital image processing system for left/right or upside/down image reversal. In situations where the instruments are facing the laparoscope instead of pointing in the same direction the image can be reversed for easier manipulations.

Endoscopic 3D systems have two optical channels, each equipped with its own video camera. With the help of a specialised stereoscopic image-processing hardware, 3D images are displayed onscreen on a single video monitor. The disadvantage is that the surgeon must still wear glasses during the whole procedure, which sometimes may cause a headache or nausea. On the other hand, one of the main problems in laparoscopic surgery, the lack of depth perception, is eliminated. Second-generation video stereoscopes with viewing systems, such as head-up displays or viewing boxes, are currently under development. Hopefully in the future shutter goggles will not be required any more.

Imaging Documentation

The video monitor must generate high-resolution images and offer a S-VHS connection. The size of the screen should be chosen according to the distance from the surgeon (diagonal 22, 36 or 52 cm), but should not be too small.

Recording can be achieved with a VHS, S-VHS, U-Matic (low or high band/SP) or Betacam recorder. S-VHS offers the advantage of a good imaging quality at a reasonable price, and is therefore the method of choice for documentation of routine procedures.

Photographs can be obtained either by endo-photography or with a video printer. The best quality is achieved with endo-photography. A specially adapted camera is mounted on the laparoscope (Fig. 4). It is connected with an electronically regulated endo-flash. The high light intensity allows a very short exposure time thereby avoiding blurring by movement. It is advisable to use high-resolution (200-400 ASA) daylight films.

Because endo-photography is a very time-consuming procedure, documentation during routine operations is easier using a colour video printer.

HF equipment for electrocoagulation

Most of the available devices are designed for monopolar coagulation. Theoretically, the use of monopolar electrocoagulation presents the risk of heat-related tissue necrosis in remote parts of the body caused by a high intensity of current in these areas. Although this danger has been proven by physical laws, its clinical relevance remains unclear. Despite the growing number of laparoscopic operations, little evidence can be found of complications due to monopolar electrocoagulation.

Bipolar electrocoagulation is an alternative to the monopolar technique. The currents are between the two electrodes at the tip of the bipolar instrument. Because the surface of these electrodes is very small, the intensity of the current is sufficient to achieve coagulation or cutting. An involuntary effect of the electric current passing throughout the body is avoided. Because of the short distance between the two electrodes, only a very low HF power is needed to achieve the desired ef-

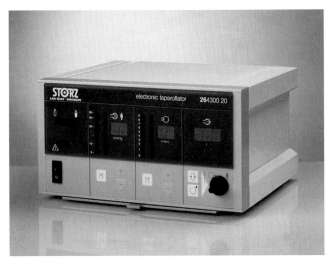

Fig. 5. Laparoscopic carbon dioxide insufflator: The desired intra-abdominal pressure and flow rate can be preselected

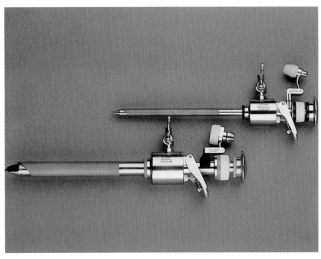

Fig. 7. Reusable trocars (K. Storz GmbH, Tuttlingen, Germany)

fect. To obtain coagulation the tissue must be seized between the tips of the instrument. Whenever this is not possible, i.e. when hemorrhage occurs on larger surfaces of a parenchymatous organ, such as the liver or kidney, monopolar coagulation or a hemostyptic collagen sheet (TachoComb®, Nycomed, München) must be used.

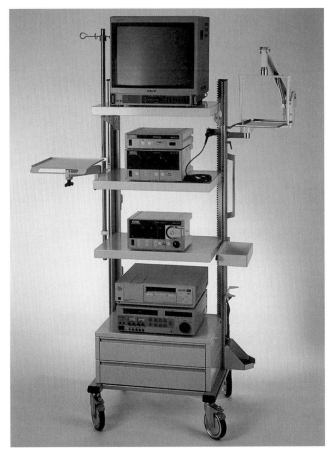

Fig. 6. The material is arranged on a video cart to be moved from one operating room to another

Insufflation Devices

To guarantee a smooth operative course, the maintenance of a pneumoperitoneum with constant intra-abdominal pressure is of essential importance. It is achieved with a pressure- and volume-regulated insufflator. These insufflators show the preselected and actual intraabdominal pressure, the total amount of insufflated CO_2 and the flow (Fig. 5). An integrated acoustic and visual alarm is activated as soon as the intra-abdominal pressure exceeds the preselected setting, e.g. due to contraction of the abdominal muscles by the patient.

The irrigation and aspiration device may be integrated in the insufflator or separated from it. Aspiration should be around 0.6 bar. A video cart helps in arranging all necessary material so that it is mobile and can easily be moved from one operating room to another (Fig. 6).

Operative Instruments

Insufflation Cannulas

The pneumoperitoneum is created by puncture of the abdominal wall with an insufflation cannula. Mostly, a Veress needle is used. It is made of a sharp-tipped cannula that contains a spring-activated blunt obturator with an opening for gas insufflation on the side. During puncture of the abdominal wall, the blunt obturator is pushed back while the sharp cannula perforates fascia and peritoneum. After penetration of the abdominal cavity, the obturator is pushed forward by the spring mechanism to protect intra-abdominal organs. Before starting insufflation, it is mandatory to check the free intraperitoneal position of the needle with the usual safety tests.

Trocars

Access to the thoracic or abdominal cavity for endoscopic procedures is gained through trocar sheaths that are introduced with the help of sharp- or blunt-tipped trocars (Fig. 7). For abdominal procedures sharp-tipped trocars present the advantage that less uncontrolled strength is applied, and therefore risk of injury to intra-abdominal organs is reduced.

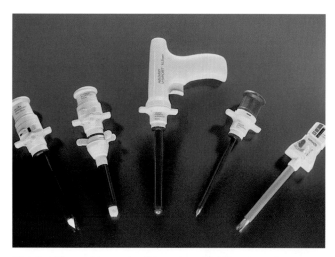

Fig. 8. Disposable trocars (from left to right): Surgiport, Surgispike, Visiport, Bluntport and Versaport (USSC, Norwalk, CT)

For thoracoscopy, trocars with a blunt tip are preferred to avoid lesion to the lung parenchyma. To keep up the intracavitary pressure, trocars are equipped with a valve. Different types of valve mechanisms are available:

1. Trumpet valve: A spring system closes the valve and must be held open for introduction of instruments. The construction is simple and works very well. A disadvantage is that if the valve is not opened completely, the sharp edges of the valve may damage the shaft of the instruments, particularly when those are insulated with a plastic cover.
2. Flap valve: They open and close automatically with passage of the instrument. The flap held in place by a magnet guarantees a smooth opening.

Trocars may be reusable or disposable. Reusable trocars spare the environment and are less expensive, but require manpower for cleaning. Disposable trocars are more expensive, but have a radiotranslucent sheath that does not impair cholangiography. Their tip is always sharp and they are provided with a safety shield or with a retractable tip to avoid organ injury.

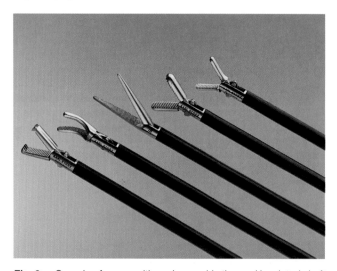

Fig. 9. Grasping forceps with exchangeable tips and insulated shaft (K. Storz GmbH, Tuttlingen, Germany)

Special Trocars

Visiport (Fig. 8). This 10-mm trocar consists of an optical obturator, encompassing a blunt clear window at the distal end, along with a crescent-shaped blade. When the trigger is pulled, the blade extends 1 mm and immediately retracts. This permits a controlled sharp dissection of tissue layers and access to the abdominal or thoracic cavity under visual control.

Versaport (Fig. 8). This disposable trocar contains an internal seal accomodating instruments ranging from 5 to 12 mm without loss of pneumoperitoneum or the need to change any adapter.

Grasping Instruments

Graspers are used laparoscopically to hold tissue and spread it during dissection. All graspers are now available as "take apart instruments" (K. Storz GmbH, Tuttlingen, Germany, Fig. 9). Their 360° rotating shafts are protected by an insulation highly resistant to chipping. Their tip is made of inserts that can be individually replaced or exchanged.

To hold the tissue, graspers with traumatic and atraumatic jaws are available (Figs. 10 and 11). For extraction of resected organs, such as the gallbladder, a strong, sharp forceps has proved to be useful (Fig. 12).

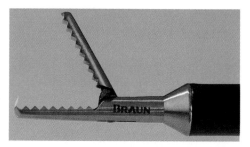

Fig. 10. Traumatic grasper with a rotatable shaft (B. Braun-Dexon GmbH, Spangenberg, Germany)

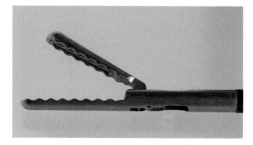

Fig. 11. Atraumatic grasper (B. Braun-Dexon GmbH, Spangenberg, Germany)

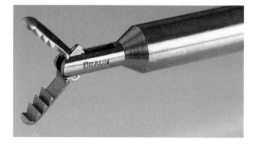

Fig. 12. Sharp grasping forceps for extraction of specimen

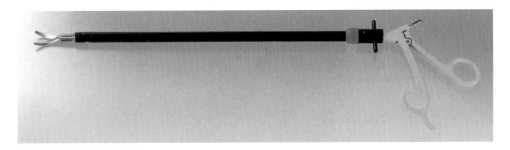

Fig. 13. A 10-mm Metzenbaum scissors with rotatable shaft (B. Braun-Dexon GmbH, Spangenberg, Germany)

Scissors

Different types and sizes of scissors are available. The choice depends on the anatomical situation. Scissors with curved blades have the advantage that the tip of the blades can always be seen during dissection (Fig. 13). Straight scissors are best suited for dissection of the peritoneum (Fig. 14). Most scissors can also be used for coagulation, but this makes the blades blunt very quickly so that if reusable, they need to be resharpened. In this case scissors with an exchangeable tip are useful (Fig. 15).

Needle Driver

Laparoscopic needle drivers are available with a straight or curved tip (Fig. 16). The variety of handles satisfies every ergonomic demand (Fig. 17). Although laparoscopic sutures are

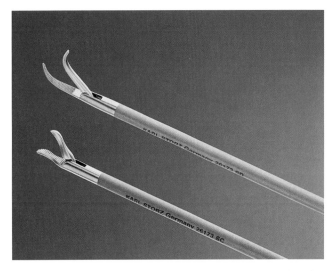

Fig. 16. Beaked needle drivers facilitate intracorporeal knotting (K. Storz GmbH, Tuttlingen, Germany)

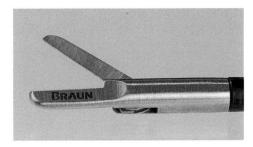

Fig. 14. Straight scissors for peritoneal transection (B. Braun-Dexon GmbH, Spangenberg, Germany)

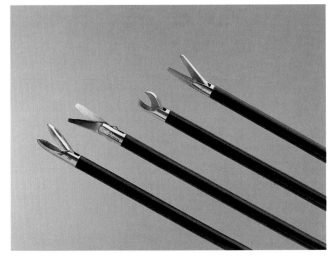

Fig. 15. Variety of scissors with exchangeable tips. "Take apart" instruments can be quickly dismantled and reassembled for safer sterilisation (K. Storz GmbH, Tuttlingen, Germany)

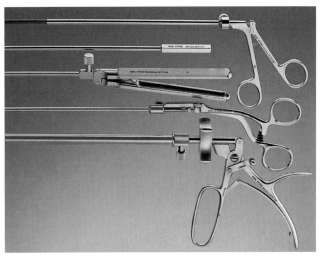

Fig. 17. The choice of needle driver handles satisfies every ergonomic requirement (K. Storz GmbH, Tuttlingen, Germany)

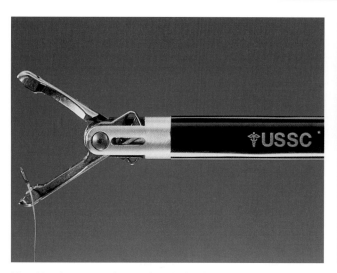

Fig. 18. Laparoscopic suturing device (Endo-Stitch, USSC, Norwalk, CT) armed with a sutured needle

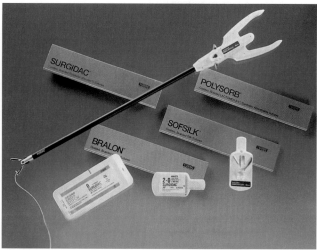

Fig. 19. A variety of sutures are available for the Endo-Stitch (USSC, Norwalk, CT)

available, any suture as used in open surgery is sufficient, except for rip-off needles.

A disposable laparoscopic suturing device with two jaws and a sutured needle has been developed (Fig. 18). The needle can be passed from one jaw to the other by closing the handle and flipping the toggle levers. Different sutures are available for the Endo-Stitch (Fig. 19).

Other Instruments

Although the general operative steps are the same in laparoscopy as in open surgery, the dissection technique may be somewhat different, because some devices do not exist in open surgery but have been specially developed for laparoscopy. One of these instruments is the electrical hook (Figs. 20

and 21). It is made of an angled wire that is used for dissection. The tissue is charged on the hook, then coagulated and transsected. This instrument is frequently used for dissecting the gallbladder from the liver bed. If the hook is combined with a suction/irrigation device, time can be spared because repeated exchange of instruments may be avoided (Figs. 22 and 23).

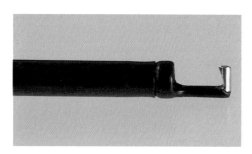

Fig. 20. Laparoscopic hook coagulator (B. Braun-Dexon GmbH, Spangenberg, Germany)

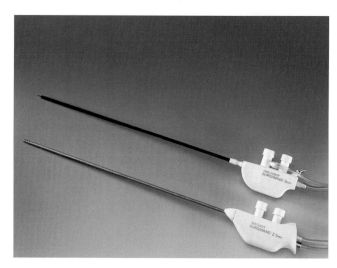

Fig. 22. The disposable 5-mm suction/irrigation device (Surgiwand, USSC, Norwalk, CT) can accomodate a laser probe up to 2.4 mm diameter

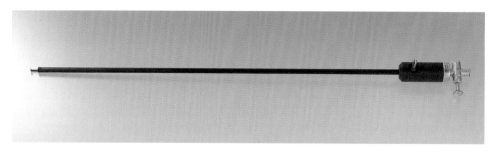

Fig. 21. Laparoscopic hook coagulator (B. Braun-Dexon GmbH, Spangenberg, Germany)

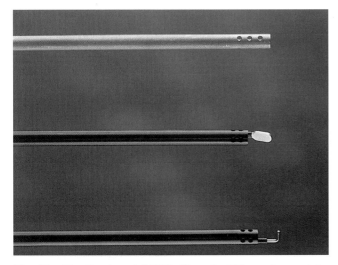

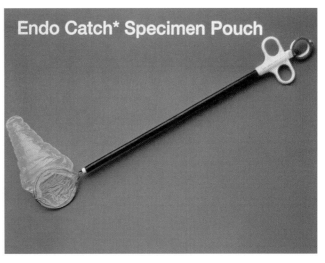

Fig. 23. The Surgiwand (USSC, Norwalk, CT) can be used for suction/irrigation only or equipped with a spatula or hook at the tip

Fig. 24. Polyurethane retrieval bag (Endo-Catch, USSC, Norwalk, CT) for specimen extraction

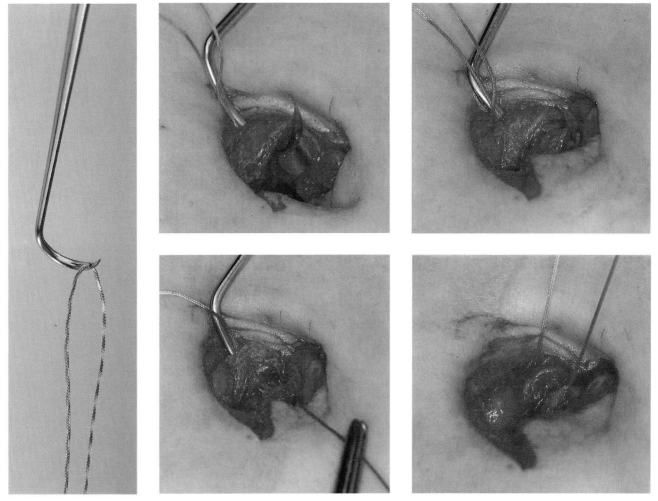

Figs. 25–29. Device for closure of the small fascia incision according to the Deschamps principle (B. Braun-Dexon GmbH, Spangenberg, Germany)

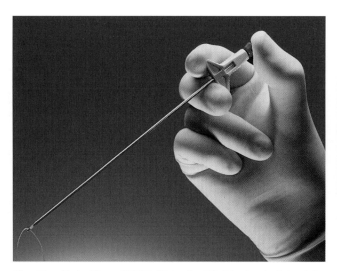

Fig. 30. Endo-Close (USSC, Norwalk, CT): The hooked tip of the device holds the suture

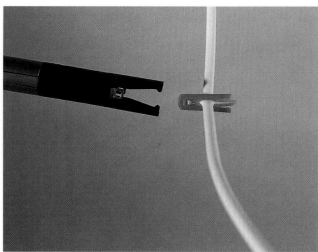

Fig. 32. The Laparoclip (B. Braun-Dexon GmbH, Spangenberg, Germany) is an absorbable clip made of two different polymers and can be placed safely with a reusable clip applier

Retrieving the resected specimens from the abdominal cavity through the small incisions is one of the specific problems of laparoscopy. To avoid contamination of the abdominal wall with bile, intestinal contents or tumor cells, the specimen should be extracted in an impermeable polyurethane bag that is introduced into the abdominal or thoracic cavity (Fig. 24) through a 15-mm trocar.

Trocar incisions of 10 mm or more must be closed with sutures of the fascia to avoid herniation. A specially designed device according to the Deschamps principle (Figs. 25–29) allows to get hold of the fascia without the danger of seizing intra-abdominal organs. The incision can also be closed with an Endo-Close (USSC*, Norwalk, CT): this suturing device is equipped with a spring-loaded, blunt-tipped stylet bearing a notched end to hook suture (2–0 to 0; Fig. 30).

*United States Surgical Corporation, Norwalk, CT

Clip Appliers

Larger vessels as well as the cystic duct or the ureter may be closed with clips. These clips are available in different sizes and may be absorbable or non-absorbable. The clips can be mounted one by one in a reusable clip applier (Fig. 31). Although this costs a little more time because the applier must be reloaded one by one, it is more economic for routine operations such as cholecystectomy where only 6–8 clips are needed. The disposable multifire clip appliers (Endo-Clip II, USSC, Norwalk, CT) contain 20 titanium clips and have a 10-mm diameter. They help in reducing operative time in more important procedures (i.e. colonic resections, fundoplication) where a larger number of clips are needed because they can be recharged automatically without having to be taken out of the abdomen.

Because it is not recommended to apply any non-absorbable suture or clip to the cystic duct stump, the newly devel-

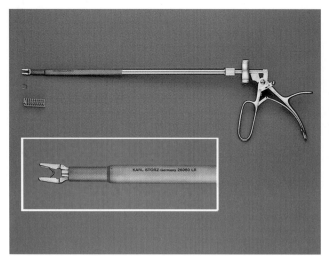

Fig. 31. Reusable clip applier (K. Storz GmbH, Tuttlingen, Germany)

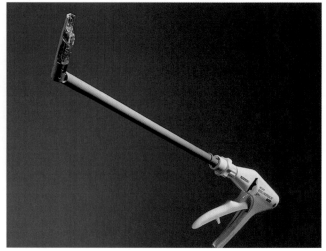

Fig. 33. The Endo-Universal 65 (USSC, Norwalk, CT) contains ten titanium single staples

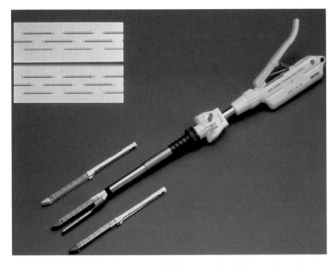

Fig. 34. The Endo-GIA 50 (USSC, Norwalk, CT) stapling device transsects the tissue between two triple staggered rows of titanium staples

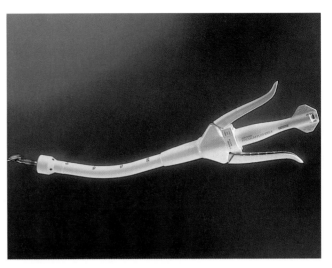

Fig. 36. The Premium Plus CEEA (USSC, Norwalk, CT) is introduced transanally for intra-abdominal anastomosis after resection of the left colon

oped Laparoclip (B. Braun-Dexon GmbH, Spangenberg, Germany), which is made of two different polymers, may be used. It adds to safety by locking at the tip (Fig. 32).

The staples of the Endo-Universal 65 (USSC, Norwalk, CT) (Fig. 33) have the mechanical function of an interrupted suture. They have been developed for the fixation of mesh and closure of the peritoneum at laparoscopic hernia repair. These staplers are provided with a 60 ° bendable tip and have a 360 ° rotating shaft to accomodate access from all angles.

Staplers

The development of laparoscopic stapling devices allowed a wide range of gastro-intestinal, pulmonary and other procedures associated with resection and/or reconstruction to be performed by laparoscopy.

The Endo-GIA 60 (USSC, Norwalk, CT) is a disposable 15-mm-diameter stapler (Fig. 34). It places two triple staggered

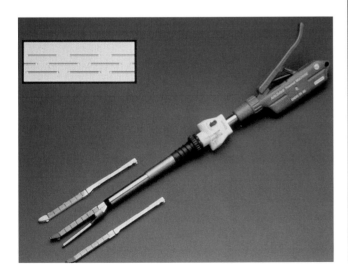

Fig. 35. The Endo-TA 60 (USSC, Norwalk, CT) places three staggered rows of titanium staples

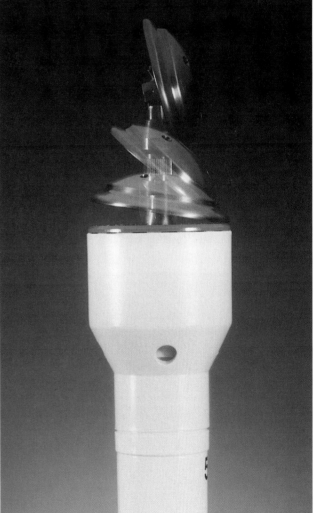

Fig. 37. The anvil of the Premium Plus CEEA can be tilted for easier placement in the proximal colon stump

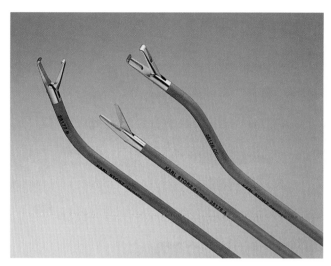

Fig. 38. Thoracoscopic instruments are provided with curved tips for better visualisation in the rigid thoracic cage (K. Storz GmbH, Tuttlingen, Germany)

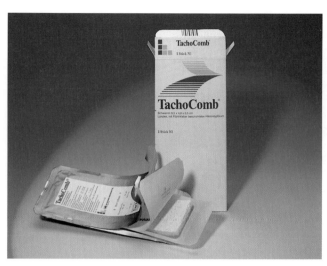

Fig. 40. Hemostyptic collagen sheet covered with fibrin glue for application on the surface of parenchymatous organs for hemostasis after resection (TachoComb™, Nycomed, München)

rows of titanium staples over a length of 6 cm and simultaneously divides the tissue between the two innermost rows, leaving three rows of staples on each side of the transsection.

The Endo-GIA 30 (USSC, Norwalk, CT) can be used through a 12-mm trocar and has a jaw length of 3 cm. Both instruments have a 360 ° rotatable shaft. Different staple sizes are available and must be chosen according to the tissue thickness, which must be evaluated with an Endo-Gauge (USSC, Norwalk, CT) prior to application of the stapler. The Endo-TA 60 (USSC, Norwalk, CT) places three rows of titanium staples and does not transsect tissue (Fig. 35).

Laparoscopic intra-abominal anastomosis after resection of the left colon is performed best with a transanally introduced circular stapler (Figs. 36 and 37). The Premium Plus CEEA (USSC, Norwalk, CT) is provided with a tiltable anvil. It places a circular, double staggered row of titanium staples. Immediately after staple formation, the instruments knife blade resects the excess tissue, creating a circular anastomosis.

Thoracoscopic Instruments

Because the thoracic cage is very rigid, unlike the abdominal wall, thoracoscopic instruments with curved tips have proved useful (Figs. 38 and 39). For parietal pleurodesis, a disposable cotton swab affixed to a 5-mm shaft (Endo-Peanut, USSC, Norwalk, CT) is available.

Miscellaneous

For hemostasis of diffuse hemorrhage from the surface of a parenchymatous organ, the application of a collagen sheet covered with a layer of the solid components of fibrin glue (human fibrinogen, bovine thrombin and aprotinin) has proved to be very useful (Fig. 40). The collagen sheet (TachoComb™, Nycomed, München) is introduced into the abdominal cavity with an applicator and spread onto the bleeding surface with slight pressure. It combines a tamponade effect with hemos-

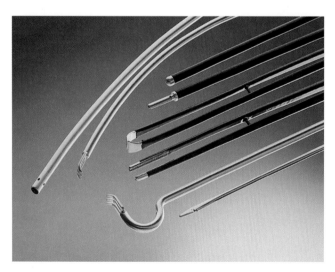

Fig. 39. A set of thoracoscopic instruments (K. Storz GmbH, Tuttlingen, Germany)

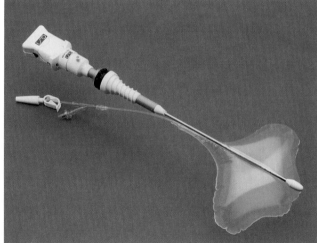

Fig. 41. Balloon dissector for creation of an operative space in extraperitoneal operations (Spacemaker II, GSI, Palo Alto, California)

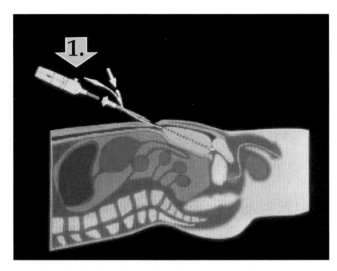

Fig. 42. Illustration of creation of the space for extraperitoneal hernia repair with the Spacemaker (GSI, Palo Alto, California)

typtic activity and allows fast and efficient control of the bleeding without excessive use of electrocautery and the dangers associated with it.

With development of endoscopic techniques, indications have been extended to the extraperitoneal space. In extraperitoneal inguinal hernia repair, nephrectomy or sympathectomy, space for operative manipulations can be created by tissue dissection with a balloon dissector (Figs. 41 and 42). The device consists of a cannula equipped with an inflatable balloon. The cannula is introduced through the skin incision and the balloon is filled with saline solution up to 600-700 ml, thereby creating the space for CO_2 insufflation. The 10-mm cannula remains in place and accomodates the laparoscope.

5. | Antibiotics in Laparoscopy

K. T. Hell-Türler

Introduction

In surgery antibiotics are used for therapy or prophylaxis depending on the clinical circumstances. Where possible, preoperative infection is treated with an appropriate antibiotic, whereas infection diagnosed during surgery generally requires postoperative therapy against the causative organism(s) ideally with laboratory confirmation of pathogen susceptibility. Prophylaxis, given in the absence of preoperative bacterial infection, is defined as perioperative cover against the major potential pathogens beginning immediately prior to surgery and continued for no more than 24 h.

Both therapeutic and prophylactic applications are guided by the clinicians' personal experience and controlled clinical efficacy studies, allied to theoretical contributions from the fields of pharmacology and pharmacokinetics, bacteriology and epidemiology. However, neither prophylaxis nor therapy are successful without competent surgery, a term which encompasses prior treatment, indication, timing, operative strategy and technique, and postoperative management.

The goal of antimicrobial prophylaxis is to achieve sufficient antibiotic tissue concentrations to prevent the growth of potential pathogens throughout the early perioperative risk period. Timing of administration is critical especially with short-acting antibiotics [2, 9].

Perioperative antibiotic prophylaxis found few proponents until the early 1960s. It subsequently gained worldwide acceptance after multiple studies in an increasing number of indications showed that appropriate antibiotic cover significantly reduced the infection rate in clean/contaminated operations. No colorectal resection would be performed presently without appropriate antibiotic cover.

Prophylaxis has also proved effective in an increasing number of clean procedures as well as in foreign body implantation (e.g. prosthetic hip, artificial heart valve, mesh for hernias, etc.) [27]. In fact, the clean vs contaminated dichotomy has been superseded by the concept of the overall risk of infectious complications, which, in turn, is determined by multiple risk factors dependent on the patient (age, coexisting disease, e.g. diabetes, general health, immune status, etc.), operating room conditions, procedure (elective or emergency), pre- and postoperative care, and also to a great extent on the surgeon's skill, knowledge and experience, procedure duration and tissue handling (traumatic or atraumatic) [10].

Perioperative mortality is much more dependent on pneumonia and septicaemia than on the subcutaneous wound infection often used as the sole yardstick of prophylactic efficacy. However, whereas respiratory and urinary tract infections cannot be eliminated by prophylaxis covering only 2-3 h [15, 22], cover exceeding 24 h postoperatively is not only unnecessary, but also potentially dangerous, in that it may select resistant bacteria.

Laparoscopic abdominal surgery has expanded exponentially in the past few years in the range of indications and number and nature of procedures. Its main advantage lies in the reduction of access trauma resulting in immediate postoperative mobilization, a lower rate of postoperative wound infection and a significantly shorter hospital stay [8]. When first employed the technique was always performed under perioperative antibiotic cover, particularly in the United States, to avoid unnecessary disrepute from an increased sepsis rate. Thus, randomized double-blind studies on the efficacy of prophylaxis are lacking, and now that perioperative cover has become standard for most laparoscopic intra-abdominal procedures, prospectively randomized comparative studies vs placebo would now generally be regarded as difficult. Evaluation of antibiotic prophylaxis in laparoscopic operations must therefore be based on analogies with conventional surgery.

Application Modalities

The choice of prophylactic antibiotic is influenced by the pharmacological and microbiological data, clinical experience and cost effectiveness. The agent selected should have a reasonable spectrum of activity against prospective pathogens with kinetics ensuring adequate serum and tissue levels throughout the risk period [12]; it should be well tolerated with proven clinical efficacy (preferably bactericidal with good tissue penetration). Cephalosporins (except those causing bleeding problems [31]) are currently the first-line choice, due to their low toxicity. Nephro- and ototoxic antibiotics, or those inducing frequent side effects, should not be used without compelling reasons.

Administration should be parenteral, rather than oral or topical, because the antibiotic must reach its target sites at high concentrations [19] and oral intake is not advised perioperatively. Beta-lactamase-resistant broad-spectrum antibiotics (e.g. third-generation cephalosporins) are more likely to prevent (Gram-negative) sepsis particularly in procedures in potentially contaminated sites.

Prophylaxis should cover the shortest period possible compatible with efficacy to minimize the risk of adverse events and inhibit the development of bacterial resistance. Wherever possible single drug is preferable to combination prophylaxis to avoid additional side effects. Protection against all conceivable pathogens is unnecessary. Assuming at least equal clinical efficacy, single-shot prophylaxis offers the following major advantages over multidose regimes:

1. Economy (reduced costs of purchase, labor, storage, transport, preparation and disposal)
2. Reduced administration errors (fewer forgotten or delayed doses) [23, 30]
3. Fewer side effects [12]
4. Greater compliance

For all these reasons the goal is single-shot prophylaxis provided it guarantees sustained antimicrobial activity throughout the risk period. In long-lasting procedures, short-acting antibiotics must be repeated to sustain adequate tissue levels at the pertinent site for the entire duration of the procedure [13, 14]. Failure to cover the whole period is associated with higher failure rates [17, 28].

Thus, the longer a surgical procedure lasts, the longer appropriate antibiotic tissue levels must be maintained, either by repeated administration or by a single dose of a suitable long-acting antimicrobial. It would be irrational to give less antibacterial protection per unit time to patients at a significantly higher risk of infectious complications due to longer-lasting operations. Most conventional cephalosporins have a half-life of only 0.5 - 2.5 h [6]. For periods exceeding 1-3 h, long-acting cephalosporins are indicated in single-dose prophylaxis provided they meet the criteria of clinical and cost-effectiveness: A single dose covers the entire perioperative risk period even allowing for long lasting surgery, making repeated administration not only unnecessary, but also impossible to forget (a great advantage in the everyday working situation). Single-dose prophylaxis with a long-acting broad-spectrum antibiotic also compares favorably in cost-benefit analyses, because it significantly reduces the rate of postoperative pneumonia and urinary tract infection [23].

Individual Laparoscopic Procedures

Biliary Surgery

A review of 15,914 laparoscopic cholecystectomies performed in 1990-1992 (with no details of the type of antibiotic prophylaxis) found an average wound infection rate of 1.3% (maximum: 11.9%) [32]. However, these results cannot be compared with conventional open cholecystectomy, because there were differences in patient selection, and approximately 4% of cases were converted to open cholecystectomy. In acute cholecystitis a 27% conversion rate of laparoscopic to open cholecystectomy has been reported with 16.9% overall operative morbidity [35].

Up to 70% of patients undergoing biliary surgery have pathogenic bacteria in the bile (mixed flora, with a predominance of Escherichia coli and Klebsiella). Thus, even faultless laparoscopic technique may not always avoid contaminating the peritoneum or abdominal wall along the instrument tract (implantation metastases) particularly when dividing the cystic duct, performing cholangiography, draining the bile ducts or during the dissection and removal of the gallbladder. Prophylaxis is therefore indicated with a broad-spectrum antibiotic active also against Gram-negative species.

Prolonged antibiotic therapy is required in suppurative cholangitis and septic cholecystitis, failure to retrieve gallstones lost in the abdominal cavity and transient abdominal fistulation of infected bile to avoid subhepatic, subphrenic and intra-abdominal abscesses (together with appropriate surgical measures, e.g. peritoneal lavage, bile duct drainage, etc.).

Most conventional cephalosporins are not excreted in bile. There is a definite advantage to using an agent that achieves high bactericidal levels of broad-spectrum antibiotic in bile as well as tissue, as does ceftriaxone even in obstructive jaundice [3, 4].

Gastro-intestinal Resection

All procedures in which the gastrointestinal tract is opened carry a high risk of infection particularly in the colon, which contains up to 10^{13} bacteria/g feces. The risk is multiplied by obstruction (irrespective of cause: cancer, adhesions, impaction, foreign body or inflammation), which prevents adequate preoperative bowel preparation. In ileus or shock the risk is compounded by stasis and impaired microcirculation. To prevent intestinal contents from contaminating the abdominal cavity, the current practice is to staple the bowel segment prior to resection. However, this is not anatomically possible at all sites. It is also often necessary to open the viscus (e.g. stomach) in order to insert the stapler arms, thereby forcing some degree of contamination. Antibiotic prophylaxis is mandatory in all such cases, and likewise in all forms of immunodeficiency.

A literature review of prospective controlled randomized studies in colonic surgery suggests that third-generation cephalosporins are clinically more effective than their first- or second-generation counterparts (wound infection rates: 7.9% vs 14.8%) [34].

It used to be thought that antibiotic cover was necessary only from the start of the operation until skin closure. However, 24 h cover in colon resection is markedly more effective than prophylaxis for 4 - 6 h [18], because the anastomotic suture or staple line will not prevent bacterial invasion for several hours. For this reason only long-acting antibiotics should be used in single-shot colonic prophylaxis [16].

Because of the high proportion of anaerobes in the colon, combination therapy with a beta-lactamase-resistant broad-spectrum antibiotic and a nitroimidazole (e.g. metronidazole) is often recommended. However, controlled studies in colorectal surgery have shown that perioperative prophylaxis with an antibiotic combination does not always protect against Gram-negative pathogens. Because such cover is essential, third-generation cephalosporins are now used - with or without metronidazole - in preference to their first-generation relatives [21]. Antibiotic cover is also mandatory in laparoscopic appendectomy [29].

Gynaecological Surgery

Laparoscopic gynaecological surgery has a relatively long history compared with laparoscopic digestive surgery. A recent compilation of more than 145,000 diagnostic and therapeutic laparoscopic gynaecological procedures showed 0.10% mortality and less than 4% laparoscopic-related morbidity. The incidence of death from cardiovascular and pulmonary complications was remarkably low, probably because the vast majority of procedures were performed in younger women [1].

However, a relatively large proportion of laparoscopic gynaecological surgery is infection-related (adnexitis, salpingitis, pelvic inflammatory disease) and may involve opening of an infected section of the genital tract. Such cases almost always require (combination) broad-spectrum antibiotic therapy [20, 26]. The flora is usually a mixture of aerobes and anaerobes, as in the colon, but with the addition of sexually transmitted disease pathogens particularly (since 1976) beta-lactamase-producing penicillin-resistant gonococci; current treatments of choice for the latter include ceftriaxone, which - alone or in combination with metronidazole - is highly effective in surgical prophylaxis [5, 7, 25, 33].

Foreign-Body Implants

Despite various attempts at laparoscopic herniorrhaphy without the use of foreign material, it is now standard practice to insert an extraperitoneal mesh using a trans- or extraperitoneal approach. Infection around a foreign-body implant not only destroys the point of surgery, but also complicates antibacterial therapy at substantial cost. All procedures involving foreign-body implants (prosthetic hip, heart valve surgery, etc.) should therefore always be carried out under antibiotic cover, although the sepsis rate is low and the efficacy of antibiotic prophylaxis remains unproven.

Other Laparoscopic Operations

Where the risk of operative infection can be excluded for practical purposes, as in elective clean procedures under optimum conditions, perioperative antibiotic prophylaxis is not required. All high-risk procedures and patients, on the other hand, require single-shot prophylaxis with an appropriate antibiotic, because the potential benefits greatly outweigh the effort, cost and minimal side effects involved.

References

1. BAILEY RW: Complications of laparoscopic general surgery. In: Zucker KA (ed.): Surgical laparoscopy. Quality Medical Publishing Inc, St Louis, Missouri (1991) 311-342.
2. BERGAMINI TM, POLK JR JC: The importance of tissue antibiotic activity in the prevention of operative wound infection. J Antimicrob Chemother 23 (1989) 301-313.
3. BIRKNER B, ADAM D, KAESS H: Elimination von 1 g Ceftriaxon i.v. in die Galle bei mechanischem Verschlußikterus. Z antimikrob antineoplast Chemother 7 (1989)103-107.
4. BROGARD JM, JEHL F, PARIS-BOCKEL D et al.: La ceftriaxone, cephalosporine à forte élimination hépatique. Schweiz Med Wochschr 117 (1987) 1549-1559.
5. CARDAMAKIS E et al.: Ceftriaxone versus cefotaxime as single-dose prophylaxis in gynecological operations. Intl J Exp Clin Chemother 4 (1991) 94-99.
6. CHRIST W: Pharmacological properties of cephalosporins. Infection 19 (1991) (Suppl 5) 244-252.
7. DECAVALAS G et al.: Comparative study of ceftriaxone versus cefamandole for pre-operative prophylaxis of infections in patients undergoing cesarean section or vaginal hysterectomy. J Chemother 1 (1989) (Suppl 4) 1048-1050.
8. FAUST H, LADWIG D, REICHEL K: Die laparoskopische Cholecystektomie als Standardeingriff bei symptomatischer Cholecystolithiasis (Erfahrungen bei 1277 Patienten). Chirurg 65 (1994) 194-199.
9. GALANDIUK S, POLK JR HC, JAGELMAN DG, FAZIO VW: Re-emphasis of priorities in surgical antibiotic prophylaxis. Surg Gynecol Obstet 169 (1989) 219-222.
10. GEROULANOS S, HELL K: Risk factors in surgery. Editiones Roche 1994, ISBN 3-907770-04-8.
11. HELL K: How to choose antimicrobials for surgical prophylaxis. J Chemother 1 (1989) 24-29.
12. HELL K: Single dose versus multiple dose prophylaxis in surgery. 28th World Congress of the International College of Surgeons, Cairo, Egypt, November 16-21, 1992. Monduzzi Editore (1993) 379-384.
13. HIRSCHMAN JV: Controversies in antimicrobial prophylaxis. Chemiotherapia 6 (1987) 202-207.
14. HOLLENDER LF, MINCK R, POTTECHER T, GARCIA-CASTELLANOS J: Der aktuelle Stand der perioperativen Antibiotikaprophylaxe in der kolorektalen Chirurgie. Zentralbl Chir 112 (1987) 896-908.
15. JONES RN et al.: Cefotaxime single-dose surgical prophylaxis in a prepaid group practice. Comparison with other cephalosporins and ticarcillin/clavulanic acid. Drugs 35 (1988) (Suppl 2) 116-123.
16. JONES RN: Antibiotic prophylaxis for surgical infections: summation. Am J Surg 164 (1992) (Suppl 4a) 4849.
17. KAISER AB, HERRINGTON JR JL, JACOBS JK, MULHERIN JR JL, ROACH AC, SAWYERS JL: Cefoxitin versus erythromycin, neomycin, and cefazolin in colorectal operations: importance of the duration of the surgical procedure. Ann Surg 198 (1983) 525-530.
18. KARRAN S et al.: Short-course antibiotic prophylaxis is inferior to a 24-hour cover in elective colorectal surgery. In: 6th Mediterranean Congress of Chemotherapy, Florence. Il Sedicesimo (1988) 161.
19. KIFF RS, LOMAX J, FOWLER L, KINGSTON RD, HOARE EM, SYKES PA: Ceftriaxone versus povidone iodine in preventing wound infections following biliary surgery. Ann Royal Coll Surg Engl 70 (1988) 313-316.
20. KOUTOULAS IG, CARDAMAKIS E, MICHOPOULOS J ET AL.: Comparison of ceftriaxone plus ornidazole, ceftazidime plus ornidazole, and ornidazole in the treatment of pelvic inflammatory disease (PID). Intl J Exp Clin Chemother 5 (1992) 159-164.
21. LUMLEY JW, SIU SK, PILLAY SP, STITZ R, KEMP RJ, FAOAGALI J ET AL.: Single dose ceftriaxone as prophylaxis for sepsis in colorectal surgery. Aust N Z J Surg 62 (1992) 292-296.
22. MCDONALD PJ, SANDERS P, TURNIDGE J, HAKENDORF P, JOLLEY P, MCDONALD H, PETRUCCO O: Optimal duration of cefotaxime prophylaxis in abdominal and vaginal hysterectomy. Drugs 35 (1988) (Suppl 2) 216-220.
23. MORRIS WT: Ceftriaxone prophylaxis in surgery. N Z Med J 103 (1990) 26.
24. MORRIS WT: Prophylaxis against sepsis in patients undergoing major surgery. World J Surg 17 (1993) 178-183.
25. PETERSEN EE et al.: Antibiotika-Prophylaxe bei Hysterektomie. Geburtshilfe Frauenheilkd 8 (1983) 481-532.
26. PETERSEN HB, GALAID E, ZENILMAN JM: Pelvic inflammatory disease: review of treatment options. Rev Infect Dis 12 (1990) (Suppl 6) 656-664.
27. PLATT R, ZALEZNIK DF, HOPKINS CC, DELLINGER EP, KARCHMER AW, BRYAN CS, BURKE JF, WIKLER MA, MARINO SK, HOLBROOK KF et al.: Perioperative antibiotic prophylaxis for herniorrhaphy and breast surgery. N Engl J Med 322 (1990) 153-160.
28. POLK JR HC, TRACHTENBERG MA, GEORGE CD: A randomized, double-blind trial of single dose piperacillin versus multidose cefoxitin in alimentary tract operations. Am J Surg 153 (1986) 517-521.
29. PUTZ A, BOGESITS R, MULLER W, WERNER C: Die laparoskopische Appendektomie als Routineeingriff. Infection 21 (1993) (Suppl 1) 54-58.
30. SCHWEIZER H, STRIFFELER H, LÜDI H, FRÖSCHER R: Single-Shot Prophylaxe in der Abdominalchirurgie. Helv Chir Acta 60 (1994) 483-488.
31. SHEVCHUK YM, CONLY JM: Antibiotic-associated hypoprothrombinemia: a review of prospective studies, 1966-1988. Rev Infect Dis 12 (1990) 1109-1126.
32. SIEWERT JR, FEUSSNER H, SCHERER MA, BRUNE IB: Fehler und Gefahren der laparoskopischen Cholecystektomie. Chirurg 64 (1993) 221-229.
33. SPITZER D ET AL.: Perioperative Antibiotikaprophylaxe bei vaginaler Hysterektomie. Therapiewoche Österreich 6 (1991) 270-276.
34. WITTMAN DH, CONDON RE: Prophylaxis of postoperative infections. Infection 19 (1991) (Suppl 6) S337-S344.
35. ZUCKER KA, FLOWERS JL, BAILEY RW et al.: Laparoscopic management of acute cholecystitis. Am J Surg 165 (1993) 508-514.

Biliary Tract Surgery

Critical Comments

C. K. McSherry

The chapters that deal with biliary tract surgery are from France, Germany and the United States and present an excellent summary of the current status of laparoscopic techniques in the management of diseases of the gallbladder and common bile duct. This assessment is timely in view of the remarkable changes that have taken place since laparoscopic cholecystectomy was introduced in France in 1989. Although there are minor variations in technique attributed to local custom and individual preferences, the approach to calculous disease is quite similar in both Europe and the United States.

The chapter from Germany by Ungeheuer and Brune documents their experience with 1.821 patients subjected to laparoscopic cholecystectomy in Munich. The authors estimate that currently 80 % of patients in need of cholecystectomy undergo the laparoscopic technique. Conversion to open cholecystectomy occurred in 3 % of the patients, and there were 5 (0.27 %) bile duct injuries. Although laparoscopic choledochoscopy was possible in 21 patients (1.1 %), the authors preferred ERCP and endoscopic papillotomy before or after laparoscopic cholecystectomy for the management of common duct stones.

The chapter by Jacques Périssat provides an excellent review of the evolution of intraoperative cholangiography and choledochoscopy. This information is helpful in understanding the "French" approach to common duct stones. Although the author prefers ERCP and endoscopic papillotomy for the treatment of common duct stones, he describes his experience with 176 patients with common duct stones. Transcystic exploration of the common duct as well as laparoscopic choledochotomy were utilized successfully. Less frequently a transcystic, transpapillary probe was placed at operation to facilitate a subsequent ERCP and papillotomy.

Dr. Birkett's chapter describes his current method for laparoscopic common duct exploration. His technique for performing intraoperative cholangiography and gaining access to the common duct via the cystic duct is detailed and well written. Dr. Birkett advocates fragmentation of common duct stones by electrohydraulic lithotripsy or preferably, the pulsed dye coumarin laser. In preference to extracting stones through the cystic duct and risking potential tears, he elects to fragment the stone and then dispose of the fragments by irrigating them into the duodenum.

It is evident that the laparoscopic techniques applied to biliary tract surgery are still evolving. The percentage of patients with gallstones subjected to open cholecystectomy continues to decrease but at a much slower rate. As experience grows, the number of patients considered to be poor candidates for laparoscopic cholecystectomy have diminished. Patients with prior operations in the upper abdomen and with mild degrees of acute cholecystitis are now successfully operated upon by laparoscopic techniques. It is difficult to track the incidence of bile duct injuries, but I have the sense that there has been a slight decrease in their frequency. Formerly, bile duct injuries were attributed to the "learning curve", but now many are related to efforts to perform the procedure in patients with acute cholecystitis. These injuries will continue until surgeons accept the limitations of their skills and adopt a greater willingness to convert to open cholecystectomy when confronted with problems.

The management of common bile duct stones continues to be controversial. As experience with laparoscopic surgery and intraoperative cholangiography increases, more surgeons are attempting laparoscopic common duct exploration with increasing success. ERCP and endoscopic papillotomy will always have a significant role in the management of common duct stones, but this technique will be utilized less frequently in future decades.

The degree of enthusiasm for laparoscopic common duct exploration depends on a variety of factors such as the operative case load of the individual surgeon, his technical skills, the availability of expensive technology and access to expert endoscopists. The latter is quite variable, and most are concentrated in large urban areas and teaching hospitals. Success rates with ERCP and papillotomy as well as their morbidity are comparable to open and laparoscopic choledocholithotomy. Thus the impetus for surgeons to adopt laparoscopic common duct exploration is very variable.

Optimal techniques for laparoscopic common duct exploration need further study. The technique as well as the extent of cystic duct dilation possibly needs to be resolved. Mechanical vs. electric or laser fragmentation of large stones is a fertile area of investigation. The technique of "pushing" or irrigating stone fragments into the duodenum is not without the hazard of postoperative pancreatitis. Laparoscopic choledochotomy has only been attempted to date by relatively few surgeons.

Despite the above uncertainties, it is clear that the role of laparoscopic techniques will expand in coming years, particularly in relation to choledocholithotomy.

6. | Laparoscopic Cholecystectomy

A. UNGEHEUER AND I. B. BRUNE

Introduction

In 1882 Carl Langenbuch performed the first successful removal of a gallbladder for cholelithiasis. Over the years both the morbidity and mortality for cholecystectomy have decreased because of the improvements in operative technique, anesthesia and the use of antibiotics, and as a result open cholecystectomy became the gold standard for the treatment of gallbladder stone disease [37]. Despite the excellent results reported by McSherry [21, 22], access to the gallbladder was still quite invasive. Therefore, a variety of other therapeutic options, such as dissolution, lithotripsy and endoscopic techniques, were tried. Although they were less invasive, they were also found to be less effective and they were only applicable to limited subgroups of patients [12, 26]. Also, the main cause of the gallstone disease, the gallbladder, was not removed, and this led to stone recurrence.

In 1989 laparoscopic cholecystectomy emerged from France as a procedure that combined the effectiveness of the open operation and a minor access method of reaching the gallbladder [2, 9, 13, 27, 28]. Initially, only the easiest cases were selected, but with growing experience laparoscopic cholecystectomy was performed in the majority of patients with results and complication rates that equalled those of the open procedure [1, 10, 34, 36, 38]. This technique soon became the method of choice for treatment of symptomatic, uncomplicated gallbladder stones.

Indications and Contraindications

The indications for cholecystectomy, either open or laparoscopic, are the presence of symptomatic gallstones. Asymptomatic gallstones are not an indication for laparoscopic cholecystectomy. Unlike open cholecystectomy, the laparoscopic procedure is still limited by a few contraindications.

At the beginning of the learning curve, severe inflammation of the gallbladder or the presence of common bile duct (CBD) stones that could not be endoscopically removed were indications for an open cholecystectomy: however, in experienced hands they are no longer absolute contraindications.

Laparoscopic cholecystectomy should not be performed when a gallbladder carcinoma is suspected, when the patient is suffering from portal hypertension associated with impaired coagulation or when the cardiopulmonary situation is such that general anesthesia and a pneumoperitoneum cannot be tolerated.

Preoperative Work-up

General preparations include patient history, clinical examination, ECG, a chest X-ray, blood tests and an ultrasound of the gallbladder, liver and bile ducts. Ultrasound gives a precise assessment of gallbladder size, thickness of the wall and identifies the presence of stones thereby making the diagnosis. The common bile duct is inspected and its diameter is measured because a dilated duct is the principal indirect sign of common bile duct stones.

If the patient presents with a history of jaundice, abnormal liver function tests or a dilated common bile duct on ultrasonography, an endoscopic retrograde cholangiopancreatography (ERCP) is performed. A study performed on 250 patients [24] showed that patients without one of these three criteria are prone to have CBD stones in only 2.5 %. Because the clinical relevance of these stones has yet to be defined, routine ERCP does not seem justifiable. Although laparoscopic common bile duct exploration is becoming used more commonly (see Chap. 7 and 8), we still prefer endoscopic papillotomy and stone extraction prior to laparoscopic cholecystectomy. Whenever a gallbladder carcinoma is suspected, a computer tomography (CT) scan should be performed because this may provide valuable information.

In the early phase of the learning curve, preoperative i.v. cholangiography was used to image the bile ducts to define the anatomy and identify bile duct stones [5, 15]. With growing experience in laparoscopic dissection techniques and widespread use of intraoperative cholangiography, this diagnostic test is no longer performed.

Operative Technique

The operation is performed under general anaesthesia with the patient in the supine position, the legs apart for those surgeons who prefer to operate from between the patient's legs ("French position") or stretched out if the surgeon stands on the patient's side. The table is tilted in a reverse Trendelenburg position and slightly to the left. A gastric tube is inserted to completely empty the stomach and reduce the chances of injury from the Veress needle or first trocar and to improve the view of the gallbladder during the laparoscopy.

The laparoscopic literature describes a variety of different positions for trocar placement and placement of the surgeon and assistants around the operating table. There is no uniformity and most of the variation is surgeon-dependent. The

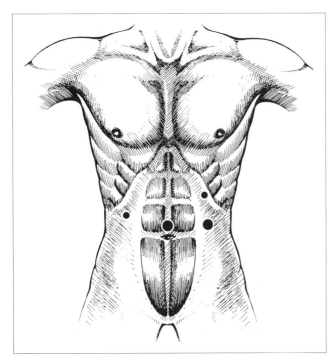

Fig. 1. Trocar placement for laparoscopic cholecystectomy

troduction of the first trocar, the other trocars are placed under direct vision to avoid intra-abdominal injury. Diaphanoscopy through the abdominal wall may help to avoid perforation of the epigastric vessels.

After lifting of both lobes of the liver to expose the gallbladder adhesions to the omentum, duodenum or transverse colon are lysed (Fig. 2). The infundibulum is grasped with forceps and retracted away from the hepatoduodenal ligament holding the cystic duct under tension. The peritoneum is incised over the cystic duct, which is dissected from the infundibulum towards the common bile duct (Fig. 3). It is important to proceed with the dissection in this direction to avoid mistaking the common bile duct for the cystic duct, thus preventing common bile duct injury [14]. Once the cystic duct and artery have been identified (Fig. 4) and exposed, the cystic artery is triple clipped, two clips proximally and one distally, and divided with scissors (Fig. 5).

most important fact is that the surgeon must operate in a direction that is parallel to the laparoscope and must face the video screen. Usually, four trocars are required: two 10-mm trocars for the laparoscope and clip applier and two 5-mm trocars for the dissection instruments, graspers, scissors and cautery hook (Fig. 1).

The Veress needle is inserted through the umbilical region and a pneumoperitoneum is created to 12-14 mmHg. If intra-abdominal adhesions are suspected because of previous abdominal operations, the Veress needle is introduced into the peritoneal cavity through the left upper quadrant of the abdomen where there are likely to be fewer adhesions, or an open access can be achieved using the Hasson technique. After in-

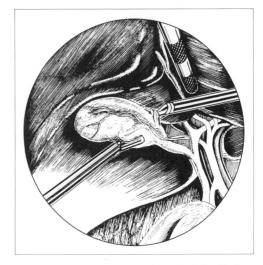

Fig. 3. Dissection of the cystic duct from the infundibulum towards the common bile duct

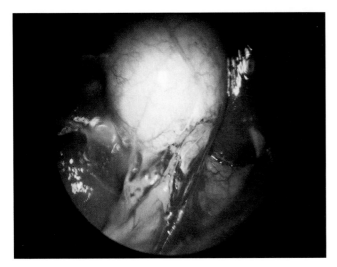

Fig. 2. Adhesions with the gallbladder are dissected

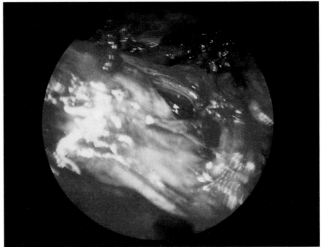

Fig. 4. Cystic artery (in the back) and cystic duct (in the front) have been identified

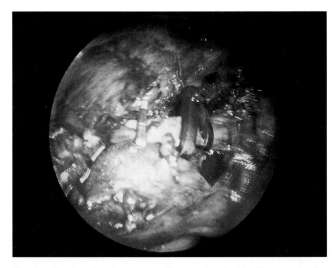

Fig. 5. Cystic artery is closed with two absorbable clips proximally, a Titanium clip distally and transsected with scissors

A cholangiogram, if it is to be performed, is the next step. The completely dissected (Fig. 6) cystic duct is closed just under the infundibulum with a clip and opened with scissors (Fig. 7). If there is no flow of bile, cystic duct occlusion by a stone should be suspected. A cystic duct stone should be milked towards the gallbladder and the opening in the cystic duct and extracted with a forceps. A cholangiogram catheter is introduced into the cystic duct either through one of the 5-mm trocars or through direct puncture of the abdominal wall. The catheter is held in place by a self-retaining mechanism (balloon) (Fig. 8), a clamp or a clip. If duct stones are found, an attempt can be made to extract them laparoscopically with baskets or by fragmentation with laser lithotripsy (Chap. 7 and 8).

Cholangiography also helps to delineate ductal anatomy in difficult cases such as those with dense adhesions or severe inflammatory disease. It can also demonstrate abnormal accessory ducts .

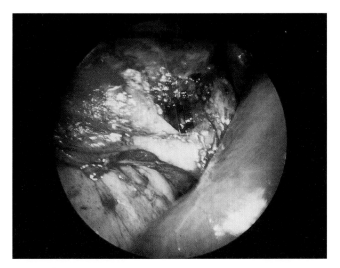

Fig. 6. Completely dissected cystic duct

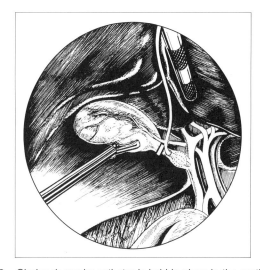

Fig. 8. Cholangiography catheter is held in place in the cystic duct with a self retaining balloon mechanism

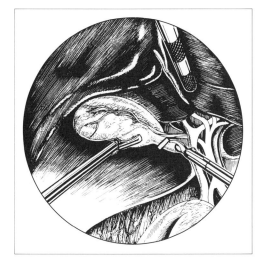

Fig. 7. Cystic duct is closed with a clip at the infundibulum and opened with scissors for cholangiography

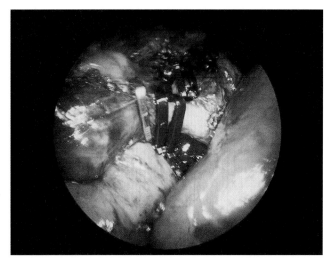

Fig. 9. Cystic duct is double clipped proximally and closed with a single clip towards the infundibulum

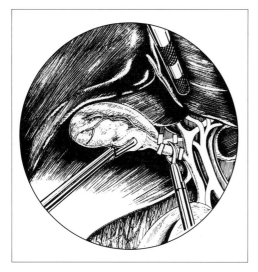

Fig. 10. Cystic duct is transsected with scissors between clips

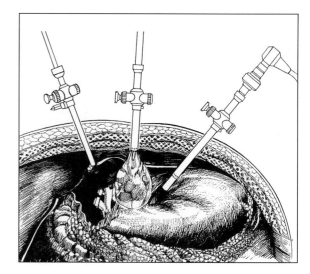

Fig. 13. Gallbladder is grasped at the infundibulum and pulled into the umbilical trocar

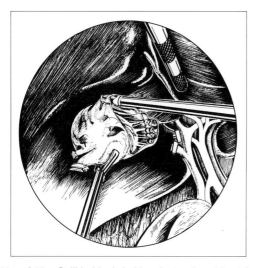

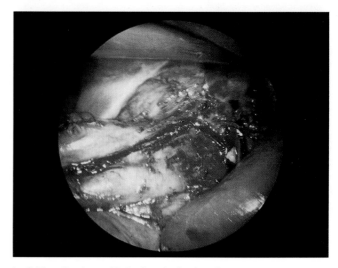

Figs. 11 and 12. Gallbladder is held under tension at the infundibulum to divide adhesions with the liver bed using electrocautery

The cholangiogram catheter is removed and the duct is double-clipped (Fig. 9) and divided with scissors (Fig. 10). Just as in an open operation, it is advisable to avoid the application of non-absorbable material on the cystic duct stump, and therefore absorbable clips are preferred. The gallbladder is grasped by the infundibulum and held under tension while the adhesions to the liver bed are divided by cautery to completely detach the gallbladder from the liver (Figs. 11 and 12).

After thorough irrigation of the liver bed, any bleeding is controlled with the cautery. In acute cholecystitis or empyema of the gallbladder, the plane of dissection may be hard to define resulting in dissection of the liver parenchyma. If there is difficulty in obtaining haemostasis, it may be necessary to introduce a collagen sheet covered with fibrin glue (Tacho-Comb®, Nycomed; see also Chap. 4) through one of the trocars and apply it to the liver bed with slight pressure. In addition to the haemostyptic effect a tamponade is achieved and small bile leaks can be prevented.

The gallbladder is grasped at the infundibulum by a strong forceps passed through one of the 10-mm trocars and partly pulled into the trocar (Fig. 13), which is then removed from the abdominal cavity. Once outside the abdominal cavity, the infundibulum is opened and the bile aspirated from the gallbladder. The stones are fragmented and extracted (Fig. 14) so that the empty gallbladder can then be removed through the small incision. When the stones are very large or the gallbladder is very thickened the skin incision may have to be enlarged.

If perforation of the gallbladder occurs during dissection or extraction of the gallbladder, bile may be spilled and stones lost. This is no reason to convert to an open operation, but every effort must be made to pick up all the stones and the abdominal cavity must be thoroughly irrigated to prevent the development of an abdominal abscess. The stones are collected and placed in a small extraction bag to avoid contamination of the abdominal wall and loss of stones in the subcutaneous tissue during extraction.

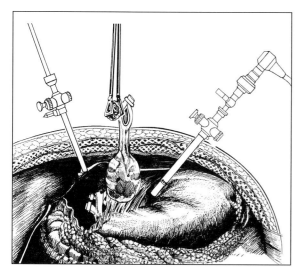

Fig. 14. Stones are fragmented and extracted with a forceps

At the end of the procedure the operative field is irrigated and inspected for haemostasis. If necessary, particularly in the case of acute cholecystitis or empyema, a drainage may be introduced through one of the 10-mm trocars and placed in the gallbladder bed. The carbon dioxide is completely evacuated and the fascia of the incisions 10 mm or larger are closed with sutures, whereas 5-mm incisions only require skin closure.

Postoperatively, the patients are allowed liquids on the evening of the day of operation. A regular diet is taken up on postoperative day 1, when most patients are discharged from hospital. Because the risk of severe postoperative hemorrhage is highest (1 %) within the first 24 h, it is advisable to observe patients for the first postoperative night in a hospital setting [39].

Intraoperative Problems

Bile Duct Injury

One of the major intraoperative problems of laparoscopic cholecystectomy is injury to the common bile duct or one of its branches. The injury rate for open cholecystectomy is low, but not zero [37]. In the laparoscopic setting all efforts must be made to avoid injury and keep it at least as low as in the open situation, because the complications of duct injury may result in lifelong problems.

If dissection is carried out cautiously, the risk of common bile duct injury is minimized. Preparation of the cystic duct should always be started at the infundibulum and be taken down as close as possible to the hepatoduodenal ligament without damaging the common duct. The most frequent mistake during laparoscopic biliary tract dissection is to mistake the common bile duct for the cystic duct and transect it. A clear identification of the junction between the cystic and common bile duct helps to avoid this problem. Whenever there is doubt about the anatomy of the biliary tree a cholangiogram should be performed because it may prevent a transection of the common duct that was mistaken for the cystic duct. Inadvertent coagulation injury of the common bile duct can

be avoided by careful use of the cautery and at the same time dissecting the cystic duct bluntly avoiding excessive coagulation.

Conversion to Laparotomy

Conversion to laparotomy should not be considered a complication, but a wise and necessary precaution to avoid undue risk to the patient. The decision whether to carry on laparoscopically or convert to laparotomy depends on the patience of the surgeon and must be influenced by the degree of his laparoscopic skills and experience. Reasons for conversion may be due to extensive adhesions or injury to the common bile duct or duodenum, which can only be repaired by open surgery.

Severe haemorrhage may require an immediate laparotomy, but unless caused by an injury to a very large vessel, it usually can be controlled laparoscopically with sufficient laparoscopic experience. Accumulation of large quantities of blood in the abdominal cavity impairs the view by both coating the tip of the laparoscope and the absorbing of light by the blood. Therefore, it is important to use a highly performant suction/irrigation device to maintain control of the situation.

Haemostasis

Smaller vessels can be grasped with forceps and coagulated, whereas large vessels must be controlled with clips or ligatures. Diffuse bleeding from the liver bed can also be stopped by coagulation if it is superficial. Deeper liver lesions of the liver bed that might also cause bile leakage are best controlled by spreading a collagen sheet covered with fibrin glue on the damaged area. This is the most effective way of achieving fast and safe haemostasis and preventing biliary leaks without the danger of uncontrolled extensive use of electrocautery.

Results

Between July 1990 and May 1995, 1821 laparoscopic cholecystectomies have been performed at the Department of Surgery of the Technical University of Munich. For the first few years the number of cholecystectomies performed each year increased, and has stabilized over the past few years at around 400-450 per year. The percentage of patients treated by laparoscopic cholecystectomy as compared with open cholecystectomy has gradually increased over the years and currently stands above 80 %.

The rate of conversion to open operation was 3.0 % (n = 56). The reasons for conversion were difficult anatomy in 34 patients (1.9 %) and complications in 22 patients (1.2 %).

Intraoperative cholangiography was performed in 64 patients (3.5 %) with 12 (0.6 %) patients found to have common bile duct stones that were removed postoperatively by ERCP. Laparoscopic intraoperative cholangioscopy with a flexible laparoscopic cholangioscope was possible in 21 patients (1.1 %).

There was no mortality. Postoperative complications occurred in 59 patients (3.2 %). Biliary complications accounted for 1.4 % (n = 27) including 5 patients (0.27 %) with a common bile duct injury. Postoperatively,12 patients (0.6 %) presented with missed or retained common duct stones that had not been found either pre- or intraoperatively. Of these patients, 11 underwent successful endoscopic removal and 1 patient underwent lithotripsy. Complications and their therapy are described in Table 1. The mean overall hospital stay was 3.1 days.

Table 1. Complications after 1821 laparoscopic cholecystectomies (n = 59; 3.2 %)

Complication	Therapy
Biliary (n = 27; 1.4 %)	
Common bile duct lesion (n = 5; 0.27 %)	Tangential injury [n = 4: suture, drain (intraoperative)] Resection [n – 1: hepato-jejunostomy (reoperation)]
Cystic duct leakage (n = 5; 0.27 %)	Nasobiliary drainage (n = 4) Reoperation and ligature (n = 1)
Leakage add. bile ducts (n = 5; 0.27 %)	Nasobiliary drainage (n = 4) Reoperation (n = 1)
Retained CBD stone (n = 12; 0.65 %)	EPT, endoscopic stone extraction (n = 11) Lithotripsy (n = 1)
Other complications (n = 32; 1.8 %)	
Intestinal injury (n = 3; 0.16 %)	Suture (n = 2) Resection (n = 1)
Bleeding (n = 5; 0.27 %)	Reoperation (n = 5; liver bed = 3, trocar incision = 2)
Haematoma of the liver (n = 3; 0.16 %)	Percutaneous drainage (n = 2) No therapy (n = 1)
Retroperitoneal haematoma (n = 1; 0.05 %)	No therapy
Pancreatitis (n = 1; 0.05 %)	Medical treatment
Deep vein thrombosis (n = 1; 0.05 %)	Medical treatment
Hernia trocar incision (n = 4; 0.2 %)	Hernia repair
Wound infection (n = 14; 0.76 %)	Local therapy

Discussion

Of all the laparoscopic procedures that have been described, laparoscopic cholecystectomy is the procedure that has most readily been accepted due to the obvious advantages of better cosmesis, less pain, a shorter hospital stay and recovery time. The procedure has spread rapidly throughout the surgical world [16, 20].

There were early concerns about the widespread clinical application of this procedure before experimental data were available. However, large studies have proven that after a learning curve the complication rates of laparoscopic cholecystectomy are no higher than that of open operation [1, 10, 17, 34, 36, 38]. Yet there are still problems to be addressed. The management of common bile duct stones in laparoscopic surgery is not as easy as during an open operation. Because the complications following operative removal of bile duct stones are no lower than after endoscopic papillotomy and stone extraction [8, 18, 30, 31], and because laparoscopic common bile duct exploration is still quite a demanding proce-

dure (see Chap. 7 and 8), we prefer treating duct stones with endoscopic papillotomy. Whenever common bile duct stones are identified preoperatively, we favour endoscopic papillotomy with stone extraction followed by laparoscopic cholecystectomy. Although this policy means that the patient has to undergo two procedures and requires a readily available experienced endoscopist, the results are excellent and the complication rate is low [3, 4, 25, 40]

If a common bile duct stone is recognized intraoperatively, the patient is referred to endoscopic papillotomy in the postoperative period. Only in some rare cases when endoscopy might be impossible (i. e. after previous gastric resection with reconstruction in a Roux-en-Y technique) will an attempt at laparoscopic common bile duct exploration or even conversion to an open operation be considered.

Another concern is the incidence of common bile duct injury. Large series have shown that the overall rate of common bile duct lesions is, after getting over the learning curve, no higher than for open surgery but the pattern of biliary injury is a different one [10, 11, 34]. Whereas at open operation, common bile duct injury is usually partial and mostly recognized intraoperatively, at laparoscopic cholecystectomy the most common complication is mistaking the common bile duct for the cystic duct which, resulting in resection of the duct, leaves a defect that is often unnoticed during the procedure and requires a secondary laparotomy for reconstruction. Also, stricture of the common bile duct can result from a clip of the cystic duct stump that catches part of the common duct [5]. Careful attention to the technical aspects of dissection of the cystic duct as described above [14] and performing an intraoperative cholangiography whenever there is doubt about the biliary anatomy will help to reduce the common bile duct injury rate to an acceptable level.

Intraoperative cholangiography as a routine procedure is advocated by some authors [7, 29, 32, 35, 41], whereas others prefer intraoperative sonography of the CBD or selective cholangiography [19] to detect common bile duct stones. Choledochoscopy can be added when laparoscopic stone extraction is planned [7]. The incidence of "silent" stones that are not suggested by patient history, cause pathological laboratory findings or a sonographically dilated common duct larger than 7 mm in diameter is very low and around 3.2 % [24, 25]. Their clinical relevance still remains to be ascertained. As a result, we do not recommend routine intraoperative cholangiography to detect common bile duct stones. In our experience, the rate of retained/missed common duct stones after laparoscopic cholecystectomy was 0.6 % [24, 25]. All of these stones could be removed postoperatively by endoscopic papillotomy.

Complication rates after laparoscopic cholecystectomy are no higher than after open cholecystectomy [1, 10, 34, 35, 38]. Wound-related complications seem to be less frequent in patients undergoing a laparoscopic procedure. Lethality is somewhat lower, but this may be due to a lower mean age among laparoscopically treated patients [17].

Another change that was induced by laparoscopic cholecystectomy is a reduction in postoperative hospital stay. Because postoperative recovery is less painful and easier, patients can be dismissed much earlier than after a conventional operation. However, we do not on the whole favour laparoscopic cholecystectomy as an outpatient procedure. About 1 % of serious complications, such as haemorrhage or bile leak, are likely to occur within the first 24 h after operation. Therefore, we prefer to observe our patients in hospital for one night. Only a very small selected patient population (young patients without concomitant disease or acute inflammation and with a family setting that assures adequate home care in the first days after the operation) can be operated on on an outpatient basis.

In conclusion, it seems that once through the initial learning curve, the complication and mortality rates are no higher after laparoscopic cholecystectomy than after an open operation. The better cosmetic result, less pain and shorter hospital stay associated with laparoscopic cholecystectomy has made it the gold standard and therapy of choice for the treatment of symptomatic cholecystolithiasis.

Laparoscopic cholecystectomy should not be performed when carcinoma of the gallbladder is suspected, in a patient with portal hypertension associated with impaired coagulation or in patients with a cardiopulmonary status that precludes general anaesthesia or a pneumoperitoneum.

References

1. BARKUN GS, BARKUN AN, MEAKINS JC, GROUP MGT: Laparoscopic versus open cholecystectomy: the Canadian experience. Am J Surg 165 (1993) 455-458.
2. BERCI G, SACKIER JM: The Los Angeles experience with laparoscopic cholecystectomy. Am J Surg 161 (1991) 382-384.
3. BOECKL O, SUNGLER P, HEINEMANN PM, LEXER G: Choledocholithiasis – therapeutic splitting. Chirurg 65 (1994) 424-429.
4. BRODISH RJ, FINK AS: ERCP, cholangiography and laparsocopic cholecystectomy: The Society of American Gastrointestinal Endoscopic Surgeons (SAGES) opinion survey. Surg Endosc 7 (1993) 3.
5. BRUNE IB, SCHÖNLEBEN K, OMRAN S: Complications after laparoscopic and conventional cholecystectomy: a comparative study. HPB Surgery 8 (1994) 19-25.
6. BRUNE IB, SCHÖNLEBEN K: Entscheidung laparoskopische oder konventionelle Cholecystektomie anhand der präoperativen Diagnostik. In: Häring R(ed.) Diagnostik und Therapie des Gallensteinleidens. Blackwell, Berlin (1992) 113-123.
7. CARROLL BJ, FALLAS MJ, PHILLIPS EH: Laparoscopic transcystic choledochoscopy. Surg Endosc 8 (1994) 310-314.
8. COTTON PB: Endoscopic retrograde cholangiopancreaticography and laparoscopic cholecystectomy. Am J Surg 165 (1993) 474-478.
9. CUSHIERI A et al.: The European experience with laparoscopic cholecystectomy. Am J Surg 161 (1991) 385-387.
10. DEZIEL DJ, WILLIKAN KW, ECONOMON SG et al: Complications of laparoscopic cholecystectomy: a national survey of 4292 hospitals and analysis of 77 604 cases. Am J Surg 165 (1993) 6.
11. GEBHARD C, MEINL P: Gallenwegsläsionen bei der offenen Cholecystektomie. Chirurg 65 (1994) 741.
12. GILLILAND TM, TRAVERSO LW: Modern standards for comparison of cholecystectomy with alternative treatments for symptomatic cholelithiasis with emphasis on long-term relief of symptoms. Surg Gynecol Obstet 170 (1990) 39-44.
13. GRAVES HA, BALLINGER JF, ANDERSON WJ: Appraisal of laparoscopic cholecystectomy. Ann Surg 213 (1991) 655-664.
14. HUNTER JG: Avoidance of bile duct injury during laparoscopic cholecystectomy. Am J Surg 162 (1991) 71-76.
15. LÄMMER-SKARKE I, HELMBERGER H, UNGEHEUER A, FEUSSNER H, GERHARDT P: Die Rolle der i.v. Cholangiographie und der Sonographie in der präoperativen Diagnostik vor laparoskopischer Cholecystektomie.Fortschr Röntgenstr161 (1994) 133-138.
16. LARSON GM et al.: Multipractice analysis of laparoscopic cholecystectomy in 1983 patients. Am J Surg 163 (1992) 221-226.
17. LEE VS, CHARI RS, CUCCHIARO G, MEYERS WC: Complications of laparoscopic cholecystectomy. Am J Surg 165 (1993) 527-532.
18. LENNERT KA, MÜLLER V: Wie hoch ist das Risiko der offenen Behandlung der Choledocholithiasis. Chirurg 61 (1990) 376.
19. LILLEMOE KD et al.: Selective cholangiography: current role in laparoscopic cholecystectomy. Ann Surg 215 (1992) 669-676.
20. LITWIN DE et al.: Laparoscopic cholecystectomy: trans-Canada experience with 2201 cases. Can J Surg 35 (1992) 291-296.
21. MCSHERRY CK: Cholecystectomy: the gold standard. Am J Surg 158 (1989) 174-178.
22. MCSHERRY CK: Open cholecystectomy. Am J Surg 165 (1993) 435-439.
23. NENNER RP, IMPERATO PJ, ALCORN CM: Serious complications of laparoscopic cholecystectomy in New York State. NYS J Med 92 (1992) 179-181.
24. NEUHAUS M, UNGEHEUER A, FEUSSNER H, CLASSEN M, SIEWERT JR: Laparoskopische Cholecystektomie: ERCP als präoperative Standarddiagnostik? Dtsch Med Wochenschr 117 (1992) 1863-1867.
25. NEUHAUS M, HOFFMANN W, FEUSSNER H, UNGEHEUER A: Prospective evaluation of the utility and safety of endoscopic retrograde cholangiography (ERC) before laparoscopic cholecystectomy. Gastrointest Endosc 38 (1992) 7.
26. O´DONNELL LD, HEATON KW: Recurrence and re-recurrence of gall stones after medical dissolution: a long-term follow-up. Gut 29 (1988) 655-658.
27. OLSEN DO: Laparoscopic cholecystectomy. Am J Surg 161 (1991) 339-344.
28. PÉRISSAT J et al.: Die laparoskopische Cholecystektomie – Operationstechnik und Ergebnisse der ersten 100 Operationen. Chirurg 61 (1990) 723-728 .
29. PHILLIPS EH: Routine versus selective intraoperative cholangiography. Am J Surg 165 (1993) 505-507.
30. PITT MA: Role of open choledochotomy in the treatment of choledocholithiasis. Am J Surg 165 (1993) 483-486.
31. RIEGER R, SULZBACHER M, WOISETSCHLÄGER R, SCHRENK P, WAYAND W: Selective use of ERCP in patients undergoing laparoscopic cholecystectomy. World J Surg 18 (1994) 900-904.
32. ROSENTHAL RJ, STEIGERWALD SD, IMIG R, BOCKHORN H: Role of intraoperative cholangiography during endoscopic cholecystectomy. Surg Lap Endosc 4 (1994) 171-174.
33. ROSSI RL, SCHIRMER WJ, BRAASCH JW, SANDERS LB, MUNSON L: Laparoscopic bile duct injuries – risk factors, recognition and repair. Arch Surg 127 (1992) 596.
34. SIEWERT JR, FEUSSNER H, UNGEHEUER A: Fehler und Gefahren bei laparoskopischer Cholecystektomie. Chirurgie 64 (1994) 221.
35. SOPER NJ, DUNNEGAN DL: Routine versus selective intraoperative cholangiography during laparoscopic cholecystectomy. World J Surg 16 (1992) 1136.
36. SOPER NJ, FLYE MW, BRUNT LM, STOCKMAN PR, SICARD GA, PICUS D, EDMUNDOWICZ SA, ALIPERTI G: Diagnosis and management of biliary complications of laparoscopic cholecystectomy. Am J Surg 165 (1993) 663-669.
37. TREDE M, SCHAUPP W: Ein Plädoyer für die Cholecystektomie – "Goldstandard der Gallensteintherapie". Chirurgie 61 (1990) 365.
38. TREDE M, TROIDL H, HERFARTH C, BEGER HG, FEUSSNER H: Ist die laparoskopische Cholecystektomie bereits als Goldstandard bei der blanden Cholecystolithiasis anzusehen? Langenbecks. Arch Chir 377 (1992) 190.
39. UNGEHEUER A, FEUSSNER H: Laparoskopische Cholezystektomie – ein tageschirurgischer Eingriff? Langenbecks Arch Chir Suppl II 167 (1995).
40. VITALE GC, LARSON GM, WIEMAN TJ, CHEADLE WG, MILLER FB: The use of ERCP in the management of common bile duct stones in patients undergoing laparoscopic cholecystectomy. Surg Endosc 7 (1993) 9.
41. WIEDEN TE, ABOUSAIDY F, LEORHO G, WEISER HF: Laparoskopische Cholecystektomie – Stellenwert der intraoperativen Cholangiographie. Minimal invasive Chirurgie 1 (1992) 86-90.

7. | Laparoscopic Treatment of Common Bile Duct Stones

J. PÉRISSAT

Introduction

The laparoscopic approach of common bile duct (CBD) stones emerged as soon as the first laparoscopic cholecystectomies (LC) were performed. This was for two obvious reasons, which are linked to the characteristics of gallbladder lithiasis and have been long known:

1. There are no CBD stones without gallbladder lithiasis, because the gallbladder is the formation site of the stones.
2. Asymptomatic CBD stones, also called silent stones (SS), are found in 6–10 % of patients with gallbladder lithiasis. Should they be overlooked during LC, they may create an unpleasant surprise when the symptoms appear a few months later.

Throughout the years these notions have been carefully analyzed and have led to this very simple golden rule applied in open surgery: *"Any operation performed on a lithiasic gallbladder must be accompanied by systematic exploration of the CBD in order to detect possible silent stones".* This is how intraoperative cholangiography (IOC) triumphed.

Born in Argentina in the hands of Mirizzi [22], it conquered the world gradually thanks to people such as Caroli in Paris [4], Mallet-Guy in Lyon [21], Tondelli in Switzerland [34], Cuschieri in Great Britain [9], and Berci in the United States [3], who were not only stubborn, but also convincing promoters who kept simplifying the technique until it eventually became a quick, precise, routine procedure. In the 1960s it was no longer conceivable to perform biliary surgery in an operating room that was not also equipped for IOC. The rate of residual stones decreased from 10 % to less than 1 %. This rate dropped again when intraoperative choledochoscopy appeared. Nothing is easier than to carry out these procedures through laparotomy, which provides a wide approach of the biliary tract. Apparently, the problem was solved, because until 1970 open surgery remained the only adequate and final cure for cholelithiasis whatever its location. In 1972 the first endoscopic retrograde cholangiopancreatography (ERCP) followed by an endoscopic sphincterotomy (ES) were performed [7]. After 10 years of steady progress, improvement and expansion, ES provides a worthy alternative to choledochotomy through laparotomy [27]. Ultrasonic imagery is making progress [1, 19] and so is the analysis of cholestatic biological markers [16].

In the 1980s [10, 14, 15] several studies were published concerning with the preoperative predictive criteria of silent CBD stones. They seem so accurate [17] that some authors do not hesitate to disregard the principle of "no cholecystectomy without IOC". They advocate a return to selective IOC, which would be performed only when the preoperative assessment suggests a possible SS presence. When no doubt remains, the technique of cholecystectomy is simplified by suppressing IOC, thus making it possible to choose a narrower and aesthetically more satisfactory approach called *minilaparotomy* [11]. After 1980, in view of the remarkable success obtained through ES in the major teams of biliary endoscopic gastroenterologists [8, 13, 23, 29–33], the growing tendency was towards a course of therapy in which endoscopy played a decisive part:

1. When CBD stones were clinically evident, ERCP was performed, followed by ES, whereas cholecystectomy was either postponed or not performed at all according to whether secondary cholecystitis appeared.
2. When gallbladder lithiasis was not accompanied by clinically obvious CBD stones, a systematic search was launched. If the predictive assessment leaned towards stone presence, the previous course of action was taken. If the predictive assessment was negative, cholecystectomy is performed through minilaparotomy without IOC. Although it was widely disputed, especially for young patients, this alternative treatment was used increasingly more often, and with indisputable success for the treatment of CBD stones, which, as a consequence, were treated increasingly less often by open surgery.

Has LC opened new prospects in the field? The answer is *yes*. Performing LC makes it necessary to approach the CBD in order to locate it and avoid injuring it. "See it in order not to touch it" was our objective when we started performing LC [24]. One should remember that in 1988, Ph. Mouret, F. Dubois [12] and myself were still treading virgin land. Not to touch the CBD implied the certainty that no stone would be left there. Our selection was therefore pitiless. A patient whose case history in the recent past or in the preceding year allowed us to suspect the presence of a CBD stone, or who was suffering from acute cholecystitis, would not be operated upon laparoscopically.

Preoperative Work-up

As for the other patients, the preoperative assessment included the measuring of cholestatic enzymes, ultrasonography of the biliary tract, X-ray opacification of the biliary tract through cholangiography, either intravenous with tomography, or through ERCP if ultrasonography revealed a wide CBD, or if the images obtained through intravenous cholangiography were not of good enough quality. The consequence of this strict selection was that in the beginning we only treated 25–30 % of gallbladder stones laparoscopically. As we became more experienced with the laparoscopic technique [25], we became able to perform laparoscopic IOC and difficult dissection of inflamed or badly infected gallbladders.

Laparoscopy offers the same range of operating techniques as open surgery. We extended our indications to all anatomopathological forms of gallbladder lithiasis and increasingly had to face the problem of silent CBD stones when the urgency of the situation did not allow an accurate preoperative checkup. This is how, under the pressure of urgency, we approached the CBD laparoscopically. This technical achievement allows us now to consider treating CBD stones laparoscopically, thus starting the competition with ERCP + SE. The decision which approach is the method of choice has not been made yet, and will depend on the conclusions of the current controlled studies.

Operative Technique

Common bile duct stones can be removed laparoscopically through two different approaches: (a) through the cystic duct (transcystic approach), and (b) via a choledochotomy. Whatever approach is chosen, it always comes after laparoscopic cholecystectomy, whose basic principles should first be recalled.

The "French" technique, developed by Ph. Mouret, F. Dubois and myself, has basic distinctive features, which concern the position of the patient and of the operating team, the way to display the triangle of Calot and the way to perform intraoperative cholangiography.

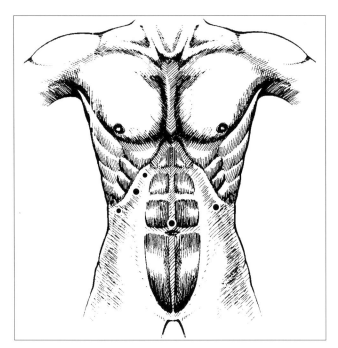

Fig. 1. Position of the trocars for laparoscopic common bile duct (CBD) exploration

Position of Patient and of Operating Team

The patient lies supine with legs spread out resting on straight supports, the surgeon sitting or standing between the patient's legs. The first assistant is on the patient's left, and the video monitor and equipment are at the right of the patient's head. The instrument table and scrub nurse are on the patient's right. The mobile X-ray equipment is rolled in to the left of the patient for the intraoperative cholangiography.

How to Display the Triangle of Calot

The trocars are placed as follows (Fig. 1):
1. A 10-mm trocar is inserted through the umbilicus for the laparoscope and the camera (I).
2. A 5-mm trocar (III) is placed 1 cm from the right costal edge directly above the lower edge of the liver and the gallbladder neck, through which the irrigation/aspiration equipment will be inserted. It will be used to lift up the lower aspect of the liver and display the gallbladder.
3. Another 5-mm trocar (II) is placed in the right hypochondrium opposite the gallbladder fundus. It will receive the grasping forceps, which holds the gallbladder neck and pulls it to the right and slightly down.

The combined actions of the instruments placed in II and III open up widely the anterior side of the triangle of Calot. A specific instrument is used to lift up the lower aspect of the liver. This is different from the "American" technique, in which the lower aspect of the liver is lifted together with the gallbladder, by means of a grasping forceps applied to the fundus of the gallbladder, which pulls it upwards and to the outside. The traction exerted here counteracts the action of the other grasping forceps, which grips the gallbladder neck and may prevent the triangle of Calot from being exposed properly (Fig. 2).

In the same way, in the "French" technique, the trocar, which is used to insert instruments for dissection, haemostasis, and clips or ligatures if necessary, is placed in the left hypochondrium. This is in agreement with what is considered in laparoscopic surgery as the adequate positioning for instruments: The instrument used to hold, and the one used to dissect, should be diametrically opposed and perpendicular to the axis of the laparoscope.

Intraoperative Cholangiography

The technique may vary according to the objective. If the aim is to clarify a confusing anatomy, it may be performed through direct puncture of the gallbladder or of the main bile duct. If the aim is to locate a silent CBD stone, it should be performed by introducing the catheter into the cystic duct once the latter has been identified with absolute certainty. It then represents the beginning of the transcystic approach of the CBD.

Transcystic Approach of the CBD

Transcystic approach of the CBD can be performed once the triangle of Calot has been dissected and the cystic artery clamped or ligated. A clip is placed at the junction of the cystic

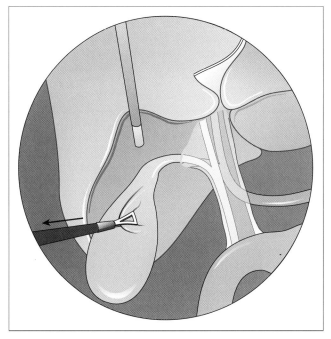 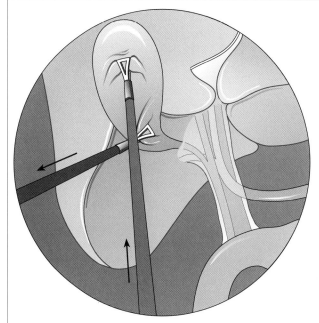

Fig. 2.   Exposure of the triangle of Calot

duct and gallbladder neck. Scissors are inserted through trocar IV, which allows lateral opening of the cystic duct, against the clip. A clamp is introduced through trocar IV, which will be used to gently milk the cystic duct from its junction with the common bile duct, and towards the partial opening of the cystic duct. This allows to clear any stones that may have migrated into the distal segment of the cystic duct. It also prevents the cholangiography catheter from pushing them into the common bile. Even if no stone is found, bile will appear, which is a good test in itself. The clamp in trocar IV is used to lift up the liver, thus replacing the irrigation/aspiration device, which has been removed from trocar III and replaced by a Reddick-Olsen clamp, which allows insertion of a ureteric catheter into the cystic duct. This clamp is closed around the cystic duct, to prevent contrast medium leakage. This allows visualization of the anatomy of the cystic duct and of the CBD, and to detect possible CBD stones, their number, shape and location.

Stone removal through the cystic duct will depend on the latter's diameter and anatomy: A short cystic duct lying perpendicular to the CBD provides ideal conditions, whereas a long cystic duct running parallel to the CBD, and implanted at an acute angle, offers the worst conditions. Usually, only stones that lie in the CBD downstream from the cystic/common duct junction can be removed through the cystic duct.

Under favourable conditions they are extracted by inserting a Dormia probe instead of the Olsen forceps in trocar III (Fig. 3), or sometimes through direct puncture of the abdominal wall. Stone capture and removal are performed blindly. Another cholangiogram is then carried out to make sure that no residual stones have been left in the CBD. If the cystic duct is too narrow, it may be dilated with a balloon probe. Removal by means of a Dormia basket is worth trying, but may not always be successful. Should it fail, one must try to either remove the stone under visual control or fragment the CBD stones and flush them through the sphincter of Oddi with irrigation.

This is performed with a choledochoscope of an appropriate diameter equipped with an operating and an irrigation channel. The ideal instrument should be less than 4 mm wide, bendable, with a 1.2-mm operating channel for the insertion of the flexible electrohydraulic lithotriptor or of the pulsed laser fibre. The choledochoscope is inserted through trocar III or through an additional trocar (V). As it is pushed slowly down the CBD, it allows to locate the stones, and to direct their capture with the Dormia basket (Fig. 4). Once a stone

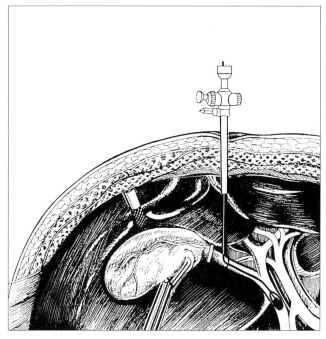

Fig. 3.   Blind extraction of a CBD stone with the Dormia basket

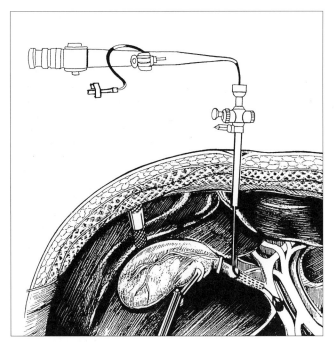

Fig. 4. Catching of a stone under visual control through the choledochoscope

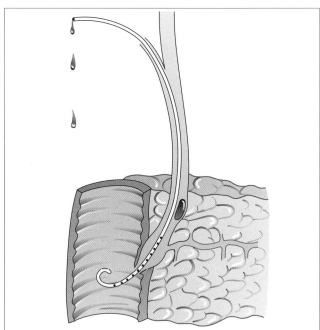

Fig. 5. Transcystic transpapillary probe left in place after failure of transcystic CBD clearance

has been caught, the Dormia basket and the endoscope are pulled out slowly. The same procedure will be repeated for each stone.

If the stones are too bulky and cannot be removed transcystically, or if it is impossible to get hold of them, the choledochoscope allows to bring the fibre of a pulsed laser or the tip of an electrohydraulic lithotriptor in direct contact with them. The stones are then fragmented, and the fragments are washed through the papilla into the duodenum under pressure of the constant irrigation, which is needed to have a clear view of the operating field throughout the fibroscopy. A narrow papilla may be dilated by means of a balloon probe of the same type as is used to dilate the cystic duct. This is a delicate, lengthy and sometimes risky procedure. It can be performed through trocars III or V, the location of the latter being chosen according to the angle of access to the cystic duct.

In particular, the angle of attack must be worked out carefully depending on the angle of the cystic/common duct junction. Any problems that may arise will be encountered at the cystic/common duct junction, which should always be approached very carefully to avoid tearing or perforation in this area. Any damage to the posterior aspect will be difficult to detect. It may pass unnoticed during the operation and become symptomatic later due to a bilioma. Each time a transcystic procedure has been unusually long, it is wise to leave a subhepatic drain for 48 h. Altogether, the laparoscopic approach of CBD stones is successful when the anatomopathological conditions found in the area are favourable, and when fairly sophisticated equipment, such as a small-diameter fibroscope, is available. This approach should be reserved for small stones lying in a narrow CBD (6–8 mm). If, under those conditions, the transcystic approach is not successful, it must be given up. Rather than performing choledochotomy on a narrow CBD, it is better to place a transcystic probe for temporary external biliary drainage (Fig. 5), which can also pro-

vide guidance for the endoscopist who will perform ERCP or ES in the postoperative course. Injection of physiological saline solution through the probe during the duodenoscopy allows easy location of the papilla and facilitates catheterism. We are currently developing a new drain to be inserted transcystically, which will descend into the CBD through the papilla and into the duodenum. This transcystic transpapillary probe (TTP) may serve as a guide wire for a subsequent ERCP + ES. Because endoscopic sphincterotomy can mostly be performed postoperatively, the presence of a small stone in a narrow choledocus duct should not lead to desperate attempts to remove it transcystically.

Laparoscopic Choledochotomy

Laparoscopic choledochotomy should be performed only if the CBD is at least 10 mm in diameter. An additional trocar (V) must be inserted right away, positioned directly above the CBD, whose orientation will allow to either descend towards the papilla or go up towards the junction of right and left hepatic duct. This 10-mm trocar should be flexible to avoid damage to the protective sheath of the fibre-choledochoscope. A scalpel is inserted through trocar V and a choledochotomy is performed lengthwise, level with the cystic/common duct junction (Fig. 6). A plastic bag is inserted into the peritoneal cavity and unrolled in the subhepatic space for retrieval of the stones. Laparoscopic extraction is performed with a Dormia basket or a forceps specially designed for this purpose, previously inserted in trocar V. Transcystic cholangiography as described allows to count the stones and locate them with great accuracy. After stone extraction, total clearance of the CBD is checked with choledochoscopy. If residual stones are found, the choledochoscope must be used to remove them under visual control. This implies that the CBD can receive a

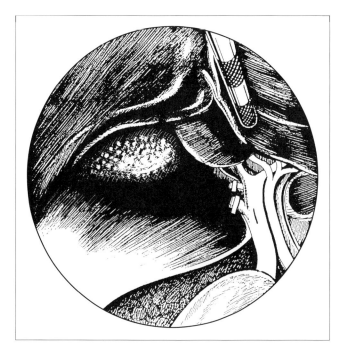

Fig. 6. On a wide CBD, choledochotomy is performed at the level of the cystic duct junction

standard-diameter choledochoscope with an operative channel through which the Dormia basket can be introduced. Once choledochoscopy has proved that the CBD is empty, passage of the papilla is checked by varying irrigation pressure. The choledochoscope can be advanced into the duodenum. The procedure ends with installation of external biliary drainage, either by inserting a T-tube into the choledochotomy or by leaving a transcystic drain of the largest possible diameter. The choledochotomy is then closed with an absorbable suture (4-O Maxon). Postoperative cholangiography is performed on the seventh day. The drain is then clamped gradually and will eventually be withdrawn once a 24-h clamping is tolerated without any signs of cholestasis.

Results and Decisional Tree

Our personal experience is based on the treatment of 176 cases of CBD stones discovered during a series of 1450 LCs. Up to now, we have consistently favoured ES, because two members of our team have an excellent command of this technique.

If the preoperative assessment suggests stone presence in the CBD, three alternatives are possible (Fig. 7):

1. The patient is over 70 years, his CBD is 10 mm or more in diameter and he suffers from cholangitis. Endoscopic sphincterotomy is undoubtedly the adequate treatment, and LC will be performed later if acute cholecystitis appears.
2. The patient is aged 50–70 years, his CBD is 10 mm or more in diameter and he does not have cholangitis. We can choose between SE and laparoscopic choledochotomy. Only a controlled study will allow determination of which solution is best.

3. The patient is under 50 years with a narrow CBD without cholangitis. We choose the laparoscopic approach and remove the CBD stones transcystically.

If the stones cannot be extracted laparoscopically, we end the procedure either by converting to laparotomy, if we are determined to perform the whole treatment in a single session, or by installing a TTP, which will serve as a guide for endoscopic sphincterotomy, postponed to a later second session. In three cases we attempted to perform ES in the same session as LC, but too many difficulties arose, which deterred us from going any further. It is difficult to perform ES on a patient lying supine, and it is difficult to perform laparoscopic procedures when the digestive tract has been insufflated with the duodenoscope.

If the preoperative assessment, which routinely includes patient history, clinical examination, sonography and liver chemistry, is negative, we perform LC with IOC. When SS are found we make an attempt to remove them laparoscopically through the transcystic route. If the attempt fails, we revert to the same course of action as described previously, namely, conversion to open surgery or placement of a TTP in view of a secondary ES. Our own results are listed in Table 1. There was no mortality. There were five complications (2.8 %): An acute pancreatitis occurred twice after ES. One pulmonary embolism and one wound infection were observed after laparoscopic transcystic approach. One retained stone had to be extracted after laparoscopic choledochotomy.

Table 1. Treatment of 176 CBD stones found in 1450 patients (12 %) undergoing laparoscopic cholecystectomy at the University Hospital Bordeaux

Method of retrieval	Clinically silent stones	Clinically evident stones	Total
ERCP + ES	41	74	115 (65 %)
Prior to LC	28	71	99
During LC	3	0	3
After LC	10	3	13
	(8 TTP)	(2 TTP)	(10 TTP)
Laparoscopic approach	8	37	45 (26 %)
Transcystic	7	11	18
Choledochotomy	1	26	27
Open surgery	9	7	16 (9 %)
Total	58 (33 %)	118 (67 %)	176

Conclusion

The laparoscopic approach of CBD lithiasis is still at a very early stage. The value of laparoscopy compared with the fibre-endoscopic approach still remains to be defined. Because no controlled study comparing the two methods is available, the choice is mostly being made according to the individual experience of the surgical team. Most authors still prefer ES [2, 18, 35]. However, important series on laparoscopic common bile duct exploration are beginning to be published. Some authors [26, 28] show that they have deliberately preferred the laparoscopic approach and disregarded ES. The results of a multicentre study including 681 patients with CBD

Laparoscopic Cholecystectomies (LC) and Common Bile Stones (CBDS)

Intraoperative Cholangiogram (IC)
Transcystic Transpapillary-Probe (TTP)

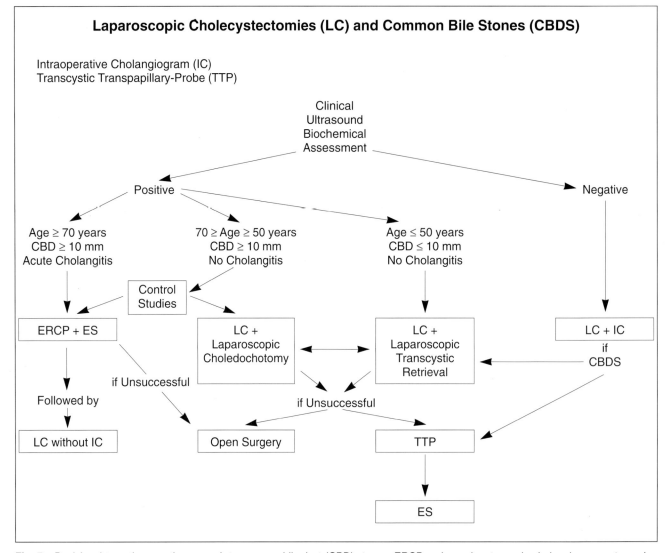

Fig. 7. Decisional tree: therapeutic approach to common bile duct (CBD) stones. ERCP endoscopic retrograde cholangiopancreatography; ES endoscopic sphincterotomy; LC laparoscopic cholecystectomies; TTP transcystic transpapillary probe

stones carried out within the FDCL and the SFCERO (presented at the 4th World Congress of Endoscopic Surgery, Kyoto 1994), are shown in Table 2. Fifty-six of 306 laparoscopic attempts (18.3 %) failed and resulted in 32 conversions to open surgery and postoperative ERCP and ES in 24 patients. The complication rate was 4.5 % (n = 14) with a mortality of 0.3 % (n = 1).

However, the decision tree proposed is only valid here and now, and will evolve with the creation of new instruments. An example can be seen in the refining and popularization of duodenal echoendoscopy for preoperative assessment, in the creation of fibroscopes less than 3 mm in diameter, equipped with an operating channel, which allows entry into very narrow cystic ducts. The individual decision will also depend on the availability of ERCP and its success rate in the different centres.

The treatment of CBD residual stones after cholecystectomy presents specific problems. We favour ES. However, if the papilla cannot be catheterized for anatomical reasons (patient with a Billroth II or total gastrectomy), we try the laparoscopic

approach using "the open laparoscopy technique". If laparoscopic dissection turns out to be too difficult or too risky, we convert to laparotomy. If the patient cannot withstand deep,

Table 2. Treatment of 681 CBD stones: results of a study of the FDCL (Fondation pour le Développement de la Chirurgie Laparoscopique) and SFCERO (Société Francaise de Chirurgie Endoscopique et de Radiologie Opératoire)

Treatment	N	%
ERCP + ES	352	51.7
Laparoscopic approach	306	45.0
Transcystic	182	
Choledochotomy	124	
Open surgery	23	3.3
Total	681	100

prolonged general anaesthesia, we refer him to the interventional radiologist for a percutaneous transhepatic approach of the CBD. This approach allows endoscopy of the CBD with a fibroscope, and fragmentation of the residual stone (or stones) through intracorporeal lithotripsy under visual control. The fragments are then flushed out through the papilla by the irrigation fluid.

Presently, thanks to the combination of ERCP + ES, followed by laparoscopic cholecystectomy, 95 % of patients with cholelithiasis can be treated purely endoscopically, regardless of stone location, in two sessions only a few days apart. The exact indication for a laparoscopic approach of the CBD still remains to be determined. Only operating teams with a wide experience in laparoscopic surgery can have a good command of the laparoscopic approach of the CBD. The development of new instruments, such as thin, bendable fibroscopes with an operating channel, pulsed laser and the adaptation of open-surgery biliary instruments to laparoscopic application, will help to promote this new type of surgery. Multicentre controlled surveys on the "laparoscopic approach of the CBD vs ERCP + ES" will hopefully soon become available. They may lead to the conclusion that cholelithiasis can be treated routinely in a single session of laparoscopic surgery.

References

1. ANCIAUX ML, PELLETIER G, ATTALI P, MEDURI B, LIGUORY C, ETIENNE JP: Prospective study of clinical and biochemical features of symptomatic choledocholithiasis. Dig Dis Sci 31 (1986) 449–453.
2. ARREGUI M, DAVIS C, ARKUSH A, NAGAN R: Laparoscopic cholecystectomy combined with endoscopic sphincterotomy and stone extraction or laparoscopic choledochoscopy and electrohydraulic lithotripsy for management of cholelithiasis with choledocholithiasis. Surg Endosc 6 (1992) 10–15.
3. BERCI G, HAMLIN JA: The fluorocholangiogram. In: Operative biliary radiology. Williams and Wilkens, Baltimore (1981) 63–109.
4. CAROLI J: La radio manométrie biliaire. Études techniques. Semaine des Hôpitaux de Paris 21 (1945) 1278–1282.
5. CARR-LOCKE DL, COTTON PB: Endoscopic surgery: biliary tract and pancreas. Br Med Bull 42 (1985) 257–264.
6. CARROL BJ, FALLAS MJ, PHILLIPS EH: Laparoscopic transcystic choledochoscopy. Surg Endosc 8 (1994) 310–314.
7. CLASSEN M, DEMLING L: Endoskopische Sphinkterotomie der Papilla Vateri. Dtsch Med Wochenschr 99 (1974) 496–497.
8. COTTON PB, VALLON AG: British experience with duodenoscopic sphincterotomy for removal of bile duct stones. Br J Surg 68 (1981) 369–370.
9. CUSCHIERI A: Cholangiomanometry. Br J Surg 68 (1981) 369–370.
10. DEL SANTO P, KAZARIAN KK, FORBES-ROGERS J, BEVINS PA, HALL JR: Prediction of operative cholangiography in patients undergoing elective cholecystectomy with routine liver function chemistries. Surgery 98 (1985) 7–11.
11. DUBOIS F, BERTHELOT G: Cholécystectomie par coelioscopie. Nouv Press Méd 11 (1982) 1139–1141.
12. DUBOIS F, BERTHELOT G, LEVARD H: Cholecystectomie par coelioscopie. Press Méd 18 (1989) 980–982.
13. ESCOURROU J, CORDOVA JA, LAZORTHES F et al.: Early and late complications after endoscopic sphincterotomy for biliary lithiasis. Gut 25 (1984) 598–602.
14. GERER A, APT MK: The case against routine operative cholangiography. Am J Surg 143 (1982) 734–736.
15. GREGG RO: The case for selective cholangiography. Am J Surg 155 (1988) 540–544.
16. HAUER-JENSEN M, KARESEN R, NYGAARD K, SOLHEIM K, AMLIE E, HAVIG O, VIDDAL KO: Predictive ability of choledocholithiasis indicators. Ann Surg 202 (1985) 64–68.
17. HUGUIER M, BORNET P, CHARPAK Y, HOURY S, CHASTANG C: Selective contraindications based on multivariate analysis for operative cholangiography in biliary lithiasis. Surg Gynecol Obstet 172 (1991) 470–474.
18. INOUE H, MURAOKA Y, KOBORI Y, HIRATA R, TAKESHITA K, GOSEKI N, YONESHIMA H, ENDO M: Combination therapy of laparoscopic cholecystectomy and endoscopic transpapillary lithotripsy for both cholecystolithiasis and choledocholithiasis. Surg Endosc 6 (1992) 246–248.
19. JAKIMOWICZ JJ, HARM-RUTTEN PD, JÜRGENS PJ, CAROL EJ: Comparison of operative ultrasonography and radiography in screening of the common bile duct calculi. World J Surg 11 (1987) 628–634.
20. MCSHERRY CK: Cholecystectomy. The gold standard. Am J Surg 158 (1989) 174–178.
21. MALLET-GUY B: Value of preoperative manometric and roentgenographic examination in the diagnosis of pathologic changes and functional disturbances of the biliary tract. SGO 94 (1952) 385.
22. MIRIZZI PL: La cholangiografia durante las operaciones de las vias biliaires. Bull Soc Cir 16 (1932) 1133.
23. NEOPTOLEMOS, JP, CARR-LOCKE DP, FRASER I, FOSSARD DP: The management of common bile duct calculi by endoscopic sphincterotomy in patients with gallbladders in situ. Br J Surg 71 (1984) 69–71.
24. PÉRISSAT J, COLLET D, BELLIARD R: Gallstones: laparoscopic treatment, intracorporeal lithotripsy followed by cholecystostomy or cholecystectomy. A personal technique. Endoscopy 21 (1989) 373–374.
25. PÉRISSAT J, COLLET D, BELLIARD R, DESPLANTEZ J, MAGNE E: Laparoscopic cholecystectomy: the state of the art. A report on 700 consecutive cases. World J Surg (1992) 1074–1082.
26. PETELIN JB: Laparoscopic approach to common bile duct pathology. Surg Laparosc Endosc 1 (1991) 33–41.
27. SAFRANY L: Endoscopic treatment of biliary tract diseases. Lancet (1978) 983–985.
28. SACKIER J, BERCI G, PAZ-PARTLOW M: Laparoscopic transcystic choledocholithotomy as an adjunct to laparoscopic cholecystectomy. Am Surg 12 (1990) 792.
29. SEIFERT RE: Long-term follow-up after endoscopic sphincterotomy. Endoscopy 20 (1988) 232–235.
30. SEIFERT RE, GAIL K, WEISSMÜLLER J: Langzeitresultate nach endoskopischer Sphinkterotomie: follow-up Studie aus 25 Zentren in der Bundesrepublik. Dtsch Med Wochenschr 107 (1982) 610–614.
31. SIVAK MV: Endoscopic management of bile duct stones. Am J Surg 158 (1989) 228–240.
32. STAIN SC, COHEN H, TSUISHYSHA M, DONOVAN AJ: Choledocholithiasis. Endoscopic sphincterotomy of common bile duct exploration. Ann Surg 213 (1991) 627–633.
33. TESTONI PA, TITTOBELLO A: Long-term efficacy of endoscopic papillo-sphincterotomy for common bile duct stones and benign papillary stenosis. Surg Endosc 5 (1992) 135–139.
34. TONDELLI P, ALLGÖWER M: Gallenwegschirurgie. Springer Verlag, 1990.
35. VITALE GC, LARSON GM, WIEMAN TJ, CHEADLE WG, MILLER FB: The use of ERCP in the management of common bile duct stones in patients undergoing laparoscopic cholecystectomy. Surg Endosc 7 (1993) 9–11.

8. Laparoscopic Biliary Endoscopy and Laser Lithotripsy during Laparoscopic Cholecystectomy

D. H. BIRKETT

Introduction

Langenbuch performed the first successful cholecystectomy in 1882 [10], and several years later Courvoisier added common duct exploration for the simultaneous treatment of common duct stones. This remained the gold standard for the management of gallstone disease; however, recently laparoscopic cholecystectomy, with its wide acceptance, has become the gold standard for the treatment of gallbladder stone disease [17]. However, the simultaneous management of common duct stones at the time of laparoscopic cholecystectomy, although not yet routine practice, is being performed more often, and is beginning to replace their treatment by endoscopic papillotomy, either before or after the cholecystectomy, or conversion to open common duct exploration.

During open cholecystectomy there is a 15–20% incidence of common duct exploration. As surgeons become more comfortable with the use of laparoscopic instruments, there is increasing use of intraoperative laparoscopic cholangiography [1, 15]. This has resulted in the finding of common duct stones, and has precipitated the introduction of laparoscopic methods to manage these stones at the time of laparoscopic cholecystectomy. Stoker et al. advocate the use of laparoscopic choledochotomy, endoscopy, stone extraction and T-tube placement [18]. This approach requires considerable dexterity and experience, and, at the moment, adds a considerable amount of time to cholecystectomy. Quattlebaum and Flanders advocate a small choledochotomy and the placement of a small straight rubber tube after basket extraction [16]. Hunter et al. [7] and Petelin, [13, 14] advocate basket extraction of stones using the cystic duct as the portal of entry to the biliary system. Phillips et al. advocate transcystic duct choledochoscopy and basket extraction of the stones [15]. However, for the extraction of some stones, particularly large stones, it may be necessary to dilate the cystic duct to permit extraction [4, 13, 14], but this could result in duct rupture and may pose a problem when treating large stones. Helms and Czarnetzki point out that with the current small endoscopes there is no need to dilate the cystic duct larger than 5 mm, thereby reducing the chance of duct rupture, because large stones can be fragmented using laser or electrohydraulic lithotripsy [6]. Swanstrom points out that with the improvement in technology, particularly the development of smaller endoscopes, the transcystic approach to the common bile duct is here to stay [19].

Fragmentation of stones reduces the need for the cystic duct to be equal to or greater than the size of the stone(s) to be removed; it only has to be the size of the instruments being passed. The two flexible stone fragmentation techniques are electrohydraulic lithotripsy and laser shock-wave lithotripsy. Laser lithotripsy has been shown in the experimental setting to be safer than electrohydraulic lithotripsy [3]. However, the equipment is larger, it requires more specialized personnel to run it, and it is more expensive to buy and maintain.

We have used choledochoscopy and laser lithotripsy via the cystic duct to treat common duct stones found at the time of laparoscopic cholecystectomy.

Methods of Lithotripsy

Fragmentation of biliary stones can be achieved through small flexible choledochoscopes using two techniques, electrohydraulic lithotripsy [8] and laser lithotripsy [5, 9, 11, 20]. Electrohydraulic lithotripsy is the passage of an electrical current between two electrodes on the end of a fine flexible probe, which generates an underwater shock wave resulting in stone fragmentation. In laser lithotripsy optical energy generates a plasma at the stone surface which, on contraction, causes a mechanical shock wave and stone fragmentation.

The first report of laser lithotripsy was using a continuous wave Nd:YAG laser. A variety of wavelengths have been used in both the pulsed and Q-switched mode. Nishioka et al. investigated wavelengths from 450 to 700 nm and found that a pulsed dye laser operating at 504 nm was the most effective wavelength for fragmenting gallstones [12].

Laser lithotripsy fragments stones into small fine fragments or sand that can be washed away, and, therefore, is preferable to electrohydraulic lithotripsy, which fragments stones into large pieces. We compared the tissue effects of both electrohydraulic lithotripsy and laser lithotripsy using an in vitro porcine model, and found the laser lithotripsy with a 504-nm coumarin pulsed dye laser to be significantly safer [3]. In the clinical setting we also found endoscopic laser lithotripsy via a T-tube tract to be a safe and effective method of clearing the common duct of stones [9]. As a result of this work, we now use laser lithotripsy exclusively to fragment gallstones at the time of laparoscopic cholecystectomy.

Accessing the cystic duct endoscopically can be difficult at times because of the problems of manipulating a flexible endoscope with endoscopic forceps into the cystic duct opening and then advancing it down into the common duct. As a result of these frustrations, we have developed a method of access-

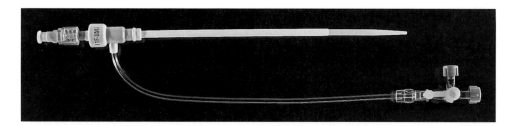

Fig. 1. The sheath and dilator through which the endoscope is passed

ing the common duct and performing laser lithotripsy using a method that circumvents the problem of manipulating a flexible endoscope [2].

Indications

The indications for this form of treatment are common duct stones whose presence is known prior to laparoscopic cholecystectomy or found on intraoperative cholangiography that cannot be basket-extracted through the transcystic duct route because of their size. The stones should preferably be in the distal biliary ductal system, as it is difficult to pass an endoscope from the cystic duct into the proximal ductal system because of the often acute angle between the cystic and common bile ducts. In approximately 40 % of patients the common duct and cystic duct join at a nonacute angle permitting passage of an endoscope into the biliary tree proximally as well as distally.

Preoperative Work-up

All patients need a preoperative ultrasound examination of the common bile duct and the intrahepatic bile ducts at the same time as examination of the gallbladder looking for intra- and extrahepatic bile duct enlargement, signs suggestive of bile duct stones. Stones themselves are rarely seen in the bile ducts on echography. In patients with a suspicion of bile duct stones, blood must be drawn for liver function studies. Patients who are jaundiced, or who have a recent history of jaundice or pancreatitis, must be worked up with extreme care because of the high incidence of duct stones in these groups of patients.

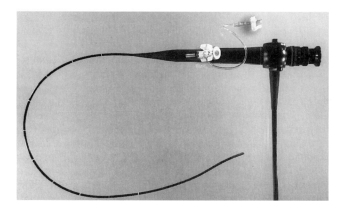

Fig. 2. The small flexible endoscope for intraoperative choledochoscopy has an instrument channel for the use of a laser fiber

Equipment

The equipment required for endoscopic common duct exploration and laser lithotripsy consists of a rigid cholangiogram catheter and introducer, a guide wire, a sheath and dilator, and a small flexible endoscope.

The cholangiogram catheter (Applied Laparoscopy Inc., Laguna Hills, CA) is rigid and self-retaining, and comes in two parts packed in one sterile package: a 13G 13-cm-long sheath mounted on a percutaneous needle and a rigid 6F cholangiogram catheter 33 cm in length. The last 3 cm of the catheter is angled at 40 °, and the tip of the catheter is tapered to 3F with a self-retaining mechanism just proximal to the tip. The mechanism is deployed by a thumb slide on the handle of the instrument. This expands a flange that occludes the cystic duct proximal to the tip, preventing reflux of contrast medium out of the cystic duct incision and allowing retention of the catheter in the cystic duct during cholangiography. The thumb slide has two ratchet positions, and the retention mechanism is 14F when fully deployed.

The guide wire is an 0.038-inch straight hydrophylic coated guide wire, 150 cm in length ("Glidewire," Microvasive Inc., Watertown, MA).

The most commonly used sheath and dilator is the 11F "Cathseal" (UMI, Ballston Spa, New York). This is an 11.5-cm sheath with a valve and a flexible dilator with a taper, which, if necessary, dilates the duct gently (Fig. 1). In some patients with small ducts, a 9F "Cathseal" is used.

Endoscopes must be small and flexible. Our preference is for the 3.2-mm Olympus choledochoscope URF P2 (Olympus Corporation, Lake Success, New York) because of its small size, large instrument channel, excellent optics, and two-way steerability (Fig. 2). If this is not available, then the Olympus P10 ureteroscope of the same diameter is excellent, but its excessive length is somewhat cumbersome. For the smaller ducts the 2.7-mm Circon/ACMI AUR8 (Circon/ACMI, Stamford, CT) is an excellent endoscope. This is also a ureteroscope and, therefore, is a little long. Its field of view is small because of its size, and it is only steerable in one direction. It will pass through a 9F sheath.

For stone fragmentation we use a 320-μm quartz fiber attached to a 504-nm coumarin pulsed dye laser with a pulse duration of 2 μs, the Pulsolith (Technomed International Inc., Danvers, MA).

Operative Technique

Once the cystic duct has been dissected out as part of a standard laparoscopic cholecystectomy, the duct is cleaned and a clip is placed just beneath the gallbladder. Using a pair of endoscopic scissors an incision is made into the duct, leaving

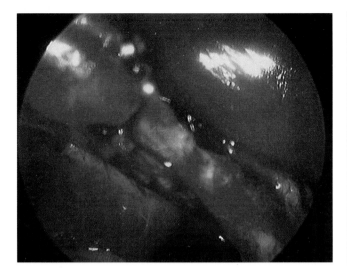

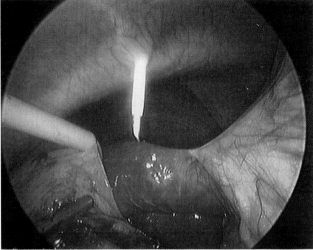

Fig. 3. The cystic duct is closed toward the gallbladder and incised for cholangiography

Fig. 4. The angiocath is introduced just above the cystic duct to permit easy cannulation

a significant amount of the back wall to permit effective gallbladder retraction for control of tension and position of the cystic duct (Fig. 3).

An intraoperative cholangiogram is an integral part of the procedure and is performed with a rigid 6F cholangiogram catheter (Applied Laparoscopy Inc., Laguna Hills, CA). A 13G angiocath and needle, 13 cm in length, are passed through the anterior abdominal wall usually just under the costal margin, to the right of the midline and to the left of the right upper quadrant 5-mm trocar. The exact position is determined endoscopically by noting the shortest and easiest line from the anterior abdominal wall to the opening in the cystic duct to permit cannulation of the duct (Fig. 4). Before passing the angiocath and needle a small skin incision is made at the predetermined site. Once the needle and angiocath are passed into the peritoneal cavity (Fig. 5) the needle is withdrawn and a rigid 6F cholangiogram catheter, with the last 3 cm of the catheter angled at 40° and a retention mechanism

on the 3F tip activated by a thumb push on the handle of the instrument, is guided into the cystic duct opening by manipulation from outside the abdomen (Fig. 6). When in position the retention is activated with the thumb to maintain the catheter's position and prevent reflux of the X-ray contrast medium around the catheter and out of the duct opening (Fig. 7). Three cholangiograms are taken with 3, 6, and 12 ml of 30 % renografin. Any cholangiogram catheter can be used. We use this particular catheter because it has become an integral part of the stone-removal technique.

After the cholangiogram the retention mechanism is released, and if stones are found or endoscopy is to be performed, the angiocath sheath is advanced over the rigid cholangiocath into the duct while the catheter is held firmly in the cystic duct (Fig. 8). The rigid cholangiogram catheter is withdrawn and an 0.038-inch "Glidewire" is passed through the angiocath sheath into the cystic duct and on into the common duct (Fig. 9). The sheath is then withdrawn over the wire. After

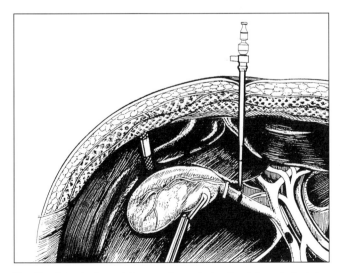

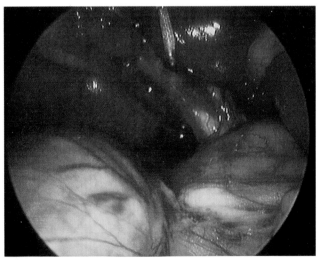

Fig. 5. Introduction of the needle and sheath at the start of the cholangiogram

Fig. 6. Placement of the cholangiogram catheter into the cystic duct

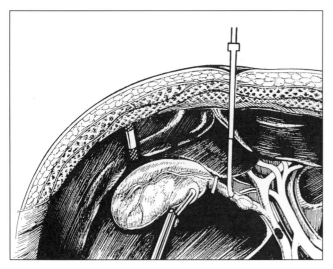

Fig. 7. The retention flange maintains the catheter in position and prevents reflux of X-ray contrast medium

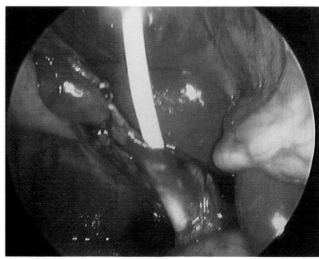

Fig. 8. After cholangiography, the angiocath sheath is advanced over the rigid cholangiocath into the duct

increasing the skin incision, the dilator/introducer of an 11F "Cathseal" is passed over the "Glidewire" into the cystic duct and into the common duct to dilate the abdominal wall tract and the cystic duct. The introducer is withdrawn over the "Glidewire", placed inside the 11F sheath, and repassed over the wire into the cystic duct and on into the common duct (Fig. 10). The "Glidewire" and introducer are removed leaving the sheath in the common duct. A flexible fiberoptic choledochoscope, 3.2 mm in diameter with a second television camera attached, is prepared for passage into the common duct by attaching a "Sureseal" valve (Applied Urology Inc., Laguna Hills, CA) to the instrument channel through which the 320-μm quartz fiber of the Pulsolith, a 504-nm coumarin pulsed dye laser (Technomed International Inc., Danvers, Mass.), is passed and advanced until it is flush with the end of the choledochoscope. The fiber is held firmly in place by the Iris valve so that it will not move while passing the choledochoscope. It is necessary to pass the fiber before passing the

choledochoscope into the common duct, because the slightly rigid and sharp quartz fiber will not always pass around the curve of the instrument channel of a deflected choledochoscope. Under a continuous irrigation of pressurized normal saline through the instrument channel and after flushing out all air bubbles, the choledochoscope is passed through the "Cathseal" sheath and advanced into the common duct (Fig. 11). The saline, pressurized to 300 mmHg by a pressure cuff applied to a liter bag, is needed to distend the duct and wash away debris and stone fragments. The rigidity provided by the sheath allows the choledochoscope to be manipulated easily from outside the body.

With the stone in sight the quartz lithotripsy fiber is advanced out of the choledochoscope, and, under direct vision, is placed in direct contact with the surface of the stone. The stone is fragmented by discharging the laser at 100-120 mJ at a repetition rate of 5 HZ until the stone is completely fragmented. Any large fragments that break off the stone are

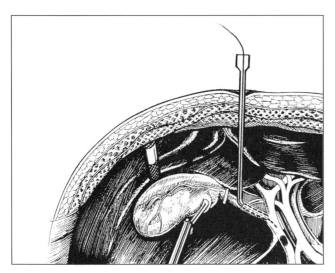

Fig. 9. The "Glidewire" is passed through the cholangiogram sheath into the common duct to maintain common duct access prior to dilatation and endoscopy

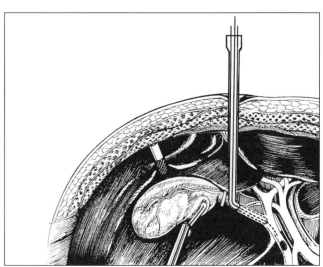

Fig. 10. Introduction of the 11F sheath and dilator into the common duct

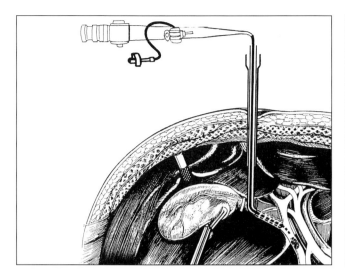

Fig. 11. The choledochoscope is being passed through the sheath into the common bile duct

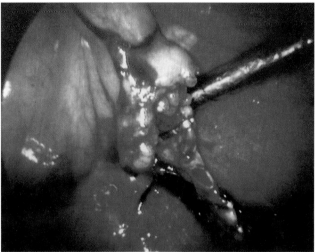

Fig. 12. The cystic duct is double-clipped and divided

fragmented until they are of a size that washes through the sphincter of Oddi into the duodenum. After the common bile duct has been cleared of stones the sphincter of Oddi is inspected for stone fragments by passing the choledochoscope through the sphincter into the duodenum. The choledochoscope is then removed along with the sheath, and the cystic duct is double-clipped and divided (Fig. 12). The operation to remove the gallbladder is continued in the usual manner.

Endoscopic examination of the common duct without laser lithotripsy can be performed quickly to examine the distal biliary tree when the cholangiogram is equivocal.

We prefer this technique because it is simple and quick. If desired the endoscope can be passed through a right upper quadrant port and advanced into the duct using laparoscopic forceps. We find manipulating the endoscope into the cystic duct and advancing it down the common duct using laparoscopic forceps to be time-consuming and difficult.

Difficulties and Problems

As with all techniques there are limitations, and this is no exception. The inability to examine the proximal biliary tree via the cystic duct is a severe handicap that is due to the cystic duct joining the common bile duct at an acute angle, which prevents the deflection of a choledochoscope and even a guide wire proximally into the common hepatic duct from the cystic duct.

A small cystic duct does present a problem, because it is necessary to pass an endoscope down the duct to perform lithotripsy. This can be overcome in two ways. In those ducts that are too small to accept an 11F sheath, it may be possible to pass a 9F sheath and use a smaller endoscope such as the AUR8 ureteroscope (Circon/ACMI Inc., Stamford, CT). This instrument will pass through a 9F sheath, but it does have a smaller field of view and lower light-carrying capacity, and a smaller instrument channel, and, therefore, a slower rate of saline irrigation around the fiber, which is important for washing the stone fragments through the sphincter of Oddi into the duodenum. This lack of adequate irrigation makes it extremely difficult to wash the duct clear

of fragments and permit good visual control of fragmentation.

The second option is to dilate the cystic duct up to a size that will accept a sheath. This is done by passing a balloon dilator (Microvasive Inc., Watertown, MA) over the guide wire and dilating the cystic duct up to 6 mm before passing the sheath over the guide wire. This cannot be done if the cystic duct is too small.

Intraoperative and Postoperative Complications

Although no complications have been reported to date, there are potential complications that must be discussed. These can be divided according to the different stages of the procedure.

The passage of a guide wire down the cystic duct could potentially perforate the cystic duct or the common duct. To reduce the chance of this happening we use a floppy-tipped 0.038-inch hydrophilic coated "Glidewire" that passes easily down the duct, requires a minimum of force, and reduces the chance of pushing a guide wire through the wall of the cystic or common duct.

Tearing or splitting of the cystic duct due to excessive dilatation is a distinct possibility particularly if the cystic duct is small. It is not yet known how much a cystic duct can be dilated, particularly a small duct. If the incision is made too large, it can thin the back wall of the duct at the site of the incision causing the duct to tear in half making the passage of an endoscope down the duct difficult, because the gallbladder counter traction, an essential part of the procedure, is lost. Shearing and tearing of the duct is a possibility when passing the dilator, sheath, or endoscope. To reduce the chances of this happening these instruments must be advanced carefully without excessive force.

Laser perforation of the common bile duct due to inadvertent discharge of the laser against the wall of the duct has not been reported. In our experience with 504-nm coumarin pulsed dye laser lithotripsy, either at the time of laparoscopic cholecystectomy or for the treatment of retained common duct stones via the T-tube tract, we have had no duct perforations. As mentioned previously, we have shown the coumarin pulsed dye laser in an in vitro porcine model to be extremely safe [11].

Results

We routinely perform cholangiography with this catheter in all laparoscopic cholecystectomies. In ten patients stones were clearly seen or the cholangiography was equivocal and suggestive of stones. In all patients endoscopy was performed, and stones were found in four patients. Three of the patients were cleared of stones, with incomplete stone fragmentation in the fourth patient because of a poor saline flow down the small endoscope. It was necessary to convert to an open operation in this patient to clear the biliary tract completely of stone fragments.

Because laser lithotripsy is demanding on the operating room staff, because of equipment maintenance and cost, and the ease with which a basket can be passed transcystically for stone removal with or without accompanying choledochoscopy, we feel that transcystic basket extraction with or without choledochoscopy should be the primary method of treating common duct stones. We reserve laser lithotripsy for stones that for technical reasons cannot be basket-extracted or are too large for cystic duct extraction.

Discussion

Although laparoscopic cholecystectomy is now the gold standard for the treatment of gallstone disease, it is rarely combined with laparoscopic common duct exploration to treat common duct stones found on intraoperative cholangiography. The more common method of performing two procedures, laparoscopic cholecystectomy and pre- or postoperative endoscopic retrograde papillotomy, must be considered a passing phase until there is more widespread use of the variety of different laparoscopic methods of common duct exploration.

One of the advantages of endoscopic laser lithotripsy via the cystic duct is that the access route is independent of the size of the stone. The incision in the cystic duct or a common duct incision does not have to be made to a size through which a large stone can be removed. The cystic duct incision must be large enough or dilated only to the size of the endoscope. A further advantage of the transcystic duct approach is the lack of necessity for T-tube placement in a choledochotomy, which clearly adds to the morbidity of common duct stone removal. The cystic duct can be clipped off or, if preferred, ligated as soon as the endoscope is removed. Cystic duct endoscopy without laser lithotripsy is an excellent and direct method of answering the questions raised by an equivocal intraoperative cholangiogram without subjecting the patient to a negative common duct exploration and T-tube placement.

There are deficiencies with this approach to the treatment of common duct stones, however. In the majority of patients (approximately 60 %) it is not possible to examine the proximal biliary tree because of the acute angle between the cystic and common bile ducts. This means that in order to screen the biliary tree completely cholangiography must be an integral part of cystic duct endoscopy not only to demonstrate anatomy, but also to pick up stones adequately in the proximal as well as distal ducts. Fortunately, the majority of biliary stones are in the distal biliary tree. Our experience has shown us that laser lithotripsy is an excellent and safe method of fragmenting and removing common duct stones found at the time of laparoscopic cholecystectomy, but there are disadvantages to this technique. The equipment is large, heavy, and bulky, its operation requires considerable expertise from the operating room staff, and it takes some time to set up once it is determined to be necessary. A further disadvantage is the cost of the laser; however, it is an instrument with multidisciplinary usefulness, which, in a variety of settings, can be used for stone fragmentation not only by gastrointestinal surgeons, but also urologists and gastroenterologists.

We feel that other methods of common duct exploration, such as transcystic basket extraction preferably with choledochoscopy, should be tried first, and laser lithotripsy should be reserved for failures of basket extraction or for the extraction of large stones.

References

1. BERCI G, SACKIER JM, PAZ-PARTLOW M: Routine or selected intraoperative cholangiography during laparoscopic cholecystectomy? Am J Surg 161 (1991) 355–360.
2. BIRKETT DH: Technique of cholangiography and cystic duct choledochoscopy at the time of laparoscopic cholecystectomy. Surg Endosc 6 (1992) 252–254.
3. BIRKETT DH, LAMONT JS, O'KEANE JC et al.: Comparison of a pulsed dye laser and electrohydraulic lithotripsy on porcine gallbladder and common duct in vitro. Lasers Surg Med 12 (1992) 210–214.
4. CARROLL BJ, PHILLIPS EH, DAYKHOVSKY L, GRUNDFEST WS et al.: Laparoscopic choledochoscopy. An effective approach to the common duct. J Laparoend Surg 2 (1992) 15–21.
5. ELL CH, LUX G, HOCHBERGER J, MULLER D AND DEMLING L: Laser lithotripsy of common bile duct stones. Gut 29 (1988) 746–751.
6. HELMS B, CZARNETZKI HD: Strategy and technique of laparoscopic common bile duct exploration. Endosc Surg Allied Technol 1(3) (1993) 117–124.
7. HUNTER JG: Laparoscopic transcystic common bile duct exploration. Am J Surg 163 (1992) 53–58.
8. JOSEPHS LG, BIRKETT DH: Electrohydraulic lithotripsy (EHL) for the treatment of large retained common duct stones. Am Surg 56 (1990) 232–234.
9. JOSEPHS LG, BIRKETT DH: Laser lithotripsy for the management of retained common duct stones. Arch Surg 127 (1992) 603–605.
10. LANGENBUCH C: Ein Fall von Exstirpation der Gallenblase wegen chronischer Cholelithiasis. Berl Klin Wochenschr 18 (1882) 725.
11. LUX G, ELL C, HOCHBERGER J, MÜLLER D, DEMLING L: The first endoscopic retrograde lithotripsy of common bile duct stones in man using a pulsed neodymium YAG laser. Endoscopy 18 (1986) 144–145.
12. NISHIOKA NS, LEVINS PC, MURRAY SC, PARRISH JA, ANDERSON RR: Fragmentation of biliary calculi with tuneable dye lasers. Gastroenterology 93 (1987) 250–255.
13. PETELIN JB: Clinical results of common bile duct exploration. Endosc Surg Allied Technol 1(3) (1993) 125–129.
14. PETELIN JB: Laparoscopic approach to common duct pathology. Surg Lap Endosc 1 (1991) 33–41.
15. PHILLIPS E, DAYKHOVSKY L, CARROLL et al.: Laparoscopic cholecystectomy: instrumentation and technique. J Laparoend Surg 1 (1990) 3–15.
16. QUATTLEBAUM JK, FLANDERS HD: Laparoscopic treatment of common duct stones. Surg Lap Endosc 1 (1991) 26–32.

17. SOPER NJ, STOCKMAN PT, DUNNEGAN DL, ASHLEY SW: Laparoscopic cholecystectomy: the new "gold standard"? Arch Surg 127 (1992) 917–923.
18. STOKER ME, LEVEILLEE RJ, McCANN JC JR, MAINI BS: Laparoscopic common bile duct exploration. J Laparoend Surg 1 (1991) 287–293.
19. SWANSTROM LL: Laparoscopic approaches to the common bile duct stone: transcystic bile duct exploration, choledochotomy and stone fragmentation. Baillieres Clin Gastroenterol 7(4) (1993) 897–919.
20. WENK H, THOMAS ST, SCHMELLER N, LANGE V, SCHILDBERG FW: Percutaneous transhepatic cholecysto-lithotripsy. Endoscopy 21 (1989) 221–222.

Oesophageal and Gastric Surgery

Critical Comments

J. R. Siewert

Thoracoscopic esophagectomy

As the data currently reported in the literature shows, thoracoscopic esophagectomy has failed to find wide acceptance. At a consensus conference in Milan in 1995, experts in the field agreed that thoracoscopic esophagectomy presently has no recognizable value in the management of esophageal carcinoma.

What were the reasons for this decision?
1. Thoracoscopic esophagectomy (TE) has just as many anesthesiological requirements as the open procedure, including unilateral ventilation. The significantly longer operation time required by TE is another negative aspect.
2. Regarding radical resection according to established oncological principles, TE is unsatisfactory in many respects. In particular, it could never be shown that thoracoscopy was able to achieve the goal of en bloc mediastinectomy.
3. In TE it is difficult to recover the organ through the narrow intercostal spaces. This makes it necessary to perform at least a small thoracotomy.
4. On the whole, the theoretically postulated prediction that thoracoscopic esophagectomy would provide benefits similar to those achieved in other thoracoscopic procedures (shorter hospitalization times, improved pulmonary function, etc.) could not be fulfilled.

Where can thoracoscopy play a role in the treatment of esophageal carcinomas in the future?
First, in endodissection for the purpose of mediastinal staging and, perhaps, to achieve a better view of the upper mediastinum. The preliminary results of endodissection in this case are quite convincing. However, endodissection is useful only in patients with a healthy esophagus, that is, in those where the tumor is located outside of the endoscopic field of dissection.

Useful applications may also arise for the diagnostic thoracoscopy. Staging of lymph node involvement in patients with esophageal cancer is still extremely difficult – as is often the case in other gastrointestinal tumors. Therefore, the reliability of diagnostic staging is only around 65 to 70 %. Thoracoscopic lymph node biopsy or lymph node excision might be useful in this case. Such diagnostic thoracoscopies have already been performed in patients with esophageal cancer (Baltimore). The preliminary results indicate that this method of diagnosis is technically feasible and that it is a low-stress procedure for the patient. However, the question as to which therapeutic consequences can be initiated once evidence of lymph node involvement has been obtained, still remains unclear. At present the ruling opinion is that, in view of the extremely high rate of lymph node metastases, this finding is not eo ipso a contraindication for esophagectomy. Compared to diagnostic laparoscopy, findings such as pleural carcinosis are extremely rare and, therefore, should not be used as an argument for diagnostic thoracoscopy.

The current and even more, the future situation regarding the management of benign esophageal diseases is totally different. Benign tumors such as leiomyomas can be excised with good results via thoracoscopy. Thoracoscopic myotomy in achalasia is likewise generally accepted. Extensive myotomy in patients with diffuse spasms is also conceivable.

Myotomy for treatment of achalasia

Laparoscopy is particularly useful in cases where the effects of creating an access for open surgery far exceed the expected benefits of the procedure. Helleris operation is a typical example of this. In this case, the effects of creating a wide abdominal access are out of proportion to the small incision that must be made in the esophageal wall. Laparoscopic myotomy was therefore quick to gain wide acceptance. The technique is on its way to becoming a standard procedure, particularly when combined with endoluminal endoscopy for quality control. This applies even more so when laparoscopy is also able to fulfill the demands of open surgery, for instance the simultaneous performance of antireflux operations such as fundoplasty. Therefore this procedure has now become widely recognized as one of the best examples of an appropriate indication for laparoscopic surgery.

A current topic of debate is the question as to which access is better – the laparoscopic or the thoracoscopic access?
One advantage of the laparoscopic access is that it is easy to carry out antireflux surgery during the same session. Antireflux surgery is much more difficult when the thoracoscopic access is used. A frequently mentioned advantage of thoracoscopic myotomy is that the Willis loop is less compromised and reflux therefore induced less often. Besides preventing reflux, transabdominal fundoplasty also fulfills other useful roles, such as holding open the myotomy and preventing periesophageal scars that could lead to cicatricial stenosis subsequent to myotomy.

Vagotomy

An outdated and no longer indicated surgical procedure does not become any more attractive just because it can be performed through a smaller access and thus, perhaps, less invasively. In view of the present understanding of the pathogenesis of ulcer disease it does not appear that surgical procedures can be applied to the advantage of these patients. Therefore, any attempt to revive a past surgical procedure via the laparoscopic approach is not likely to be successful in the future. Financial considerations brought forward repeatedly in these discussions also do not seem to provide hope for laparoscopy, as the increasing propagation of proton-pump inhibitors and a related drop in procedural costs can be expected. In addition, antibiotic therapy to eradicate Helicobacter colonization is becoming more and more effective, thus requiring less and less cost and effort. Furthermore, Helicobacter eradication seems to be gaining significance in the prevention of gastric carcinoma. It does not appear that the eradication concept will be abandoned in the future. Even the greatest optimist must admit that there is no apparent future for vagotomy.

Laparoscopy may be able to gain a certain degree of acceptance in the management of ulcer complications. It already plays a role in the management of acute perforating ulcers. The repair of cicatricial pyloric or postpyloric stenosis via the laparoscopic approach may be possible in the near future. Although laparoscopic management of bleeding ulcers does not appear prudent at present, encouraging developments are to be expected soon. For instance, if endo- and extraluminal procedures can be combined successfully, it may one day become possible to achieve hemostasis endoscopically while simultaneously performing extraluminal vessel ligature through the laparoscopic approach. The field for the application of laparoscopic techniques in the management of ulcer complications will further expand in the future.

Fundoplication

In contrast to ulcer disease, reflux disease is still a mainly peptic and primarily pH-dependent disease. Furthermore, the pathogenetic significance of biliary reflux is still unclear. More and more findings indicate that its significance is greater than originally assumed, particularly regarding the development of relevant complications of reflux disease (Barrett's ulcer, Barrett's carcinoma, etc.). It can therefore be expected that surgical management of reflux disease will gain more significance in the future. As far as medical management is concerned, the pathogenetic principle of reducing the rate of acid secretion seems to be the only helpful approach.

Of the various techniques for surgical management of reflux disease, fundoplication is currently the best documented and longest tested method. The advances made in open fundoplication during the past few years due to intensive work on the technique should also be integrated into the laparoscopic procedures. Negative trends on the other hand, include the attempts of some surgeons to ignore the rules applying to open antireflux surgery when performing the procedure via the laparoscopic approach, and the attempts of others to revive long abandoned surgical procedures only because they can be more easily performed by laparoscopy.

In other words, the same technical rules must apply for both laparoscopic and open fundoplication. The goal of fundoplication is to create a loose, short cuff from the anterior wall of the stomach. The available reports indicate that laparoscopy is well capable of achieving this goal. Under these circumstances it can be said that laparoscopic fundoplication is now the best principle of management for reflux disease. Any deviation from this principle must be viewed as an experimental therapeutical approach requiring renewed and very careful clinical evaluation and documentation.

Still, fundoplication does not appear to be the end of the development of laparoscopic surgery and open antireflux surgery. Fundoplication is subject to potential cuff complications that can lead to undesirable effects that may outweigh the primary problem of reflux. It is obvious that further development will take place in this field, whereby the primary goal will be the prevention of cuff complications. The use of the gastric fundus as the foundation of the wrap will be challenged, possibly leading to new surgical techniques that may just be best achieved by the laparoscopic approach.

Any such new minimally invasive technique would then receive more recognition amongst the various antireflux techniques.

Gastric anastomosis and resection

Laparoscopy always plays an important role in cases where the effects of creating an access for open surgery are out of proportion with the expected benefits. This is especially true in palliative surgery, where extensive laparotomy can often lead to longer hospitalization times and undesirable side effects. This reduces the quality of life in patients who already have a short survival time. Therefore, laparoscopic gastroenterostomy has meanwhile gained a secure position in the management of inoperable carcinoma of the pancreatic head. However, the basic principles of open surgery must also be followed during laparoscopy. For example, gastroenterostomy should always be performed on the posterior wall and in a prudent manner. Even though this requires a greater amount of time and effort, it ensures the patient improved functional results.

Gastroenterostomy, however, remains a poor operation in principle, because the artificial passage becomes functionally effective only after the stomach is overfilled to a certain degree. The duodenal passage remains physiologically unchanged as long as it is still patent. Future discussions might therefore be directed at whether antrectomy and enterostomy using the residual stomach is likely to lead to better functional results than unmodified side-to-side anastomosis. Such procedures pose a challenge for laparoscopic surgeons and new techniques should be tried and tested.

This indication could become a useful application for gastric resection. The classical indication for gastric resection in the frame of ulcer disease has become extremely rare and will not come back into bloom just because gastric resection can be performed by the laparoscopic approach. That gastric resection by laparoscopy is technically possible is undisputed. However, the mere technical possibility should not be used as an excuse to create new and arbitrary indications. It is not without reason, that laparoscopic surgery is still controversial when considering established oncological principles. Laparoscopic gastric resection should only be seriously considered in benign indications. At present the only indication for distal gastric resection is complicated peptic ulcer. As long as bleeding ulcers do not comprise an indication for laparoscopy, the only possible indication would, at best be related to pyloric stenosis. The use of laparoscopic gastric resection for the management of pyloric stenosis is currently very limited.

Early-stage gastric carcinoma is a highly controversial indication for laparoscopic surgery. Japanese workers feel the procedure is indicated in early-stage carcinoma of the mucosa type. The main advantage of combining endoscopy and laparoscopy for total gastric wall excision is that the pathologist thereby obtains a complete gastric wall specimen, enabling him or her to definitively confirm the diagnosis of early carcinoma of the mucosa type. Such total gastric wall excision techniques are currently limited to easily accessible areas of the stomach (anterior wall, greater curvature, etc.). It is easily imaginable that this field of laparoscopic activity will grow eventually. However, it does not appear prudent to perform extensive gastric resections in patients with early-stage carcinoma of the mucosa type just to prove the capacity of laparoscopy. Gastric carcinoma of the submucosa type is an indication for surgery according to established oncological principles, that is, subtotal gastrectomy with D2 lymphadenectomy as the standard procedure. Laparoscopy is still unable to achieve this goal reliably enough.

9. | Thoracoscopic Oesophagectomy

J. M. WEERTS, B. DALLEMAGNE, C. JEHAES, AND S. MARKIEWICZ

Introduction

Carcinoma of the oesophagus, both squamous and adenocarcinoma, continues to have an extremely poor prognosis. The performance of a curative operation requires an extensive, wide resection because the position of the oesophagus and its rich lymphatic drainage makes an extensive node dissection necessary.

One particularity of the oesophagus is to be located in three different compartments: the neck, chest and abdomen. Any procedure intended to remove widely the oesophagus will have to be carried out in at least two of these compartments.

Despite major improvements in preoperative and intraoperative care, the morbidity is still very high in Western countries as a result of pulmonary complications [1, 4, 7, 9]: many of the patients are smokers and have suffered from "microinhalations" as a result of stasis within the oesophagus leading to chronic inflammation of the respiratory tree. Denervation and lymph node clearance may weaken the bronchi. Finally, the thoracotomy itself has its own morbidity added to the operative trauma to which the lung is exposed.

The posterior mediastinectomy performed by thoracoscopy might improve the postoperative morbidity due to the reduced thoracic trauma and allow a more rapid recovery of respiratory function postoperatively. This theoretical advantage still has to be confirmed by large-scale clinical studies [3, 4].

Indications

The only curative approach of the carcinoma of the oesophagus is oesophagectomy with a posterior mediastinectomy, clearing the lymphatic nodes from the posterior mediastinum and the cephalad lymph nodes of the lesser curvature with or without a preoperative neoadjuvant radiochemotherapy [3, 11, 12, 13].

The thoracoscopic approach can only be considered for a tumor appearing to be resectable on the preoperative assessment: no invasion of the aorta, the trachea or the bronchi, or the pericardium; no distant metastasis. This assessment requires an endoscopy, a computed tomography (CT) scan of the chest and abdomen, an echoendoscopy and a bone scan.

Any previous thoracic surgery will be a contraindication, as well as previous right chest pleuritis, because of the possibility of severe adhesions between the pleura and the lung.

Preoperative Work-up

To exclude irresectability a full work-up is mandatory requesting:

1. An upper gastrointestinal (GI) tract endoscopy with biopsies
2. A bronchoscopy to rule out invasion of the posterior wall of the trachea or of one of the bronchi, and to identify any bronchial synchronous tumor
3. A CT scan of the chest and abdomen
4. A bone scintigraphy
5. An ear, nose and throat examination
6. A respiratory function test
7. An oesophageal endoluminal ultrasound

The latter examination is probably the most accurate investigation presently to assess depth of invasion and infiltration of the adjacent organs. At the same time the cardiovascular system has to be fully investigated.

In some patients the stomach may not be used to replace the oesophagus, and colonoscopy should always be part of the preoperative work-up to exclude any colonic disease. The colon is prepared preoperatively by an orthograde lavage.

When the tumor is located in the lower third of the oesophagus and endosonography and CT scan reveal an advanced tumor stage, diagnostic laparoscopy for exclusion of intra-abdominal disease, especially of peritoneal carcinosis, may be indicated.

Our extensive work-up allows precise pretherapeutic staging. This has become very important with development of multimodal treatment in oncology. Because the decision whether to proceed directly to an operation, submit the patient to a neoadjuvant radiochemotherapy followed by an operation, to a palliative radiation with chemotherapy, or to no treatment at all, depends on the stage of the disease at diagnosis, an exact evaluation has become mandatory.

The operation is a three-stage procedure where the oesophagus is dissected through a thoracic approach, and a gastric tube is created in the abdomen and brought up to the neck where the cervical oesogastric anastomosis is performed [1, 11, 13].

The procedure can be partially endoscopic: A thoracoscopy is done and a laparotomy will give the access to the abdomen. It can also be fully endoscopic with a thoracoscopy and a laparoscopy.

Operative Technique

General Considerations

Selective ventilation of the left main bronchus is required to allow complete collapse of the right lung during thoracoscopy. A Carlens™ tube is the most commonly used. Postoperative analgesia can be provided by an epidural catheter in patients undergoing laparotomy, because this facilitates postoperative physiotherapy.

It is generally unnecessary to use CO_2 insufflation during thoracoscopy, but at the start, a slight increase in pressure from CO_2 in the pleural cavity is useful to obtain a rapid collapse of the lung. It is useful to allow air entry during the thoracoscopic dissection to maintain the lung collapsed especially when suction is used.

The cervico-abdominal stage is best performed with two surgical teams working simultaneously. This way dissection of the neck can be started while the gastric tube is prepared allowing a considerable saving of time.

Positioning of the Patients

For the thoracoscopic stage the patient is placed in the left lateral decubitus position with the right arm lifted on an arm support. The surgeon is placed facing the video monitor located on the left side of the patient. One assistant will be standing on each side of the surgeon.

For the cervico-abdominal stage the patient is in the supine position with the head turned towards the right. If a laparotomy is performed, the patient is to lay flat, but the legs are to be set apart and elevated if a laparoscopy is to be performed.

The surgeon is to then stand between the legs with the monitors on either the right or the left side of the patient's head. One assistant is to stand on each side.

Thoracoscopy

A first 10-mm trocar is inserted in the sixth intercostal space on the axillary line. If any pleural adhesions are suspected, the placement should be done under direct vision. A 0° or a 30° scope is introduced in the pleural cavity and the exploration is started. Gradually, the right lung will deflate, more quickly if a small amount of CO_2 is insufflated. Any hyperpressure must be avoided in the right chest, and the insufflation can be stopped once the lung is completely collapsed.

Under vision four other trocars are inserted; the positioning might have to be modified according to the patient's anatomy. Two trocars (5 and 10 mm) are placed on the anterior axillary line and two others (10 and 12 mm) on the posterior axillary line. By using several 10-mm trocars the camera can be moved easily from one side to the other. The 12-mm trocar is needed for the use of staplers (Fig. 1).

An atraumatic forceps and scissors with diathermy are introduced through the posterior trocars. The camera is held by the right or the left assistant depending on the side of the chest where the dissection occurs. The anterior and inferior trocars are used for a suction device, because a permanent oozing might require continuous suction and aspiration. The last anterior trocar is needed for the introduction of a lung retractor (usually a 10-mm instrument).

Oesophageal Dissection

A careful investigation of the right chest will exclude any secondaries on the pleura or on the right lung. The inferior pulmonary lobe is retracted after dividing the right triangular ligament. Dissection is carried out along the mediastinal pleura towards the right inferior pulmonary vein removing all lymph nodes. After incision of the mediastinal pleura (Fig. 2), the oesophagus is identified and the tumor palpated with one of the instruments. One should check that the tumor appears to be resectable at this stage.

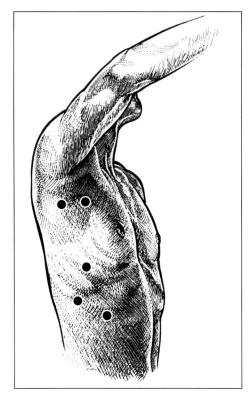

Fig. 1. Trocar placement for thoracoscopic dissection of oesophagus

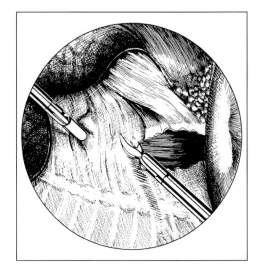

Fig. 2. Incision of mediastinal pleura along anterior surface of oesophagus

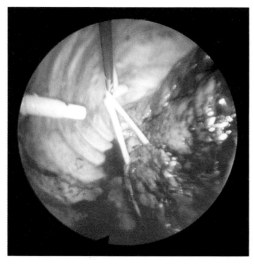

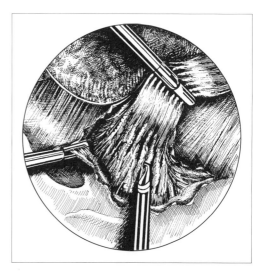

Fig. 3. To facilitate dissection, the oesophagus can be held up with a rubber band

Fig. 4. Posterior dissection of oesophagus

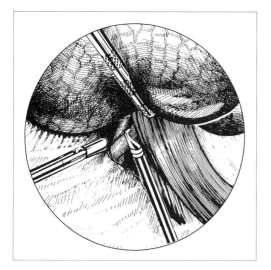

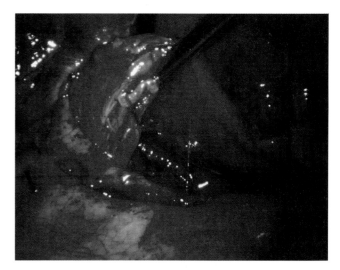

Figs. 5 and 6. Dissection of azygos vein up to the junction with the superior vena cava

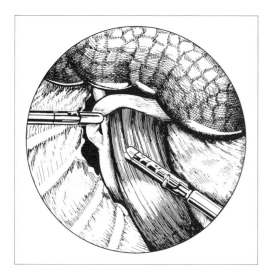

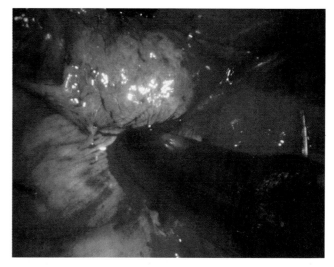

Figs. 7 and 8. Transection of azygos vein with an Endo-GIA using a 30-mm vascular cartridge

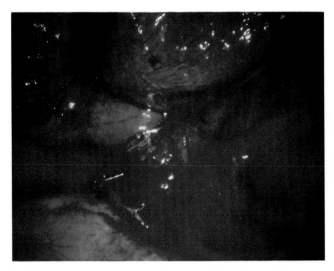

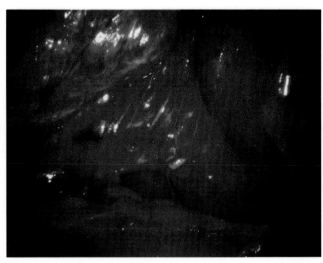

Fig. 9. Azygos vein is secured on both sides with a triple row of staples at transection

Fig. 10. Lymph node dissection in the intertracheobronchial space

The pleura is dissected towards the hiatus and the inferior vena cava is identified. The pleura should be removed around the hiatus. The azygos vein is dissected and ligated just above the diaphragm. The intercostal veins are transected between clips as the dissection moves up cephalad.

The aorta is cleared from all lymph nodes and nervous tissue. This dissection helps progressively mobilizing the oesophagus. For an easier atraumatic handling of the oesophagus, a rubber band can be placed around it (Fig. 3).

On the posterior side dissection is carried out towards the azygos vein (Fig. 4), transecting the various intercostal branches and finally the azygos vein itself as close as possible to the superior vena cava (Figs. 5 and 6). Usually, an Endo-GIA (USSC) 30-mm vascular device is used for this purpose (Figs. 7–9). The dissection will end at the apex where the subclavian and jugular veins meet.

On the anterior side, once the inferior pulmonary vein has been identified and dissected, a careful lymph node clearance

will be obtained by removing all the intertracheobronchial space (Fig. 10). This stage is difficult especially if large nodes are present. The membranous wall of the bronchi is very thin particularly on the left side where the bronchus is dilated by an intraluminal balloon. There is usually a permanent oozing, and a continuous suction is needed. Bronchial branches of the vagus nerves are transected at this stage of the dissection.

On the lateral sides the left pleura is identified and a complete clearance is performed (Figs. 11 and 12). The thoracic duct is divided between clips as it enters the thorax (Fig. 13). Once the aortic arch is reached, special attention must be paid to the left recurrent nerve. The oesophagus will be completely separated from the posterior wall of the trachea. At this stage a full mobilization has been obtained together with a full lymph node clearance of the posterior mediastinum (Figs. 14 and 15).

The pleural cavity is washed with large amounts of warm saline and a chest tube is inserted after a careful check

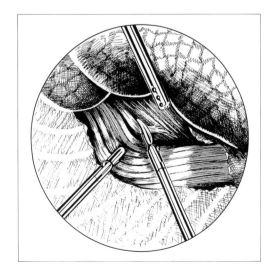

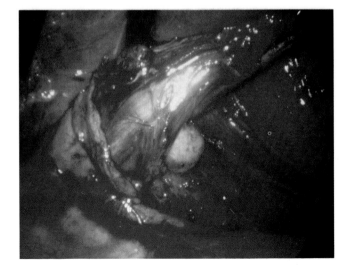

Figs. 11 and 12.   Dissection of oesophagus from the left pleura en bloc with lymph nodes

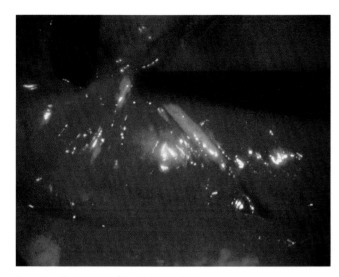

Fig. 13. Dissection of the thoracic duct

for hemostasis. The right lung must be reinflated gently under direct vision. All the ports are removed and the openings are closed.

Abdominal and Cervical Dissection

The positioning of the patient depends on the chosen approach.

Laparotomy
The patient lies flat in the supine position. A median or a transverse incision is done. A careful exploration is carried out with eventually an intraoperative ultrasound investigation of the liver. Care is taken to inspect the stomach and make sure the gastric tube can be brought up to the neck. The lymph node clearance will remove the nodes of the coeliac axis as well as those along the lesser curvature of the stomach.

The gastrolysis is started by the opening of the lesser sac, dividing the gastrocolic ligament. The vascular supply of the greater curvature must be carefully preserved. The short gastric vessels are divided as close as possible to the splenic hilum to preserve as much vascularization as possible.

The mobilized stomach can then be lifted up and the left gastric artery and vein are isolated and transected through the lesser sac. The left gastroepiploic artery is divided close to the splenic artery. The stomach is then almost totally mobilized and freed from attachments, the vascularization being maintained by the pyloric artery and the right gastroepiploic vessels.

The gastric tube can be created either by hand or with the help of staplers. The stomach is stretched as much as possible to give enough length to bring the tube up for the cervical anastomosis. The tube is started at the arch of the stomach removing the lesser curvature with the lymph nodes and going upwards towards the fundus.

Cervicotomy
While the gastrolysis is done and the tube is created, a second team starts the cervical stage: Through a left cervical incision anterior to the sternocleidomastoid muscle the exposure of the cervical oesophagus is obtained.

Attention is paid to the recurrent nerves. The oesophagus is dissected and divided 2–3 cm below the superior oesophageal sphincter. A nasogastric tube is fixed to the oesophagus and the whole specimen is removed from the abdomen, pulling the nasogastric tube down. The gastric tube is then attached to the nasogastric catheter and is pulled up to the cervical incision.

The oesogastric cervical anastomosis is performed using continuous or separate sutures. A drain is left in the cervicotomy and the various layers are closed.

Before closing the laparotomy, a pylorotomy or a pyloroplasty is done. To avoid any tension on the gastric tube, a Kocher manoeuvre can be of help. After drainage, the laparotomy is closed in layers. It is obvious that if for any reason the stomach cannot be used (previous gastric resection, invasion of the upper part of the stomach, etc.), the use of the right or left colon is recommended.

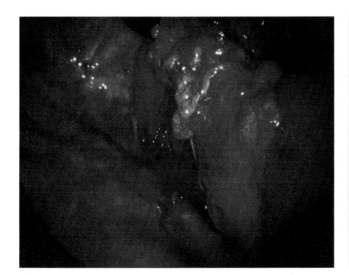
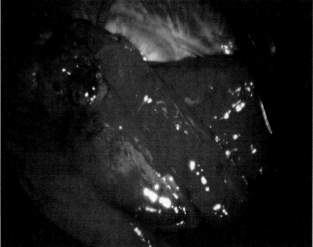

Figs. 14 and 15. Oesophagus is completely mobilized en bloc with dissected lymph nodes

Laparoscopy

As has already been stated, the laparotomy stage can also been done by laparoscopy. The patient is then placed in a lithotomy position with the legs apart. The surgeon stands between the legs with one assistant on each side and facing the video monitor(s) at the patient's head. The head of the patient is slightly turned to the right and the abdomen, chest and neck are prepared for surgery. The pneumoperitoneum is created with a Veress needle inserted in the left hypochondrium. A permanent control of the insufflation pressure is of course mandatory.

A first 10- to 11-mm trocar is then placed slightly above the umbilicus, and a careful inspection of the abdominal cavity is done for potential secondaries.

Four other trocars are inserted according to the laparoscopic approach of the upper abdominal cavity (Fig. 16). A 5-mm trocar is placed in the left hypochondrium on the anterior axillary line, and a second 5-mm trocar on the midline just under the xyphoid process. A 10-mm trocar is inserted in the right hypochondrium and is used for the liver retractor; the last 10-mm trocar is placed in the left hypochondrium midway between the umbilicus and the costal margin (Fig 16). Laparoscopic ultrasonography (see Chap. 23) can be performed to exclude liver metastasis before starting the dissection. The various following steps of the laparoscopic stage resemble those of the laparotomy.

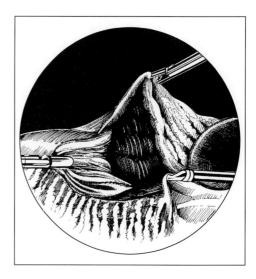

Fig. 17. Opening of lesser sac with transection of short gastric vessels between clips, close to the spleen

Gastrolysis

The lesser sac is opened (Fig. 17) through the great omentum, which is divided and separated from the stomach taking care not to harm the vascular arcade of the right gastroepiploic vessels. The dissection can be done either with a hook or scissors. Transection of the short gastric vessels is then carried out using clips as close as possible to the spleen. It is important not to dissect and open the hiatus at this stage, to prevent any loss of the pneumoperitoneum into the chest.

Dissection of Left Gastric Artery

The stomach is lifted up and the left gastric artery and vein are exposed and dissected through the lesser sac (Fig. 18). The lymph node clearance is done while dissecting towards the diaphragm without opening the hiatus again.

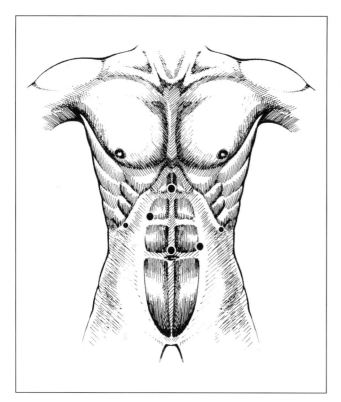

Fig. 16. Trocar placement for laparoscopic abdominal dissection of gastric tube

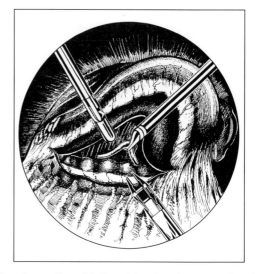

Fig. 18. Transection of left gastric artery between clips through lesser sac

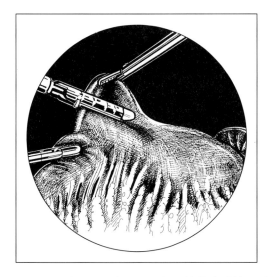 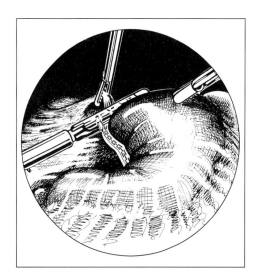

Figs. 19 and 20.   Creation of gastric tube with Endo-GIA stapler

Creation of Gastric Tube

At this stage an extra trocar is inserted: A 12- or 15-mm trocar is placed in the epigastric area slightly to the right (Fig. 16). The small omentum and the inferior branches of the left gastric artery are divided by the application of a 30-mm Endo-GIA with a vascular cartridge (USSC) just below the fourth inferior branch of the left gastric artery. The tubulization is then performed by several applications of Endo-GIA staplers along the greater curvature. One must remain at 3 cm from the edge of

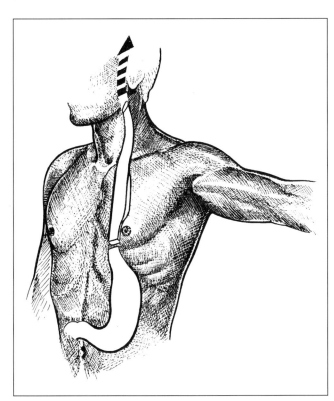

Fig. 21.   Extraction of specimen through cervical incision

the stomach to maintain the vascular supply. A certain tension must be kept on the stomach to obtain the sufficient length (Figs. 19 and 20).

Opening of Hiatus

Once the gastric tube is ready, the hiatus is dissected and finally opened. One will easily find the dissection planes from the thoracoscopic stage. It is very important at this stage to monitor very closely the patient's hemodynamic condition as well as the ventilation. The gas redistribution due to the opening of the hiatus could lead to some hemodynamic disturbance.

Removal of Specimen

The gastric tube is fixed to the proximal side of the stomach using a stitch. The whole specimen is then pulled up through the cervicotomy (Fig. 21). At the same time the gastric tube is brought up to the neck where the oesogastric anastomosis is performed. During the manoeuvre the laparoscope can check the correct position of the tube in the abdomen and the chest, thereby avoiding any twisting. The abdominal cavity is then rinsed extensively with warm saline and checked for hemostasis. No drain is left, the trocars are removed and the wounds are closed.

Intraoperative Complications

Two stages of the thoracoscopic dissection can be difficult: The first difficulty is the identification of the right inferior pulmonary vein, which is sometimes difficult to separate from the pericardium. The second difficulty is the lymph node dissection in the space between the bronchi. The thin posterior membrane of the left bronchus must be identified to avoid any damage especially with the inflated intraluminal balloon of the Carlens™ tube. In our experience, two tears were done during this stage of the dissection, but could be immediately repaired by thoracoscopic suture.

Postoperative Course

At the end of the procedure the patient is usually transferred to the intensive care unit (ICU). Artificial ventilation is maintained until complete recovery from the anaesthesia; blood gas monitoring and chest X-rays are done regularly. If the whole procedure has been done by endoscopy, the recovery will generally be faster and the ileus shorter. Thus, the patient will be allowed to drink on the fourth or fifth postoperative day. After radiological exclusion of an anastomotic leakage with a gastrografin swallow, oral intake is increased to a normal diet. This control is done on the fourth day after a laparoscopic procedure and on the seventh day if the patient has had a laparotomy.

The patient is discharged from ICU after 48 h and returns to a normal ward. If the postoperative course is uneventful, he can be discharged on the 10th-12th postoperative day.

Postoperative Complications

As in the open operation, complications can be quite severe after minor access surgery of the oesophagus. Two types of problems can arise:

1. Complications related to the gastric tube: If the vascular supply of the gastric tube or colon replacing the oesophagus is impaired, necrosis of the stomach or bowel may occur. Another problem is the development of a fistula at the cervical anastomosis. If the leakage is well drained through the wound, it will usually resolve spontaneously. The development of an abscess in the mediastinum or an empyema of the left pleura is far more serious.
2. Pulmonary complications are usually due to the bad preoperative lung conditions of patients with oesophageal carcinoma who mostly also have been smokers. In addition to this, the trauma caused by thoracotomy and the intraoperative manipulations favour postoperative disturbance of pulmonary function. These problems theoretically might be reduced by a less invasive way of access.

Results

The first fully endoscopic procedure in our unit was done in July 1991. At the time we were very impressed by the postoperative course of this 80-year-old patient who was discharged on the ninth day. From July 1991 to December 1993, 15 patients underwent an endoscopic approach for an oesophageal cancer: 2 were done totally by videoendoscopy, and 13 partially.

There was no mortality in the fully endoscopic group. Five patients (38.5 %) died in the second group: one from a myocardial infarction on the second postoperative day, and all the others from partial necrosis of their gastric tube. Two of these patients developed a fistula between the gastric tube and the right bronchus on the 17th and 35th day, respectively. There was an 80 % morbidity due mainly to chest infection among the 8 other patients.

Discussion

Prognosis of oesophageal carcinoma is still very poor, despite all efforts of finding new therapeutic options. Surgery, together with neoadjuvant radiochemotherapy or by itself depending on the tumor stage, is still the only attempt at cure.

The high rate of complications due to the surgical procedure is due partly to the very invasive way of access. The idea to reduce these complications by diminishing the access trauma therefore seemed appealing. Unfortunately, in our limited experience, which we stopped in December 1993, videosurgery failed to prove its efficacy in controlling chest infections. However, it is obvious that our experience is too limited to assess any definitive conclusions. Several trials are actually going on in centres such as Milano (Prof. Peracchia) or Rennes (Prof. Launois). Dealing with a large number of patients, they should arrive at a definite conclusion.

Among different procedures available for the treatment of a malignant tumor of the oesophagus, the exact place of the endoscopic approach remains still to be proven. In theory the videoscopic patient should encounter fewer pulmonary problems and stay a shorter period in ICU and in the hospital. The postoperative course should be more comfortable for such a patient. We did not find these advantages in our series, but obviously multicentric studies on a larger scale should prove these theoretical advantages.

References

1. AKIYAMA H, TSURUMARU M ET AL.: Principles of surgical treatment for carcinoma of the oesophagus. Analysis of lymph node involvement. Ann Surg 194 (1981) 438–443.
2. BAKER JW, SCHECHTER GL: Management of paraoesophageal cancer by blunt dissection without thoracotomy and reconstruction with the stomach. Ann Surg 203 (1986) 491–499.
3. BOLTON JS, OCHSNER JL, ABDOH AA: Surgical management of esophageal cancer: a decade of change. Ann Surg 219 (1994) 475–480.
4. BUESS GF ET AL.: Endoscopic oesophagectomy without thoracotomy. Probl Gen Surg 8 (1991) 478–486
5. DALLEMAGNE B, WEERTS JM ET AL.: Case report: subtotal oesophagectomy by thoracoscopy and laparoscopy. Min Inv Therapy 1 (1992) 183–185.
6. DEMEESTER T, KLEIN HJ: Surgical therapy for cancer of the oesophagus and the cardia. In: Castell O (ed.) The oesophagus. Little, Brown and Company, Boston (1992).
7. KIPFMÜLLER K, NAHRUN M ET AL.: Endoscopic microsurgical dissection of the oesophagus: results in an animal model. Surg Endosc 3 (1989) 63–69.
8. LEWIS I: The surgical treatment of carcinoma of the oesophagus with a special reference to a new operation for the growth of the middle third. Br J Surg 34 (1946) 18–25.
9. NAGAWA H, KOBORI O, MUTO T: Prediction of pulmonary complications after transthoracic oesophagectomy. Br J Surg 81 (1994) 860–862.
10. ORRINGER MB, SLOAN H: Esophagectomy without thoracotomy. Thorac Cardiovasc Surg 76 (1978) 643–654.
11. RAHAMIM J, CHAM CW: Oesophagogastrectomy for carcinoma of the oesophagus and cardia. Br J Surg 80 (1993) 1305–1309.
12. RICHELME H, BAULIEUX J: Le traitement des cancers de l'oesophage. Monographies de l'AFC 1986.
13. SKINNER DB, LITTLE AG ET AL.: Selection of operations for oesophageal cancer based on staging. Ann Surg 204 (1986) 391–401.
14. SWEET RH, SOUTAR L ET AL.: Muscle wall tumors of the oesophagus. J Thorac Surg 27 (1954) 13–35.
15. TAM PC, SIU KF ET AL.: Local recurrence after subtotal oesophagectomy for squamous cell carcinoma. Ann Surg 205 (1987) 189–194.

10. Laparoscopic Heller Myotomy

A. L. DE PAULA, K. HASHIBA, M. BAFUTTO, AND C. A. MACHADO

Introduction

Esophageal achalasia is a motility disorder characterized by the absence or incomplete relaxation of the lower esophageal sphincter (LES) in response to swallowing. Its etiology can be primary or idiopathic, or secondary to Chaga's disease [3], to pseudointestinal obstruction [21], to surgical trauma [22], or to neoplasia [20].

Chaga's disease is the most common cause of achalasia in Brazil. In other countries, such as England, the most common cause is idiopathic, reaching a prevalence of 7–13 cases per year in a population of 100 000 inhabitants [13, 14].

In achalasia the main pathological finding is a decreased number or absence of ganglion cells especially in Auerbach's plexus. In Chaga's disease this reduction of ganglion cells is either caused directly by Trypanosoma Cruzi, by toxic substances produced by Trypanosoma, or indirectly by an immunological mechanism [3]. The consequence is a motility disorder up to the total absence of peristaltic contractions in the esophageal body or incomplete relaxation of the LES in response to swallowing.

These histological changes are followed by major pathophysiological disregulations including uncoordinated peristalsis, esophageal stasis, and progressive dilation and elongation of the esophagus [5, 15]. The typical symptoms are progressive dysphagia, regurgitation, weight loss and chest pain, or retrosternal discomfort [3]. Because the tissue damage is not reversible, treatment is limited to relief of symptoms, especially dysphagia. Therapeutic options include administration of nifedipine, endoscopic dilation of the distal esophagus, and the surgical procedure [4, 9, 10, 12]. Surgical treatment is associated with a low morbidity and mortality rate, and provides long-term relief of symptoms and therefore increased quality of life.

With technical developments in minor access surgery, achalasia became accessible to this technique. In fact, because no resection is necessary, the main problems of minimally invasive surgery, i. e., retrieval of specimen and reconstruction, do not arise. Therefore, the Heller myotomy seems to be an excellent indication for laparoscopic surgery [2, 17].

Indications

We have performed laparoscopic modified Heller's myotomy in patients with stage-one and stage-two achalasia. The laparoscopic procedure is not indicated in patients who had previous upper gastrointestinal surgery, who present a high cardiorespiratory risk, uncorrectable coagulation disorders, or an esophageal neoplasia associated with achalasia. Because of the reduction of postoperative pain and stress provided by laparoscopic surgery, patients in poor general condition who normally might have been submitted to open surgery only at a very high risk are considered more readily to be candidates for surgical treatment. This concerns mainly older, undernourished patients.

Preoperative Work-up

After patient history, clinical examination, and laboratory tests, an endoscopy of the upper gastrointestinal tract is always performed. Endoscopic findings include the typical signs of esophagitis, i. e., hyperemia, edema, a dilated esophagus with mucosal thickening, and a loss of the typical vascular pattern of the distal esophagus. The esophagitis is not caused by gastroesophageal reflux but by stasis of food in the esophagus. Usually, a slight pressure on the endoscope is sufficient to cross the LES, but in very advanced cases passage may be quite difficult. The cardia must be investigated carefully in inversion to exclude any malignancy in this area.

Esophageal manometry usually shows absence or incomplete relaxation of the LES in response to swallowing, an elevated pressure at the lower esophageal sphincter, and simultaneous low-amplitude contractions or no peristaltic activity in the body of the esophagus [5].

A barium swallow is routinely obtained. Features include esophageal dilation, narrowing at the gastroesophageal junction (Figs. 1–4), and absence of the gastric air bubble. Esophageal achalasia was classified into three types based on radiological and manometric findings [20]:
1. Initial stage: no dilation of the esophagus, a small amount of contrast medium stasis
2. Nonadvanced stage: dilated esophagus, keeping its longitudinal orientation, uncoordinated peristalsis with tertiary waves
3. Advanced stage: esophageal dilation > 7 cm, absence of peristaltic contractions, and loss of longitudinal orientation with distortion especially in the lower part ("sigmoid esophagus")

Because Chaga's disease may also cause pathology of the myocardium, extensive cardiac risk evaluation is as mandatory as precise intraoperative monitoring. In some patients a transitory pacemaker is required. Severely undernourished patients should receive hyperalimentation prior to surgery to reduce the operative risk.

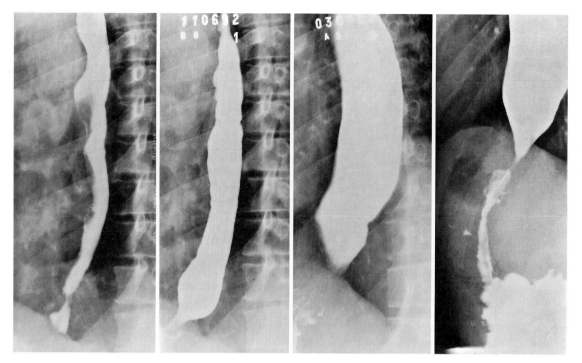

Figs. 1–4 Radiographic imaging of nonadvanced achalasia

The esophagus is emptied and irrigated through a thick nasogastric tube preoperatively to avoid aspiration at the beginning of anesthesia and to reduce the risk of intra-abdominal contamination in case of an accidental esophageal perforation during the procedure. For the last 3 days before the operation, patients are administered a liquid diet only. Peroperative antibiotic prophylaxis is given routinely.

Operative Technique

The procedure is carried out with the patient in a supine position, legs abducted and in a reverse Trendelenburg position of approximately 30°. The surgeon stands between the patient's legs with the first assistant on the patient's left. The second assistant holds the camera on the other side of the patient.

The pneumoperitoneum of 12–14 mmHg is established with a Veress needle 3–4 cm above the umbilicus and a 10-mm trocar is introduced for the 30° laparoscope. Two 5-mm trocars are placed near the right and left subcostal margins (Fig. 5) on the midclavicular line and a third one below the xiphoid. The last 10-mm trocar is introduced between the left subcostal and the supraumbilical trocar.

After retraction of the left lobe of the liver and pulling the stomach caudad, dissection is started with the division of the gastrohepatic ligament above the hepatic branch of the anterior vagus nerve. The peritoneum overlying the esophagogastric junction and the phrenoesophageal membrane are incised (Fig. 6). The right crus of the diaphragm and the anterior and posterior vagus nerves are identified. The short gastric vessels are divided between clips over a length of 6–8 cm.

A 51-F Savary-Guillard dilator is placed in the esophageal lumen. After identification of the gastroesophageal junction, the posterior aspect of the esophagus is dissected. If necessary, a Penrose drain can be passed behind the esophagus to

allow atraumatic traction. The myotomy is carried out sharply with scissors (Fig. 7) and by blunt dissection with a dissector (Fig. 8). It is continued upward 5–6 cm on the anterior surface of the esophagus (Fig. 9) and extended for 2 cm down on the stomach (Fig. 10). Cautery in this area should only be applied with great care.

Partial anterior fundoplication is routinely performed, using three rows of nonabsorbable sutures. The first row sutures

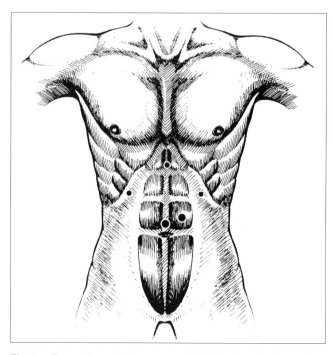

Fig. 5. Trocar placement for laparoscopic modified Heller's myotomy

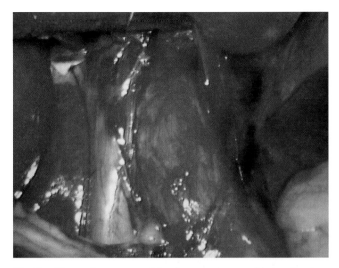

Fig. 6. The peritoneum overlying the esophagogastric junction has been incised and dissected

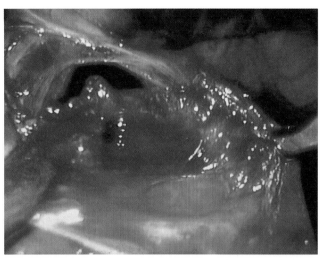

Fig. 9. The myotomy is carried out upward on the anterior surface of the esophagus

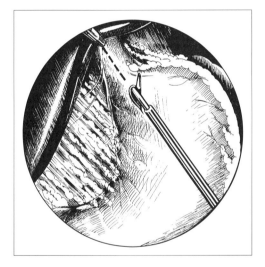

Fig. 7. The muscular layer is transected with scissors

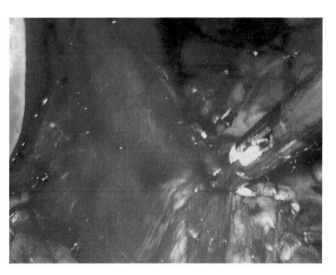

Fig. 10. The incision is taken down for 2 cm on the anterior wall of the stomach

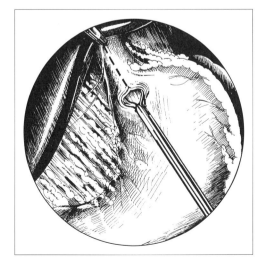

Fig. 8. The edges of the myotomy are spread apart with a dissector

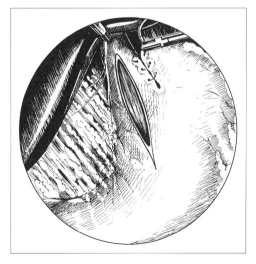

Fig. 11. The gastric fundus is attached to the posterior esophageal wall with 3–4 interrupted, nonabsorbable sutures

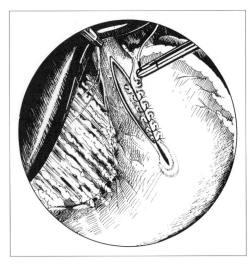

Fig. 12.   Suturing of the anterior aspect of the gastric fundus to the left-side edge of the myotomy

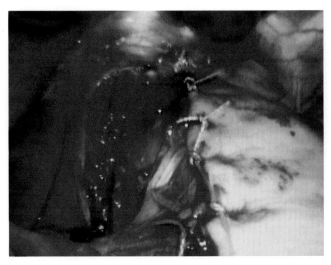

Fig. 14.   The finished partial anterior 180° fundoplication

the gastric fundus to the posterior esophageal wall (Fig. 11). The second row fixes the anterior aspect of the gastric fundus to the left side edge of the myotomy (Fig. 12) and the third one covers the myotomy by attaching the greater curvature of the gastric fundus to the right side edge of the myotomy (Fig. 13). The result is a partial, posterior-left lateral-anterior fundoplication of 180 to 270°.

Possible Complications

As Chaga's disease may also cause dilation of the colon, the danger of colonic injury, especially when creating the pneumoperitoneum, may be high. Another feature of this disease is portal hypertension, which can result in severe bleeding during dissection.

The most frequently encountered intraoperative complication is perforation of the esophageal mucosa. This happens

with an increased frequency in patients who had undergone previous endoscopic dilation. If the intra-abominal pressure is high, bulging of the mucosa can usually not be seen very well. In any case of doubt the mucosal integrity can be checked by instillation of methylene blue via the gastric tube. An accidental mucosal perforation can be repaired with interrupted nonabsorbable 4-0 sutures.

Postoperative Management

Postoperatively, all patients are given a first-generation cephalosporine and a liquid diet from the first postoperative day on. If a perforation of the esophageal mucosa has occurred, the gastric tube is left at least for 48 h with parenteral nutrition. If the postoperative course is uneventful, patients are discharged after 24 h. From the fifth postoperative day on, they can resume normal activities.

Endoscopic, radiological, and manometric controls are performed routinely after 3 and 12 months. At endoscopy care is taken to look for signs of a reflux esophagitis, which can develop as a complication after myotomy. Radiologically, the diameter of the esophagus is usually diminished and passage of the contrast medium into the stomach is unimpaired. Manometry shows a decrease in the pressure at the LES.

Results

From August 1991 to December 1993, 85 patients with esophageal achalasia were submitted to laparoscopic treatment. In 77 patients achalasia was caused by Chaga's disease and in 8 patients of unknown etiology. There were 59 men and 26 women with a mean age of 41.4 years (range 12–74 years). The mean weight was 56 kg (range 41–88 kg). The most frequent symptoms were dysphagia, regurgitation, and chest pain. A total of 53 patients had experienced weight loss. Average duration of symptoms was 7.6 years (range 2–18 years).

The mean operative time was 142 min. There was no conversion to open surgery. Laparoscopic esophageal myotomy

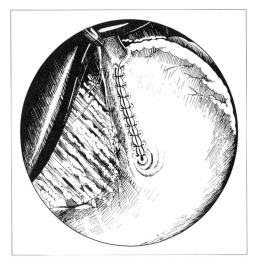

Fig. 13.   The myotomy is covered by suturing the greater curvature to the right-side edge of the myotomy

with cholecystectomy was performed in six patients, and an additional transcystic common bile duct exploration in another patient. The mean hospital stay was 30 h. On average, the patients were able to return to full activity on the eighth postoperative day. In 3 patients who all had had previous endoscopic dilation of the LES, an accidental mucosal perforation occurred and was recognized during the procedure. The lesion was sutured and covered with the fundoplication. Recovery was uneventful in all 3 patients.

Postoperative complications are shown in Table 1. One patient developed an esophageal leak and was reoperated on through open surgery on the eighth postoperative day. The perforation had gone unnoticed at surgery. Another patient who had required a transitory pacemaker was readmitted on the 17th postoperative day after having been discharged on the second postoperative day. She had suffered cardiac arrest, and after resuscitation, developed acute peritonitis, which was revealed as being due to an esophageal tear at the site of the myotomy.

Table 1. Laparoscopic esophageal myotomy (postoperative complications)

Complications	Patients	%
Costochondritis	1	1.2
Wound infection	1	1.2
Esophageal leak	1	1.2
Cardiac arrest	1	1.2
Total	4	4.8

The mean follow-up was 20 months ranging from 8 to 36 months. A total of 81 patients (95 %) were available for follow-up. Clinical evaluation is summarized in Table 2. Results were considered excellent (total relief from dysphagia) in 79.1 % of patients. Twelve patients (16.1 %) complained of occasional dysphagia without dietary restrictions. Preoperative symptoms persisted in 2 patients who were reoperated on. Inadequate myotomy was the reason for therapeutic failure. A third patient developed severe heartburn due to reflux esophagitis. Upon relaparoscopy, rupture of the fundoplication was found at the right edge of the myotomy.

Table 2. Laparoscopic esophageal myotomy (postoperative clinical results)

Results	Patients	%
Excellent (no dysphagia)	64	79.1
Good (occasional dysphagia)	13	16.0
Fair (frequent dysphagia)	1	1.2
Poor (no improvement)	2	2.5
Poor (heartburn)	1	1.2
Total	81	100

Radiological follow-up in 75 patients showed free flow of the contrast medium through the cardia. Reduction of the esophageal diameter was observed in 34 patients. Endoscopy showed reflux esophagitis in 1 patient. A total of 54 patients were submitted to postoperative esophageal manometry in a period ranging from 3 to 16 months. The mean postoperative LES pressure decreased from preoperative values of 35.6 mmHg to 15.2 mmHg. No difference in peristaltic activity was noticed.

Discussion

Esophageal achalasia is a chronic disease. The treatment involves palliative measures to relieve symptoms. Prior studies confirm that esophagocardiomyotomy is the best treatment choice, except for patients in a very advanced stage of the disease.

The most favored surgical choice has been esophagocardiomyotomy associated with an antireflux procedure [1]. Myotomy alone is followed by a gastroesophageal reflux in 20–50 % of patients [4]. The surgeons who use this procedure vary in its extension, access, and antireflux management with techniques such as Dor, Belsey, Mark IV, Thal, Hill, Lortat-Jacob, Pinotti, and "floppy" Nissen [15, 16]. Comparative studies demonstrated poor results in 16–37 % of patients who underwent esophagocardiomyotomy alone, whereas this number has dropped to 0–16 % for the procedures with added antireflux wrap. Therefore, we conclude that fundoplication can improve the results of esophagocardiomyotomy. Moreover, 24-h esophageal pH monitoring showed greater recurrence of reflux in patients without fundoplication.

Length and depth of the myotomy are very important issues. A very deep myotomy can cause mucosal perforation, whereas in a superficial and incomplete one, the achalasia will persist. Also, a very small incision can cause incomplete section of the lower esophageal sphincter and persistence of symptoms. The abdominal approach is preferred to the thoracic one in our department. It allows a better exposure of the distal esophagus and cardia, and has a reduced incidence of pulmonary complications. The results obtained in 1200 patients operated on in 25 different centers from 1980 to 1990 demonstrated success rates of 89 % (63–100 %), with a mortality of 0.3 % (0–3 %), antireflux reoperation in 3 % (0–11 %), and gastroesophageal reflux in 10 % (0–53 %) [11, 15, 16, 19].

Esophageal mucosal perforation is the most important early complication [1], which can cause fistula, abscess, or peritonitis [6]. Late complications were gastroesophageal reflux, which usually occurred in patients submitted to myotomy alone, and recurrent dysphagia, due to poor surgical indication or inappropriate technique.

Experience with the laparoscopic approach demonstrated that the exposure of the distal esophagus is facilitated due to the patient's position and pneumoperitoneum. The easier access to the operative site and a magnified view can make the myotomy more adequate by allowing a more precise division of the muscle layers as well as sufficient extension.

All the aspects mentioned herein, which at the moment are presented as advantages of laparoscopic surgery, do not take away the important role of open surgery, the most established procedure. Nevertheless, open surgery would hardly be able to offer advantages such as minimal postoperative discomfort, early discharges, 24-h hospitalization and a rapid return to full activities. It is possible that the indication for laparoscopic treatment will surpass dilatation procedures, if we consider that 10–40 % of the patients submitted to the latter have had recurrent dysphagia and 3–22 % needed surgical treatment after dilation [9]. However, the laparoscopic approach does not seem to have reduced the incidence of esophageal mucosal perforation during myotomy. Due to positive intra-abdominal pressure, the mucosal bulging is less evident, therefore, impairing the definition of muscular layers. The use of an intraluminal balloon or Savary dilator made this step safer. Manometric postoperative evaluation proved the efficacy of the laparoscopic approach by decreasing considerably the LES pressure.

Finally, we concluded that laparoscopic esophagocardiomyotomy is the best alternative to open surgery in the treatment of nonadvanced esophageal achalasia, because it provides the same safety and efficiency as the open Heller myotomy. Furthermore, patients are provided with the advantages of minor access surgery such as less postoperative discomfort, shorter hospitalization, rapid return to full activities, and better cosmesis.

References

1. ANDREOLO NA, EARLAM RJ: Heller's myotomy for achalasia: Is an added antireflux procedure necessary? Br J Surg 74 (1987) 765.
2. ANSELMINO M, HINDER R, FILIPI CJ, WILSON P: Laparoscopic Heller cardiomyotomy and thoracoscopic esophageal long myotomy for the treatment of primary esophageal motor disorders. Surg Laparosc Endosc 3 (1993) 437–441.
3. BETTARELO A, PINOTTI HV: Oesophageal involvement in Chagas' disease. Clin Gastroenterol 5 (1956) 107.
4. BORTOLOTTI M, LABO G: Clinical and manometric effects of nifedipin in patients with oesophageal achalasia. Gastroenterology 80 (1981) 39.
5. COHEN S, LIPSHUTZ W: Lower oesophageal sphincter dysfunction in achalasia. Gastroenterology 61 (1971) 814.
6. CSENDES A, BRAGHETTO I, CORTES C: Late results of a prospective randomized study comparing forceful dilatation and oesophagomyotomy in patients with achalasia. Gut 30 (1989) 299–304.
7. DEPAULA A, HASHIBA K, BAFUTTO M: Laparoskopische modifizierte Oesophagusmyotome nach Heller. In: Brune, I (ed.): Laparo-Endoskopische Chirurgie, Hans Marseille Verlag (1993).
8. DIAS JCP, DOENTA DE CHAGAS EM BAMBUI MG: Brasil. Estudo clinicoepidemiológico a partir da fase aguda, 1940-1982. Tese Faculdade de Medicina Univ. Fed. Minas Gerais, Belo Horizonte. 1982.
9. Ellis FH, Kiser JC, Schlegal JF et al.: Esophagomyotomy for achalasia: experimental, clinical and manometric aspects. Ann Surg 166 (1967) 645.
10. FELLOWS IW, OGILVIE AL, ATKINSON M: Pneumatic dilatation in achalasia. Gut 24 (1983) 1020.
11. FERGUSON KM: Achalasia: current evaluation and therapy. Ann Thorac Surg 52 (1991) 336.
12. GOULBOURNE IA, WALDBAUM PR: Long term results of Heller`s operation for achalasia. J R Coll Surg Edinb 30 (1985) 101.
13. MAYBERRY JF, ATKINSON M: Studies of incidence and prevalence of achalasia in the Nottingham area. Q J Med 56 (1985) 451.
14. MAYBERRY JF, ATKINSON M: Variations in the prevalence of achalasia in Great Britain and Ireland: an epidemiological study based on hospital admissions Q J Med 62 (1987) 67.
15. MURRAY GF, BUTTAGLINI JW, KEUGY BA ET AL.: Selective application of fundoplication in achalasia. Ann Thorac Surg 37 (1984) 185.
16. NELEMS JMB, COOPER JD, PEARSON FG: Treatment of achalasia: esophagomyotomy with antireflex procedure. Can J Surg 23 (1980) 588.
17. PELLEGRINI C, WELTER LA, PATTI M, LEICHTER R, MUSSAN G, MORI T, BERNSTEIN G, WAY L.: Thoracoscopic esophagomyotomy. Initial experience with a new approach for the treatment of achalasia. Ann Surg 216 (1992) 291–299.
18. PINOTTI HW, NASI A, CECONELLO I, ZILBERSTEIN B, POLLARA W: Chagas' disease of the esophagus. Dis Esoph 1 (1988) 65.
19. REES JR., THORBJARNARSON B, BARNES ACHALASIA WH: Results of operations in 84 patients. Ann Surg 171 (1970) 195.
20. REZENDE JM., LAUAR KM, OLIVEIRA AR: Aspectos clinicos e radiológicos da aperistalsis do esôfago. Rev Bras Gastroenterol 12 (1960) 247–262.
21. SCHUFFLER MD, POPE CE: Esophageal motor dysfunction in idiopathic intestinal pseudoobstruction. Gastroenterology 70 (1976) 677.
22. SHARP JR: Mechanical and neurogenic factors in postvagotomy dysphagia. J Clin Gastroenterol 1 (1979) 321.
23. TUCKER HJ, SNAPE WJ, COHEN S: Achalasia secondary to carcinoma. Manometric and clinical features. Ann Intern Med 89 (1978) 315.

11. Laparoscopic Vagotomy

R. W. BAILEY

Introduction

The recent popularity of laparoscopic cholecystectomy has lead to the adaptation of other routine surgical procedures to a minimally invasive approach. One of the more exciting areas has centered around the development of a laparoscopic approach to the treatment of peptic ulcer disease.

A thorough understanding of the epidemiology and pathophysiology of peptic ulcer disease is essential to an effective and well-planned approach to its management. Peptic ulcer disease continues to be a major health care problem in the United States. Approximately 500,000 new cases are reported every year [43, 44]. The incidence of peptic ulcer disease, however, appears to have declined over the last 20–30 years [43]. Although this decline appears to have preceded the introduction of H-2 receptor antagonists into widespread clinical practice, surgery for intractable ulcer disease has been largely replaced by pharmacologic management. Furthermore, the recent identification of Helicobacter pylori as an etiologic factor in the development of peptic ulcer disease has virtually eliminated the need for elective ulcer surgery [11]. Some physicians have even voiced the opinion that elective vagotomy for the treatment of ulcer disease will soon be of historical interest only [1]. The decline in elective ulcer surgery may also be attributed to the fact that both physicians and patients alike have been content, in the past, to continue medical therapy when faced with the alternative of major abdominal surgery, even if pharmacologic management provides only partial or temporary relief of symptoms.

Indications and Contraindications

Laparoscopic management of peptic ulcer disease is reserved, for the most part, for those individuals who have failed medical management or require indefinite drug therapy to control their symptoms. A laparoscopic approach to patients presenting with bleeding or gastric outlet obstruction has been successfully completed but only in a few isolated situations [26, 39]. Laparoscopic closure of acute duodenal perforations have also been reported but a simultaneous anti-ulcer operation is usually not performed [8, 34]. Due to the large percentage of patients with peptic ulcer disease who present with duodenal perforation, it is anticipated that with further experience such conditions may be routinely managed via a minimally invasive approach in the future.

Patients with pre-pyloric or gastric ulcers are not considered ideal candidates for a highly selective vagotomy. Previ-

ous studies with open highly selective vagotomy [20], as well as our own initial experience has shown that these individuals are at a much higher risk for recurrence. Other contraindications to the performance of a laparoscopic vagotomy include pregnancy, morbid obesity, extensive prior upper abdominal surgery, and irreversible coagulopathies.

Choice of Operative Procedure

The last one hundred years have witnessed a profound evolution in the surgical treatment of peptic ulcer disease. Truncal vagotomy combined with pyloroplasty, gastrojejunostomy, or antrectomy has remained one of the most effective forms of surgical treatment. Unfortunately, this procedure is associated with undesirable side effects such as dumping and diarrhea. For this reason, the introduction of highly selective vagotomy has had an enormous impact on the current surgical treatment of peptic ulcer disease [9, 17–19]. A review of the literature reveals this procedure to be extremely safe and effective, with a mortality rate of 0–0.3 %, a recurrent ulcer rate in the ranging from of 3–30 %, with over 85 % of patients reporting a good to excellent outcome [9, 17–19]. Despite the availability of this procedure, the majority of operations for peptic ulcer disease are being performed on an urgent or emergent basis for acute hemorrhage, perforation, or obstruction [43]. Furthermore, even though the overall rate of elective ulcer surgery may be decreasing, patients presenting with such emergent conditions appear to be older and sicker, thereby accounting for a persistently high morbidity and mortality rate [43].

Since it is impossible to identify a single operation that is applicable to all patients requiring surgery for peptic ulcer disease, a surgeon must be aware of the numerous factors which will influence the choice of operative procedure (Table 1)

Table 1. Factors influencing choice of operation

Experience and personal preference of surgeon

Indications for surgery and the urgency of operation

Clinical Presentation of Patient (Age, sex, nutritional status, body habitus, associated medical illnesses, presence of shock or peritonitis)

Characteristics of Ulcer Diathesis (Chronicity of disease, location and size of ulcer, responsiveness to medical therapy)

Use of ulcerogenic drugs or the presence of ulcerogenic endocrine disease (i.e., gastrinoma or hyperparathyroidism)

Modified from Stabile BE. Current Surgical Management of Duodenal Ulcer. Surg Clin N Am. 72:335–356, 1992.

[43]. These factors, especially the experience and personal preference of the surgeon, will have an important impact on determining the surgical approach to a patient with peptic ulcer disease. These factors play an even greater role when considering a laparoscopic or thoracoscopic approach because each individual surgeon's experience will substantially affect the outcome of the operation.

A minimally invasive approach to the surgical treatment of peptic ulcer disease was first conceptualized and performed in the clinical setting in 1989. It has been demonstrated that bilateral truncal vagotomy may be safely and quickly accomplished via a thoracoscopic or laparoscopic approach [10]. Unfortunately, bilateral truncal vagotomy usually necessitates a gastric drainage procedure and is associated with several disadvantages, including delayed gastric emptying, postoperative diarrhea, and the dumping syndrome. Due to the technological and skill limitations during the early development of laparoscopic general surgery, the performance of a drainage procedure or antrectomy under laparoscopic guidance was extremely difficult and time consuming. For this reason, alternative means of establishing effective gastric drainage were considered. Balloon dilation has been used successfully to perform an "endoscopic" pyloromyotomy. Prior experience with this procedure, however, had been reserved for patients presenting with pyloric stenosis and not for patients undergoing elective ulcer surgery. Therefore, this technique has not been widely adopted as an alternative means to provide adequate gastric drainage. As the equipment, instrumentation, and training available for advanced laparoscopic procedures has improved, so has the ability to safely and quickly perform a hand sewn pyloroplasty or stapled antrectomy under laparoscopic guidance. Over the next 5 years the quantity and complexity of upper abdominal laparoscopic surgery will certainly increase substantially.

Similarly, due to an early lack of surgeon experience and appropriate laparoscopic instrumentation, early attempts at a conventional highly selective vagotomy were technically difficult and often led to excessively long operative times. Highly selective vagotomy, if it is to be effective, is, by definition, a meticulous and time consuming procedure. Due to the disadvantages of a bilateral truncal vagotomy, and because a conventional highly selective vagotomy was initially very difficult to perform under laparoscopic guidance, several modifications of standard ulcer operations were proposed [3, 15, 22].

During the preliminary clinical trials of laparoscopic ulcer surgery, one of the most commonly performed modification consisted of a posterior truncal vagotomy combined with some type of highly selective denervation of the anterior stomach. The rationale for performing this type of procedure is that an intact vagal nerve supply to the anterior aspect of the antrum appears to be sufficient to allow for normal gastric emptying [48]. This thereby obviates the need for performing a drainage procedure and decreases the risk of postoperative diarrhea and dumping.

A posterior truncal vagotomy is easily and quickly accomplished under laparoscopic guidance. The *anterior* highly selective denervation may be accomplished by one of several techniques: individual ligation of the neurovascular bundles along the lesser curve of the stomach (highly selective vagotomy) [3], by a seromyotomy [22], or by interruption of the nerve fibers with an endoscopic stapling device (linear gastrectomy) [15]. Amongst these options, an anterior highly selective vagotomy has met with a substantial degree of popu-

larity. This procedure is very similar in concept to an open technique described in 1978 by Hill and Barker [16].

Many surgeons who first began to contemplate the performance of a laparoscopic anti-ulcer procedure recognized that some of these modifications might have definite advantages if performed under laparoscopic guidance. These advantages included a decreased operative time and improved technical ease of the procedure. Although laparoscopic posterior truncal vagotomy combined with an anterior highly selective vagotomy represents a viable alternative to more standardized procedures [16], such procedures (whether performed open or laparoscopically) have not gained much clinical popularity. The last five years have witnessed a revolution in the development of new laparoscopic instrumentation and procedures. As overall surgical experience with laparoscopic general surgery has increased, there has been a simultaneous trend toward the performance of more standardized procedures. A recent survey of prominent laparoscopic surgeons indicates that nearly all surgeons currently favor a standard highly selective or bilateral truncal vagotomy over that of one of the above-described modifications (unpublished data). The author agrees with this approach to peptic ulcer disease and now performs only recognized, conventional anti-ulcer procedures.

Preoperative Work-up

The preoperative evaluation is very similar to that for patients being considered for conventional ulcer surgery (Table 2). All patients are subjected to a routine history, physical examination, and laboratory evaluation. Patients with atypical presen-

Table 2. Preoperative evaluation

History
Physical Examination
Laboratory Studies (+/– Serum Gastrin)
Endoscopy (+/– UGI contrast study)
Acid secretion studies
Gastric emptying scan

tations of ulcer diathesis should also undergo a work-up to exclude gastrinoma. All patients should undergo upper gastrointestinal endoscopy to exclude malignancy as well as contrast studies to determine the extent and severity of disease. In addition, to evaluate the effectiveness of this procedure, patients should have determinations of their acid secretion (basal and pentagastrin stimulated) and gastric emptying capacity. Repeat studies are performed between one and six months after surgery to confirm the effectiveness of the procedure. A thorough assessment of the patient's operative risk should also be made, similar to patients undergoing any major abdominal operation.

Operative Technique

Patient Positioning

The patient should be positioned in the modified lithotomy position which will allow the surgeon to stand between the patient's legs, in excellent position to perform the operative dissection of the distal esophagus and stomach (Fig. 1).

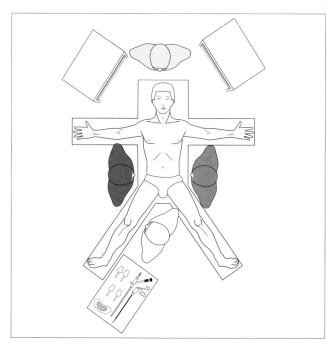

Fig. 1. The modified lithotomy position is employed during laparoscopic vagotomy. In allows the surgeon to stand in an optimal position during the operative dissection

When placing the patient in the lithotomy position, the proper precautions must be taken to prevent neurovascular compromise of the lower extremities. "Booted" stirrups should be used to elevate the lower extremities and appropriate padding placed to protect the calf. An alternative to the lithotomy position is to use a "split-leg" orthopedic table. This will allow the patient's legs to remain flat but apart so as to allow easy access for the surgeon between the patient's legs.

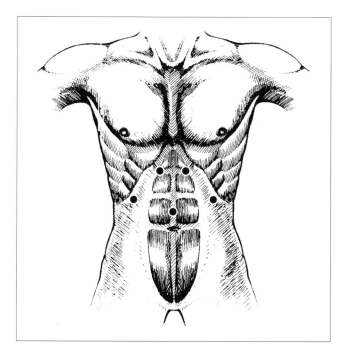

Fig. 2. A total of five trocars, usually 10 mm in diameter, are routinely used during laparoscopic vagotomy

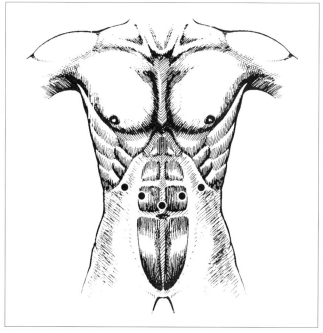

Fig. 3. The placement of the operating ports should be modified if access to the pylorus is required. The surgeon should consider the placement of an additional port if necessary

It is important to insert a nasogastric (or orogastric) tube and a urinary catheter as soon as possible to decompress the stomach and bladder. The gastric tube may subsequently be replaced with a large esophageal tube (Maloney dilator) or a flexible gastroscope to distend the distal esophagus and facilitate its identification during the early stages of the operative dissection. However, due to the inherent limitations of laparoscopic surgery, care must be taken to assure proper retraction of the stomach during the passage of any large esophageal tube. Careful coordination between the anesthesiologist and the surgeon during this process will avoid inadvertent perforation of the stomach or esophagus.

Trocar Placement

A total of five primary laparoscopic cannulas are employed in most cases (Fig. 2). The ports should be placed as evenly as possible across the abdominal wall. If the ports are located too close together they will tend to interfere with each other. This will severely hamper the ease with which the operative dissection is completed.

The trocars should be placed as high as possible in the upper abdomen to facilitate dissection of the gastroesophageal junction. If manipulation of the pyloric region is needed then one or both of the operating ports may be placed more caudally, toward the level of the umbilicus (Fig. 3). This will make the operative approach to the antrum and pylorus easier than if the ports remain in a more cephalad location.

A 30–45 ° angled laparoscope should be used in all cases, as this will facilitate examination of the distal esophagus and hiatus. The surgeon and other operating room personnel should be aware that some of the angled laparoscopes substantially reduce the amount of light being transmitted from the light source. This will diminish the overall illumination of the peritoneal cavity and cause the operative field to appear

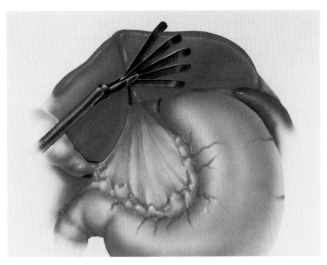

Fig. 4. An atraumatic liver retraction is used to elevate and retract the liver away from the anterior wall of the stomach. Care must be taken to avoid "spearing" of the liver with the retractor

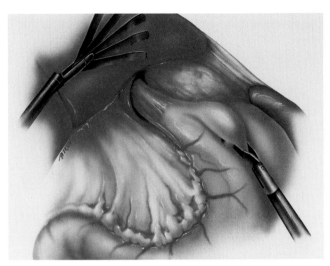

Fig. 6. Exposure of the distal esophagus is best achieved by left-lateral and caudal retraction of the body of the stomach. Atraumatic grasping forceps should be used which will help avoid injury to the stomach wall

dim. The surgeon should "test" the angled scope that will be used during the laparoscopic vagotomy prior to the actual procedure. Additional equipment and instrument considerations are listed in (Table 3).

The laparoscope is inserted through a 10 mm port placed in the midline, approximately 6–8 cm above the umbilicus. Two

Table 3. Equipment and instrumentation considerations for laparoscopic vagotomy

Angled (30–45°) laparoscope
Large (21–25") video monitor
"Booted" stirrups
"Convertor-less" Trocars
Atraumatic liver retractor
Atraumatic stomach retractor (Babcock)
Scissors, Dissector, Grasper
Tapered esophageal dilator

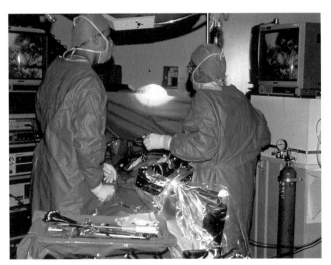

Fig. 5. Picture of a fully automated robotic device that attaches to the laparoscope and allows the surgeon to control its movement

retraction ports are placed along the right and left anterior axillary lines, just below the costal margin. The right subcostal port will provide access for the liver retractor. Retraction of the stomach and esophagus is accomplished through the left subcostal port. The operative dissection is accomplished through two operating ports placed in the right and left mid-epigastric region, approximately 2–4 cm below the costal margin. An optional sixth puncture should be readily considered if additional retraction of the stomach, liver, or surrounding adipose tissue is necessary.

The size of the laparoscopic trocars will depend on the surgeon's preference and the instrumentation to be used during the procedure. Currently, 10.5 mm trocars seem to be the best choice for all five ports. This gives the surgeon greater versatility during the operation to exchange instruments (clip applier, laparoscope, etc.) from one port to another. Furthermore, newly released trocars (Premium Surgi-Port, United States Surgical Corporation, Norwalk, CT) are equipped with a universal adaptor that allows for the interchange of instruments ranging in size from 3–12 mm without the need for using a converter.

Retraction of the Left Lobe of the Liver

Almost all anti-ulcer procedures will require dissection of the distal esophagus. In order to provide adequate visualization of this area, the left lobe of the liver must be retracted away from the anterior surface of the stomach. A 10 mm, atraumatic liver retractor appears to best serve this purpose. It is inserted through the right sub-costal cannula and opened carefully within the abdomen, just underneath the edge of the liver. This will allow the surgeon to elevate and retract the left lobe of the liver toward the right side of the patient (Fig. 4). Care must be taken not to "spear" the liver with the tip of the retractor during its insertion underneath the liver. The liver retractor, once properly positioned, may be held in place by the camera operator or by a robotic "arm" (Computer Motion, Inc., Goleta, CA) (Fig. 5). It is not usually necessary to divide the left triangular ligament in order to gain adequate exposure of the gastroesophageal junction. This technique may be helpful however in situations where the left lobe of the liver is found to be enlarged.

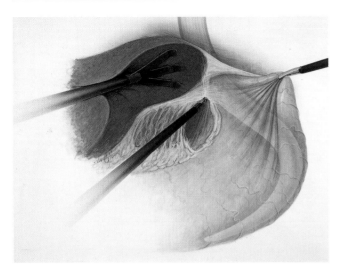

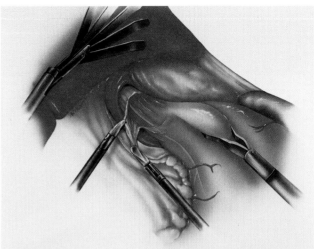

Fig. 7. The initial approach to the distal esophagus is made by opening a window through the lesser omentum

Fig. 9. Operative dissection of the stomach and esophagus should be performed utilizing a two-handed technique

Dissection of the Distal Esophagus and Proximal Stomach

To provide adequate exposure around the esophageal hiatus, the greater curvature of the stomach is pulled caudally and to the patient's left side with an atraumatic Babcock forceps (Fig. 6). This maneuver facilitates the initial approach to the distal esophagus. The posterior aspect of the distal esophagus may be approached through a window made in the lesser omentum (Fig. 7) or by directly incising the phreno-esophageal ligament overlying the proximal stomach and distal esophagus (Fig. 8 A and 8 B). The latter is the preferred method of approach as it should help to avoid injury to the hepatic branch of the anterior vagus nerve.

The initial opening of the peritoneum should be made directly over the distal esophagus. The dissection along the upper stomach is best performed with dissecting forceps using a "two-handed" operating technique (Fig. 9). Patients with large amounts of adipose tissue surrounding the gastroesophageal junction and greater curvature pose a difficult task to the operating surgeon during dissection of the esophagus.

A large esophageal tube or gastroscope may be inserted into the stomach to facilitate early visual identification of the distal esophagus. The placement of an esophageal tube to guide the initial dissection, however, becomes less and less necessary as the experience of the surgical team increases.

The right crus of the diaphragm is an important landmark and should be quickly identified (Fig. 10). It may be retracted away from the esophagus with one blade of the liver retractor if necessary. A plane is then developed between the right crus and distal esophagus and continued in a posterior direction, behind the esophagus. Once a small portion of the distal esophagus is clearly identified, the Babcock clamp on the upper stomach is repositioned to the gastroesophageal junction to allow for improved retraction. A previously placed esophageal dilator or gastroscope must be withdrawn at this point to permit adequate retraction of the esophagus. Small blood vessels and adhesions should be dissected free and controlled with clips or with the judicious use of electrocautery. The surgeon should try to limit the amount and frequency of irrigation when dissecting around the esophageal hiatus. As is the case with open sur-

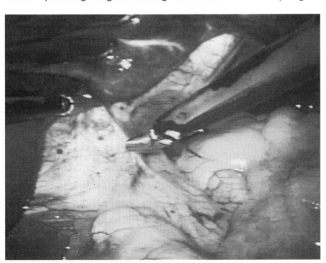

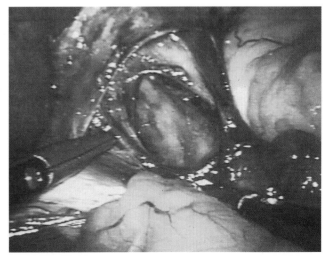

Figs. 8 A, B. Opening of phreno-esophageal ligament directly over top of the distal esophagus. **A.** initial incision. **B.** completed incision

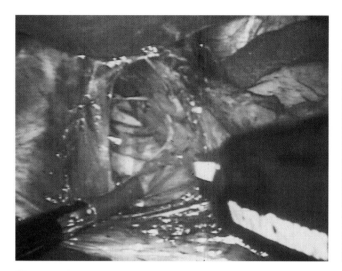

Fig. 10. Continued dissection around the gastroesophageal junction will identify the right crus of the diaphragm and the esophageal wall

gery, irrigation fluid tends to "pool" around the distal esophagus, thereby obscuring the operative exposure in this region.

The posterior trunk of the vagus nerve is usually found along the right posterior aspect of the esophagus. Further anterior and left-lateral retraction of the distal esophagus will help to visualize the posterior aspect of the esophagus. Continued dissection in this area will lead to identification of the main posterior vagal trunk (Fig. 11). When performing a truncal vagotomy, the posterior vagus is usually quite prominent and can be easily ligated between clips and divided (Fig. 12). An extensive skeletonization of the distal esophagus should be performed, with dissection of the posterior trunk away from the esophagus for a distance of at least 6–7 cm (Fig. 13). This should be performed regardless of the type of vagotomy (truncal or highly selective) to be performed. This will help identify secondary or "criminal" branches of the vagus nerve, thereby increasing the effectiveness of the operative procedure. When performing a truncal vagotomy, it is important to identify and transect this nerve as high as possible within the dia-

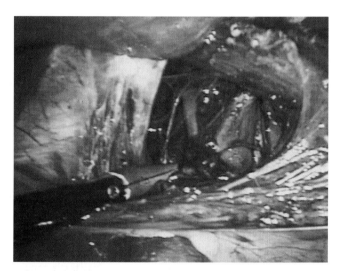

Fig. 12. Once identified, the vagal trunk is dissected free from the esophagus and ligated with clips

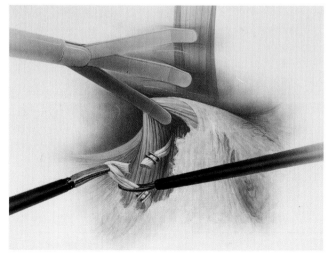

Fig. 13. Intraoperative view showing completed dissection of the distal esophagus from a distance of 5-7 cm

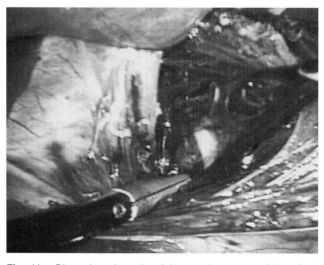

Fig. 11. Dissection along the right-posterior aspect of the distal esophagus will routinely identify the right vagus nerve

Fig. 14. Once ligated, a segment of the posterior nerve should be excised and sent for histologic confirmation

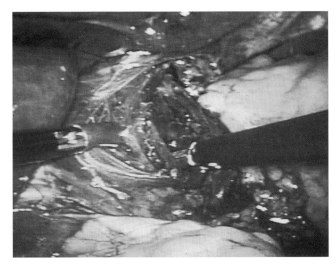

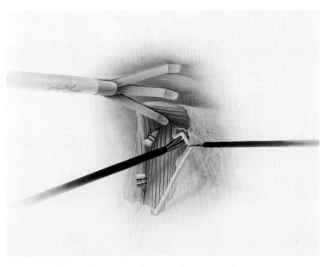

Fig. 15. The anterior nerve is identified as it courses along the antero-lateral wall of the distal esophagus. The anterior trunk is located just at the tip of the dissector on the right side of the image

Fig. 17. Dissection of anterior vagal nerve trunk to begin anterior highly selective vagotomy

phragmatic hiatus. This will also help to assure that a complete vagotomy is obtained. A short segment of the transected nerve should be excised and sent for histologic confirmation (Fig. 14). If a highly selective vagotomy is to be performed, the operator should next turn his attention to dissection of the anterior nerve (see below). The operative field, especially the posterior aspect of the distal esophagus is carefully inspected to confirm completeness of vagotomy and adequate hemostasis.

Dissection of the Anterior Vagus Nerve

Following complete dissection of the posterior vagal trunk, the surgeon must next identify the anterior vagus nerve. This may have already been accomplished during the initial, anterior dissection of the distal esophagus. If not, the opening in the phreno-esophageal membrane is carefully extended towards the patient's left side using both sharp and blunt dissection. This dissection should be continued until the left crus of the

diaphragm and the Angle of His has been completely identified. Care must be taken during this portion of the operation to avoid inadvertent injury to the spleen and/or short gastric vessels. The management of capsular tears to the spleen is much more difficult under laparoscopic guidance and has a high probability of leading to conversion.

The anterior vagus nerve is usually smaller than the posterior trunk and care must be taken to avoid inadvertent injury. The anterior vagus is usually found within the fatty connective tissue overlying the anterior aspect of the distal esophagus, towards the patient's left side (Fig. 15). However, it is not unusual for the nerve trunk to be closely adherent to the superficial muscle fibers of the esophageal wall, thereby making its identification difficult. The anterior nerve trunk may also be found along the left postero-lateral aspect of the distal esophagus. Once identified above the gastroesophageal junction, the anterior nerve may be either ligated (Fig. 16) to complete the bilateral truncal vagotomy or, if a highly selective vagotomy is to be performed, it should be carefully dissected away

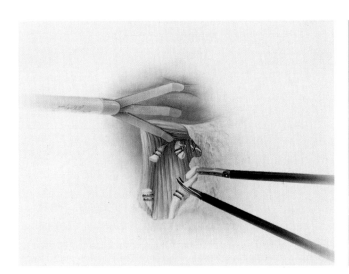

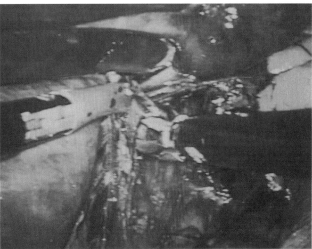

Fig. 16. Ligation of anterior vagal nerve to complete a bilateral truncal vagotomy

Fig. 18. The anterior nerve is dissected free from the esophageal wall and mobilized toward the right side of the esophagus

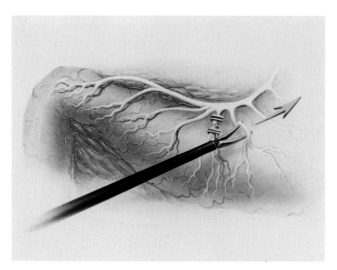

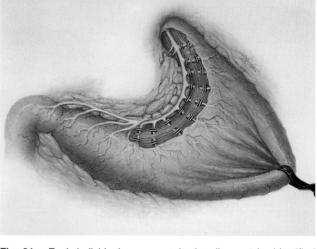

Fig. 19. The anterior highly selective vagotomy is begun near the first branch of the Crow's post along the lesser curve of the stomach. Each neurovascular bundle must be carefully dissected free from the underlying stomach wall and ligated with clips

Fig. 21. Each individual neurovascular bundle must be identified and controlled with either electrocautery or surgical clips

from the esophageal wall (Fig. 17). As the dissection is carried distally, mobilization of the anterior nerve trunk should proceed in a left to right fashion, sweeping the nerve away from the lesser curvature of the stomach. The hepatic branch of the anterior vagal nerve should be identified and preserved whenever possible. This is best accomplished by beginning the operative dissection in a cephalad location, near the diaphragmatic hiatus.

Highly Selective Vagotomy

The initial dissection of the anterior vagus is perhaps the most difficult portion of the operative dissection. The anterior nerve must be gently dissected away from its normal anatomic location along the left anterior esophagus and mobilized toward the right side of the esophagus (Fig. 18). This will allow the

surgeon to continue his operative dissection down along the lesser curvature of the stomach without fear of injury to the nerve trunk. The operative dissection is usually performed with a curved dissecting forceps. Direct grasping of the nerve trunk should be avoided at all times. Branches of the anterior vagus which are identified in this region are ligated with clips and divided. Approximately 6–7 cm of intra-abdominal esophagus is eventually dissected free from its surrounding tissue to ensure that any proximal branches from the anterior vagal trunk have been identified and divided.

Once the esophageal dissection is completed, the highly selective vagotomy is continued in a caudal direction along the lesser curvature of the stomach. Initially, the anterior vessels with their accompanying nerves are identified, isolated and controlled. This may be accomplished with either clips, an ultrasonic dissecting instrument (Ultracision, Inc., Smithfield,

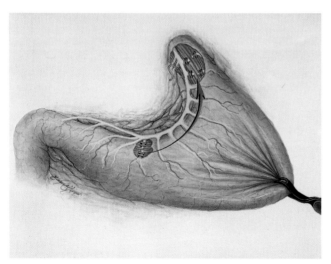

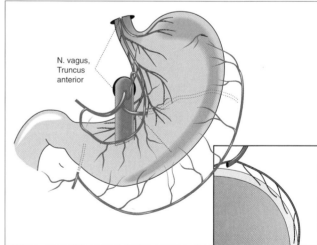

Fig. 20. The dissection along the lesser curvature is continued in a cephalad direction until the region of the previous proximal dissection is reached

Fig. 22. An extensive dissection of the anterior lesser curve must be performed to assure a complete vagotomy. The surgeon must realize that the small nerve branches enter the body of the stomach at different levels. Inset: Cross-sectional view of lesser curvature demonstrating that the small vagal fibers enter the stomach at different levels

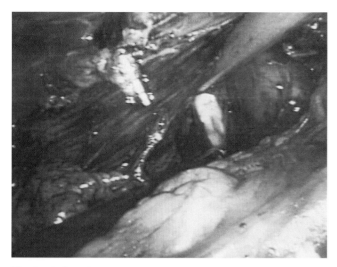
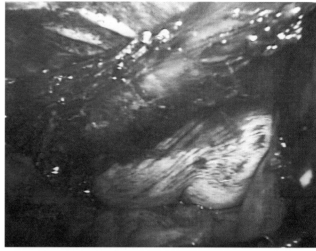

Figs. 23 A, B.   The posterior dissection is continued until the posterior peritoneal attachments are divided and the lesser sac is entered. **A.** Initial opening into lesser sac. **B.** complete view of lesser sac and posterior wall of stomach

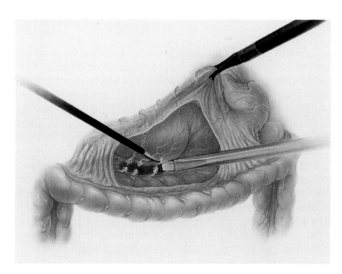

Fig. 24.   Retrogastric approach to stomach through gastro-colic omentum

RI), or electrocautery, depending on their size. The dissection is continued caudally, toward the antrum, until the mid-portion of the greater curvature is reached. The dissection should be stopped at this junction and attention turned toward the antrum and pylorus.

The pylorus is identified by both visual inspection and by palpation with the tip of the dissecting instrument. A distance of 6 cm is measured proximal to the pyloric sphincter complex. The "Crow's foot" branches of the Nerve of Latarjet are visually identified in this region. The most proximal 1–2 branches of the Crow's foot are identified and the operative dissection is restarted at this location. These first branches of the Crow's foot, along with their accompanying blood vessels, are dissected away from the underlying gastric wall, ligated with clips, and then divided with scissors (Fig. 19). The operative dissection then continues along the lesser curvature in a cephalad manner, away from the Crow's foot, until the previous area of dissection has been reached (Fig. 20). If only an anterior highly selective vagotomy is to be performed (i.e., a posterior truncal vagotomy has been accomplished), then the

operative dissection is stopped (Fig. 21). Prior to termination of the operation, the surgeon must assure that a complete and thorough vagotomy of the anterior aspect of the stomach has been achieved. It is somewhat difficult, however, to determine precisely when this goal has been accomplished. The small branches of the vagal nerves entering the lesser curve of the stomach do not enter in a discrete layer, but rather at multiple levels and locations (Fig. 22). The surgeon must completely dissect around the anterior portion of the lesser curve, toward the posterior leaflet, to assure that an adequate anterior vagotomy has been performed. This extended dissection led us to recognize that it is not substantially more demanding, from a technical standpoint, to perform a standard (anterior and posterior) highly selective vagotomy under laparoscopic guidance.

If a standard highly selective vagotomy is to be performed, then the dissection along the lesser curvature is continued in a more posterior direction, around the stomach. This dissection is continued until the posterior peritoneal attachments are divided and the lesser sac is entered (Figs. 23A and 23B). This signifies that the operative dissection has been completed in this area. This dissection is continued along the entire length of the lesser curvature until all of the posterior attachments are divided. The dissection should also be continued up to and toward the cardia of the stomach, with identification and division of the attachments in this region. Usually, the completed dissection during a highly selective vagotomy can be accomplished entirely from an anterior approach along the lesser curvature of the stomach. However, if there is concern as to the completeness of vagotomy, the posterior aspect of the stomach can also be exposed by making an opening through the gastro-colic omentum (Fig. 24). Additional dissection of the epiploic vessels is at the discretion of the surgeon but should be considered.

Having completed the highly selective vagotomy, the operative field is copiously irrigated with saline and carefully inspected to ensure adequate hemostasis. The stomach wall along the lesser curve and the distal esophagus should be inspected for signs of ischemia or perforation. Care must be taken not to accidently dislodge any of the previously placed clips during this final inspection process.

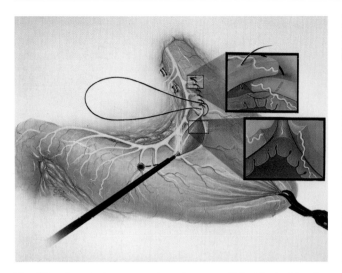

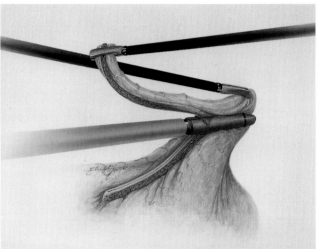

Fig. 25. An anterior seromyotomy is accomplished by incising the gastric wall along the lesser curve, approximately 1.5 cm away from the anterior vagal trunk. The incision is carried down to the level of the gastric mucosa, thereby interrupting the small vagal fibers to the anterior portion of the stomach

Fig. 27. Sequential firing of the stapler along the lesser curve of the stomach is performed in a cephalad direction. Care must be taken to avoid injury to the main trunk of the anterior vagus nerve

Miscellaneous Operative Techniques

Most of the laparoscopic procedures share many technical aspects and some of these key features have already been discussed. Nonetheless, all laparoscopic anti-ulcer procedures will have their own specific considerations, some of which are discussed below.

Posterior Truncal Vagotomy and Anterior Seromyotomy

An operation to treat patients with intractable ulcer disease which has been popular in Europe for the past two decades is a posterior truncal vagotomy combined with anterior seromyotomy [36, 46, 47, 49]. This procedure has been popularized by the work of Taylor and colleagues from the United Kingdom. The small gastric branches of the anterior vagus nerve course obliquely through the seromuscular layer of the stom-

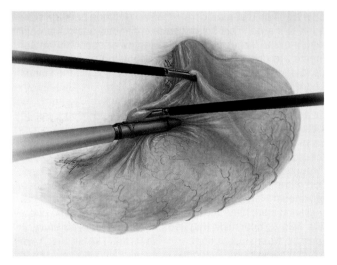

Fig. 26. An anterior linear gastrectomy may be performed to achieve a highly selective vagotomy of the anterior stomach. A 3 cm laparoscopic stapling device is used to perform this technique

ach before reaching the acid secreting mucosal layer. Dividing the seromuscular layer interrupts these small branches, thereby accomplishing a highly selective vagotomy of the anterior aspect of the stomach (Fig. 25 – lower inset). Ongoing clinical investigation by Taylor and others have shown that posterior truncal vagotomy and anterior seromyotomy does not significantly alter gastric motility or emptying and therefore a gastric emptying procedure is not necessary [48].

The seromyotomy may be performed using either an electrocautery (hook-spatula) probe, LASER, ultrasonic dissection, or sharp dissection with scissors. Care must be taken not to penetrate the mucosa or to cause extensive thermal damage with the electrocautery or laser modalities. It appears that small perforations of the mucosa are not uncommon following this technique but they can be easily repaired under laparoscopic guidance. To avoid a "missed" perforation, the seromyotomy is completed by adding a running, "overlapping" suture which approximates the cut edges of the gastric muscular layer (Fig. 25, top inset). This will adequately seal any small, "missed" gastric perforations. The important factor is to assure that such perforations do not go unrecognized at the time of surgery. The stomach should be distended with a methylene blue/saline solution at the end of the case, to exclude the presence of a gastric leak.

Posterior Truncal Vagotomy and Anterior Linear Gastrectomy

Recently a group of surgeons in Mobile, Alabama have developed a modification of the anterior seromyotomy which utilizes a laparoscopic stapling instrument [15]. In this procedure, Hannon and colleagues perform a posterior truncal vagotomy but complete an anterior highly selective denervation by dividing the fundic branches of the anterior vagus nerve with a' laparoscopic stapling device.

Following ligation and division of the posterior vagus nerve the remainder of the distal esophagus is carefully dissected to assure completeness of vagotomy. The course of the anterior vagus is then identified in order to avoid subsequent injury with the stapler. A stapled division (and simultaneous reanas-

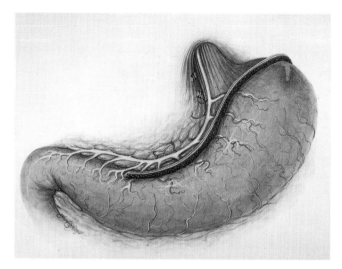

Fig. 28. The final result is a completed full-thickness excision of the anterior surface of the stomach along the lesser curvature

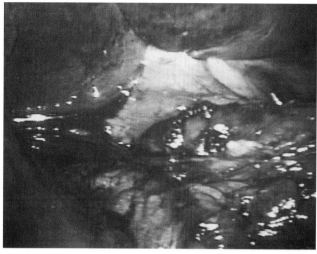

Fig. 29. Operative view of a completed laparoscopic pyloromyotomy. Note the presence of the "bulging" mucosa in the pyloric region

tomosis) of the anterior wall of the stomach is then accomplished by firing of a 3 cm laparoscopic GIA (Fig. 26). A long strip of gastric wall, approximately 1.5 cm from the lesser curvature, is then divided with serial applications of the laparoscopic GIA in a cephalad manner (Fig. 27). The resulting staple line extends from the proximal antrum in a cephalad direction to the gastric cardia and then continues over the top of the cardia, onto the posterior aspect of the stomach (Fig. 28).

Although clinical experience with this technique is extremely limited, early results have been encouraging. The use of the laparoscopic GIA allows the procedure to be completed in far less time then previously described methods and the stapled anastomosis appears to eliminate the risk of unrecognized gastric perforation. This technique, however, may have several disadvantages. It creates a gastric staple line (or anastomosis) which is subject to all of the recognized risks of any intestinal anastomosis. Bleeding, dehiscence, or ischemic necrosis may develop following any such procedure. Furthermore, the effects of this type of transection of the stomach wall on gastric motility are not yet clearly defined. From a technique standpoint, it must also be noticed that safe and correct placement of the staples may be difficult, especially in the obese patient. In fact, it may be difficult to place the staples close enough to assure a complete anterior vagotomy without injuring the anterior trunk.

Table 4. Endoscopic procedures for the management of intractable ulcer disease

Standard Procedures
Highly selective vagotomy
Bilateral truncal vagotomy and Drainage (pyloroplasty, pyloromyotomy, or gastrojejunostomy)
Bilateral truncal vagotomy and Resection (Billroth I or II)

Modifications
Posterior truncal vagotomy and anterior highly selective vagotomy
Posterior truncal vagotomy and anterior seromyotomy
Posterior truncal vagotomy and anterior linear gastrectomy
Bilateral truncal vagotomy and endoscopic pyloric dilation
Thoracoscopic truncal vagotomy and endoscopic pyloric dilation

Drainage Procedures

A drainage procedure is recommended when performing a bilateral truncal vagotomy or, in some cases, when performing a highly selective vagotomy. The same considerations for performing a drainage procedure during open surgery should be used to determine when one is required during a laparoscopic vagotomy. A large variety of techniques are available to accomplish effective gastric drainage (Table 4).

n general, the surgeon should perform the same operation that he would attempt during open surgery. A sutured pyloroplasty is perhaps the most commonly performed technique and can be readily accomplished under laparoscopic guidance. The performance of a pyloromyotomy has proven to be difficult from a technical standpoint, mostly due to a lack of direct tactile sensation. A properly created pyloromyotomy requires division of the sphincter muscles without entering the duodenal or gastric lumen (Fig. 29). This requires very precise control of the depth of the myotomy incision which is extremely difficult to obtain under laparoscopic guidance. In addition, the surgeon needs to make sure that a complete division of the pyloric sphincter complex has been achieved. This also requires a substantial degree of tactile sensation which is diminished during laparoscopy. In cases where a pyloromyotomy is attempted, experience has shown that it is not unexpected to enter the lumen of the duodenum, thereby necessitating the performance of a formal pyloroplasty. The use of the ultra-sonic tissue dissector has proven useful in this situation. If the surgeon is not comfortable with the performance of a hand-sewn pyloroplasty under laparoscopic guidance then a laparoscopic pyloromyotomy should not be attempted.

The use of "traction and counter-traction" is required to maintain proper tension on the pylorus and duodenum while performing a pyloroplasty. It may be necessary to insert an additional trocar if adequate exposure cannot be maintained with the existing ports (Fig. 3). A standard Heineke-Mikulicz pyloroplasty is then begun by making a longitudinal incision across the pylorus. The incision should extend from a point 2 cm proximal to the pylorus and continue onto the duodenum for another 1–2 cm. Laparoscopic Metzenbaum scissors (with attached electrocautery) should be used to make this incision.

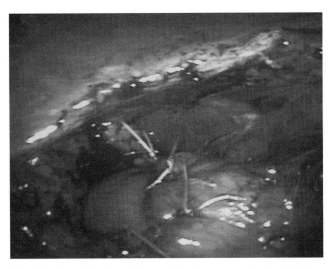

Fig. 30. Operative view of a completed laparoscopic pyloroplasty

As with open surgery, care should be taken to avoid injury to the posterior wall of the stomach or duodenum. The pyloroplasty is then fashioned by closing this incision in a horizontal fashion using 5 or 6 interrupted sutures of 0 or 2-0 nonabsorbable material (Fig. 30). The surgeon must be extremely facile with laparoscopic suturing techniques before attempting a hand-sewn closure of a pyloroplasty incision under laparoscopic guidance. A nasogastric tube can be passed under direct vision and manipulated with graspers either through or just proximal to the suture line.

Other more complex procedures, such as antrectomy, are performed on a less frequent basis than a standard pyloroplasty [13]. Although these more complex procedures are being increasingly reported in the literature, the equipment, instrumentation, and technical skill required to safely perform such techniques is not readily available at all centers. However, there can be little doubt that as our laparoscopic experience continues to grow during the next five years, that these procedures will become more commonplace.

Postoperative Care

The laparoscopic instruments, liver retractor and cannulas are removed and the carbon dioxide is evacuated from the abdomen. An attempt is made to close all of the fascial defects with an interrupted suture of 0-vicryl. The skin edges are reapproximated with skin staples or subcuticular sutures and sterile dressings are applied.

The urinary catheter is usually removed in the recovery room and the nasogastric tube is placed on low, intermittent suction for 6–12 hours. The tube may be removed the night of surgery (or the following morning if the operation was finished late in the day). Most patients are able to tolerate a liquid diet the morning after surgery which may then be advanced as tolerated. The patient may be discharged in the afternoon on the first postoperative day or in the morning of the second postoperative day. Patients are continued on a mild acid-reducing regimen (ranitidine) as well as a promotility agent (metoclop-ramide or cisapride) for 1–2 weeks after surgery. Most patients are able to return to normal activity within 7–10 days. Repeat endoscopy, pH testing, and gastric empty-ing studies are performed between 1 and 3 months after surgery.

Complications

Complications from laparoscopic anti-ulcer procedures are to be expected, just as they would with any surgical operation, regardless of whether it is performed open or under laparoscopic guidance.

Role of Proper Patient Selection

Laparoscopic (or thoracoscopic) management of peptic ulcer disease is usually indicated for those individuals who have failed medical management or require indefinite drug therapy to control their symptoms. A surgeon with limited laparoscopic experience should try to avoid complex clinical situation such as patients presenting with acute bleeding, gastric outlet obstruction, or duodenal perforation. Unfortunately, most patients requiring surgery today usually present with one of these urgent conditions. Although a few isolated case reports have appeared in the literature, experience with these difficult cases still remains limited. Perhaps, in the near future and with further refinement of surgical techniques and instrumentation, such conditions may be routinely managed via a minimally invasive approach.

Other contraindications to the performance of a laparoscopic vagotomy include extensive prior upper abdominal surgery, obesity, and bleeding disorders. For patients with chronic peptic ulcer disease who have undergone a previous abdominal procedure for a perforated ulcer or intractable ulcer diastasis, a thoracoscopic vagotomy should be considered. This will allow the surgeon to provide definitive treatment without incurring the risks and difficulties associated with re-operative upper abdominal surgery.

Morbidly obese patients also pose a challenge to the surgeon from several standpoints. First, "correct" trocar placement is essential in order to minimize the deleterious effects of a thick abdominal wall which can severely limit the mobility of the laparoscopic instruments. Additionally, substantial amounts of intraabdominal fat around the gastroesophageal junction will make the operative dissection extremely difficult. Even minor bleeding during this dissection can very quickly obscure the operative field, making progress slow and frustrating. The surgeon must proceed diligently and make frequent adjustments of the liver and gastric retractors to maintain adequate exposure in these difficult cases.

Preoperative Evaluation

A thorough preoperative evaluation is perhaps one of the most important means to avoid many of the peri-operative complications that may develop in patients undergoing surgery for peptic ulcer disease. The surgeon should not "cut corners" in the standard pre-operative evaluation just because the procedure is to be performed under laparoscopic guidance. Unfortunately, such poorly conceived preoperative planning has led to undesirable outcomes for many patients.

Anesthetic Considerations

The surgeon and anesthesiologist should be aware of all of the potential risks associated with laparoscopic surgery, especially as they pertain to the presence of pneumoperitoneum and other unique aspects of laparoscopic surgery. During the performance of most laparoscopic anti-ulcer procedures, a thorough dissection of the gastroesophageal junction must be completed in order to assure a complete vagotomy. As such, the surgeon must complete a thorough dissection across the diaphragmatic hiatus, into the mediastinum. This dissection creates the possibility of inadvertent entrance into the pleura, usually on the left side. This may lead to the rapid development of a tension pneumothorax as a result of the positive pressure intraabdominal CO_2 insufflation. Fortunately, this situation has not been observed clinically on a regular basis, even if the pleura is opened. In fact, centers reporting on their large experience (> 350 cases) with laparoscopic anti-reflux procedures have observed a very low incidence of peri-operative pneumothoraces.

The most plausible physiologic explanation for this phenomena is that the intrathoracic pressure created by positive-pressure, mechanical ventilation is higher than the intra-abdominal pressure created by the CO_2 pneumoperitoneum. This finding is not unexpected, as normal airway pressures often are in the range of 20–25 mmHg, somewhat higher than the usual 10–12 mmHg achieved with standard CO_2 pneumoperitoneum. Even if the pleura is violated during dissection of the hiatus, it is not always necessary to insert a chest tube. Once the procedure is completed, the pneumoperitoneum can be completely evacuated and several forceful, manual breaths can be delivered by the anesthesiologist to clear any remaining CO_2 from the pleural cavity. As long as an airway leak is not present, a postoperative pneumothorax should not develop. This can be confirmed by a post-operative chest x-ray which can be obtained prior to extubation, if so desired. Aside from the above description, other complications such as subcutaneous emphysema or gas embolism may develop during laparoscopic vagotomy that will require expertise on the part of the anesthesiologist.

Equipment and Instrumentation

A tapered, as opposed to a blunt-"tipped" esophageal dilator should be employed when intubating the esophagus (Fig. 31). A blunt tip dilator may tend to get "hung-up" at the gastroesophageal junction, especially if significant distortion of the distal esophagus is present. A tapered tip will allow the dilator to slip easily into the stomach and should help minimize the risk of esophageal or gastric perforation.

The surgeon should also be familiar with all of the new and innovative instruments being designed for abdominal laparoscopic procedures. Atraumatic liver retractors, grasping forceps, powerful suction/irrigation devices are just a few of a vast array of the innovative instruments recently available to the laparoscopic surgeon.

Bleeding Considerations

Intraoperative hemorrhage during laparoscopic vagotomy usually occurs from one of two sources; from the left lobe of the liver during its retraction or during dissection of the esoph-

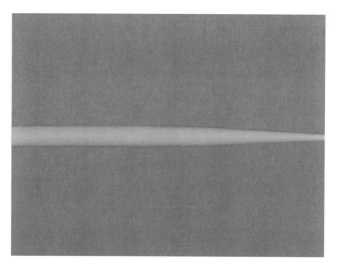

Fig. 31. A tapered esophageal dilator should be used when intubating the esophagus and stomach. The tapered tip will help to guide it across the gastroesophageal junction into the stomach

agus and stomach. Major hemorrhage from the vena cava, aorta, or major branches of the celiac axis is extremely unusual. Similarly, trocar injury to the epigastric artery is unusual during upper abdominal procedures. However, if such an injury does occur, it should be managed by one of several available techniques, including suture ligation performed either open or under laparoscopic guidance.

Hepatic Bleeding

In order to provide adequate visualization of the distal esophagus and stomach, the left lobe of the liver must be retracted in a cephalad and right-lateral direction. Injury to the liver is most likely to occur during insertion and positioning of the retractor. An atraumatic "fan-like" retractor appears to be best suited to avoid this complication. Nonetheless, small lacerations and hematomas do occur during routine retraction of the liver. Fortunately, bleeding that does occur is usually minimal and self-limiting. Conversion to laparotomy to control such bleeding is usually unwarranted. The most disadvantageous result from such an injury is that blood will tend to "pool" in the exact area of the operative dissection. This will severely hamper visualization and frustrate the operating surgeon during dissection in this area.

The surgeon must also be aware that the liver is also at risk for injury when introducing instruments through the centrally located operating ports. As our overall experience with laparoscopic surgery has increased, surgeons have developed the skill to insert and withdraw instruments into the abdomen without having to watch their entire path of entry. Unfortunately, the retracted surface of the left lobe of the liver is usually in close approximation to the tip of the operating sheaths. Therefore, the surgeon should always pay close attention while introducing any instruments through these ports. If any resistance is met during the insertion of an instrument, the surgeon should not attempt to force the instrument in through the trocar. Rather, the surgeon should retract the laparoscope and attempt to view the end of the operating sheath as the instrument enters the abdomen. This should help prevent "spearing" of the liver with one of the operating instruments.

Dissection of the Esophagus

Bleeding may also occur during the operative dissection of the stomach and esophagus. Caudal retraction of the stomach should be maintained at all times. A two-handed operative technique should be used to perform all tissue dissection. This will allow the surgeon to provide precise traction and counter-traction at the site of operation. The dissection should also be carried out in a gentle and meticulous manner. The numerous small blood vessels along the lesser curve and around the distal esophagus can be easily torn during blunt dissection. Gentle, repetitive spreading with a laparoscopic dissector will allow for safe identification of each individual vessel. Once identified, small vessels can usually be controlled with electrocautery alone. Larger vessels may require the placement of clips or a suture ligature. Fortunately, if bleeding does occur from one of these small vessels, it is usually self-limiting. Patience on the part of the surgeon is the best policy in the event of minor bleeding. Gentle irrigation and the avoidance of "blind" clipping into a "puddle" of blood should yield superior results.

Visceral Injury

Gastric and Esophageal Injury
The surgeon must also be constantly aware of the risk of visceral injury during laparoscopic vagotomy. Perforation of the stomach or esophagus may occur as a result of passage of a large dilator or secondary to direct operative trauma from the dissecting or retracting instruments. Passage of an esophageal dilator is usually performed for the sole purpose of guiding the surgeon's initial dissection around the gastroesophageal junction. As each surgeon's experience increases, the need for placing such a tube decreases and should be avoided whenever possible. Direct operative injury can be avoided by using only atraumatic grasping forceps to retract the stomach or esophagus. Laparoscopic Babcock forceps were initially designed in the exact same fashion as "open" Babcock forceps. These were found to be extremely traumatic and have resulted in gastric and esophageal tears. Newly modified Babcock clamps with "paddle"-shaped tips seem to provide stable retraction without causing trauma to the gastric or esophageal wall (Fig. 32). Injury to the esophagus or stomach may also occur from excessive use of electrocautery during dissection and can result in a thermal injury. Direct injury may also occur from the dissecting instruments themselves if the plane of dissection becomes obscured.

Vagal Nerve Injury
Injury to the vagal nerves is best avoided by definitive identification of the main nerve trunk early in the operative dissection. The posterior trunk of the vagus nerve is usually found along the right posterior aspect of the esophagus. It may be necessary to elevate the distal esophagus anteriorly and rotate it to the patient's left side in order to visualize the main trunk. If an esophageal dilator or gastroscope has been previously placed, it must be withdrawn into the mid-to-upper esophagus, away from the gastroesophageal junction, to permit adequate retraction of the esophagus. The posterior trunk should be gently dissected away from the posterior wall of the esophagus. The anterior vagal trunk usually travels along the left anterior aspect of the distal esophagus until it crosses the

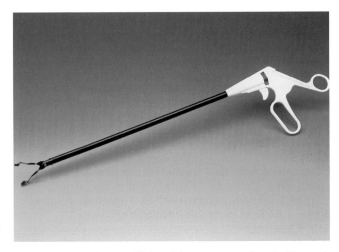

Fig. 32. Newly designed Babcock forceps are equipped with a paddle-shaped tip which allows for safe, atraumatic retraction of the stomach or esophagus

gastro-esophageal junction towards the right side of the patient. The nerve then travels caudally along the lesser curvatures of the stomach. Direct grasping of the vagal nerve trunks should be avoided at all times unless a bilateral or a posterior truncal vagotomy is to be performed. Similarly, the surgeon should not use energy modalities such as electrocautery or laser in close proximity to the main vagal nerves. If direct retraction of a vagal trunk is required it should be done with a blunt probe or an atraumatic curved laparoscopic retracting instrument.

Splenic Injury
The surgeon must also be aware that any complication that can occur during an open vagotomy procedure such as an injury to the spleen can also develop during the performance of its laparoscopic counterpart. Complications such as recurrent ulceration, gastric ischemia, inadequate drainage, incomplete vagotomy, or delayed gastric emptying are always possible. Whether or not the incidence of such complications is less, more or the same as following open surgery has not yet been elucidated. Initial reports, however, do not demonstrate an unusual rate of any specific complications.

Current Results

Published reports on the laparoscopic treatment of peptic ulcer disease remain extremely limited. To date, limited retrospective studies involving small numbers of patients or isolated case reports comprise the majority of the published clinical reports on laparoscopic vagotomy [2–5, 12, 14, 15, 22, 24–28, 30, 33–35, 42]. In fact, a large proportion of the published literature on these techniques involves animal studies [21, 40, 41, 38, 50]. Unfortunately, the decreasing incidence of patients requiring elective surgery for peptic ulcer disease has limited the performance of prospective, randomized trials evaluating the effectiveness of laparoscopic anti-ulcer procedures.

Amongst the options available to the surgeon, bilateral truncal vagotomy with and without drainage, highly selective vagotomy, and several modifications of these standard procedures (Table 4) have been described in the surgical literature.

Dr. François Dubois in France has presented results from bilateral truncal vagotomy in over 20 patients [10]. This procedure has been associated with effective control of ulcer disease and surprisingly, the incidence of delayed gastric emptying is only 10 % in his experience. Based on this information. Dr. Dubois does not advocate the routine performance of a drainage procedure at the time of truncal vagotomy. He recommends close clinical observation during the post-operative period and performs endoscopic balloon dilation of the pylorus for those patients who develop evidence of gastric outlet obstruction.

The posterior truncal vagotomy/anterior seromyotomy technique is an accepted "open" procedure in Europe [36, 46, 47, 49]. It was quite logical, therefore, for surgeons in Europe to adapt the open seromyotomy procedure to a laparoscopic approach. The largest published experience appears to be that from the University of Nice and their initial results are encouraging [22, 32, 33].

Drs. Mouiel and Katkhouda have reported on 36 patients with peptic ulcer disease treated by laparoscopic surgery. Thirty-four underwent posterior truncal vagotomy plus anterior seromyotomy and two patients underwent bilateral truncal vagotomy with endoscopic balloon dilation of the pylorus. The average operative time was 90 minutes and the average hospital stay was 3–5 days. (One must recognize that the need for early discharge does not exist in Europe as it does in the United States). Post-operative endoscopic evaluation revealed healing of the ulcers in 33 of 36 patients. They also demonstrated a 78/83 % decrease in BAO/MAO, respectively. Two patients manifested evidence of delayed gastric emptying secondary to bezoars and one patient was re-operated for severe, intractable gastroesophageal reflux disease. Otherwise, overall patient outcome was excellent and without evidence of ulcer recurrence during follow-up.

Laws and McKernan have reported on 17 patients who underwent surgery for peptic ulcer disease, either alone or in combination with surgery for gastroesophageal reflux disease [26]. Eight patients had a posterior truncal vagotomy combined with a highly selective vagotomy and eight patients had a standard highly selective vagotomy. One patient had an omentopexy for perforated ulcer disease. Patients were discharged from the hospital between 1–5 days and major complications were seen in four patients, and included temporary fluid overload. Other post-operative complications included marginal ulceration and dysphagia in two patients following Nissen fundoplication.

Kum and Goh reported on 12 patients who underwent various anti-ulcer procedures including: posterior truncal vagotomy plus anterior highly selective vagotomy – 6 patients; bilateral truncal vagotomy with endoscopic dilation – 3 patients; posterior truncal vagotomy plus anterior seromyotomy – 2 patients; and bilateral truncal vagotomy with gastrojejunostomy – 1 patient [25]. The average operating time was 150 minutes and they documented substantial post-operative decreases in BAO (14.6 to 4.1 mmole/L) and MAO (47.4 to 16.5 mmole/L). Patients were discharged on post-operative day four. One patient presented with post-operative evidence of delayed gastric emptying. Otherwise, their early experience was encouraging and without major complications.

Hannon and colleagues have described their experience with posterior truncal vagotomy plus anterior linear gastrectomy in two patients [15]. Their ongoing experience in more than 10 patients has also been encouraging.

The surgical literature also includes numerous case reports describing other anti-ulcer procedures such as vagotomy and antrectomy, posterior truncal vagotomy plus anterior highly selective vagotomy, posterior truncal vagotomy plus anterior seromyotomy, highly selective vagotomy, pyloroplasty, and thoracoscopic vagotomy [2–5, 12–15, 22, 24–28, 30, 33–35, 42]. The initial experience in all of these areas appears to be promising.

Discussion

The overwhelming success of laparoscopic biliary tract surgery has encouraged many surgeons to investigate a laparoscopic approach for the treatment of peptic ulcer disease.

The choice of the operative approach and the indications for surgery, however remain controversial. Already, all of the procedures previously available for open surgery have been successfully completed under laparoscopic guidance. Early laparoscopic clinical trials were directed at the use of modified selective procedures to manage patients with intractable peptic ulcer disease. As the overall laparoscopic experience of general surgery has increased, so has the ability to perform more complex and sophisticated operative procedures. Currently, it is feasible for a surgeon to perform anyone of several anti-ulcer procedures, including a highly selective vagotomy, truncal vagotomy with drainage or, if necessary, a gastric resection.

Although a bilateral truncal vagotomy may be easily accomplished under laparoscopic guidance, the need for a drainage procedure will result in a significant incidence of postvagotomy diarrhea and dumping. This has led many surgeons to explore other surgical options. Except for a few European centers, clinical experience with the performance of a posterior truncal vagotomy with an anterior seromyotomy for the "open" treatment of peptic ulcer disease is not widespread. Surgeons in the United States, therefore, initially favored performance of a laparoscopic posterior truncal vagotomy with an anterior highly selective vagotomy. The anterior vagotomy is accomplished by individual ligation of the neurovascular bundles along the lesser curvature of the stomach. This is similar to the technique employed during open highly selective vagotomy [16]. Although clinical experience with posterior truncal vagotomy/anterior highly selective vagotomy performed via a laparotomy is limited, on a theoretical basis it should provide similar results to the seromyotomy technique. Both procedures involve a posterior vagotomy (which may be confirmed by histologic examination) and an anterior highly selective denervation of the stomach. Experience with conventional highly selective vagotomy is extensive and widespread [9, 17–19, 29]. Modifying a conventional highly selective vagotomy to include a posterior truncal vagotomy should, if anything, improve the acid-reducing potential of the procedure. Unfortunately, definitive data in support of this theory is lacking and, given the decreasing incidence of surgery for peptic ulcer disease, it is unlikely that such evidence will be forthcoming in the near future.

As laparoscopic skills and technology has increased so has the complexity of the operative procedures. The performance of an extensive dissection along the lesser curvature of the anterior stomach wall has led to the recognition that a standard (anterior and posterior) highly selective vagotomy could be reliably accomplished. Currently, this is our preferred procedure for the elective surgical management of chronic peptic ulcer disease. On occasion, there will be certain clinical circumstances such as severe gastric outlet obstruction that will require a truncal vagotomy with drainage or gastric resection. However, given their inherent postoperative disadvantages, such procedures are being performed less frequently.

The recent data surrounding Helicobacter pylori have also had an enormous impact on the current medical management of peptic ulcer disease. This has certainly affected the rate at which patients have been referred for surgical treatment. In fact, whether or not vagotomy should be performed anymore is being extensively debated [23, 31, 37]. The recent decrease in the prevalence of peptic ulcer disease, combined with the vast improvements in medical therapy, will have other significant implications for the future of minimally invasive surgery for peptic ulcer disease. It will be much more difficult for surgeons to overcome the learning curve if patients presenting for surgery are encountered on an increasingly infrequent basis. Despite the initial enthusiasm for such minimally invasive procedures, patient referrals for laparoscopic vagotomy are becoming more and more uncommon. This will result in a much slower rate of adoption for laparoscopic anti-ulcer procedures as compared to other more commonly performed procedures such as laparoscopic cholecystectomy or Nissen fundoplication.

Despite the lack of prospective data, it has not been difficult for surgeons to recognize the potential advantages of a minimally invasive approach to the treatment of peptic ulcer disease. This type of approach has allowed patients to return home within 24–48 hours and resume normal activities within 7–10 days. If it can be shown that effective, long-term control of acid secretion can also be achieved in these patients, then a minimally invasive approach to peptic ulcer disease might become a more attractive alternative to life-long medical therapy [3 ,6, 7, 45]. Certainly, from the standpoint of long-term health care costs, this would seem logical.

Regardless of each surgeon's preference, the preliminary reports on these techniques have been encouraging and in the near future a minimally invasive approach may become the preferred modality to manage, at the very least, the few remaining patients requiring surgery for peptic ulcer disease.

References

1. ALEXANDER-WILLIAMS J: A requiem for vagotomy [editorial] [see comments]. Br Med J 302 (6776) (1991) 547–548.
2. AXFORD TC, CLAIR DG, BERTAGNOLLI MM, ET AL.: Staged antectomy and thoracoscopic truncal vagotomy for perforated peptic ulcer disease. Ann Thorac Surg 55 (1993) 1571–1573.
3. BAILEY RW, FLOWERS JL, GRAHAM SM, ET AL.: Combined laparoscopic cholecystectomy and selective vagotomy. Surg Laparosc Endosc 1 (1991) 45–9.
4. CHISHOLM EM, CHUNG SCS, SUNDERLAND GT, ET AL.: Thoracoscopic vagotomy: A new use for the laparoscope. Br J Surg 79 (1992) 254.
5. CORBELL JL JR, CORBELLE JL: Indication for thoracoscopic truncal vagotomy. Surg Laparosc Endosc 3 (1993) 395-7.
6. CUSCHIERI A: Laparoscopic vagotomy – gimmick or reality? Surg Clin N Amer 72 (1992) 357–367.
7. CUSCHIERI A: The spectrum of laparoscopic surgery. World J Surg 16 (1992) 1089–1097.
8. DARZI A, CAREY PD, MENZIES-GOW N, MONSON JRT: Preliminary results of laparoscopic repair of perforated duodenal ulcers. Surg Laparo Endosc Vol. 3 (3) (1993) 161–163.
9. DONAHUE PE, RICHTER NM, LIU KJ, ET AL.: Experimental basis and clinical application of extended highly selective vagotomy for duodenal ulcer. Surg Gynec Obst 176 (1) (1993) 39–48.
10. DUBOIS F: Invited Presentation. SAGES Postgraduate Course, Monterey, California (1991).
11. FALLAHZADEH H: Elective procedure for peptic ulcer: a disappearing operation. Am Surg 59 (1) (1993) 20–22.
12. FRANTZIDES CT, LUDWIG KA, QUEBBEMAN EJ, ET AL.: Laparoscopic highly selective vagotomy: Technique and case report. Surg Laparosc Endosc 2 (4) (1992) 348–352.
13. GOH P, TEKANT Y, ISAAC J, ET AL.: The technique of laparoscopic Billroth II gastrectomy. Surg Laparosc Endosc 2 (3) (1992) 258–260.
14. GOMEZ-FERRER-BAYO F: A new technique for the treatment of chronic duodenal ulcer [letter]. Int Surg 77 (4) (1992) 317.
15. HANNON JK, SNOW LL, WEINSTEIN LS: Linear gastrectomy: Endoscopic staple assisted anterior highly selective vagotomy combined with posterior truncal vagotomy for treatment of peptic ulcer disease. Surg Laparosc Endosc (in press).
16. HILL GL, BARKER CJ: Anterior highly selective vagotomy with posterior truncal vagotomy: A simple technique for denervating the parietal cell mass. Br J Surg 65 (1978) 702–705.
17. HOFFMANN J, OLESEN A, JENSEN HE: Prospective 14- to 18-year follow-up study after parietal cell vagotomy. Br J Surg 74 (11) (1987) 1056–1059.
18. JOHNSTON D: Operative mortality and postoperative morbidity of highly selective vagotomy. Br Med J 4 (1975) 545–547.
19. JOHNSTON GW, SPENCER EF, WILKINSON AJ, ET AL.: Proximal gastric vagotomy: follow-up after 10–20 years. Br J Surg 78 (1) (1991) 20–23.
20. JORDAN PH JR: Surgery for peptic ulcer disease. Curr Probl Surg 28 (1991) 265–330.
21. JOSEPHS LG, ARNOLD JH, SAWYERS JL: Laparoscopic highly selective vagotomy. J Laparosc Endosc Surg 2 (3) (1992) 151–153.
22. KATKHOUDA N, MOUIEL J: A new technique of surgical treatment of chronic duodenal ulcer with laparotomy by videocoelioscopy. Am J Surg 161 (3) (1991) 361–364.
23. KILBY JO: Laparoscopic vagotomy. Ann R Coll Surg Engl 75 (6) (1993) 448.
24. KUM CK, GOH P: Laparoscopic posterior truncal vagotomy and anterior highly selective vagotomy – a case report. Singapore Med J 33 (3) (1992) 302–303.
25. KUM CK, GOH P: Laparoscopic vagotomy: a new tool in the management of duodenal ulcer disease [letter]. Br J Surg 79 (1992) 977.
26. LAWS HL, MCKERNAN JB: Endoscopic management of peptic ulcer disease. Ann Surg 217 (5) (1993) 548–556.
27. LAWS HL, NAUGHTON MJ, MCKERNAN JB: Thoracoscopic vagectomy for recurrent peptic ulcer disease. Surg Laparosc Endosc 1 (1) (1992) 24–28.
28. LIRICI MM, BUESS G, BECKER HD: The laparoscopic approach to modified taylor's procedure in the treatment of chronic duodenal ulcer: an improved technique. Surg Laparosc Endosc 2 (3) (1992) 199–204.
29. MACINTYRE IM, MILLAR A: Highly selective vagotomy a safe operation for duodenal ulcer. Immediate and long-term complications and sequelae in 500 patients. Eur J Surg 157 (4) (1991) 261–265.
30. MCDERMOTT EWM, MURPHY JJ: Laparoscopic truncal vagotomy without drainage. Br J Surg 80 (1993) 236.
31. MOONT M: Laparoscopic vagotomy for chronic duodenal ulcer [letter; comment]. Med J Aust 156 (2) (1992) 139–140.
32. MOUIEL J, KATKHOUDA N: Laparoscopic truncal and selective vagotomy. In: Zucker KA, Bailey RW, Reddick EJ (eds): Surgical Laparoscopy. St. Louis, Quality Medical Publishing, (1991) 263–279.
33. MOUIEL J, KATKHOUDA N: Laparoscopic vagotomy for chronic duodenal ulcer disease. World J Surg 17 (1993) 34–39.
34. MOURET P, FRANCOIS Y, VIGNAL J, BARTH X, LOMBARD-PLATET R: Laparoscopic treatment of perforated peptic ulcer. Br J Surg 77 (1990) 1006.

35. Nottle PD: Laparoscopic vagotomy for chronic duodenal ulcer: Med J Austr 155 (1991) 648.
36. Oostvogel HJM, van Vroonhoven Th JMV: Anterior lesser curve serotomy with posterior truncal vagotomy versus proximal gastric vagotomy. Br J Surg 75 (2) (1988) 121–124.
37. Orr KB: Laparoscopic abdominal surgery. Reservations about the revolution. Med J Aust 155 (4) (1991) 273–274.
38. Pietrafitta JJ, Schultz LS, Graber JN, et al.: Laser laparoscopic vagotomy and pyloromyotomy: Gastrointest Endosc 37 (3) (1991) 338–343.
39. Reddick EJ: Personal Communication. (1991).
40. Schneider TA II, Wittgen CW, Andrus CH: Comparison of minimally invasive methods of parietal cell vagotomy in a porcine model. Surgery 112 (4) (1992) 649–655.
41. Shapiro S, Gordon L, Dayhkovsky L, et al.: Development of laparoscopic anterior seromyotomy and right posterior truncal vagotomy for ulcer prophylaxis. J Laparoendosc Surg 1 (5) (1991) 279–286.
42. Snyders D: Laparoscopic pyloroplasty for duodenal ulcer [letter]. Br J Surg 80 (1) (1993) 127.
43. Stabile BE: Current surgical management of duodenal ulcers. Surg Clin N Am 72 (1992) 335–356.
44. Sturdevant RAL: Epidemiology of peptic ulcer. Am J Epidemiol 104 (1976) 9–14.
45. Taylor TV, Bhandarkar DS: Laparoscopic vagotomy: An operation for the 1990s? Ann R Coll Surg Engl 75 (6) (1993): 385–386.
46. Taylor TV, Gunn AA, Macleod DAD, et al.: Anterior lesser curve seromyotomy and posterior truncal vagotomy in the treatment of chronic duodenal ulcer. Lancet 2 (1982) 846–848.
47. Taylor TV, Gunn AA, MacLeod DAD, et al.: Mortality and morbidity after anterior lesser curve seromyotomy with posterior truncal vagotomy for duodenal ulcer. Br J Surg 72 (12) (1985) 950–951.
48. Taylor TV, Holt S, Heading RC: Gastric emptying after anterior lesser curve seromyotomy and posterior truncal vagotomy. Br J Surg 72 (1985) 620–622.
49. Taylor TV, Lythgoe JP, McFarland JB, et al.: Anterior lesser curve seromyotomy and posterior truncal vagotomy versus truncal vagotomy and pyloroplasty in the treatment of chronic duodenal ulcer. Br J Surg 77 (1990) 1007–1009.
50. Voeller GR, Pridgen WL, Mangiante EC: Laparoscopic posterior truncal vagotomy and anterior seromyotomy: A porcine model. J Laparosc Surg 1 (1991) 375–378.

12. | Laparoscopic Nissen Fundoplication

J. G. Hunter and J. K. Champion

Introduction

Gastroesophageal reflux disease (GERD) with its resultant symptoms of heartburn and indigestion is a common disorder accounting for three quarters of all esophageal dysfunction [10]. In the United States alone 60 million people are affected and one third of those require medication [12]. Initial therapy has traditionally been medical and centered around lifestyle changes (diet, elevation of the head of the bed) and treatment with acid-reducing agents such as antacids, H_2 receptor antagonists, and proton pump inhibitors [13]. Open surgical correction of GERD has actually declined over the last few decades as fundoplication was maligned for reported adverse side effects and patients' refusal to accept the expense, discomfort, and prolonged recovery associated with this procedure [4]. Surgery was reserved for those patients who had failed prolonged medical therapy or developed reflux complications. Surgical outcomes were often adversely affected by periesophagitis, strictures, and esophageal shortening associated with advanced GERD. Laparoscopic Nissen fundoplication offers the opportunity for correction of the underlying anatomic and functional defect associated with GERD with lessened discomfort and hospitalization, and rapid recovery [21].

Indications and Contraindications

Laparoscopic Nissen fundoplication is indicated in those patients with documented gastroesophageal reflux whose symptoms are refractory to medical therapy or who develop a complication of reflux such as esophageal stricture, Barrett's mucosa, or recurrent aspiration (Table 1) [1]. Although there are no absolute contraindications, there are several relative contraindications to operation that merit technical considera-

tion before attempting a laparoscopic antireflux procedure (Table 2) [7]. Fundoplication in patients with previous hiatal or upper abdominal surgery may be difficult, due to scarring or adhesions. Patients with an enlarged left lobe of the liver, due to fatty infiltration, present a challenge to operative exposure. A shortened esophagus may be difficult to mobilize sufficiently to bring 2–3 cm of distal esophagus back into the abdomen. A laparoscopic Collis lengthening procedure is technically feasible and may offer promise in the future. In patients with nonspecific motility disturbances, the Toupet partial 270° fundoplication may be performed laparoscopically. Bremner et al., however, reported no increased dysphagia when they utilized a standard Nissen in this population [2]. Aperistalsis of the esophagus may be due to a number of different underlying etiologies (achalasia, scleroderma, or end-stage GERD), which would be poorly served by Nissen fundoplication [23].

The laparoscopic Nissen procedure is a technically demanding operation that requires an extensive two-handed dissection and advanced suturing skills. It should only be performed after careful preoperative evaluation by surgeons with prior experience in managing GERD who demonstrate by observation and in-depth training an expertise in this procedure [1, 21].

Preoperative Work-up

Appropriate preoperative evaluation of esophagogastric function is essential prior to performing laparoscopic fundoplication. Failure of surgery to control symptoms in up to 10 % of cases is a reflection that antireflux surgery has been inadvertently utilized for unrecognized cardiac, hepatobiliary, esophageal, or gastric etiologies [20]. In addition, patients with documented reflux may have secondary surgical contributors to their symptoms such as cholelithiasis, esophageal motility

Table 1. Indications for laparoscopic antireflux surgery

Refractory to medical therapy
    Symptoms present after 12 weeks of medical therapy
    Noncompliance with therapy

Development of complications and/or symptoms
    Stricture
    Bleeding
    Barrett's mucosa
    Aspiration

Table 2. Relative contraindications to laparoscopic antireflux surgery

Previous hiatal/upper abdominal surgery

Morbid obesity with left hepatomegaly

Shortened esophagus

Aperistalsis of esophagus
    Achalasia
    Scleroderma
    End-stage GERD

disorders, or gastroparesis. Waring et al. reported that 13 % of the patients in their series underwent an alteration of their planned surgery due to associated findings on preoperative evaluation [28].

Table 3. Preoperative evaluation of GERD

Mandatory
   Esophagogastroduodenoscopy with or without biopsy
   Esophageal manometry

Selective
   Barium swallow
   24-h pH monitoring
   Gastric studies

Preoperative evaluation can be divided into mandatory and selective tests (Table 3). Evaluation must include esophago-gastroduodenoscopy and esophageal manometry. During endoscopy the presence of esophagitis is recorded and graded by the Savary-Miller score. Biopsies may be performed and complications (esophagitis, ulceration, stricture, Barrett's esophagus) are documented [1]. The length of the esophagus and presence of hiatal hernia are noted. Routine manometry will demonstrate lower esophageal sphincter (LES) dysfunction and characterize esophageal motility disorders [31]. A defective LES exhibits low resting pressure, shortened length, or an intrathoracic location. Impaired esophageal peristalsis (less than 70 %) or diminished esophageal body contraction amplitude (less than 30 mmHg) indicate a motility disturbance [28]. The differentiation between nonspecific motility disturbances and aperistalsis is imperative to direct surgical therapy. The nonspecific motility disturbances do not contraindicate antireflux surgery. Aperistalsis, however, may dictate another procedure such as myotomy or esophageal resection particularly if a stricture is present [30].

Esophageal pH monitoring may be performed in selected patients when the diagnosis is in doubt [28]. In symptomatic patients with endoscopically documented esophagitis the pH study may be omitted. However, in the absence of esophagitis 24-h pH monitoring is the best diagnostic indicator of reflux [11]. Reflux occurs when the pH drops below 4, and abnormal reflux is defined as a total reflux time greater than 4.2 % of the study [18]. Barium swallow is selectively utilized in patients with a history of stricture or dysphagia. Additionally, if the EGD was performed outside our institution, a barium swallow is performed to confirm the reported findings. Gastric studies to rule out gastroparesis, gastric acid hypersecretion, or duodenal gastric reflux are indicated only in the patient with symptoms or signs of gastric disease or frequent vomiting [28].

Operative Technique

The patient is admitted on the morning of surgery. No prophylactic antibiotics are utilized. The patient is placed in the supine position under general anesthesia. A Foley catheter and nasogastric (NG) tube are inserted. Pneumatic compression hoses are applied and the legs are separated in a Y configuration to allow the surgeon to operate from between the legs. Initially during draping and trocar insertion the surgeon stands to the patient's right. The first assistant is on the patient's left and the camera operator stands between the patient's legs.

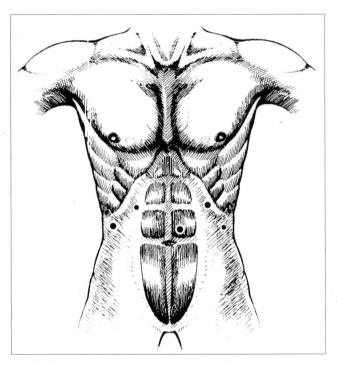

Fig. 1. Trocar insertion sites for laparoscopic Nissen fundoplication

Five trocars are routinely utilized with three 10- and two 5-mm ports. A 15-mmHg pneumoperitoneum is obtained by puncture of the abdominal wall at the umbilicus and the initial trocar is inserted through the left rectus muscle, 15 cm below the xiphoid (Fig. 1). Trocars are tunneled and are obliquely passed through the fascia to minimize the risk of trocar site herniation. An angled 30 or 45 ° video laparoscope is inserted through the first trocar to give direct access to the hiatus. An angled scope is mandatory for this procedure to adequately visualize the posterior esophagus and fundus during dissection [16]. It also allows instruments to pass below the oblique-viewing lens preventing instrument overcrowding in the shallow operative field. The second 10-mm trocar is inserted along the left costal margin 10 cm from the xiphoid. A blunt instrument is inserted in this trocar and used to elevate the falciform ligament to expose the right upper abdominal wall. The third 10-mm trocar is then inserted along the right costal margin 15 cm from the xiphoid. An expandable fan retractor is inserted via the third trocar and used to elevate the left lobe of the liver. The triangular ligament to the left lobe is not divided, because it aids in exposure with this technique. Utilization of a mechanical arm to secure the fan retractor minimizes liver trauma [20]. A fourth trocar (5 mm) is inserted just below the left lobe of the liver medial to the falciform ligament. The fifth trocar (5 mm) is inserted along the left costal margin 20 cm from the xiphoid (Fig. 1). The surgeon then moves to between the patient's legs and the camera operator stands to the patient's right. The assistant provides retraction on the GE junction via the left lower trocar and the surgeon utilizes the upper two trocars to begin a two-handed dissection. With the stomach under traction the lesser omentum is opened above the hepatic branch of the anterior vagus nerve exposing the caudate lobe of the liver (Figs. 2 and 3). Dissection and division of the gastrohepatic ligament is carried to the left until the right crus is identified. The peritoneum and phrenoesopha-

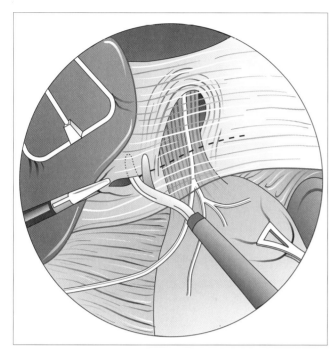

Fig. 2. With the gastroesophageal junction under tension the lesser omentum is opened and the line of dissection is carried across the left crus

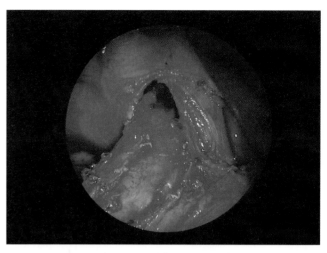

Fig. 4. Anterior exposure of the right and left crus after division of the peritoneum overlying the anterior esophagus

geal ligament overlying the abdominal esophagus are divided until the left crus is identified (Fig. 4). The gastrophrenic attachments along the left crus are mobilized and then the dissection returns to the right side. The right crus is exposed, and utilizing blunt dissection a window between the crus and esophagus is developed (Fig. 5). The hepatic branch of the anterior vagus is swept inferiorly, and any vessels are coagulated using electrocautery or the harmonic scalpel. The blunt dissection proceeds posteriorly under direct visualization with the angled scope. The NG tube is retracted above the hiatus during the posterior dissection to minimize the risk of perforation, which can occur if the esophagus is fixed by a dilator or NG tube. The posterior vagus, when encountered, is allowed

to reside in its natural state. Usually it will separate from the esophagus and lie along the diaphragm; however, if it stays with the esophagus, it will be included within the floppy wrap. Posterior dissection proceeds until the left crus is visualized (Fig. 6). The remaining retroesophageal tissue is divided, usually from the right side, but occasionally some left-sided dissection is necessary. The grasper is placed behind the esophagus and a quarter-inch Penrose drain is passed around the esophagus (Fig. 7). The drain is secured by approximating the arms with a metal clip (Fig. 8). Care must be taken not to clip the Penrose too close to the esophagus, or this will cause angulation. Passage of the large Bougie will then be difficult and may precipitate a perforation. The assist-

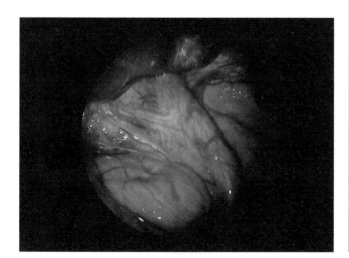

Fig. 3. The gastrohepatic ligament between the liver and right crus is the point of the initial dissection

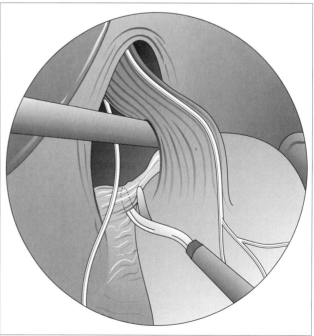

Fig. 5. Posterior dissection exposing the posterior vagus from the right side of the esophagus

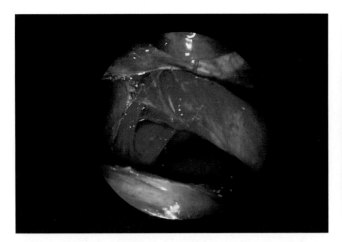

Fig. 6. Posterior dissection and window developed with both crura exposed. The esophagus is at top of photo

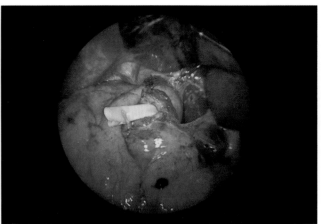

Fig. 8. The Penrose is secured with a metal clip and used for atraumatic esophageal retraction

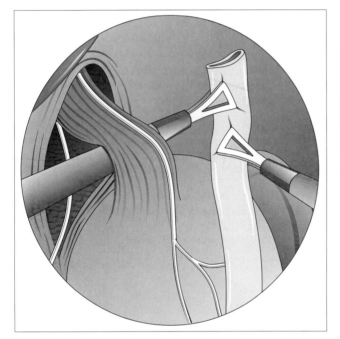

Fig. 7. A quarter-inch Penrose is passed posteriorly to encircle the esophagus and is used for retraction

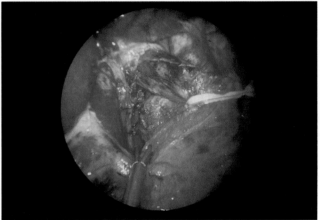

Fig. 9. Retraction of the esophagus with the Penrose and closure of the crura with 2–3 nonabsorbable sutures

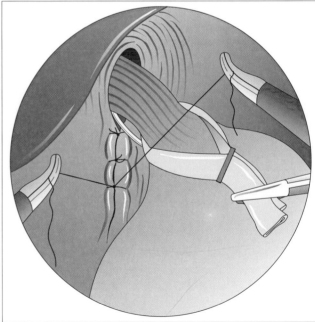

Fig. 10. Closure of the crura with 2–3 sutures of nonabsorbable suture

ant now grasps the Penrose and retracts the esophagus to the left and inferiorly. The posterior window is further opened to expose the entire length of left and right crura posteriorly to their junction. At least 3 cm of the esophagus must be mobilized into the abdomen to ensure adequate intra-abdominal length for fixation. At this point, if a hiatal hernia is present, the crura are reapproximated with 2–3 sutures of 0-nonabsorbable suture (Figs. 9 and 10). Extracorporeal or intracorporeal suturing may be utilized. Pledgets may be utilized if either crus is attenuated. The gastric fundus is further mobilized at this point by dividing all gastrophrenic attachments from the angle of His to the tip of the spleen (Fig. 11). The short gastric vessels are next routinely divided along the upper one third of the stomach to ensure a floppy wrap with no tension. The lesser sac is entered inferiorly and a right angle dissector is

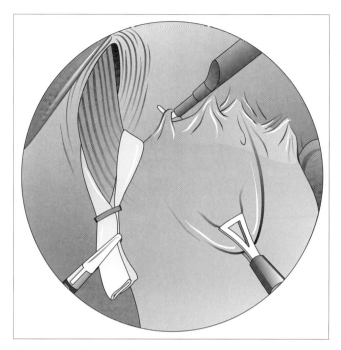

Fig. 11. Mobilization of the posterior fundus under direct vision with the angled scope

utilized to isolate each vessel (Figs. 12 and 13). It may then be clipped and divided or coagulated with the harmonic scalpel. Ligation and division of the short gastric vessels should begin distally and proceed over the fundus to ensure adequate visualization and mobilization. With the fundus mobilized it can be passed behind the esophagus (Fig. 14) and will remain in place without being grasped (Fig. 15). A 60F Bougie dilator is next carefully passed into the distal esophagus. If a stricture is

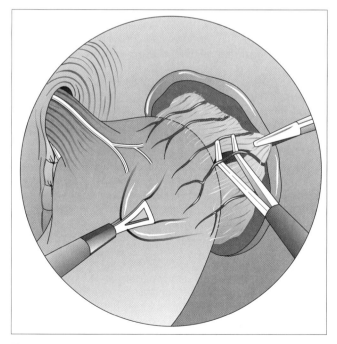

Fig. 12. Division of short gastric vessel beginning inferiorly and proceeding over the fundus

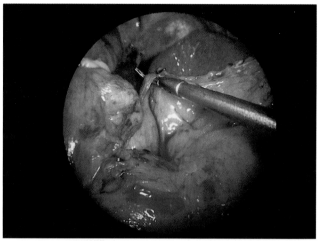

Fig. 13. Isolating the short gastric vessels for ligation

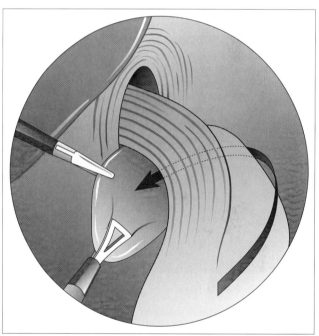

Fig. 14. Passing the fundus posteriorly to fashion the wrap

present, a dilator the size used for dilatation is utilized. A 2-cm wrap is then sutured intracorporeally utilizing three 2–0 nonabsorbable sutures (Fig. 16). Extracorporeal sutures in this location tend to saw through the esophagus, and it is hard to assess the amount of tension on the suture during tying. Large bites of tissue must be obtained with each suture, and the esophagus is incorporated into the wrap to prevent slippage. Although advocated by some, pledgets are not necessary in this position. The dilator is removed and the wrap may be sutured to the diaphragm at 11, 2, and 7 o'clock to prevent intrathoracic migration (Figs. 17 and 18). An NG tube is used to aspirate the stomach and is then removed. The abdomen is irrigated and the liver retractor and trocars are removed under visualization to rule out bleeding. A chest X-ray is obtained in the recovery room to exclude a pneumothorax.

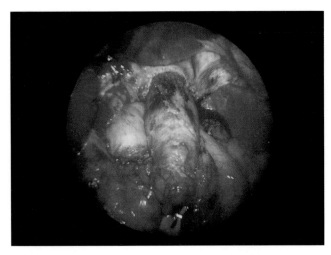

Fig. 15. The fundus should remain in place when released by the grasper; if not, then further mobilization is necessary

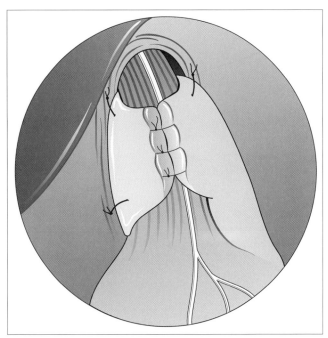

Fig. 18. The completed wrap sutured to the diaphragm at 7, 11, and 2 o'clock to prevent herniation

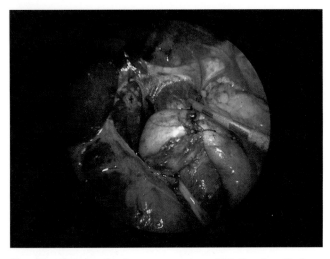

Fig. 16. Suturing the 2-cm wrap over a 60F Bougie with three nonabsorbable sutures incorporating the esophagus with each bite

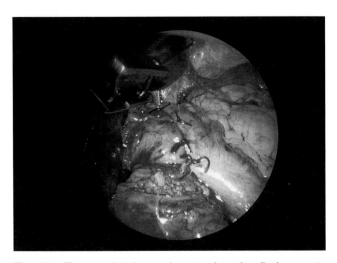

Fig. 17. The completed wrap is sutured to the diaphragma to prevent herniation

Postoperative Care

Postoperatively patients are begun on clear liquids the day of surgery and placed on a mechanical soft diet the following day. The average length of stay is 2 days. Upon discharge patients remain on the mechanical soft diet for 3 weeks and begin solids in the fourth week. They are allowed to return to work when they are ready. They return to our outpatient clinic in the fourth week and are assessed. If doing well, they are seen yearly with appropriate monitoring, selectively ordered to follow any complications of GERD (Barrett's, stricture, etc.). Selected tests may also be ordered to evaluate persistent symptoms. Initially, routine postoperative pH monitoring and manometry was performed as a quality-control measure, but after near-uniform correlation of symptoms and objective results were discovered consistently, these tests became selectively used only.

Complications

The complications of laparoscopic Nissen fundoplication may be divided into two categories, intraoperative and postoperative complications, which are listed in Table 4. With intraoperative complications, conversion to open laparotomy is in itself not a complication, but rather an exercise in sound surgical judgment in most instances. Conversion may be required due to adhesions, difficult exposure secondary to a large left lobe of the liver, uncontrolled bleeding, or to repair certain perforations [29]. Visceral perforations occur equally with open or laparoscopic techniques, and may be the result of periesophagitis or adhesions. Anterior perforations can usually be repaired laparoscopically, but posterior perforations may require conversion to open repair [6]. Coverage of the repair with the fundoplication is ideal when technically feasible [29]. The incidence of perforation can be minimized by attending to several principles of dissection:

Table 4. Complications of laparoscopic Nissen fundoplication

Intraoperative complications

Visceral perforation
  Esophageal
  Gastric
  Diaphragmatic
Bleeding
Pneumothorax
Emphysema/pneumomediastinum
Vagal injury

Postoperative complications

Wrap disruption (slippage)
Thoracic
  Pulmonary (atelectasis, pneumonia, effusion)
  Pericardial effusion
Dysphagia
Gas bloat
Vagal neuropraxia
  Diarrhea
  Gastroparesis
Persistent symptoms

1. Dissect only under direct vision (an angled scope is mandatory)
2. Dissect the crura and the esophagus will dissect itself
3. Do not grasp the esophagus
4. Do not dissect around the esophagus with a Bougie or NG tube in place
5. Ensure that there is no angulation of the esophagus when the dilator is passed
6. The anesthesiologist must pass the Bougie slowly while the surgeon watches the gastro-esophageal junction for signs of the dilator becoming lodged or kinked

Bleeding (greater than 250 cc) is frequent, but rarely requires transfusion. The most common sources of bleeding are small periesophageal and peridiaphragmatic vessels, which can be controlled with meticulous use of electrocautery during dissection [18]. Metal clips, bipolar electrocautery, and the harmonic scalpel may be utilized to control the short gastric vessels. Splenic injuries are rare, but may occur and may necessitate open splenectomy. Pneumothorax is frequently seen on chest X-ray, but rarely requires a chest tube [15]. Pneumomediastinum and cervical subcutaneous emphysema are routinely noted, but there have been no reports of resultant adverse effects [6].

Among postoperative complications (Table 4), wrap disruption or slippage have been associated with violent retching or increased intraabdominal pressure in the early postoperative period, and may necessitate secondary surgical correction [15]. Technical keys to minimize this serious complication are:
1. Mobilize the esophagus such that 3 cm of distal esophagus will reside in the abdomen without tension.
2. Close the crura snugly posterior to the esophagus. Subsequent dilator passage will keep this closure from being too tight.
3. Take large, full-thickness bites of the stomach with each suture.
4. Fix the fundoplication to the esophagus with each suture.
5. Fix the completed fundoplication to the undersurface of the diaphragm with interrupted sutures. We generally use two or three sutures at the 11-, 2-, and 6-o'clock positions (Figs. 17 and 18).

Pulmonary complications (fever, atelectasis, pneumonia) still occur with laparoscopy, but should be rare when compared with open techniques. Dysphagia, the most common complication, is usually short term, may be secondary to wrap edema or hematoma, and will usually resolve in 3–6 weeks with expectant therapy [16, 29]. Occasional postoperative dilatation may be necessary particularly if a stricture was present preoperatively. Early postoperative dysphagia was reduced from 54 to 17 % in our experience by modifying the operation to include routine division of the short gastric vessels [15]. Creation of a loose, short (less than 2.5 cm) wrap is critical to minimize iatrogenic dysphagia. Long-term dysphagia was seen in only 4 % of our series [15]. Gas bloat syndrome has been reported, but is minimized with a floppy or partial fundoplication [1, 6, 21]. Vagal neuropraxia may result in diarrhea or delayed gastric emptying in a small number of patients.

Clinical Outcomes and Results

Early reports indicate favorable morbidity and mortality figures for laparoscopic antireflux procedures compared with open surgery (Table 5 and 6). Symptomatic and physiologic results are also equivalent between the laparoscopic and open antireflux procedure [6, 29]. Short-term follow-up (less than 2 years) indicates that laparoscopic techniques yield symptomatic success in greater than 90 % of cases [6, 15, 29]. Postoperative assessment with endoscopy, pH monitoring, and manometry has been reported by several authors in postoperative volunteers to document the physiologic effects of the laparoscopic Nissen [6, 29]. Cuschieri et al. reported endoscopic and pH-monitoring follow-up in 92 of 116 patients [6]; 65 patients had complete healing on EGD and 19 were improved. The pH monitoring was normal in 88 of 92 patients. Weerts et al. reported 40 postoperative EGDs and 32 manometry studies in their series of 132 patients [29]. The EGD was normal in 39 of 40, and manometry revealed mean LES was increased from 4.6 mmHg preoperatively to 24.5 mmHg postoperatively with a laparoscopic Nissen. These short-term physiologic reports of laparoscopic antireflux surgery will continue to be monitored to establish long-term effects of the laparoscopic approach.

Table 5. Clinical outcome of laparoscopic antireflux surgery

No. cases	Mortality	Morbidity %	Excellent/good symptom relief (%)
175 (93 Nissen, 82 Toupet)*	0	12	93
132 (all Nissen)**	0	7.5	94

*From Ref. 15 **From Ref. 29

Table 6. Clinical outcome of open antireflux surgery

No. cases	Mortality	Morbidity (%)	Excellent/good symptom relief (%)
349 (255 Toupet, 94 Nissen)*	1	17	n. n.
100 (all Nissen)**	1	13	91

*From [26] **From [8]

Discussion

There are two goals that form the foundation of current treatment of GERD: (1) relief of symptoms, and (2) prevention or correction of complications. The achievement of these goals requires the coordinated efforts of the medical and surgical specialties. The etiology of GERD is multifactorial with an extended list of possible culprits (Table 7) [17]. Factors beyond

Table 7. Etiology of GERD

Diminished pressure of LES

Hiatal hernia

Reduced esophageal motility (clearance)

Diminished gastric emptying

Iatrogenic destruction of LES (Heller myotomy, esophago gastrectomy)

the dysfunctional LES must be considered to address the 10% failure rate of traditional Nissen fundoplication [20]. There is not a single approach that can be applied to every patient. Treatment must be individualized through the team approach with careful diagnostic evaluation being the cornerstone of management. Medical therapy for GERD has undergone a reevaluation in recent years as several new concepts have come to light. Firstly, a multicenter randomized study demonstrated that open Nissen fundoplication was superior to medical therapy in long-term management of GERD [24]. This study did not include the proton-pump inhibitors, but others report an 85% relapse rate of symptoms after continuation of medication within 6 months [14]. Questions are being raised about the safety of prolonged use of potent acid-reducing medications and the associated achlorhydria [22]. Despite long-term medical therapy, 20% of patients with esophagitis develop a complication (stricture, ulcer, Barrett's), with 8% occurring within the first year [3, 19]. Another analysis reported that antireflux surgery is less expensive than long-term medical therapy [5, 23]. These shortcomings have prompted a reappraisal of surgical options.

The emergence of laparoscopic antireflux surgery presents an attractive alternative to long-term medical therapy without many of the previous drawbacks to open surgery. Although any of the open techniques (Nissen, Toupet, Belsey, Hill) can be performed laparoscopically, current opinion favors the 360° Nissen fundoplication or 270° Toupet partial fundoplication. DeMeester et al. had previously demonstrated that the open Nissen fundoplication was superior to both Belsey and Hill procedures in controlling reflux symptoms [9]. Further attention to resolving technical errors should reduce postoperative side effects: (1) take care that the wrap is properly positioned, not too long (2 cm) or too tight (60F Bougie); (2) divide the short gastric vessels and mobilize the posterior fundus routinely; and (3) close the crura and anchor the wrap to the diaphragm. Several authors have advocated utilizing the laparoscopic Toupet 270° partial fundoplication as an alternative to reduce gas bloat syndrome and dysphagia seen with early open Nissen fundoplication [1, 6, 15, 16, 21]. The only published prospective study comparing open Nissen with open Toupet technique suffers from several critical deficiencies [30]. The number of patients was small (31 patients over 5 years), and two of the three wrap disruptions occurred early

in the series. The technique of Nissen fundoplication was flawed [30]. The Nissen fundoplication was constructed to be 4 cm in length over a 40F Bougie, and no crural approximation or fixation was attempted. The short gastric vessels were routinely divided in only the Toupet group. In an analysis of gastroesophageal leaks after 1005 open antireflux procedures, there were 12 (1.2%) leaks reported [27]. Of the 12 leaks, 10 (83%) occurred in the open Toupet procedures. This raises questions concerning the safety of the Toupet partial fundoplication. The added security of covering the esophageal suture line with the gastric wrap in laparoscopic Nissen fundoplication offers a potential safety over laparoscopic Toupet procedures. The previous indication for laparoscopic Toupet by many authors was a nonspecific motility disturbance [15, 20, 21, 28]. In light of Bremner's report of the success of open modern Nissen fundoplication in the treatment of nonspecific motility abnormalities with reflux, good questions may be raised about the place of the laparoscopic Toupet procedure. We favor the laparoscopic Nissen fundoplication because of its technical ease in comparison with the Toupet and the body of literature that supports the open Nissen technique. The laparoscopic Nissen can be performed currently in the same manner as the open procedure with less discomfort, shorter hospitalization, and quicker resumption of normal activity [6, 21, 29]. These improvements resolve many of the objections voiced concerning open surgery. Early reports indicate low morbidity and mortality, and the symptomatic and physiologic results of laparoscopic antireflux surgery are comparable to the open fundoplication [6, 15, 29]. The laparoscopic Nissen offers promises in establishing itself as an accepted standard in the management of GERD if long-term follow-up continues to document the initial short-term success.

References

1. BORDELON BM, HUTSON WR, HUNTER JG: Laparoscopic approaches to gastroesophageal reflux disease. Gastrointest Endosc Clin North Am 3 (1993) 309–317.
2. BREMNER RM, DeMEESTER TR, CROOKES PF et al.: The effects of symptoms and nonspecific motility abnormalities on outcomes of surgical therapy for gastroesophageal reflux disease. J Thorac Cardiovasc Surg 107 (1994) 1244–1249.
3. BROSSARD E, MONNIER PH, OLLYO JB et al.: Serious complications – stenosis, ulcer and Barrett's epithelium – develop in 21.6% of adults with erosive reflux esophagitis. Gastroenterology 100 (1991) A36.
4. Centers for Disease Control (CDC), Rockville, Maryland. Surgical Statistics 1985 and 1989.
5. COLEY CM, BARRY MJ, SPECHLER SJ et al.: Initial medical vs surgical therapy for complicated or chronic gastroesophageal reflux disease. Gastroenterology 104 (1993) A5 (abstract).
6. CUSCHIERI A, HUNTER J, WOLFE B et al.: Multicenter prospective evaluation of laparoscopic antireflux surgery. Surg Endosc 7 (1993) 505–510.
7. CUSCHIERI AE: Hiatal hernia and reflux esophagitis. In: HUNTER JG, SACKIER JM (eds.): Minimally invasive surgery. McGraw-Hill, New York (1993) 87–111.
8. DeMEESTER TR, BONAVINA L, ALBERTUCCI M: Nissen fundoplication for gastroesophageal reflux. Ann Surg 204 (1986) 9–20.
9. DeMEESTER TR, JOHNSON LF, KENT AH: Evaluation of current operations for the prevention of gastroesophageal reflux. Ann Surg 180 (1974) 511–525.
10. DeMEESTER TR, STEIN HJ: Surgical treatment of gastroesophageal reflux disease. In: Castell DO (ed.): The esophagus. Little Brown, Boston (1992) 579–625.

11. Fuchs KH, DeMeester RT, Albertucci M: Specificity and sensitivity of objective diagnosis of gastroesophageal reflux disease. Surgery 102 (4) (1987) 575.
12. Gallup Survey on Heartburn Across America. Princeton, The Gallup Organization. March 28, 1988.
13. Havelund T, Laursen LS, Skoubo-Kristensen E et al.: Omeprazole and ranitidine in the treatment of reflux esophagitis: double blind comparative trial. Br Med J 269 (1988) 89–92.
14. Hetzel DJ, Dent J, Reed WD et al.: Healing and relapse of severe peptic esophagitis after treatment with omeprazole. Gastroenterology 95 (1991) 903–912.
15. Hunter JG, Waring P, Oddsdottir M, Swanstrom L: Complications and early symptoms following laparoscopic antireflux surgery. World Congresses of Gastroenterology 1994.
16. Hunter JG: Antireflux surgery. In: Griffith Pearson F (ed.): Esophageal surgery. Churchill Livingstone (1995) 795–798.
17. Jamieson GG, Duranceau A: Pathogenic mechanisms associated with GERD. In: Gastroesophageal reflux. W. B. Saunders Co., Philadelphia (1988) 19.
18. Johnson LF, DeMeester TR: Twenty four hour pH monitoring of the distal esophagus. Am J Gastroenterol 62 (1974) 325–332.
19. Lanspa SJ, Spechler SJ, DeMeester TR et al.: Incidence of esophageal stricture formation in patients with complicated GERD. Gastroenterology 100 (1991) A–7.
20. Laycock WS, Hunter JG: Laparoscopic management of esophageal disease. In: Brookes DC (ed.): Current techniques in laparoscopy, 2nd edn (1995) 98–111.
21. McKernan JB, Laws HL: Laparoscopic Nissen fundoplication for the treatment of gastroesophageal reflux disease. Am Surg 60 (1994) 87–93.
22. Omeprazole. Med Lett Drugs Ther 32 (1990) 19–21.
23. Richter JE: Surgery for reflux disease – reflections of a gastroenterologist. NEJM 326 (1992) 825–827.
24. Spechler SJ: Comparison of medical and surgical therapy for complicated gastroesophageal reflux disease in veterans. NEJM 326 (1992) 786–792.
25. Thor KBA, Silander T: A long-term randomized prospective trial of the Nissen vs. Toupet technique. Ann Surg 210 (1989) 719–724.
26. Urschel JD: Complications of antireflux surgery. Am J Surg 165 (1993) 68–70.
27. Urschel JD: Gastroesophageal leaks after antireflux procedures. Ann Thorac Surg 57 (1994) 129–1232.
28. Waring JP, Hunter JG, Oddsdottir M et al.: The preoperative evaluation of patients considered for laparoscopic antireflux surgery. Am J Gastroenterology 90 (1) (1995) 35–38.
29. Weerts JM, Dallemagne B, Hamoir E et al.: Laparoscopic Nissen fundoplication: detailed analysis of 132 patients. Surg Lap Endosc 3 (1993) 359–364.
30. Zaninotto G, DeMeester TR et al.: Esophageal function in patients with reflux induced strictures and its relevance to surgical treatment. Ann Thorac Surg 47 (1989) 362–370.
31. Zaninotto G, DeMeester TR et al.: The lower esophageal sphincter in health and disease. Am J Surg 155 (1988) 104.

13. | Laparoscopic Gastroenterostomy and Billroth II Gastrectomy

P. Goh and D. J. Alexander

Introduction

The minimally invasive technique of laparoscopic gastroenterostomy offers a very attractive and less traumatic alternative
to the same bypass performed at laparotomy. As might be expected the laparoscopic technique results in significantly less
wound-associated morbidity, the patients are able to ambu-
late independently within 24 h and are often able to go home
within 4–5 days. The beneficial effects of surgery without the
requirement of laparotomy and the resulting quicker rehabilitation may also suggest a reduced risk of chest infection and
deep vein thrombosis. The laparoscopic technique involves
less bowel handling, thus resulting in a shorter post-operative
intestinal ileus, as has been the experience in some studies
on laparoscopic colectomy.

Although these benefits can be enjoyed by all patients, it is
perhaps in those patients that are undergoing palliative surgery that the results of less operative morbidity and a quicker
return to full mobility are best appreciated, since their life expectancy is very short.

Historical Perspective

The value of laparoscopy in the diagnosis and management
of pancreatic carcinoma was established by Cuschieri in 1978
[3] in a study of 23 patients in whom laparoscopy provided
useful information in the diagnosis of disease, in the assessment of operability and in the retrieval of material for histological confirmation of pancreatic cancer. In particular, an infra-
gastric laparoscopic method for inspection of the body and tail
of the pancreas was described with the hope that the technique might allow earlier detection of neoplasms in that region. Ishida and colleagues [8], approximately 3 years later,
confirmed the potential accessibility to the pancreas by laparoscopy using a supra-gastric approach through the lesser
omentum, thus allowing direct pancreatic biopsy.

Developments in this field largely rested at diagnosis until
the recent explosion of laparoscopy in the field of general surgery. This has resulted in a dramatic proliferation of laparoscopic alternatives to many general surgical operations. The
benefits of exchanging a laparotomy incision against between
three to five 1-cm laparoscopic port incisions are evident, and
indeed the first two reported laparoscopic gastroenterosto-
mies were in the palliation of patients with malignant gastric
outflow obstruction. In 1992 Wilson and Varma [16] reported
on two elderly patients, one with an obstructing carcinoma of

the third part of the duodenum, and the other with extrinsic
compression of the third and fourth parts of the duodenum, in
whom laparoscopic gastroenterostomy was successfully performed [16]. Full diet was tolerated within 4 days, postoperative pain was controlled with oral analgesia and both patients
were discharged home within 5 days. Also in 1992 Katkhouda's
group [14] reported on two patients in whom duodenal and biliary obstruction secondary to advanced pancreatic carcinoma
were relieved by the combination of endoscopic biliary stenting and laparoscopic gastroenterostomy. This latter paper
concluded that patients with a limited life expectancy benefit
greatly from the shortened hospital stay and convalescence
that this manner of treatment offers.

Indications for Laparoscopic Gastroenterostomy

Advanced Pancreatic or Duodenal Carcinoma Resulting in Gastric Outflow Obstruction

Once the decision has been made that curative surgery is impossible the advantages of the laparoscopic approach in a
patient group whose median survival is likely to be 6 months
or less are self-evident. It is unusual for a patient with advanced pancreatic carcinoma to present with the symptoms of
jaundice and gastric outflow obstruction simultaneously, and
in such circumstances we would palliate jaundice by endoscopic biliary drainage using a stent and gastric outflow obstruction by laparoscopic gastroenterostomy, as it has been
described by Mouiel et al. [14]. However, we have had occasion to perform laparoscopic gastroenterostomy for gastric
outflow obstruction in a patient with advanced pancreatic carcinoma in whom we had performed laparoscopic cholecys-
toenterostomy several months earlier at the time of their original presentation with obstructive jaundice. Although the patient had initially been managed successfully by endoscopic
stenting, the stent became obstructed and the patient elected
to have laparoscopic bypass.

Antral Carcinoma Resulting in Gastric Outflow Obstruction

Although we believe that gastric resection provides a better
quality of palliation than gastric bypass in distal tumours, we
would consider laparoscopic gastroenterostomy if the presence of distant metastases were proven pre-operatively and
the tumour was sufficiently distally placed to allow a satisfactory bypass. The prognosis of patients with liver secondaries

resulting from a gastric primary is very poor, and again the benefits of the laparoscopic approach in producing a faster convalescence are likely to outweigh the fact that it may be a technically more inferior form of palliation than a sub-total gastrectomy. In the present context a palliative laparoscopic gastric resection is worth considering.

Indications in Conjunction with Truncal Vagotomy

It is our practice to repair perforated duodenal ulcers laparoscopically. We would consider laparoscopic truncal vagotomy with either pyloroplasty or gastroenterostomy in some patients with a chronic history of duodenal ulcer and minimal peritoneal soiling.

Benign Pyloric Stenosis

Benign pyloric stenosis is handled in conjunction with truncal vagotomy.

Contra-indications

If there is a contra-indication to general anaesthesia.

Preoperative Work-up

As with open surgery, haematological, biochemical and clotting profiles, chest X-ray and ECG are obtained. The patient should be grouped and saved, although there is seldom a need for transfusion with laparoscopic gastroenterostomy alone.

Operative Technique

Operating Room Set-up and Anaesthesia

Surgery is performed under general anaesthesia with a nasogastric tube in situ. If the diagnosis is of gastric outflow obstruction, it is vitally important that the stomach is washed out thoroughly in the 48 h prior to surgery. This is important in open surgery, but even more so in the laparoscopic approach, because it is much more difficult to prevent peritoneal contamination from gastric and bowel contents. End-tidal carbon dioxide is monitored. Antibiotic prophylaxis, a single intravenous dose of a third-generation cephalosporin, is given at the induction of anaesthesia. The patient is positioned with legs apart, but in the same plane as the rest of the body, with a minor degree of reverse Trendelenburg tilt. This provides the option of allowing the operator to stand between the patient's legs. The operating room set-up is shown in Figure 1. The precise technique of anastomosis dictates the best positions for the surgeon and assistants during the procedure. To begin the operation the operator stands between the patient's legs with one assistant on either side of the patient. The camera operator stands on the surgeon's right and two video monitors are used, both placed obliquely over the patient's shoulders.

Surgical Technique

The closed technique of establishing a pneumoperitoneum using a Veress needle is used unless the patient has had previous abdominal surgery, in which case an open introduction is employed. Insufflation of the abdomen is produced and maintained using a Semm's automatic pneumoinsufflator.

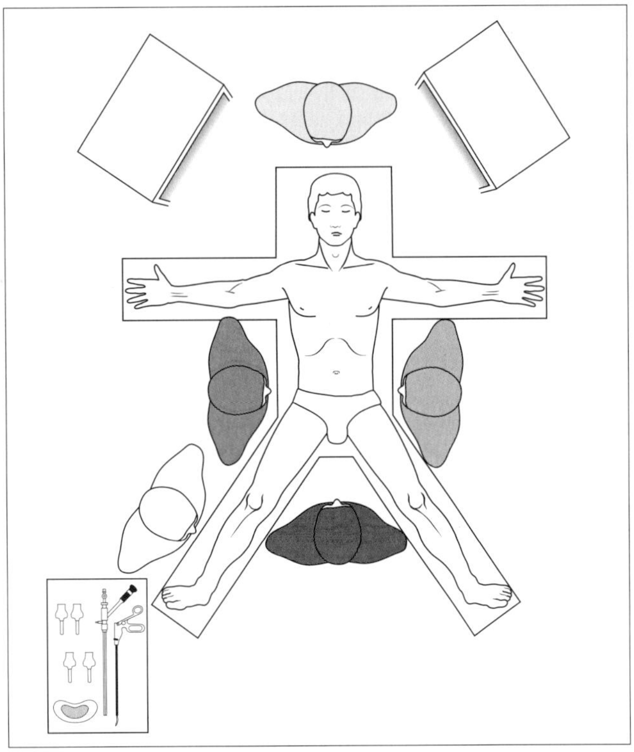

Fig. 1.   Operating room set-up for laparoscopic gastric procedures

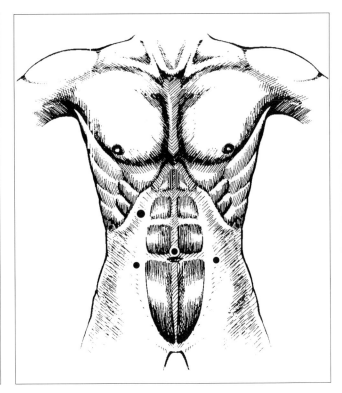

Fig.2.   Trocar positions for laparoscopic gastrojejunostomy

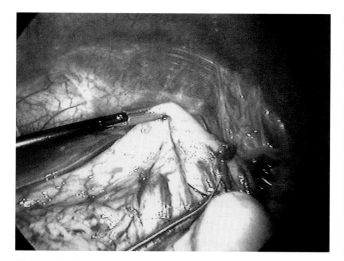

Fig. 3. The first mobile jejunal loop is brought up in an antecolic way to the greater curvature of the stomach

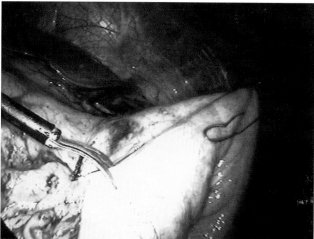

Fig. 5. The incisions for the stapler jaws are made in the jejunum and stomach using diathermy scissors

This instrument has a flow indicator and a pressure gauge that continuously monitors intra-abdominal pressure. A 10-mm trocar is inserted at the sub-umbilical position through which the three-chip endocamera is placed. A general laparoscopy is performed and the diagnosis is confirmed. Accessory ports are then positioned under direct vision as shown in Figure 2. The iliac fossae ports are used for suturing, and it is therefore not mandatory to use larger port sizes here; however, we prefer the greater flexibility that the 10- to 11-mm port provides. Of more vital importance is the use of a 12-mm port in the right hypochondrium to permit use of an endoscopic stapling device.

The first step is to identify the duodeno-jejunal (DJ) flexure with the ligament of Treitz. This is most easily achieved with the patient in the head-down position and then sweeping the transverse colon cephalad and anteriorly with a blunt forceps. A loop of small bowel is selected in the upper left quadrant and followed proximally, using atraumatic bowel clamps, to the junction of duodenum and jejunum. Having thus established the position of the DJ flexure, the jejunum

is traced down to a point approximately 35–45 cm from the DJ flexure and a 20-cm segment is selected. The patient is then placed in the head-up position and the selected segment of small bowel is gently manipulated in front of and above the transverse colon, and brought to lie along the inferior margin of the greater curve of the stomach (Fig. 3). The anastomosis may be either iso- or anti-peristaltic; however, we feel that by positioning the gastroenterostomy such that the afferent loop is on the lesser curve side of the stomach (efferent loop on greater curve side) the likelihood of significant narrowing of the efferent limb of the anastomosis is reduced (see Peri-operative Complications). Thus, we prefer the anti-peristaltic arrangement. The jejunum is initially held in position with an Endo-Babcock forceps and then fixed using an intracorporeal technique of knot tying with two 3-0 absorbable sutures (Fig. 4), one at either end of the proposed gastroenterostomy, fixing the anti-mesenteric aspect of jejunum to the juxtapyloric anterior surface of the stomach. The suture ends are left long and can thus be used for retraction.

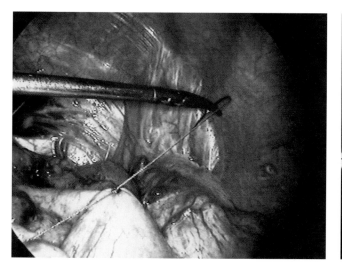

Fig. 4. The stay suture adapting the jejunum to the stomach is tied intracorporeally

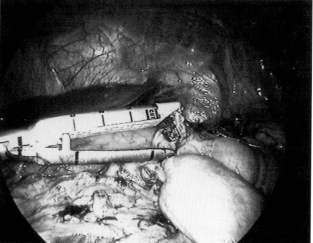

Fig. 6. The 30-mm Endo-GIA is introduced through the 12-mm trocar in the right upper quadrant of the abdomen

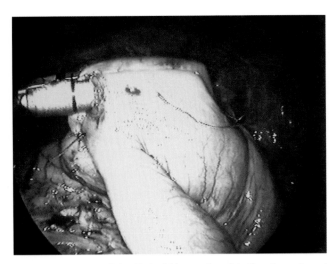

Fig. 7. The jaws of the Endo-GIA are placed in the stomach and anti-mesenteric side of the small-bowel wall

Stapled Anastomosis

The surgeon is placed best on the patient's right to allow easy insertion of the stapling device while the camera operator moves to between the patient's legs and the first assistant is on the patient's left. The stapled anastomosis is begun by creating two stab incisions using the diathermy scissors (Fig. 5), one each on the stomach and the jejunum, on the right side of the proposed anastomotic line. The two incisions must be adjacent to one another. While maintaining traction on the stays, the jaws of an Endo-GIA 30 stapler are inserted (Fig. 6) via the 12-mm right hypochondrial port into the formed enterotomies so that the Endo-GIA is inserted in the direction lesser curve to greater curve of the stomach and has one jaw within the stomach and the other within the jejunum (Fig. 7). The device is closed, and having checked that the posterior and inferior surfaces are free, it is fired. It is not always easy to place the jaws of the stapler into the enterotomies, and this step can be facilitated by the placement of an additional stay suture, placed in order to join the bottom of the two holes,

which has the effect of keeping them close together. A second firing of the GIA at the apex of the newly created gastroenterostomy results in an anastomosis of approximately 6-cm length. During this step it is important to pull the stab-wound margins against the hilt of the stapler to maximize the anastomotic length.

Although the single firing of a 60-mm stapler to create the enterostomy would seem logical, there are practical problems associated with inserting the larger 60-mm stapler through a left upper quadrant port, because there may be difficulty in opening the stapler as the distance from the abdominal wall to the greater curve of the stomach may be too short to allow complete opening of the stapler itself. The same problem is encountered at laparoscopic gastrectomy, and although insertion of the 60-mm stapler through a left lower quadrant port has been used, the resulting angle tends to produce a more vertical anastomotic line than is ideal with the risk of narrowing or kinking of one of the loops. A side-viewing [14] or flexible laparoscope can be used for inspection of the gut lumen and stapled edges for bleeding at this stage.

The resulting enterotomy can be closed using a continuous 2-0 vicryl suture on a 30-mm needle mounted on a 5-mm endoscopic needle holder, in two layers, or by application of the Endo-TA having again used two stay sutures to hold up the edges of the defect. It is important to staple or suture this defect transversely to create a "plasty" effect in order to prevent the narrowing that would occur by simple longitudinal opposition. It is equally important to pick up as little excess tissue as possible in stapling this defect, and hand suture, although slower, is less likely to result in narrowing (Fig. 8). Because of the position of the common stab wound, any narrowing resulting from its closure is likely to affect the afferent limb only, and to be of less significance; hence, our preference for the "anti-peristaltic" gastroenterostomy with the technique described.

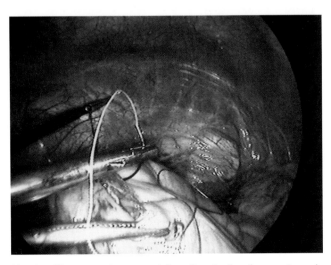

Fig. 8. The enterostomy remaining after stapling the anastomosis is closed by manual suture

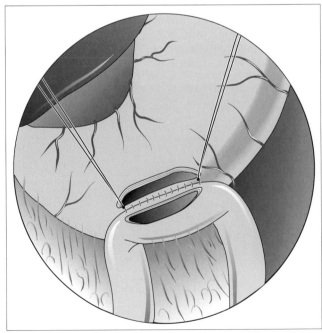

Fig. 9. After a continuous posterior seromuscular suture, the gastrotomy and enterotomy are created with electrocoagulation

Hand-sutured Anastomosis

Although a less convenient and more time-consuming alternative, it is significantly less expensive to perform a hand-sutured anastomosis. We perform a "continuous" two-layered sutured gastrojejunostomy using the Szabo-Berci "parrot beaked" needle holder and "flamingo-beaked" knot-tying forceps. The initial step is the placement of two vicryl stay sutures at either end of the proposed gastroenterostomy, as already described. A continuous posterior seromuscular layer is then fashioned after which the full-length gastrotomy and enterotomy are created using a combination of hook and scissors with coagulative diathermy (Fig. 9). Bleeding from the gastrotomy is usually worse than that from the enterotomy, and it is therefore important to carefully diathermy the serosal stomach wall at the proposed site of enterostomy prior to gastrotomy, and to precisely pick up tiny bleeding points with fine forceps. The right iliac fossa and right hypochondrial ports are used for the stitching instruments with the surgeon placed on the patient's right and the first assistant between the patient's legs, following the thread using a grasping forceps passed through the left iliac fossa port. The posterior inner full-thickness layer is then completed (Fig. 10), followed by the anterior inner full-thickness layer, and finally the anterior outer seromuscular layer. In each case it is ergonomical to suture towards oneself, and thus four separate sutures are used (3-0 vicryl). The time-consuming process of laparoscopic knotting may be obviated by using absorbable suture clips. One clip is used to hold the proximal starting end of a continuous suture and the suture line is secured with a second clip at the end.

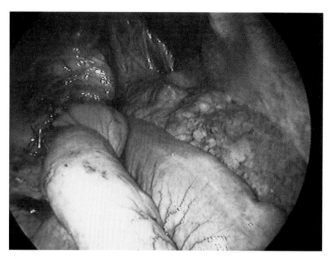

Fig. 11.   Afferent and efferent loop of jejunal anastomosis

Checking the Anastomosis

The anastomosis must be checked endoscopically for leakage as well as patency. The patient is tilted head down about 20 °. The anastomosis is flooded with saline. A gastroscope is passed into the stomach and air is blown under pressure to distend the stomach. The absence of bubbling confirms competency of the anastomotic line. The scope should also visualize the opening of both the efferent and afferent loops of the jejunal anastomosis (Fig. 11). It is possible to gently pass the scope into both loops.

Drainage and Closure

The operating field is irrigated with sterile saline and free fluid aspirated. It may occasionally be necessary to use a 5-mm suction drain if there has been significant soiling or bleeding, and this may be introduced through the right hypochondrial port. The pneumoperitoneum is fully evacuated and the fascial defects are closed with 0-vicryl suture. The wounds are infiltrated with long-acting anaesthetic (bupivacaine) to give immediate post-operative pain relief, and the skin is closed with 3-0 prolene.

Postoperative Management

An additional two doses of prophylactic antibiotics are given. Postoperative ileus would seem to be shorter in this laparoscopic approach, probably because there is less bowel handling and it is not uncommon for the patient to be up to free fluids within 48–72 h and taking some diet by the third postoperative day. Patients who have had relatively long-standing gastric outflow obstruction may take longer to resume normal diet; however, the major benefit of the laparoscopic approach is seen in the early mobility of these patients who are able to walk unaided on the day following surgery. It is therefore possible to discharge patients within 5–7 days of surgery. Because this operation is most often a palliative procedure, it is even more important that the patient is able to recover as quickly as possible and obtain a significant benefit from the surgery.

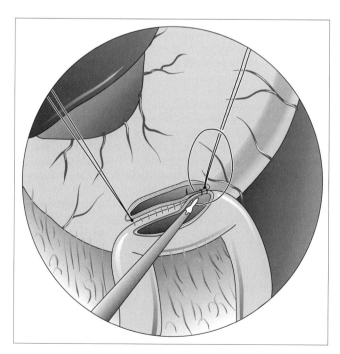

Fig. 10.   Suture of posterior full-thickness layer

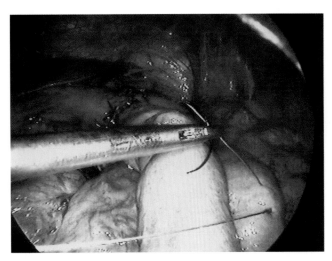

Fig. 12. The afferent and efferent loop are adapted with a stay suture for enteroenterostomy

Perioperative Problems

Bleeding

Hemorrhage from the gastrotomy can be very troublesome. The bleeding points must be carefully identified and coagulated with fine forceps, because it is vital to keep a clear field. Bleeding results in absorption of light, which darkens the field of view.

Anastomotic Leaks

Anastomotic leaks may result from either inadequate suture or a misfire of the stapling device. The defect should be obvious at the time of anastomotic testing, and further direct suture of any observed deficiency can be performed.

Narrowing of Gastrojejunal Anastomosis

Narrowing of the gastrojejunal anastomosis is most likely to occur at the site of the common stab wound in a stapled anas-

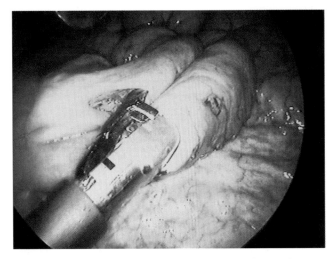

Fig. 13. Creation of enteroenterostomy with Endo-GIA stapler

tomosis. Because it is more important to have a widely patent efferent loop (c. f. afferent loop which is only required to drain bile) we have found it better to position the gastrojejunal anastomosis such that the afferent loop is on the side of the lesser curve of the stomach and the efferent loop is on the greater curve side (anti-peristaltic). This means that the common stab wound is on the side of the afferent loop, using the technique we have just illustrated. Any narrowing of the lumen caused by subsequent closure of the common stab wound is thus likely to involve only the afferent loop and hopefully be of little significance. Should this complication occur it can be dealt with using laparoscopic enteroenterostomy (Figs. 12 and 13).

Retrocolic Gastroenterostomy

In most instances our indication for laparoscopic gastroenterostomy has been in the management of malignant duodenal obstruction, usually secondary to pancreatic carcinoma, and thus an antecolic gastroenterostomy has been fashioned. Retrocolic gastroenterostomy is technically a little more difficult, because the colon must be retracted superiorly to reveal the window to the left of the middle colic artery through which the jejunum can be brought. Having identified and created this window it is easier to complete the anastomosis above the transverse colon, rather than perform it below the mesocolon. Once the anastomosis has been completed using the technique described, the colon is retracted superiorly, the anastomosis is gently manipulated through the mesocolonic window and two vicryl stay sutures are inserted between mesocolon and anastomosis to prevent herniation, as in open surgery.

Laparoscopic Billroth II Gastrectomy

The totally intra-abdominal laparoscopic Billroth II gastrectomy offers a minimally invasive option for gastric resection that is remarkably less traumatic and more patient friendly. Initial experience with this operation around the world has largely concentrated on resection for benign gastric ulcer, but recently the indications have been extended to both benign and neoplastic lesions of the stomach. Experience with a small experimental series of 18 cases showed that this operation has many advantages over open surgery in terms of less postoperative pain, quicker mobilization, fewer wound problems, better cosmesis and quicker discharge. The main problem remains the cost of disposable stapling devices. Better suturing instrumentation and techniques will impact significantly in making the operation less expensive and more accessible to cost-conscious medical infra-structures.

Development

On 29 January 1881 Christian Albert Theodor Billroth (1829–1894) performed the first successful gastric resection for cancer at the Allgemeine Krankenhaus in Vienna [1]. The patient, a 43-year-old housewife, lived 4 months and succumbed to metastatic disease. The remaining stomach was anastomosed directly to the duodenum with 50 silk sutures. The operation came to be known as the *Billroth I gastrectomy*. On 15 January 1885 Billroth performed the first gastrectomy where both the stomach and duodenal stump were closed off and an anterior gastrojejunostomy was constructed. This form of reconstruction came to be known as the *Billroth II gastrectomy* [5]. Between 1881 and his death in 1894, at the age of 65 years, Billroth performed 24 gastrectomies for gastric carcinoma. The Billroth II operation became the prototype for all operations for distal carcinoma of the stomach, although more recently the importance of extensive nodal clearance has been emphasized especially by surgeons in Asia [2, 9]. The development of staplers has made the operation quicker and easier [15]; however, it did not make the operation any more patient friendly in terms of reducing the pain, morbidity and fairly long recovery and hospitalization associated with major stomach resection performed by open surgery.

The advent of laparoscopic cholecystectomy in 1987 [4] prompted many surgeons to look for more challenging applications of the new minimally invasive surgical technology. The first successful totally intra-abdominal laparoscopic Billroth II gastrectomy was performed on February 10, 1992 by our group [7] in Singapore. The patient was a 76-year-old Chinese man with a 2-year history of gastric ulcer who presented with bleeding from the ulcer. The operation took 4 h and consumed 17 Endo-GIA staplers. The patient was walking on the first postoperative day, taking liquids on the third, solid food on the fourth and discharged on the fourth postoperative day. The operation was subsequently emulated by surgeons in about a dozen countries. The description in this chapter is a modification of the original technique using the improved instrumentation now available. The technique described is suitable for a gastrectomy for benign gastric ulcer at the incisura of the stomach, antrum or pre-pyloric region.

Anatomy

A precise appreciation of the anatomy of the stomach and its attachments is necessary in understanding the concept of the operation and is the key to success in this demanding laparoscopic procedure (Fig. 14).

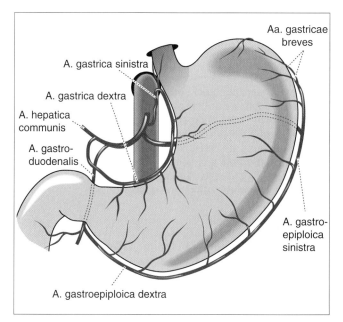

Fig. 14.   Anatomy of vascular supply of stomach

Vascular Arcade of Greater Curvature of the Stomach

This area is important in the initial mobilization of the greater curvature, which is the first part of the dissection. The proximal limit of the dissection is the first short gastric vessel which comes from the spleen. The distal dissection extends down to the first part of the duodenum. In a patient with a very fat omentum the best strategy is to keep the dissection as close to the stomach as possible. In a thinner individual it is possible to choose the most avascular plane, i. e. the one requiring the least dissection and clipping of omental vessels and curve in towards the stomach wall only at the point of proximal gastric transection.

Vascular Attachments of the First Part of the Duodenum

The level of the pylorus externally can be identified by the vein of Mayo, which runs across it. If this is obscure, gastroscopic localization should be done to determine the exact level of the pylorus. The first part of the duodenum must be mobilized sufficiently to apply the Endo-GIA stapler to transect it cleanly just distal to the pyloric ring. The vascular supply of the duodenum comes in from three directions: superiorly, inferiorly and posteriorly. These vascular attachments are very fragile and must be carefully dissected, clipped and transected. The position of the supra-duodenal bile duct should be ascertained to prevent accidental stapling of this structure. The origin of the right gastroepiploic vessel is inferior to the duodenum, but can usually be avoided.

Occasionally, it is in the way and has to be clipped or ligated and transected. The duodenum is attached to the pancreas inferiorly by some fine small vessels. These must be individually coagulated before transection; otherwise, they may cause troublesome bleeding. Vessels larger than 1 mm should be clipped.

Vascular Attachment of the Lesser Curvature

Branches of the left and right gastric artery and their accompanying veins run along the lesser curve of the stomach. There is an avascular area in the lesser omentum above this vascular arch that facilitates the dissection. It is not advisable to dissect between the arcade and the stomach. The gastric ulcer is usually located at the incisura, which may be difficult to localize externally. If the ulcer has been chronic, there is usually a patch of inflammatory tissue in the lesser omentum just adjacent to the ulcer.

Left Gastric Pedicle

The left gastric pedicle is located about two thirds up along the lesser curve. It is seldom necessary to dissect out this vessel unless operating for cancer or in a high lesser-curve ulcer. There is usually an accompanying large vein and several smaller vessels around it.

Duodenal–jejunal Junction

The identification of this point is important in selecting a loop of small bowel for anastomosis. This is best found by sweeping the transverse colon cephalad and anteriorly. A loop of small bowel is selected in the upper left quadrant and followed proximally to the junction.

Indications

The laparoscopic Billroth II gastrectomy is performed mainly for benign chronic gastric ulcer. The indications for surgery are as follows:

1. Resistant or recurrent ulcer disease after a suitable course of medical treatment (3 months)
2. Bleeding gastric ulcer that is resistant or recurs after endoscopic hemostasis
3. Perforated ulcer with minimal soilage
4. Palliative resection for cancer of the stomach

The patient must be fit for general anaesthesia. Age itself is not a contra-indication, but the operation should not be considered in patients with concomitant medical problems who are above 75 years of age. Previous upper abdominal surgery is not an absolute contra-indication, because the operation is still possible for instance after a previous cholecystectomy or repair of a perforated duodenal ulcer. The presence of adhesions does make the operation more difficult and is a contra-indication if there are also other concomitant medical problems such as coagulopathy.

Contra-indications

The only absolute contra-indication is a patient who is unfit for general anaesthesia. Presently, we do not perform this operation for cancer of the stomach if there is a chance for cure or benefit from extensive lymph node dissection. A meticulous lymph node dissection is presently still too daunting to perform by the laparoscopic route. Other workers have, however, already performed the operation for pre-pyloric cancer of the stomach. This operation would be reasonable for early gastric cancer or for cancer with metastasis where the gastrectomy is done for palliation of bleeding or obstruction.

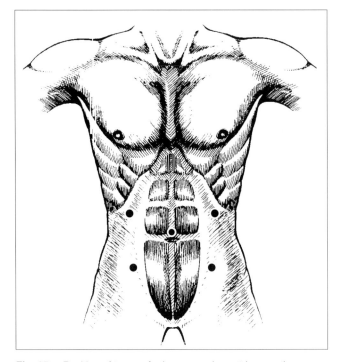

Fig. 15.   Position of trocars for laparoscopic gastric resection

Preoperative Work-up

The patient should have upper GI endoscopy and the ulcer should be biopsied. Standard preoperative work-up, i. e. hematology, electrolytes, coagulation, electrocardiogram and chest X-ray , are all that is required. Other investigations are ordered only if there are concomitant medical problems. Blood should be matched and available. The stomach should be washed out if pyloric stenosis is present.

Operative Technique

The operating room set-up and anaesthesia are the same as for gastroenterostomy. Five ports are placed in the positions shown in Fig. 15. All ports are 12 mm, except the central camera port, which is 10 mm.

Mobilization of the Greater Curve of the Stomach

A diagnostic laparoscopy is first done to orientate to the configuration of the stomach and identify the surface stigmata of the ulcer site. If the ulcer site is not obvious, on-table gastroscopy is done to identify the ulcer site and also the site of the pylorus. The greater curvature of the stomach is then picked up with two Endo-Babcock forceps, stretched out and lifted anteriorly. The individual branches of the epiploic vessels supplying the greater curvature are identified, skeletonized, clipped and transected. In thinner individuals with less fat in the greater omentum it is possible to perform the dissection outside the epiploic arcade making use of avascular planes. It is then necessary to cut in towards the stomach only at the site of the stomach resection. The dissection is carried out about two thirds up the greater curve proximally and down to the pylorus distally. In fat individuals it is more convenient to take down the epiploic attachments just next to the greater curve of the stomach wall.

Dissection of the Duodenum

The first part of the duodenum must be mobilized adequately to provide space for a safe transection with the Endo-GIA stapler. To do this it is important to identify the vein of Mayo, which marks the pylorus. If this landmark is not obvious, the pylorus must be identified by gastroscopy and the site carefully marked by diathermy on the serosal surface. Small vessels at the inferior and posterior surfaces of D1 (first part of duodenum) are connected to the pancreas and must be carefully controlled with diathermy or small clips and transected precisely without tearing. The superior angle of the duodenum can be identified by dissecting through a window of lesser omentum and creating a defect through it with endoshears and diathermy. Once this is done a stapler can be positioned to traverse the entire width of the duodenum.

Transecting the Duodenum

To transect the duodenum safely, the Endo-GIA 30 stapler is positioned transversely across the duodenum so that both blades of the stapler protrude beyond the superior border of the D1. An Endo-Babcock forceps is used to pull the duodenum against the hilt of the stapler jaws (Fig. 16). Usually, one application is adequate, but some broad duodenums require two applications for complete transection.

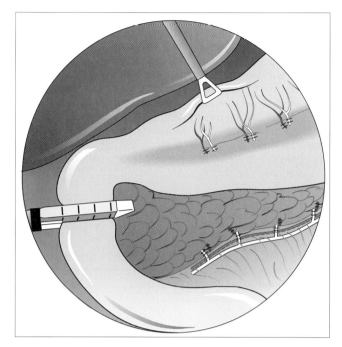

Fig. 16. Transection of duodenum with Endo-GIA stapler

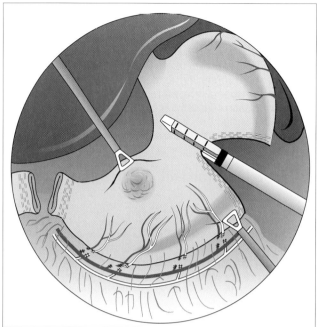

Fig. 17. Proximal transection of stomach with several stapler applications

Mobilization of the Lesser Curve

The ulcer usually causes an area of thick inflammatory tissue adjacent to it in the lesser omentum. This area is avoided and the lesser omentum is dissected through the less vascular tissue closer to the liver. More proximally it is necessary to transect the descending branches of the left gastric vessels. This thick bundle is best dealt with by transecting en bloc with the vascular Endo-GIA 30 at the point adjacent to the level of gastric resection along the lesser curvature.

Transecting the Stomach

The line of transection on the anterior surface of the stomach is marked with diathermy. The resection line should aim to leave out about one third of the stomach. Actual cutting of the stomach is done with the Endo-GIA stapler and proceeds with multiple applications from greater curvature to lesser curvature along the transection line marked out by diathermy. The 30- or 60-mm stapler can be used. The former is more ergonomic and easier to position, but requires three or four applications to transect the stomach. The stapler is inserted via a 12-mm port in the left upper quadrant of the abdomen. This port gives the best angle for application of the stapler. If the 60-mm stapler is used it usually has to be inserted in the left lower quadrant using a 15-mm port. This does not give such a satisfactory angle and there is a tendency to make the resection line too vertical resulting in narrowing of the stomach inlet. If the 60-mm stapler is inserted via the upper left port, there may be difficulty in opening the jaws, because the distance from the abdominal wall to the greater curvature of the stomach is too short to allow opening of the stapler. When making multiple applications of the stapler, subsequent applications are made exactly at the apex of the "V" of the previous

staple line (Fig. 17). Once the stomach is transected it is "parked" on top of the right lobe of the liver and only removed after the gastrojejunostomy has been completed.

Constructing the Gastrojejunostomy

The technique of performing a gastrojejunostomy after a gastrectomy does not differ from the one described in the preceding section on this operation. The anastomosis may be totally constructed with staples, partly stapled and partly sutured or totally hand sutured. Because the operation of laparoscopic Billroth II gastrectomy is fairly long, it may be easier on the surgical team to take the less time consuming option of at least doing a partially stapled anastomosis. Most operators will resort to a totally stapled anastomosis at this stage just to be able to get over with the operation. Hand suturing the anastomosis is facilitated by use of the Szabo-Berci needle driver set and is completed by continuous suture. Knotting may be avoided by using absorbable suture clips to hold the suture ends in place of knotting.

Checking the Anastomosis

The patient is gastroscoped at the end of the operation to check for anastomotic leaks and patency of the anastomosis. Both afferent and efferent openings must be visualized.

Extraction of the Stomach and Final Points

The transected portion of the stomach is grasped with a strong forceps and pulled through the left upper 12-mm port. Actually, the stomach can be pulled out through any convenient port. The trocar incision may have to be extended, but it is never necessary to make the incision more than 25 mm long. It is usually possible to remove the stomach through an 18- to

20-mm incision. The stomach is squeezed through the hole by pulling on it with a spiral twisting motion. The fluid is aspirated from the abdomen and the stab wounds in the abdominal wall are closed in two layers being careful to suture the fascia securely to prevent hernia formation. The wounds are infiltrated with long-acting anaesthetic (bupivicaine) to give immediate postoperative pain relief. Infiltrating the anesthetic under laparoscopic vision makes a difference in the post-operative pain profile. This was observed in a recently conducted randomized controlled trial in our department.

Perioperative Problems

Bleeding

Bleeding can be caused by the wrong choice of planes or the inappropriate use of the vascular Endo-GIA stapler. When mobilizing the greater and lesser curve it is best to choose avascular planes away from the stomach edge, rather than dissect close to the stomach across the vascular arcades. It is only necessary to dissect close to the stomach at the line of transection. It is tempting to use the Endo-GIA to take out large sections of mesentery, but these staplers often prove not adequately hemostatic, and much more time is then spent trying to control bleeding from the staple line. The most expedient rule would be to prevent bleeding from occurring at the start, and this can be done by meticulous dissection and control of individual vessels by ligatures or clips. Bleeding causes light absorption, which darkens the field of view.

Anastomotic Leaks

Occasionally, misfiring of staplers or inadequate suturing can lead to defects in the anastomotic line. This can occur at the duodenal stump or at the gastrojejunostomy. It is our practice to always test the latter anastomosis by performing gastroscopy and inflating the stomach after the anastomosis is complete. The test is performed with the anastomotic line submerged in saline irrigation fluid. Such defects present as a brisk stream of bubbling. The best way to mend these defects is to attempt intracorporeal suture. Therefore, the surgeon should always be familiar with laparoscopic suturing techniques.

Narrowing of the Gastrojejunostomy

When closing the common stab wound of the gastrojejunostomy with staplers it is possible to narrow either the afferent or efferent orifice of the anastomosis. This can be recognized at gastroscopy. The solution is to construct an enteroenterostomy just below the anastomosis. This can be done with the Endo-GIA or with hand-sutured anastomosis laparoscopically. A quicker, but more invasive, technique would be to make a small incision exposing the anastomosis site under laparoscopic guidance and construct the enteroenterostomy by open surgical techniques with either staplers or sutures.

Problems Encountered in Transecting the Stomach

The line of transection of the stomach must be marked out carefully so as not to compromise the inlet of the stomach or block off the esophago-gastric junction. This is a very easy mistake to make especially if 60-mm endostaplers are used. These staplers give little room for error, and because they need to be protruded fairly deeply inside the abdomen before they can be opened, they may make it necessary for one to use them through the left lower quadrant port. When used through this port the angle of transection on the stomach is fairly vertical, and one may transect higher up on the lesser curve than one realizes, thus compromising the esophageal lumen. The 30-mm staplers can be used through the upper left port giving a more horizontal and safer transection line. Furthermore, because each cut is only 30 mm, there is a margin for error and the operator can shift the angle of resection either up or down quite freely and adjust the transection line accordingly.

Malignancy in the Ulcer

Where malignancy is discovered in the ulcer after resection the surgeon is faced with a difficult problem. The best solution in such a situation is to perform a completion lymphadenectomy by open surgery to give the patient a chance for a cure. In most of these cases the cancer is early.

Results

A recent collection of data from 20 surgeons in 17 countries recorded 117 laparoscopic Billroth II gastrectomies. In 31 of these patients the indication was for gastric cancer. From February 1992 to June 1994 a total of 16 laparoscopic Billroth II gastrectomies were performed in our department. The patients were all adult males with ages ranging from 53 to 86 years (mean 65 years). The indications for operation were: gastric ulcer (14 patients), combined gastric and duodenal ulcers (1 patient) and volvulus of the stomach (1 patient). Of the patients operated on for ulcer, 13 presented with recurrent bleeding and 2 with chronic failure of medical treatment. In all patients preoperative endoscopic biopsies had excluded malignancy.

The operative time ranged from 2 h 30 min to 4 h 20 min. Mean duration was 3 h 20 min. With growing experience the operative time decreased. In the postoperative period all patients were mobilized on the first day. Fluids were allowed on the third or fourth day (mean 3.2 days) and solid food on postoperative day 4 or 5 (mean 4.6 days). Patients were usually discharged within a week (mean 7.2 days) and returned to work within a mean period of 2.3 weeks (range 0–7 weeks). The cosmetic result was excellent.

Complications

Two patients had minute foci of early gastric cancer at the ulcer edge. Both had had negative preoperative biopsies. Reoperation with lymphadenectomy was performed in both. Pathological examination showed negative lymph nodes in both cases.

In one patient immediate postoperative bleeding occurred from an uncontrolled vessel in the omentum requiring laparotomy. Another patient had an inadequate afferent loop on intraoperative endoscopy and needed an enteroenterostomy through a small incision. In one patient with a high gastrectomy, the gastro-oesophageal lumen was compromised by stapling and the operation was converted to open surgery.

There was one mortality: Our oldest patient developed a sub-hepatic collection and died during re-laparotomy from a lesion to the portal vein.

Discussion

Early experience with this operation has shown that there are certain important advantages to this approach. Firstly, the postoperative recovery is very impressive. Certainly, it holds the promise of less pain, less immobility, quicker alimentation, shorter hospitalization, less wound and respiratory complications and earlier return to normal activities. After an uneventful postoperative course, our patients are walking around on the first post-operative day, drink on the third, eat on the fourth and may even go home by the fifth day. It is the older patient who really benefits from this reduction in morbidity [6]. A similar advantage is seen in the experience with laparoscopic vagotomy for duodenal ulcer disease [11, 12]. The cosmetic appearance of the wounds, especially after 6-12 months have elapsed, is also remarkable. Most importantly, the patient is less likely to refuse the surgical option because the laparoscopic procedure is available. This is important in countries with a high incidence of early gastric cancer where benign ulcers frequently harbour foci of malignant change, and these patients may develop into advanced cancer if close surveillance is not maintained. Patient demand is likely to exert a strong demand for this procedure in Asia just as laparoscopic cholecystectomy has been driven by patient demand in the West.

The main drawback of this procedure is the cost of the endoscopic stapling devices. This is being overcome in many imaginative ways. One surgeon in China is able to modify existing staplers to fire about 10 times! The ultimate solution of course is the development of the laparoscopic suturing technique. Although still not surgeon friendly, new equipment now available makes the prospect at least worth considering. Almost all the anastomoses can be hand sutured if one is experienced with the technique. Presently, most surgeons are using a combination of stapling and suturing.

The other problem is the high degree of surgical skill required to perform the procedure. Presently, it is usually attempted by laparoscopic surgeons who are quite advanced in their development. The procedure using the present instrumentation is still fairly daunting for the average surgeon. Presently, it is only performed in about 12 advanced centres in the world. In our own experience of 18 cases, 16 were performed for gastric ulcers, 1 for combined gastric and duodenal ulcers and 1 for gastric volvulus.

The time taken for the procedure is fairly long, but well compensated for by the quicker recovery and shorter hospitalization. Our shortest operative time was 2 h 30 min, but operations have been known to go on for 5 h or more. Experience has shown, however, that the operating time steadily decreases with greater numbers.

The indication for laparoscopic resection has already been extended to operations for cancer. A group from Italy has submitted a paper on this subject for the World Congress of Endoscopic Surgery in Kyoto, Japan (June 1994). Early gastric cancer has also been resected locally under endoscopic control, and so have benign gastric tumours. With the availability of laparoscopic ultrasound dissectors it may become possible to do potentially curative resections for cancer of the stomach with wide lymph node dissection. The Asian experience has been that this form of wide clearance has improved survival significantly [10, 13]. New instrumentation and techniques have made laparoscopic Billroth gastrectomy and laparoscopic total radical gastrectomy with Roux-en-Y oesophagojej-unostomy reconstruction possible. Many laparoscopic-assisted operations are also being developed.

Presently, this operation is still at the stage of early clinical trial and can be considered reliable only for benign conditions. It may eventually replace open gastrectomy for benign conditions. Its role in the management of cancer of the stomach remains, however, to be evaluated. With better instrumentation and growing expertise it will eventually be possible to perform the wide lymph node dissection that is considered necessary to cure the disease. A major issue will be whether operative time can be brought down to reasonable limits, and whether the operation can be technically simplified so that even the surgeon with average experience in laparoscopy can perform it safely.

Conclusion

The totally intra-abdominal laparoscopic Billroth II gastrectomy is a significant step forward in the development of gastric surgery and has spawned a host of new "minimal access" approaches to gastric pathology. We now look forward to laparoscopic gastric surgery for cancer. The operation is still technically challenging and costly, but new innovations are very quickly solving many of the problems that were encountered by the early pioneers.

References

1. BILLROTH T: Über einen neuen Fall von gelungener Resektion des Carcinomatösen Pylorus. Wien Med Wochenschr 31 (1991) 1427.
2. CUSCHIERI A: Gastrectomy for gastric cancer: definitions and objectives. Br J Surg 73 (1986) 513–514.
3. CUSCHIERI A, HALL AW, CLARK J: Value of laparoscopy in the diagnosis and management of pancreatic carcinoma. Gut 19 (1978) 672–677.
4. DUBOIS F, BERTHELOT G, LEVARD H: Cholecystectomie par coelioscopie. Presse Med 18 (1989) 980–982.
5. ELLIS H: Billroth and the first successful gastrectomy. Contemp Surg 15 (1979) 63.
6. GOH P, KUM CK: Laparoscopic Billroth II gastrectomy: a review. Surg Oncol 2 (Suppl 1) (1993) 13–18.
7. GOH PMY, TEKANT Y, KUM CK, ISAAC J, NGOI SS: Totally intra-abdominal laparoscopic Billroth II gastrectomy. Surg Endosc 6 (1992) 160.
8. ISHIDA H, FURUKAWA Y, KURODA H, KOBAYASHI M, TSUNEOKA K: Laparoscopic observation and biopsy of the pancreas. Endoscopy 13 (1981) 68–73.
9. JAPANESE RESEARCH SOCIETY FOR GASTRIC CANCER: The general rules for gastric cancer study in surgery and pathology. Jpn J Surg 11 (1981) 127–145.
10. KOGA S, KISHIMOTO H, TANAKA K ET AL.: Results of total gastrectomy for gastric cancer. Am J Surg 140 (1980) 626–628.
11. KUM CK, GOH PMY: Laparoscopic vagotomy – a new tool in the management of peptic ulcer disease. Br J Surg 79 (1992) 977.
12. KUM CK, ISAAC JR, TEKANT Y, NGOI SS, GOH PMY: Laparoscopic repair of perforated peptic ulcer. Br J Surg 80 (1993) 535.
13. KITAOKA H, YOSHIKAWA K, HIROTA T, ITABASHI M: Surgical treatment of early gastric cancer. Jpn J Clin Oncol 14 (1984) 283–293.
14. MOUIEL J, KATKHOUDA N, WHITE S, DUMAS R: Endolaparoscopic palliation of pancreatic cancer. Surg Lap Endosc 2 (3) (1992) 241–243.
15. RAVITCH MM, STEICHEN FM: Techniques of staple suturing in the gastrointestinal tract. Ann Surg 175 (1972) 815–837.
16. WILSON RG, VARMA JS: Laparoscopic gastroenterostomy for malignant duodenal obstruction. Br J Surg 79 (1992) 1348.

Pancreatic Surgery

Critical Comments

M. Trede

Let me begin with two statements. First, Dr. Michael Gagner is to be congratulated on his pioneering of laparoscopic pancreatic surgery. He will be remembered as the surgeon, who took the "laparoscopic Whipple procedure" out of the realm of virtual reality, making it a matter of actual fact.

Second, most of us have "burnt our tongues" before with short-sighted comments on laparoscopic appendicectomy (when it was pioneered in 1982 by K. Semm in Kiel, Germany [5]) and laparoscopic cholecystectomy (when it was first described in 1985 by E. Mühe in Böblingen, Germany [4]).

I am not going to make the same mistake again when commenting on laparoscopic pancreatic surgery! In fact, it is safe to say that this may well be the future approach to pancreatic problems, when – and only when – a new generation of laparoscopic instruments has been developed and when a new generation of surgeons becomes skilled enough to use them.

Having said this, I do have some critical comments. First, there are general thoughts on the possible benefits of minimal access over open surgery of the pancreas. Alfred Cuschieri, one of the pioneers of laparoscopic surgery has formulated this very nicely in his State-of-the-Art Address "Whither minimal access surgery: Tribulations and expectations" [1]. He points out: "The likely benefit of minimal access surgery over conventional open surgery is dependent of the ratio of access to procedual trauma". In pancreaduodenectomy "the access trauma constitutes a relatively small component of the total operative insult. The benefit in terms of recovery, convalescence and short-term disability is non-existant. Moreover the risks of inadequate surgery and of tumor-cell dissemination by the total laparoscopic approach using the current technology are unacceptable".

Now I am going to comment on some technical aspects of Dr. Gagner's presentation.

Preoperative Work-up

Although I would agree that it is probably wise to drain obstructed bile ducts in jaundiced patients endoscopically before proceeding to pancreatectomy, I would take issue with the statement that successful biliary drainage reduces mortality to below 10 %, whereas it "may be above 80 %" if decompression fails and bilirubin levels remain high. To my knowlegde, there has been no randomized controlled study to support this contention.

The author states that laparoscopic staging enables one "to identify more than 90 % of unresectable lesions". But what of the remaining 10 %?! So far none of those experienced in laparoscopic staging (including laparoscopic sonography) have been able to dispense entirely with the findings that only surgical dissection and palpation – in particular at the mesenteric root – can provide [2].

Operative Technique

With a good preoperative ERCP, we have never had to resort to an additional intraoperative cholangiogram.

Intraoperative fine-needle aspiration is unnecessary since a negative finding is meaningless and a positive finding carries some danger of seeding malignant cells with the peritoneal cavity.

The most difficult part of any open Whipple procedure is the retropancreatic dissection, i.e., separating cleanly the uncinate process, pancreatic head and surrounding connective and lymphoid tissue from the large retropancreatic veins and superior mesenteric artery. In the laparoscopic procedure this step is of necessity simplified using two 60 mm catridges of a linear stapler. This is going to be less than adequate in the case of a malignant tumor of the head of the pancreas and it is going to be well-nigh impossible if one is dealing with chronic pancreatitis severe enough to be worth resecting.

The biliary and pancreatic anastomoses (the "Achilles heel" of any Whipple resection) are performed laparoscopically with "precise and delicate sutures". In the hands of the author "four to six sutures are positioned" for anastomosing the pancreatic duct with the antimesenteric side of the jejunum. I find it very difficult to place even three to four such sutures in a very widely dilated pancreatic duct – which is the exception in cases of pancreatic carcinoma. Futhermore, it seems an illusion to try to make assurance doubly sure by squirting fibrin glue over the anastomosis. This can never seal off a pancreatic leak. The fibrin will be digested away.

Postoperative care

I will not comment in detail on questions of postoperative care, such as routine prophylactic octreotide administration or leaving the nasogastric tube in place for seven (!) days – since these are measures that may or may not apply equally well to be conventional open procedure [7]. However, the author mentions that the average hospital stay after open pancreatoduodenectomy is 20 days (it actually is 16 days in our clinic), but he fails to mention how many pancreatoduodenectomies have so far been performed via the laparoscopic approach and how long the postoperative hospital stay was.

Comments on "Laparoscopic Treatment of Cystic Tumors and Cysts of the Pancreas"

Cystic tumors of the pancreas, even cystadenocarcinomas are among the few tumors of the pancreas with a reasonably good long-term prognosis – provided radical resection is performed according to established oncological principles. At present this is still done best and most safely by an open procedure. It seems superfluous to risk local recurrence by attempting removal of such tumors laparoscopically – not to mention the risk of implantation metastases in the abdominal wall.

Large, persistent and symptomatic pseudocysts are best drained by an open cysto-jejunostomy at the lowest point of the cyst – always including a generous biopsy of the cyst wall to exclude malignancy.

If one is anxious to avoid a laparotomy, i.e., to minimize the trauma of access, there are at least two far less invasive approaches that are safer than the laparoscopic method described above. The first is endoscopic cysto-gastrostomy (or -duodenostomy), which is an entirely endoluminal procedure that does not require the insertion of several percutaneous trocars [3].

Secondly, pseudocysts, especially if they are thin-walled or "immature" can be drained percutaneously by merely inserting a catheter under local anesthesia. Admittedly, the rate of recurrence may be high [6].

And then of course the purely expectant conservative approach is often rewarded by the gradual and spontaneous disappearance of pseudocysts, even if they exceed 6 cm in diameter.

References

1. CUSCHIERIE A, Whither minimal acces surgery: Tribulations and expectations. Am J Surgery 169 (1995) 9-19.
2. JOHN TG, GREIG GD, CARTER DC, GARDEN OJ: Carcinoma of the pancreatic head and periampullary region. Tumor staging with laparoscopy and laparoscopic ultrasonography. Ann Surg 221 (1995) 156-164.
3. MAYDEO A, GRIMM H, SOEHENDRA N: Endoscopic interventional techniques in chronic pancreatitis. In: M Trede, DC Carter (eds.): Surgery of the Pancreas. Churchill Livingstone, London (1993).
4. MÜHE E: Die Erste Cholecystektomie durch das Laparoskop. Langenbecks Arch Chir 369 (1986) 804.
5. SEMM K: Endoscopic appendicectomy. Endoscopy 15 (1983) 59-64.
6. SONNENBERG E van, WITTICH GR, CASOLA G et al.: Percutaneous drainage of infected and noninfected panreatic pseudocysts: experience in 101 cases. Radiology 170 (1989) 757-761.
7. TREDE M, SCHWALL G, SAEGER HD: Survival after pancreatoduodenectomy. 118 consecutive resections without an operative mortality. Ann Surg 211 (1990) 447-458.

14. Laparoscopic Pancreatoduodenectomy

M. GAGNER

Anatomy

The pancreas is a soft pink gland appproximately 15 cm long extending from the duodenum to the spleen hilum. The right lateral extremity from the duodenum to the mesenteric vessels consists of the head. Relations to the head of the pancreas are important for dissection. The lower part of the head has a posterior projection, which surrounds the mesenteric vessels and is called uncinate process. A groove between the neck of the gland and the head permits the location of the gastroduodenal artery. The upper border of the head of the pancreas is delineated by the first portion of the duodenum, and going laterally by the pylorus inferiorly and to the right of the mesenteric vessels, the third and fourth portion of the duodenum also come in contact with the transverse colon. Posteriorly, the head is related to the inferior vena cava, and its uncinate process lies in front of the aorta. The common bile duct is also posterior and traverses the pancreatic tissue for a short distance close to the second portion of the duodenum.

Preoperative Work-up

Among periampullary tumors, pancreatic adenocarcinoma accounts for 90 % of these tumors. Distant metastases are often found at the time of diagnosis. The most common clinical presentation is a mixture of weight loss, anorexia, jaundice, and sometimes pain and pruritus. Less frequently a tumor of the periampullary region may invade the duodenum and cause an ulceration with bleeding or an obstruction with vomiting. The jaundice is progressive and profound. Upon physical examination jaundice and weight loss are measured, and a palpable gallbladder in the right upper quadrant may be seen. Hepatomegaly, ascites, and palpable nodes are rarely seen upon examination and are the signs of unresectability. Apart from the biochemical profiles, which may reveal an elevated bilirubin, serum alkaline phosphatase, and liver enzymes, an anemia may be present on the complete blood count. A chest X-ray should be performed to eliminate pulmonary metastases. Often an inital ultrasound is performed by the referral physician and reveals some degree of bile duct distension with or without a periampullary mass. We personally prefer to obtain a CT scan of the upper abdomen to delineate the peripancreatic mass extension, look for metastatic process in the liver or peritoneal cavity, and if a portoScan is performed (intraarterial contrast into the mesenteric artery), one can determine if the portal vein is involved. An MRI scan may show approximately the same information and may not give additional information over the CT scan. The biliary tree should be delineated preoperatively to plan the operation. This may be achieved by an ERCP or a percutaneous transhepatic cholangiogram (PTC). However, ERCP is the method of choice, because endoscopy may reveal a duodenal or ampullary tumor that may be biopsied at the time of the procedure. Brushings and cytology of the lower common bile duct may be obtained as well. A cholangiogram and pancreatogram may also be obtained for anatomical purposes. During bile duct imaging a stent may be inserted and a decision for resection may be made later with a multidisciplinary consultation. If the patient is felt to be an operative candidate, a mesenteric angiogram should be performed preoperatively, because mesenteric artery or vein involvement means incurability (not necessarily unresectability).

In deeply jaundiced and malnourished patients a preoperative bile duct decompression permits an improvement of the hepatic, renal, and immunological function to sustain the operative trauma. The bilirubin response may be a prognostic factor. If there is a return to normal or near-normal bilirubin level, the mortality is less than 10 %. However, if no response of the bilirubin level occurs after decompression, the 30-day mortality may be above 80 %. Some surgeons may prefer to perform a diagnostic laparoscopy to exclude distant metastases and do a second procedure (i. e., laparotomy possibly with a Whipple procedure). It is our policy to perform a diagnostic laparoscopy first and continue the procedure if indeed the tumor is resectable during the same anesthesia. Warshaw and Castillo [4] from The Massachusetts General Hospital have found in a series of 72 patients that if CT scan, angiography, and laparoscopy were negative for tumor extension, resectability was 78 %. Peritoneal cytology can be done, but is not useful during the laparoscopy itself, because it takes some time to get the results.

Laparoscopic staging of periampullary tumors is completely different when one speaks about surgical laparoscopy. This involves doing a guided percutaneous fine-needle aspiration biopsy of the pancreatic lesion. Inspection of the body and tail of the pancreas is performed by creating a window between the transverse colon and the greater curvature of the stomach using cautery and endoscopic clips. A laparoscopic Kocher maneuver allows evaluation of the duodenal and vena caval involvement. Also, the ligament of Treitz is inspected for mesojejunal involvement; regional nodes in the periduodenal and pericholedochal areas are also sampled. Finally, one can follow a branch of the middle colic vein to the mesenteric vein with the blunt irrigation-suction probe to exclude portomesenteric vein involvement. Laparoscopic ultrasonography, if available with or without Doppler, can be used to evaluate vascular involvement. With all these maneuvers it is possible to identify more than 90 % of unresectable lesions. The list of indications and contraindications for this particular procedure is shown in Tables 1 and 2.

Table 1. Indications

Ampullary tumors
Duodenal tumors
Islet-cell tumors (head)
Distal bile duct tumors
Cystadenomas/cystadenocarcinomas (head)
Chronic pancreatitis localized to the head

Table 2. Contraindications

Liver or peritoneal metastasis, and/or positive regional nodes
Inability to localize the lesion
Pancreatic adenocarcinoma
Portal hypertension
Vascular invasion
Obesity
Coagulopathy
Previous extensive abdominal surgery

Preoperatively the bowel is prepared with 4 liters of GoLitely, and a cephalosporin is given on call to the operating room. Heparin is administered subcutaneously the day before, and 4 units of blood are cross-matched. The abdomen is shaved.

Operative Technique

There are three main steps in this operation: staging, resection, and reconstruction. The technique used is the same one used in open surgery with the modification of Longmire and Traverso, which is a pylorus-preserving pancreatoduodenectomy.

Staging

The patient is placed in a supine position with slight reverse Trendelenburg inclination with both legs abducted. The surgeon is at ease to stand between the legs of the patient for easier suturing and assistants are standing on both sides of the patient. The patient should be provided with an indwelling Foley catheter, nasogastric tube, a central venous line, and an arterial line for monotoring. The CO_2 is insufflated in the umbilical region with a Veress needle for a pneumoperitoneum of 15 mmHg. A 10-mm trocar is placed near the umbilicus and a 30 ° degree laparoscope of 10-mm diameter is inserted for a simple diagnostic laparoscopy.

If no obvious peritoneal or liver metastasis are seen, a second 10-mm epigastric trocar and a paramedian right and left trocar are inserted under laparoscopic vision. Instruments passed through these trocars permit a full evaluation of the tumor extension and the possibility of resection. Through the epigastric port a laparoscopic Babcock forceps grasps the greater curvature of the stomach. The camera is moved to the right paramedian trocar, and the surgeon works with both

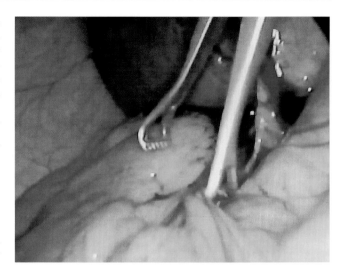

Fig. 1. Laparoscopic Kocher maneuver. Exposure of the vena cava

hands using the umbilical and paramedian left trocar. Both instruments are used to dissect the gastrocolic ligament below the gastroepiploic vessels and enter the lesser sac. Transverse branches from the gastroepiploic arcades are clipped, but the arcade itself is preserved, because this provides the blood to the pylorus and antrum. After a window of 10 cm has been created, the body and tail of the pancreas are inspected for possible seeding. It is also possible to inspect the upper part of the lesser sac by creating a window next to the left caudate lobe of the liver and assess invasion locally.

A laparoscopic Kocher maneuver is carried out by positioning the Babcock forceps on the second portion of the duodenum and lifting it upward and cephalad (Fig. 1). The dissection is then continued to separate the lateral border of the second and third duodenum from the transverse colon and vena cava. This frees the entire duodenal arcade and the posterior aspect of the head of the pancreas and uncinate process (Fig. 2). Any suspicious nodes should be biopsied with a laparoscopic biopsy forceps. When the common bile duct and common hepatic duct are identified (they are usually dilated)

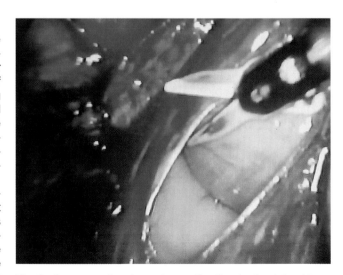

Fig. 2. Laparoscopic scissors transecting the duodenojejunal junction after full mobilization of the duodenum and pancreas superiorly

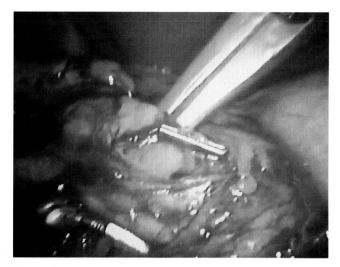

Fig. 3. Dissection of the common bile duct from the hilar structures using a laparoscopic right angle dissector

(Fig. 3), a cholangiogram can be performed directly on the anterior aspect of the duct using a 22-gauge metallic spinal needle percutaneously to better delineate the regional anatomy. Rarely, choledocholithiasis or tumor extension localized on the proximal bile duct can be found. If the gallbladder is present, it should be used for liver retraction to expose the liver hilum during the procedure and resected at the very end.

If diagnosis has not yet been confirmed, it is our policy to perform a fine-needle aspiration using a 22-gauge needle directly in the palpable mass or in the presumed area through the anterior head of the pancreas. This is easily achieved with a Franzen aspirating syringe apparatus used for cytology. Multiple biopsies are spread on the glass for microscopic examination. Finally, to complete the diagnostic work-up, a branch of the middle colic vein is identified and followed until it reaches the anterior and inferior aspect of the mesenteric vein (Fig. 4). A gentle blunt dissection with the irrigation-suction probe is used with sterile saline injected in the proper plane between the pancreatic neck and the mesenteric and portal vein (Fig. 5).

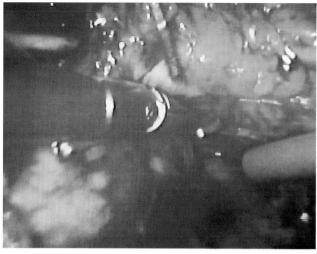

Fig. 5. Blunt dissection of the mesenteric vein inferiorly from the pancreatic neck superiorly using an irrigation-suction probe

Resection

The peritoneum covering the common bile duct is opened anteriorly and laterally so that it can be dissected free from the portal vein and the hepatic artery. Using a large curved needle, a no. 2 nylon suture is passed through the abdominal wall in the right subcostal area and passed under the bile duct to create a suspension with minimal retraction. The bile duct is transected at least 2 cm above the pancreatic border, or higher above the cystic duct junction using sharp laparoscopic scissors (Fig. 6).

Bile under pressure is aspirated and a specimen is sent for culture. The suspension suture is then removed. The next structure to be divided is the first portion of the duodenum, approximately 1 cm distal to the pylorus. The pylorus can be easily identified by looking inferiorly for the Mayo veins and by palpating a slight induration in the area. If there is any doubt, a peroperative gastroscopy could be performed and the pylorus identified by transillumination. The dissection of the gastrocolic ligament is completed and the gastroepiploic vessels

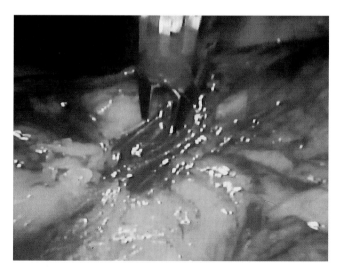

Fig. 4. Dissection of the middle colic vein up to the mesenteric vein

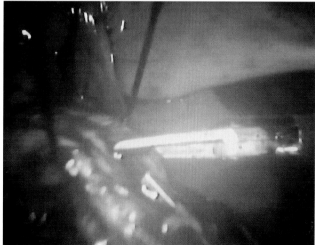

Fig. 6. Complete transection of the common bile duct using laparoscopic scissors after a bile duct suspension using nylon sutures

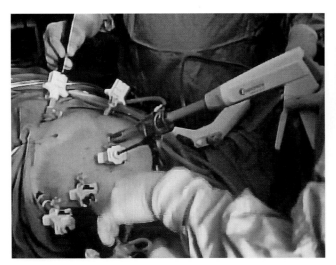

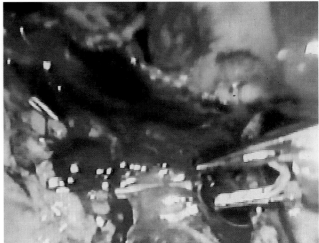

Fig. 7. External view of the six trocars' position and insertion of the endoscopic linear stapler for duodenal and jejunal transection

Fig. 9. Double ligature with titanium clips of the gastroduodenal artery

coming toward the gastroduodenal vessels are double-clipped with titanium clips. Then a right-angle dissector is easily passed under the pylorus to create a window of 1 cm and allow passage of an endoscopic linear stapler (Fig. 7).

Because a 60-mm stapler is used (Fig. 8), the umbilical trocar of 10 mm is exchanged for an 18-mm trocar by using a 10-mm plastic rod for dilation. Reducers from 18 mm to 10 mm or 18 mm to 5 mm must be used throughout the operation. Similarly, the duodenal-jejunal junction is transected as close to the proximal jejunum as possible with the same stapler, to the right of the mesenteric vessels. The proximal jejunum will retract in the retroperitoneum and will be freed at the ligment of Treitz. After transection, the gastroduodenal artery is exposed because the antrum of the stomach is pushed toward the left upper quadrant. The artery is dissected from the pancreatic neck, and more superiorly near its origin from the hepatic artery, it is double-clipped with titanium clips and divided (Fig. 9).

An endoscopic linear stapler of 30 mm with vascular staples may also be used. The pancreas above the mesenteric vein

and the portal vein is transected with scissors (Fig. 10), starting on the inferior aspect going superiorly. The inferior and superior pancreatic vascular arcades are controlled with a combination of metallic clips and cautery. The pancreatic duct is easily seen because of the magnification; it is left open and can be cannulated with a 5-F pediatric feeding tube. Once hemostasis has been achieved on the transected pancreatic planes, the uncinate process is resected from the mesenteric vessels approximately 1 cm from them using an endoscopic linear stapler with two cartridges of 60 mm length (Figs. 11 and 12).

The resected specimen is placed in a large endoscopic bag with a purse string and dropped in the lower quadrant of the abdomen for later extraction. Three forceps are needed to perform this task, one forceps on the lower lip of the bag, another one on the superior lip, and finally, one Babcock forceps to push the specimen into the bag. The closed purse-string suture avoids spilling of potentially malignant cells or gastrointestinal secretions in the abdominal cavity.

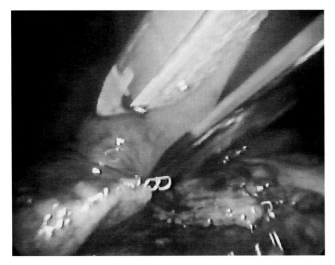

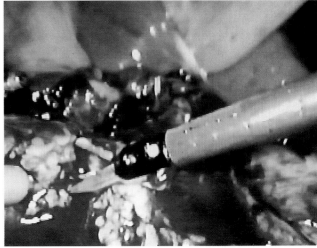

Fig. 8. Endoscopic linear stapler removal after complete transection of the first portion of duodenum 1 cm distal to the pylorus

Fig. 10. Transection of the pancreatic neck using straight endoscopic scissors over the mesenteric vein

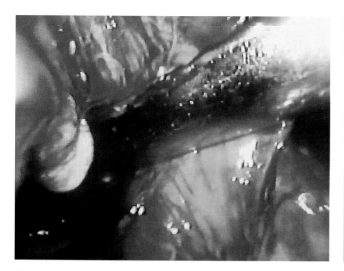

Fig. 11. Unicate process transection and stapling using a 60-mm endoscopic linear stapler

Reconstruction

Three anastomoses need to be created, and therefore a good two-hand technique with fast intracorporeal knot tying is necessary. The proximal jejunal loop is prepared for this task by further mobilization at the Treitz ligament, and several vessels are taken care of with the hook cautery and metallic clips. The loop has to be retrocolic, and a window is created in the transverse mesocolon for passage of the jejunum using soft bowel forceps. The reconstruction will replace the duodenum by performance of an end-to-end pyloro jejunostomy, an end-to-side pancreatico jejunostomy, and an end-to-side hepatico jejunostomy. However, the first anastomosis created is pancreatic (Fig. 13). Because of the need for precise and delicate sutures, it is easier to perform it with the jejunal loop still free. We have placed a stent into the pancreatic anastomosis in one patient. A 5-F pediatric feeding tube was brought outside the jejunal loop and through the right side of the abdomen. The anastomosis is created using 4-0 absorbable sutures with a semicurved needle, suturing

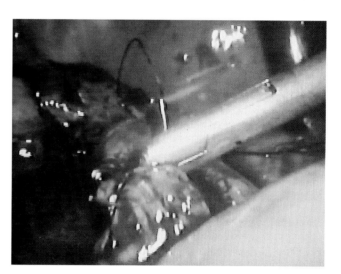

Fig. 13. Inspection of the pancreatic duct for size and consistency

Fig. 14. First anastomosis. The pancreaticojejunal anastomosis (end-to-side) is created with intracorporeal interrupted absorbable sutures

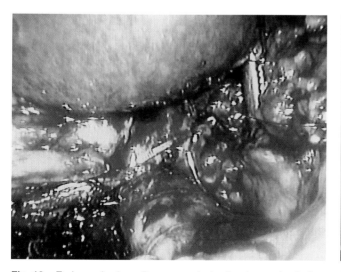

Fig. 12. Endoscopic view after pancreatoduodenal resection before reconstruction

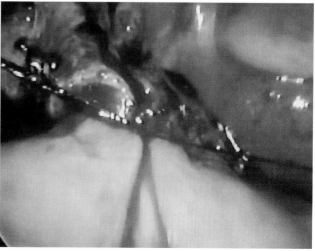

Fig. 15. Second anastomosis. The hepaticojejunal anastomosis (end-to-side) is created with intracorporeal interrupted absorbable sutures

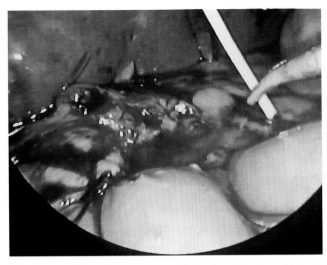

Fig. 16. Both anastomoses are sealed using fibrin glue delivered through a percutaneous catheter

the duct to the antimesenteric side of the jejunum, through the whole wall (Fig. 14). Four to six interrupted sutures are positioned starting posteriorly. We have sealed the pancreatic and the biliary anastomosis with fibrin glue after suturing (Fig. 16), which is delivered by a catheter passed through the abdominal wall. The hepatic jejunostomy is created in a similar fashion with intracorporeal sutures starting posteriorly. No stent or T-tubes are necessary (Fig. 15), and 6-10 sutures are placed. The anastomoses are at a distance of approximately 10 cm from each other. Excess of proximal jejunum and staple lines are resected, and the pyloric jejunostomy is created using a 3-0 absorbable monofilament suture with a curved needle. A posterior running suture followed by an anterior one is performed starting superiorly (Fig. 17). The gallbladder can be removed at the end, and the specimen is extracted via the largest trocar, which is the 18-mm port near the umbilicus. Two Jackson-Pratt drains are positioned below and above the anastomoses and passed through the trocar

sites in the right subcostal and right paramedian area. A feeding jejunostomy is inserted approximately 30 cm distal to the hepatic jejunostomy on the antimesenteric side of the jejunal loop via the left paramedian trocar site. The nasogastric tube is left in place and verified. All fascial wounds are closed with 2-0 absorbable sutures.

Postoperative Care

This procedure results in a major operative trauma to the patient and the postoperative morbidity is high (from 40 to 60 %). Therefore, care is extremely important. We routinely administer somatostatin analogs (octreotide 50 µcg) subcutaneously every 8 h to decrease the likelihood of pancreatic fistulas for a minimum of 7 days. Similarly, the Jackson-Pratt drains are left in place for 7 days or longer if amylase content in the drain fluid is five times greater than normal. The nasogastric tube also remains for 7 days. On the seventh postoperative day gastrografin swallow is performed to exclude an anastomotic leak at any of the three anastomoses. If no leaks are apparent, the nasogastric tube is removed and a liquid diet is started. The feeding jejunostomy is used from day 3 or 4 on and increased progressively. Total parenteral nutrition was administered in the first patient because we had omitted placement of jejunostomy. Antibiotics are usually given for 5-7 days (cephalosporin). H_2-blockers are administered intravenously postoperatively to prevent anastomotic jejunal ulcers. Prophylaxis of deep vein thrombosis is initiated preoperatively by using heparin subcutaneously and maintained until the patient is fully ambulatory. Serum glucose is checked frequently intraoperatively and postoperatively at least every 6 h, and an insulin drip may be necessary especially during nutritional support. Pulmonary physiotherapy should be aggressive in order to decrease the incidence of atelectasis and pneumonia. The pancreatic stent is left in place for 6 weeks, and most patients are able to manage this on an outpatient basis. In open surgery the average hospital stay is 20 days with a 30-day mortality of 5 %.

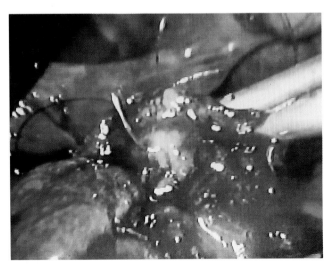

Fig. 17. Third anastomosis. The pylorojejunal anastomosis (end-to-end) is created with intracorporeal running posterior and anterior absorbable sutures

Complications

The complications encountered are essentially the same ones seen in open pylorus-preserving pancreatoduodenectomy. The delay in gastric emptying is quite frequent and occurs in about 20-35 % according to different series. Sutures between the pylorus and the jejunum should not be too tight and the antrum-pylorus area must not be devascularized. The most feared complication is a pancreatic leak, which often is due to a leakage of the pancreatic jejunostomy. It is preferable to perform a mucosa-to-mucosa anastomosis than a dunking procedure, which invaginates the transected pancreas plane into a loop of jejunum. Therefore, the laparoscopic suturing must be meticulous. Alternatively, a drain or stent can be placed in the anastomosis to drain the pancreatic flow and decrease the pancreatic juice fistula. This is more difficult to perform laparoscopically than in open surgery, because the stent of 5 F in diameter has to be inserted into the jejunal loop, into the anastomosis, and sutured at the anastomosis for slippage prevention.

Hemorrhage is another complication that may be avoided by meticulous hemostasis during the procedure and corrections of possible coagulopathy. A biliary stenosis can be prevented by meticulous suturing between the common hepatic duct and the antimesenteric side of the jejunal loop. Interrupted sutures of absorbable material should be used.

A complicated postoperative period is often related to advanced age, a long operative time, and increased operative blood loss. Intra-abdominal sepsis is seen in less than 10 % of patients and can be managed by antibiotic therapy with or without percutaneous drainage of abscesses. Biliary leaks are often associated with a pancreatic leak and can be managed conservatively.

Conclusion

An obvious selection of patients is necessary in order to decrease the likelihood of complications and to assure a successful operation. It should be performed by an experienced team of surgeons in both advanced laparoscopy and hepatopancreatic biliary surgery. This should be evident if the 30-day mortality of open Whipple operation is below 5 %. Because our policy is to perform a laparoscopic staging procedure on all potential candidates for a Whipple operation (after negative CT scan and angiogram), the laparoscopic mobilization will usually give a gradual experience to the laparoscopic surgeon to become confident one day that he can indeed perform the operation. Now that we have shown that the procedure is technically feasible in several patients, we should ask if it is desirable. Is it oncologically sound? More data need to be collected and larger series of patients are necessary to answer these questions. Maybe this intervention will be further developed and the technique may improve with new instrumentation. Also, the indications may become more precise. Whether in the future the extensive gastrointestinal reconstruction will cause such an internal trauma and stress that it will overcome the benefit of laparoscopy itself still needs to be evaluated.

References

1. ALTIMARI A, ARANHA GV, GREENLEE HB, PRINZ RA: Results of cystoduodenostomy for treatment of pancreatic pseudocysts. Ann Surg 52 (1986) 438-441.
2. ARANKA JV, PRINZ RA, ESQUERRA AC, GREENLEE HB: The nature and course of cystic pancreatic lesions diagnosed by ultrasound. Arch Surg 118 (1983) 486-488.
3. CAMERON JL: Solid and papillary epithelial neoplasms of the pancreas. Surg 108 (1990) 475-480.
4. CREMER M, DEVIERE J: Endoscopic management of pancreatic cysts and pseudocysts. Gastrointest Endosc 32 (1986) 367-368.
5. CROSS RA, WAY LW: Acute and chronic pseudocysts are different. Am J Surg 142 (1981) 660-663.
6. GAGNER M: La pancréatectomie distale par laparoscopie pour insulinomes. Réunion des endocrinologues de l'Université de Montréal, Hôpital Sacre-Coeur, Montréal, 5 avril 1993.
7. GAGNER M: Laparoscopic duodenopancreatectomy. In: Steichen F, Welter R (eds.): Minimally invasive surgery and technology. Quality Medical Publishing, St. Louis (1994) 192-199.
8. GAGNER M: Laparoscopic transgastric cystogastrostomy for pancreatic pseudocyst. Surg Endosc 8 (3) (1994) 239.
9. KARAVIAS T, DOLLINGER P, HÄRING R: Cystogastrostomy in the treatment of pancreatic pseudocysts. In: Beger HG, Bücher M, Malfertheiner P (eds.): Standards in pancreatic surgery. Springer, Berlin Heidelberg New York (1993) 540-543.
10. KERLIN DL, FREY CF, BODAI BI, TWOMREY PL, RUEBNER B.: Cystic neoplasms of the pancreas. Surg Gynecol Obstet 165 (1987) 475-478.
11. KOZAREK RA, BRAY KO, HARLEN J, SANOWSKI A, CINTORA I, KOVAC A: Endoscopic drainage of pancreatic pseudocysts. Gastrointest Endosc 31 (1985) 322-328.
12. NIELSEN OS: Bleeding after pancreatic cystogastrostomy. Acta Chir Scand 145 247-249.
13. WANDROWSKI KB, SOUTHERN JF, PINS MR, COMPUTOR CC, WARSHAW AL: Cyst fluid analysis in the differential diagnosis of pancreatic cysts. A comparison of pseudocysts, serous cystadenomas, mucinous cystic neoplasms, and mucinous cystadenocarcinomas. Ann Surg 217 (1993) 41-47.
14. WANEN WD, MARSH W, SANDUSKY W: An appraisal of surgical procedures for pancreatic pseudocyst. Ann Surg 147 (1958) 903-920.
15. WARSHAW AL, FERNANDEZ-DEL CASTILLO C: Laparoscopy in preoperative diagnosis and staging for gastrointestinal cancers. In: Zucker K (ed.): Surgical laparoscopy. Quality Medical Publishing, St. Louis (1991) 101-114.
16. WARSHAW AL, RUTLEDGE PL: Cystic tumors mistaken for pancreatic pseudocysts. Ann Surg 205 (1987) 393-398.
17. WAY L, LEGHAHA P, MORI T: Laparoscopic pancreatic cystogastrostomy. The first operation in the new field of intraluminal laparoscopic surgery. Surg Endosc 8 (3) (1994) 235.

15. Laparoscopic Treatment of Cystic Tumors and Cysts of the Pancreas

M. GAGNER

Introduction

Cystic tumors of the pancreas are rare and represent less than 1% of exocrine pancreatic malignancies. They are classified into serous or mucinous cystadenoma or cystadenocarcinoma [10], cystic papillary tumors and mucinous ductal dilatation. They must be differentiated from pseudocysts as the treatment is a different one [16]. Pancreatic pseudocysts have no wall, and no epithelial outline, and a connection with the pancreatic duct is suspected. They are usually encountered after a pancreatitis and tend to regress spontaneously within 6 weeks [5]. Whereas true cystic tumors require resection, symptomatic pseudocysts only need drainage. The use of diagnostic laparoscopy permits classification of the cystic tumor, exclusion of distant intra-abdominal metastasis, and evaluation of local resectability [7, 8,15].

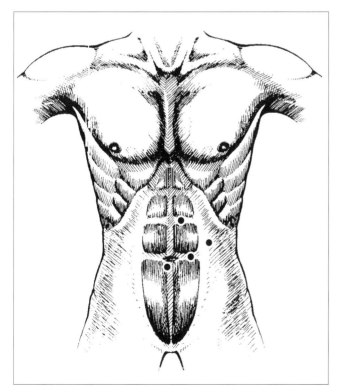

Fig. 1. Trocar placement for laparoscopic left-side pancreatectomy

Indications

The indication for laparoscopy, which in the first step will always be diagnostic, is given by the presence of a cystic tumor of the pancreas. In some cases the histological diagnosis may have been assessed preoperatively by percutaneous or endoscopic puncture. Laparoscopy may not be recommendable in patients who have been submitted to extensive abdominal surgery previously, because the adhesions may render the procedure quite time-consuming and difficult. Portal hypertension associated with an uncorrectable coagulation disorder are also to be considered a relative contraindication.

Preoperative Work-up

The preoperative work-up includes patient history, clinical examination, and laboratory tests. Percutaneous ultrasonography, CT scan of the upper abdomen, and endoscopy of the upper gastrointestinal tract should be routinely obtained. If available, endoluminal ultrasound is helpful for evaluation of infiltration into adjacent organs. For imaging of the biliopancreatic ductal system, ERCP should be performed. A preoperative mesenteric angiogram is also obtained.

Left-side Pancreatectomy

Operative Technique

The patient is placed on his right side and a pneumoperitoneum is created by insufflation with the Veress needle in the left upper quadrant of the abdomen 2 cm below the left costal margin. Four 11-mm trocars are inserted in the left abdomen as described in Figure 1.

The cystic lesion can be punctured under laparoscopic visual control for cytological analysis and assessment of CA 19-9. A biopsy can be taken for histological examination to ascertain the cystadenomatous tumor.

After extensive diagnostic laparoscopy with a 30° laparoscope, the retrogastric space is explored. A 10-mm Babcock forceps is introduced to grasp the lower side of the greater curvature, lift it up, and push it cephalad. The gastrocolic ligament is opened with a dissector and scissors, the vascular structures being transected between titanium clips. A space about 8-10 cm wide is created for exploration of the pancreatic corpus and cauda. Depending on the localization of the

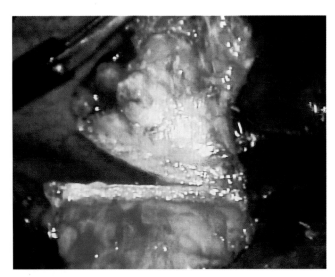

Fig. 2. Left-side resection with linear stapler

cystic tumor, a resection can be performed. We prefer a distal pancreatic resection, preserving the spleen.

Dissection starts on the inferior edge of the pancreatic cauda, which is mobilized from the splenic artery and vein. A forceps that can be bent at the tip is very useful for dissection of the transverse pancreatic vessels, which must be ligated. For good visualization of the pancreatic cauda, the left colonic angle and splenocolic ligament must be mobilized. Dissection in this area must be carried out with extreme care. In case of a hemorrhage from the splenic artery or vein, these vessels must be ligated. This can be done safely as the spleen is sufficiently vascularized by the short gastric and gastroepiploic vessels.

The pancreas is transected with a laparoscopic stapler (Fig. 2) of 30 mm (diameter 12 mm) or 60 mm (diameter 18 mm). Thereby the pancreatic duct is safely closed, but the application of the stapler may cause bleeding from the superior pancreatic vascular arcades, which then must be ligated separately. The resected specimen is placed into a bag measuring 10 x 10 cm and extracted by slightly enlarging the trocar incision used for the stapler. After thorough irrigation of the abdominal cavity and control of hemostasis, a drainage is left in place near the plane of resection of the pancreas.

Postoperative Management

Oral intake can be started much earlier after left-side gastric resection than after pancreatoduodenectomy, because no gastrointestinal reconstruction is necessary. The nasogastric tube is removed on the first postoperative day, liquids are given and gradually increased up to a normal diet. The patients are mobilized from the first postoperative day on.

Results

Our experience with laparoscopic surgery is still quite limited. Thus far we have performed three laparoscopic distal pancreatic resections. The data concerning these patients are presented in Table 1. In one patient with serous cystadenocarcinoma, we added a leftside adrenalectomy and cholecys-

tectomy during the same procedure. This patient developed an abscess that required percutaneous drainage on the 30th postoperative day.

Table 1. Laparoscopic distal pancreatic resections

Indication	Age (years)/ gender	Operative time (h)	Postoperative hospital stay (days)
Insulinoma	33/F	3.5	3
Insulinoma	30/F	4	4
Serous cyst adenocarcinoma	70/M	5	7

Laparoscopic transgastric cystogastrostomy

Two different techniques have been evaluated. For the first technique a diagnostic laparoscopy was performed through the umbilical trocar. Two additional trocars were placed to expose the pancreas in the retrogastric space. An intraoperative duodenoscopy was performed for endoscopic creation of the cystogastrostomy. An endoprosthesis or drain could be left in place especially when the posterior wall of the stomach was not visibly bulging anywhere. Laparoscopic control allows performance of the anastomosis under visual guidance and maneuver the pseudocyst as necessary (Fig. 3).

The results of this technique, which we tried in five patients, were quite deceiving: three times a conversion to open surgery was necessary because of the inability to create a safe

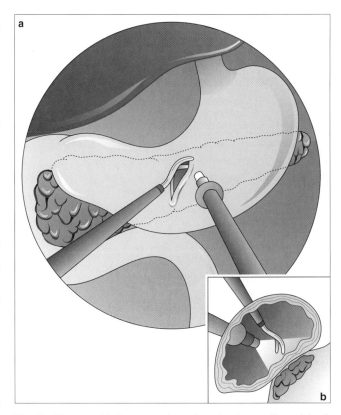

Fig. 3. Transgastric laparoscopic cystogastrostomy with endoluminal trocars

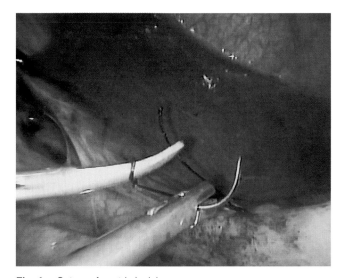

Fig. 4. Suture of gastric incisions

anastomosis between the posterior wall of the stomach and the anterior part of the pseudocyst. In two patients the pseudocyst collapsed after puncture and could no longer be adequately cannulated for the anastomosis. Because of these poor results, we abandoned this method.

The second technique was a transgastric cystogastrostomy that was realized intraluminally with special RED (Radial Expanding Dilators, InnerDyne, California) trocars [7, 8]. These trocars are provided with a balloon at the tip to fix them in the stomach so that an endoluminal laparoscopic procedure can be performed with two or three additional trocars [17]. The trocars are available with a diameter of 5 and 7 mm and therefore do not allow the use of a clip applicator or stapling device. They cause only very small perforations in the gastric wall, which can be closed by a single 2–0 suture (silk or absorbable; Fig. 4).

The patient is placed in a supine position and a pneumoperitoneum is insufflated. Three trocars are introduced in the umbilical region (11 mm), left of the midline (11 mm) and on the left side (5 mm). The first endoluminal trocar is introduced in the epigastric area, above the pseudocyst through the abdominal and the anterior gastric wall. After taking out the trocar, the balloon is inflated and pulled against the gastric wall for fixation. Intraoperative gastroscopy allows placement of a nasogastric tube and insufflation of the stomach during the whole procedure. A 5-mm 0° laparoscope is introduced to visualize the posterior aspect of the stomach. A second endoluminal trocar is placed about 8 cm lateral to the left or to the right for the hook to the irrigation/suction device (Fig. 5).

The cyst is identified with the help of a long #16 or #18 needle, which is introduced percutaneously through the anterior gastric wall and under laparoscopic endoluminal visual control into the posterior gastric wall where the cyst is suspected. The aspiration of cystic contents confirms the localization and avoids accidental vascular lesion. A posterior linear gastrostomy is performed with the hook over a length of 4–5 cm. The contents of the cyst are aspirated and the cystic cavity is cleaned and explored. A biopsy of the cystic wall is taken to exclude a cystadenomatous tumor.

A nasogastric tube is left in the stomach, the balloons at the trocar tip are deflated, and the trocars are taken out. The gastric incisions are closed with single intracorporeal 2–0 silk

sutures. A Jackson-Pratt #7 suction drainage is left next to the anastomosis for 24–48 h. A liquid diet is given from the second postoperative day on and the anastomosis is checked with a gastrografin swallow.

Results

With this technique we have performed cystogastrostomy in six patients and cystoduodenostomy in another case (Table 2). There was no lethality and no complication. The mean size of the cysts was 16 cm (6–20), and the contents were clear in 75 % and necrotic in 25 %. One procedure had to be converted to laparotomy. The mean operative time was 80 min (range 65–110 min). The mean postoperative hospital stay was 4 days (range 3–10 days).

A CT scan of the abdomen showed complete regression of the cyst in 83 % of patients after 3 months.

Table 2. Laparoscopic transgastric cystogastrostomy Technique

Cystogastrostomy	n = 6
Cystoduodenostomy	n = 1
Conversion to laparotomy	n = 1
Mean hospital stay	4 days (3–10)
Mean operative time	80 min (65–110)
Cyst diameter	12 cm (6–20)
Cyst contents	clear 75 % – necrotic 25 %

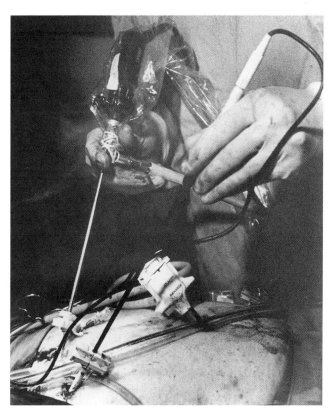

Fig. 5. Insertion of 5-mm laparoscope and hook through endoluminal trocars

Complications

The complications that may occur after laparoscopic pancreatic resection are the same ones that can happen after open surgery. The most severe complication after pancreatic resection is a pancreatic fistula, which can often be managed by percutaneous, radiologically guided puncture and drainage, but significantly delays postoperative recovery. Hemorrhage can result from insufficient control of the pancreatic vessels or a lesion to the spleen, and may require relaparoscopy or even a laparotomy.

Complications after pseudocyst drainage include leakage of the cystogastrostomy and occlusion of the anastomotic lumen impairing emptying and regression of the cyst.

Discussion

A cystadenoma can be encountered in all parts of the pancreas, whereas cystadenocarcinoma are usually located in the head of the pancreas. Still the localization as well as CT imaging cannot really give ascertain or exclude malignancy. Endoscopic retrograde pancreatography can show a connection of the cystic lesion with the pancreatic duct [3]. Analysis of the cyst contents helps to distinguish pseudocysts from benign or malignant cystic tumors [13].

Because the 5-year survival rates after resection of cystic tumors of the pancreas are around 60–90 %, the laparoscopic approach may be considered in certain selected patients.

The technique of endoluminal laparoscopic cystogastrostomy seems to be promising. The surgical principles that have been applied in open surgery for treatment of pseudocysts remain unchanged. Of pseudocysts measuring 6 cm or more after 6 weeks of observation, only 15 % regress spontaneously; therefore, the indication for surgical treatment is given [9]. In the presence of a portal hypertension this procedure is contraindicated, because the blind lesion of a collateral vessel may cause a very severe hemorrhage.

The first cystogastrostomy was described by Jedlicks in 1921 and Junes in 1932 [9]. This method was very popular until two decades ago when the potential risk of hemorrhage was mentioned [12]. Studies comparing cystoduodenostomy, cystoenterostomy and cystogastrostomy revealed similar results in the hands of experienced surgeons [1]. The rate of recidivism in open surgery is below 10 %. The endoscopic technique alone provides a success rate of 90 % but goes along with a morbidity rate of 15 % and a mortality rate of 4 % (16 A).

With careful selection of patients, some of them will probably obtain greater benefit by endoluminal surgery which allows a more precise hemostasis and gives the surgeon the possibility to realize an anastomosis of adequate size.

References

1. ALTIMARI A, ARANHA GV, GREENLEE HB, PRINZ RA: Results of cystoduodenostomy for treatment of pancreatic pseudocysts. Ann Surg 52 (1986) 438–441.
2. ARANKA JV, PRINZ RA, ESQUERRA AC, GREENLEE HB: The nature and course of cystic pancreatic lesions diagnosed by ultrasound. Arch Surg 118 (1983) 486–488.
3. CAMERON JL: Solid and papillary epithelial neoplasms of the pancreas. Surgery 108 (1990) 475–480.
4. CREMER M, DEVIERE J: Endoscopic management of pancreatic cysts and pseudocysts. Gastrointest Endosc 32 (5) (1986) 367–368.
5. CROSS RA, WAY LW: Acute and chronic pseudocysts are different. Am J Surg 142 (1981) 660–663.
6. GAGNER M: La pancréatectomie distale par laparoscopie pour insulinomes. Réunion des endocrinologues de l'Université de Montréal, Hôpital Sacre-Coeur, Montréal, 5 avril 1993.
7. GAGNER M: Laparoscopic Duodenopancreatectomy. In: Steichen F, Welter R Ed: Minimally invasive surgery and technology. QMP Inc. St.-Louis (1994) 192–199.
8. GAGNER M: Laparoscopie Transgastric cystogastrostomy for pancreatic pseudocyst. Surgical Endoscopy 8 (3) (1994) 239.
9. KARAVIAS T, DOLLINGER P, HARING R: Cystogastrostomy in the treatment of pancreatic pseudocyst. In: Beger HG, Bücher M, Mal Fertheimer P (eds.): Standards in Pancreatic Surgery. Berlin, Springer (1993) 540–543.
10. KERLIN DL, FREY CF, BODAI BI, TWOMREY PL, RUEBNER B: Cystic neoplasms of the pancreas. Surg Gynecol Obstet 165 (1987) 475–478.
11. KOZAREK RA, BRAY KO, HARLEN J, SANOWSKI A, CINTORA I, KOVAC A: Endoscopic drainage of pancreatic pseudocysts. Gastrointest Endosc 31 (1985) 322–328.
12. NIELSEN OS: Bleeding after pancreatic cystogastrostomy. Acta Chir Scand 145 (1979) 247–249.
13. WANDROWSKI KB, SOUTHERN JF, PINS MR, COMPUTOR CC, WARSHAW AL: Cyst fluid analysis in the differential diagnosis of pancreatic cysts. A comparison of pseudocysts, serious cystadenocarcinomas. Ann Surg 217 (1993) 41–47.
14. WANEN WD, MARSH W, SANDUSKY W: An appraisal of surgical procedures for pancreatic pseudocyst. Ann Surg 147 (1958) 903–920.
15. WARSHAW AL, FERNANDEZ-DEL CASTILLO C: Laparoscopy in preoperative diagnosis and staging for gastrointestinal cancers. Zucker K Ed Surgical Laparoscopy. St. Louis: Quality Medical Publishing (1991) 101–114.
16. WARSHAW AL, RUTLEDGE PL: Cystic tumors mistaken for pancreatic pseudocysts. Ann Surg 205 (1987) 393–398.
17. WAY L, LEGHAHA P, MORI T: Laparoscopic pancreatic cystogastrostomy. The first operation in the new field of intraluminal laparoscopic surgery. Surgery Endosc 8 (3) (1994) 235.

Colonic and Rectal Surgery

Critical Comments

J. A. COLLER

New operative approaches and techniques are frequently the result of breakthroughs in technological advances or transfers of technology. Sometimes these advances result in a procedure that is of such a compelling improvement that there is little problem with acceptance. Such an example was the management of colonic polyps by fiberoptic colonoscopy. This technological advance resulted in the ability to definitively manage a disease, the excision of a colon polyp, in a manner that was faster, cheaper, and far less traumatic than what was required by open operation. Similarly, two decades later, laparoscopic cholecystectomy was introduced and rapidly became the standard therapeutic modality for surgical management of diseases of the gall bladder. Once sufficient understanding and experience demonstrated the cost, comfort and physiologic benefits of this operation, it was only natural to project similar advantages for other abdominal laparoscopic procedures. However, as applied to the colon, it has become apparent that the laparoscopic approach in its current state of technological maturity has some major barriers to overcome.

Firstly, the colon is not nestled in one discrete spot within the abdominal cavity as is the gall bladder. Even when removing a very limited colon segment, a much larger dissection area must be traversed than for cholecystectomy. When performing laparoscopic cholecystectomy, the surgeon is, for the most part, converging from the work area circumference towards the central focus of the gall bladder location. By contrast, during laparoscopic colectomy, even for just a limited resection, the surgeon is working at, around, and behind the colon segment. If one is performing an extended colon resection or total colectomy, then the work area is the entire abdominal cavity. Trocar sites that are situated in an optimal location for one segment may be in poor position for another phase of the resection. Viewing angles that are in line with instrument position and video monitors may well be reversed or backwards at times during the operation. Such disorted manipulations are not particularly intuitive and require a longer learning curve.

Secondly, the redundancy and mobility of the colon often confounds the dissection process. As dissection proceeds, the liberated colon tends to get in the way of the field work. As with open surgery, the identification of structures within the mesentery is facilitated by placing the mesentery on traction. This may be difficult because of limited distensibility of a confining abdominal wall. When the lymphovascular pedicle is heavily invested with fat, and retraction exposure is limited by redundancy, it may be somewhat tedious and difficult to obtain vascular control at an optimal level. On the other hand, when removing the proximal transverse colon, the often tethered middle colic vessels limit precise dissection. These are nested within the peritoneal investments of the right margin of the lesser sac. When approached for the right side, the boundaries of dissection are somewhat ambiguous. In order to obtain a clean view of this area it is usually beneficial to approach the middle colic vessels from the left after entry into the lesser sac. Although this approach may be used during open surgery it is not as critical as it is for laparoscopic resection of the hepatic flexure and proximal transverse colon.

Thirdly, the potential for physiologic insult during colon resection, especially for complex prolonged dissection in the pelvis, is considerable. Pelvic dissection often requires extreme Trendelenburg position. When added to the pneumoperitoneum, this places further compromise on ventilatory compliance. Unless special attention is paid to respiratory function, the patient can develop a severe respiratory acidosis. The threat of this occuring can be lessened by limiting the time and depth of steep Trendelenburg to only that which is required and by keeping the pneumoperitoneum pressure at a minimal level, usually around 10 mmHg. CO_2 accumulation can be easily and inexpensively watched with the use of end-tidal monitors, allowing the anesthesiologist to make changes in ventilatory mechanics as appropriate. However, even with these preventive measures, certain patients will not tolerate prolonged procedures. In some patients with pulmonary fibrosis and compromise in gas exchange, the end-tidal CO_2 monitor will not accurately reflect the true state of acid-base balance. In such patients it is advisable to use intraoperative pH monitoring.

In order to minimize the likelihood of overextending sensible physiological limits, one should exercise judgement in both patient selection and surgical persistence. If the disease process is extensive, particulary if there is involvement with adjacent structures, the likelihood of laparoscopic completion diminishes. If, during the course of dissection, progress is stalled because of confused or unanticipated obliteration of normal tissue planes, it is usually advisable to convert to open dissection rather than persist with a technical tour de force that results in unreasonably long anesthesia.

Fourth, there is concern that the laparoscopic approach may result in an outcome disadvantage when performed for certain colon cancers. Conceptually, there is no obvious reason why laparoscopic cancer resection has to be less effective than conventional open resection. It is even possible that it offers some advantage from the cancer treatment standpoint. However, at the present time, there have been no comprehensive randomized studies that provide definitive insight into the role of laparoscopic surgery for colon cancer. A major multi-institutional study sponsored by the National Cancer Institute of the United States National Institutes of Health is underway to evaluate the treatment of colon cancer by laparoscopy.

The initial reports of cancer recurrence in port sites gives cause for concern even though there is poor data on incidence as compared to wound recurrence in standard resection. The possibility that pneumoperitoneum in itself may have adverse consequences must be considered.

The traditional ritual of manual exploration of the abdomen, although not previously subjected to the rigors of scientific study, not infrequently results in treatment change during open operation. One must consider that some findings will be lost from detection during the visual only laparoscopic approach. Whether an outcome difference will occur must be determined. One of the traditional concepts of cancer surgery is acquisition of a high ligation of the lymphovascular pedicle. If proximal and lateral margins are important in cancer surgery, then it must be ascertained that the laparoscopic approach does indeed contin-ue to at least meet these standards.

The adapation of minimally invasive surgical techniques has had a profound and beneficial effect on the management of gall bladder disease. Extension of these techniques to the management of colon disease has clearly indicated feasibility in many disease circumstances. However, there are unique technical complexities of laparoscopic colon surgery along unanswered issues that must be addressed for cancer.

16. Laparoscopic Colorectal Surgery

S. D. WEXNER, R. VERZARO, AND F. AGACHAN

Introduction

The first laparoscopic operation of the large bowel dates back to 1983 when Semm incidentally removed the appendix during a laparoscopic gynecologic procedure [84], but it is only since the early 1990s that laparoscopic surgery has been widely used to manage colorectal disorders. With the advent of minimally invasive surgery, an effort has been made to treat the entire spectrum of colorectal diseases laparoscopically with the hope that the patient could potentially benefit from less pain, shorter hospital stay, earlier return to work, and improved cosmesis as compared with laparotomy. However, unlike laparoscopic cholecystectomy, the advantages of laparoscopy in colorectal surgery were not immediately apparent and, at present, this technique is under clinical investigation and critical appraisal [34, 102].

Soon after its introduction it was apparent that laparoscopic colorectal surgery has a steep learning curve [13], requires more skill, and presents more challenging issues than does single quadrant laparoscopy. Many differences exist between colorectal surgery and all other surgical procedures performed laparoscopically. Firstly, one of the main indications for colorectal resection is malignancy, whereas other more common procedures, such as cholecystectomy, fundoplication, and herniorrhaphy are performed for benign disease. Moreover, laparoscopic "curative" resection for colorectal cancer lacks adequate follow-up and the possibility of a higher rate of locoregional recurrence and decreased 5 year survival exists [101]. Secondly, some anatomic features of the colon and rectum contribute to render the laparoscopic approach difficult. The large bowel is located in all the quadrants of the abdomen, and usually the dissection and mobilization must be accomplished in more than one region. To obtain the best operating field the surgeon often has to change the position of the camera, instruments, and even of the personnel. To aid dissection the mobilized bowel needs to be retracted; however, this maneuver is not easily accomplished within the confined space of the abdominal cavity, often resulting in long, tedious surgery. Due to the loss of tactile sensation, the site of the lesion is not easily identified, and intraoperative colonoscopy is often needed to ensure removal of the correct segment of bowel.

Other features unique to colorectal surgery are ligation of vessels and removal of a large specimen. Cholecystectomy requires division of the small cystic artery and the gallbladder, and can easily be removed through a 10-mm-port. Other procedures performed laparoscopically, such as herniorrhaphy or fundoplication, do not even require vascular ligation or speci-

men removal. On the contrary, mesenteric vessels are numerous, large, and run in a layer of opaque fat. To laparoscopically isolate, divide, and ligate these vessels is difficult and requires more time and/or money. Specifically, endoscopic vascular staplers, although expensive, usually provide rapid, safe vascular control. Pretied vessel loops are inexpensive, but require more time to be repetitively applied. Currently, existing clips are not large enough to safely secure most colorectal mesenteric vessels. In patients with inflammatory bowel disease with a delicate mesentery, these maneuvers can be extremely difficult, if not dangerous, even with modern technology.

Next, retrieval of the resected colon requires large ports with a consequent stretching of the fascia or, alternatively, a 3- to 4-cm incision, thereby limiting the cosmetic benefit. Negotiating the specimen through the wound may cause skin infection or tumor implantation, whereas attempting to remove the specimen through the anus may result in either peritoneal contamination or sphincter injury.

Fashioning of the anastomosis is another challenge of laparoscopic colorectal surgery. Significant morbidity and mortality are increased if anastomotic leakage occurs; thus, the need for a well vascularized, tension-free, and circumferentially intact anastomosis is mandatory. Achieving a perfect anastomosis in an intracorporeal fashion is sometimes very difficult as noted by Phillips and coworkers [69]. In their series anastomotic "donuts" were incomplete in 18 % of cases, a rate much higher than that seen in "open" surgery. Although it might be argued that no adverse clinical sequelae ensued, defect reinforcement requires time. Furthermore, contingent upon the patient's body habits, level of the anastomosis, and location and size of the defect, conversion to laparotomy may be required. Although conversion by no means represents failure, it is nonetheless frustrating to have spent numerous hours performing a laparoscopic anterior resection and have to then convert because of an anastomotic defect.

From this issue it is apparent that adequate training is needed for laparoscopic colorectal surgery. The Society of American Gastrointestinal Endoscopic Surgeons (SAGES) published the guidelines for credentialing and training surgeons in the art of laparoscopy. They suggested that after a period of traditional surgery training, experience in laparoscopy must be gained through diagnostic procedures, didactic courses, "hands-on" laboratory practice, and assisting surgeons already experienced in these techniques [88, 89]. Experience in other simpler laparoscopic procedures, colonoscopy, or both are essential. Moreover, expertise in "open" colorectal surgery is mandatory.

The American Society of Colon and Rectal Surgeons (ASCRS) has suggested that laparoscopic colorectal surgery should only be undertaken in a setting in which prospective data retrieval will occur [4]. This opinion is particularly important when treating colorectal cancer where a technical "success" may result, years later, in oncologic failure. An updated policy statement notes that although resection of benign pathology is acceptable, cure of carcinoma is still unproven and cannot be endorsed presently [5].

This chapter reviews and discusses common colorectal procedures – with the exception of abdominal perineal resection and rectopexy discussed in Chapters 17 and 18 – providing the reader with the main indications and contraindications to laparoscopic colorectal surgery.

Indications

Almost all colorectal surgical procedures have proven to be laparoscopically feasible [17, 69, 74, 83, 102]. Contraindications are presently relative to the experience and skill of the surgical team. As experience and technology increases, the use of the laparoscope in colorectal surgery will expand. However, several absolute contraindications exist and include advanced fecal peritonitis and unstable hemodynamics (Table

1). Relative contraindications include morbid obesity, cirrhosis, and bleeding dyscrasias or coagulopathies, severe acute inflammatory bowel disease, large abscess, phlegmon, and others (Table 1). Due to the adverse effect of the pneumoperitoneum, cardiovascular or pulmonary diseases can contraindicate a laparoscopic approach depending largely upon the surgeon's experience, patient's condition, and the proposed operation. According to the ASCRS [4, 5], malignancy should be undertaken only in a setting in which prospective data are obtained in order to prove the efficacy and safety of laparoscopy in treating colorectal cancer. For malignancy, the same oncologic surgical principles adopted in open procedures must be followed, and the procedure must be converted to a laparotomy if these principles are not satisfied. Basic surgical principles must prevail over the eagerness to laparoscopically perform a resection.

Several benign diseases have been successfully treated by laparoscopy [53, 73, 84] and currently represent the best indications for laparoscopic surgery (Table 1). In experienced hands the morbidity and mortality are low; the concern for long-term disease-free survival is virtually absent and the patient enjoys better cosmesis as compared with standard "open" surgery. In many centers laparoscopic appendectomy is now the procedure of choice to remove the inflamed appendix [70, 98]. Other minor operations, such as intestinal diversion, are now being laparoscopically performed and seem to be promising [30, 45, 95]. Although not yet proven, laparoscopic construction of an ileostomy or a colostomy may result in lesser postoperative adhesions, thus facilitating a subsequent reconstructive surgery. In the stable patient laparoscopic colonic repair for trauma can be a safe alternative to laparotomy. Table 2 shows the most commonly performed laparoscopic colorectal procedures as reported in the literature. Appendectomy represents the largest series due to its frequency. Colonic resections are the second most commonly performed operations, and in the majority of cases the indication for resection is neoplasia.

Table 1. Indications and Contraindications for Laparoscopic colorectal surgery

Indications

Benign	Malignant* (curative or palliative procedure)
Appendicitis	Carcinoma*
Diverticular disease	Other
Adenomas	
Inflammatory bowel disease	
Familial adenomatous polyposis	
Colonic inertia	
Trauma	
Volvulus	
Rectal prolapse	
Endometriosis of the colon	

Absolute contraindications

Carcinoma (for curative purpose outside of controlled studies)*
Septic Shock with Diffuse Peritonitis

Relative contraindications

Morbid obesity
Cirrhosis
Severe acute inflammatory bowel disease
Large abscess, phlegmon
Severe cardiovascular or pulmonary disease
Large abdominal aneurysm
Pregnancy
Previous laparotomy
Coagulopathy
Blood dyscrasia
Medical contraindications to laporoscopy

*Laparoscopic surgery for cure of malignancy should be undertaken only in prospective randomized trials

Table 2. Most common early laparoscopic colorectal procedures reported in the literature (1991–1994)

Procedure	No. of cases	Reference
Appendectomy	625	70
Appendectomy	465	98
Appendectomy	109	81
Right colon/transverse	10	69
Right colon/transverse	33	109
Right colon/transverse	22	77
Left colon	22	69
Left colon	22	109
Left colon	17	77
Anterior resection	7	69
Anterior resection	9	109
Anterior resection	5	77
APR*	3	69
APR*	1	109
APR*	3	77

*APR abdominal perineal resection

Equipment

Laparoscopy has made the operating room more crowded, full of monitors, devices, and new instruments. Besides a standard laparoscopy tray, other instruments are needed for laparoscopic colorectal surgery. A 10-mm, 0° laparoscope is useful for all colorectal procedures. Occasionally, a 10-mm, 30° laparoscope or a flexible laparoscope are helpful to achieve better visualization in difficult cases. Four or five 10/12-mm trocars are required for colonic resections because of the need to change positioning of the camera and instruments to access the different sectors of the abdomen. A 15- or 18-mm port is needed to allow the passage of the currently available 60-mm laparoscopic staplers, and a 33-mm port is required if the specimen must be retrieved through a port site. Several 10-mm-diameter endoscopic clamps are now available to reduce trauma to the bowel as compared with 5-mm clamps; they include Allis, Babcock, Kelly, and other adaptations of traditional grasping instruments. One must carefully and gently apply the clamps only to the section of bowel intended for resection. Alternatively, the clamps can be used in their nonracheted (open) positions for retracting other loops of bowel. An anvil clamp has been specifically designed to facilitate intracorporeal positioning of the anvil onto the circular stapler trocar, and is needed during left colonic resections. Stapling instruments are shown and described in Chap. 4. Other instruments that are helpful in colorectal surgery include the 10-mm-diameter rotating clip applier to ligate small vessels and the hernia stapler. The latter instrument facilitates mesenteric defect closure.

Preoperative Work-up

Preoperative preparation is the same as in open procedures. The patient undergoing laparoscopic surgery should be advised of the risks, benefits, potential complications, and available alternatives. An informed consent, including that for a possible laparotomy, must be obtained. Consent is also obtained from all patients for possible intraoperative colonoscopy. This latter precaution is taken in case the pathology cannot be identified by laparoscopic visualization or "palpation".

Patients scheduled for elective laparoscopic surgery should undergo a preoperative mechanical cathartic bowel preparation 24 h prior to surgery, typically with polyethylene glycol solution [100]. In addition, both oral and parenteral broad-spectrum antibiotics are administered (see Chap. 5). Patients are in the supine, modified lithotomy position in Allen Stirrups (Allen Medical, Bedford Heights, Ohio). The hips and knees are flexed gently at a maximum of a 15° angle. This position allows transanal access for both the colonoscopy and the stapling device. Moreover, the surgeon can stand between the patient's legs, a position particularly helpful during mobilization of the transverse colon. All patients must be intubated with an orogastric tube and a urinary catheter to minimize the risk of stomach or bladder injury, respectively, during trocar insertion. A steep Trendelenburg position is used to facilitate a safe insertion of the Veress needle. Elastic compression stockings are used in every patient, and subcutaneous heparin needs to be initiated in patients with an increased risk of thrombosis [34]. Ureteric stents are sometimes used to help in identification of the ureters. These stents are selectively utilized during pelvic dissection in patients wih severe inflamma-

tion or adhesions. Routine use of ureteric stents should be condemned. Insertion of ureteric catheters is an invasive, expensive, potentially morbid, and time-consuming procedure. The indications for stents must be the same whether the patient is scheduled for a laparoscopic or open procedure. The addition of stents merely to allow the procedure to be laparoscopically performed is unconscionable.

Operating Room Setup

The abdomen is prepped and draped in the standard fashion to provide wide exposure in case a laparotomy is necessary. Position of the surgeon, personnel, and equipment must be strategically planned depending on the type of surgery, patient's body habitus, and surgeon's preference. Generally, two monitors are placed toward the operating team and must always be in the line of dissection so that the eyes and hands of the surgeon work in the same direction. The surgeon usually stands opposite the lesion, changing position if the dissection takes place in different quadrants of the abdomen. Figure 1 illustrates a possible arrangement of the patient, personnel, and equipment in the operating room for right-sided pathology. A colonoscope should be available in the operating room if correct localization of the lesion is necessary. Also, a complete set of laparotomy instruments must be ready in case of rapid conversion.

Operative Technique

Major colorectal resections may be accomplished in two ways. In the majority of cases a laparoscopic-assisted technique is used. This means that the bowel is laparoscopically mobilized and is then exteriorized through a small incision to extracorporeally perform the vascular ligation, resection, and anastomosis. The other way is a complete laparoscopic approach. In such a case colonic mobilization, resection, and anastomosis are accomplished, by definition, in an intracorporeal fashion. In either procedure the first step is the same. To establish the pneumoperitoneum, the patient is placed in steep Trendelenburg position and a 1-cm incision is made just below the umbilicus and Veress needle placement is verified in four ways. Firstly, the surgeon should have a manual sensation that the needle has entered the peritoneal cavity. Secondly, an audible noise should be detected as the needle enters the abdominal cavity. Thirdly, a few cubic centimeters of sterile water are placed on top of the vertically held needle conus. By lifting the anterior abdominal wall, negative intra-abdominal pressure is created and the liquid is drawn into the abdominal cavity. Lastly, high-flow insufflation should result in a gradual rise of intra-abdominal pressure. A rapid rise in pressure or the appearance of subcutaneous crepitus indicate that the needle has been placed in the preperitoneal space. After the pneumoperitoneum is established with CO_2 to a pressure of 15 mmHg, the Veress needle is removed and a 10/12-mm port is placed through the 1-cm Veress needle incision. In case of adhesions from previous surgery, the incision for the first trocar can be done where it is convenient, or alternatively, the Hasson technique can be used [36].

A 0° laparoscope is then introduced and a thorough peritoneoscopy is undertaken to verify the diagnosis, assess other associated diseases, and, in case of malignancy, determine any metastatic dissemination of the tumor. To inspect the liver the patient is brought into a deep reverse Trendelenburg position so that the lobes of the liver are exposed. A laparoscopic ultrasound probe can be used. If the proposed operation is deemed feasible, all the subsequent maneuvers are done under direct endoscopic visualization. The majority of the laparoscopic colorectal operations require that the ports be interchangeable and, for this reason, all ports must be at least 10 mm in diameter. Port positioning should be tailored to each procedure and patient. The patient's anatomy, site of lesion, extent of the resection, and, most importantly, location of the incision or large port for specimen retrieval are all factors that dictate port placement. Standard laparoscopic instruments, for example, will not reach the pelvis in an obese patient if placed in the middle of the abdomen. If an incision is necessary to remove the specimen, one or two ports should be placed in such a way that the incision can incorporate both or at least one in order to reduce the number of scars [103]. An effort should be made to place ports where a stoma or a drain is planned. The ports must generally be close enough to easily reach the operating field, but far enough to avoid the so-called sword fighting of the instruments as they clash and obstruct each other. In order to improve cosmetic results, it is also important that the incisions for trocar placement are hidden in natural creases and folds, or made in the direction of Langers' lines. This can be easily done by marking the skin the day before the surgery with the patient sitting and standing to accentuate natural skin creases that disappear when the abdomen is expanded by pneumoperitoneum [94]. After a complete inspection of the abdominal cavity, any adhesions are lysed with the monopolar electrocautery. Additional ports are placed as necessary during the procedure. Generally, three ports are used for stoma creation, and 4–5 ports for resection and anastomosis.

The procedure usually begins with mobilization of a segment of bowel. This maneuver is accomplished by grasping the bowel and retracting it in a medial direction to facilitate exposure of the white line of Toldt. Dissection is then undertaken as in open surgery. During the mobilization of the ascending or descending colon, the ureters must be clearly visualized. Failure to identify the ureters is an indication to convert the procedure to laparotomy. Care is taken to avoid injury to the duodenum and spleen during mobilization. Meticulous hemostasis helps to obtain a clear view during mobilization.

If the site of the lesion is not easily identified after mobilization, intraoperative colonoscopy can be used to visualize the lesion and the serosal surface can be marked with clips. The maneuver is helpful to obviate removal of the wrong segment. Once the length of the colon to be resected is mobilized, the main vessels need to be ligated. Ligation can be done extracorporeally if a laparoscopic-assisted procedure is planned, or intracorporeally if the mesentery is too short or if a completely laparoscopic approach is planned. In laparoscopic-assisted procedures an incision is made to include one or two ports, the bowel is eviscerated with the mobilized mesentery, and the vessels are ligated in the normal fashion. The length of the incision required to extract the bowel is usually 2–4 cm, still much smaller than that required during standard open surgery. If an intracorporeal anastomosis is planned or if the mesentery is too short, intra-abdominal vascular division is mandatory. As in open surgery, division of the mesenteric vascular supply is facilitated by skeletonization of the vessels. Ligation is best accomplished with endoscopic

linear staplers with a vascular cartridge. However, contingent upon anatomy, vessels can be ligated or doubly clipped. Division and ligation by staplers is safer and faster, but it increases cost.

Once the mesentery is divided and the lines of resection are free of vessels, the bowel is ready to be transected. Intracorporeal resection and anastomosis can be performed with the help of endoscopic linear cutting devices (see Chap. 4). These staplers avoid peritoneal contamination during bowel transection, and their routine use has made laparoscopic colorectal surgery easier and more popular. However, expense is a limiting factor in many settings. The technique of intracorporeal anastomosis is described in this chapter, but it is too expensive and time consuming to be widely adopted. Furthermore, after numerous hours and many dollars in staplers have been spent, an incision must be made to deliver the specimen. Thus, completely laparoscopic right-sided procedures are presently illogical. Other techniques, such as the use of fibrin glue and other endoscopic staplers, are experimental. Technical difficulty in fashioning an anastomosis and the need for an incision to retrieve the specimen are the main issues that demand a combined approach.

Retrieval of the specimen can pose a problem, and presently the best solution is either a small abdominal incision or a large port. All specimens, whether benign or malignant, should be placed in a bag or withdrawn through a port or wound protector to avoid skin wound infection or tumor implantation. An attempt to extract the specimen through the anus [27, 69] after left colonic resections may result in sphincter injury, due to the unphysiologic anal dilatation [39]. Moreover, tumor seeding throughout the rectum can occur if a malignant specimen is delivered transanally. Tissue morcellators are another experimental option to avoid the need for incision; however, shattering the specimen may render the pathologic examination impossible.

After the specimen has been removed and the anastomosis has been fashioned, hemostasis is assured and the port sites are closed under direct vision using one of the port-site closure instruments if available. The trocars should be removed under direct vision to ensure that there is no bleeding or hematoma formation from the port sites. The final umbilical trocar is removed and the port-site sutures are tied. It is important to close the fascia after a 10/12-mm or larger port is used, because herniations have been reported [76].

Postoperative Management

The same criteria adopted in open surgery are used to manage the patient after laparoscopic colorectal surgery. Pain due to diaphragmatic irritation is treated with conventional analgesics. Patients will receive antibiotic therapy depending on the type of surgery performed. Many factors, such as preoperative morbid conditions, social conditions, and patient expectations contribute to determine the hospital discharge. The orogastric or nasogastric tube is usually removed at the time of surgery. The urinary catheter is removed after 4–5 days if a low pelvic dissection is undertaken, otherwise it can be removed earlier. The patient receives a clear liquid diet on the first postoperative day and, if tolerated, a regular diet on the second postoperative day. The patient is discharged on approximately the fourth to fifth postoperative day if an uneventful postoperative period has occurred.

The main laparoscopic colorectal procedures are described herein. It is evident from the previously mentioned considerations that as technology improves, indications and operative steps may change, and laparoscopic colorectal surgery will be easier and more widely used. Technology alone, however, must not change accepted surgical principles. Regardless of which operation is performed, fundamental surgical principles and basic surgical techniques must be followed as in open surgery. Maneuvers unacceptable in open surgery must also be refused during laparoscopy. Technical progresses must meet the criteria of sound and ethical surgery. If safety and efficacy is compromised, the surgeon must convert the procedure to laparotomy. Conversion to laparotomy must not be considered a failure, but rather sound judgment when taking into consideration that the meaning of successful surgery is delivery to the patient the best *short and long-term* cure with the lowest possible morbidity and mortality.

Resection of the Right and Transverse Colon

Laparoscopic resections of the right and transverse colon include the same surgical steps and technical problems; therefore, these two procedures are presented together. Indications to perform resection of the right colon or transverse colon are the same as for open surgery. A previous open appendectomy does not contraindicate a laparoscopic right colonic

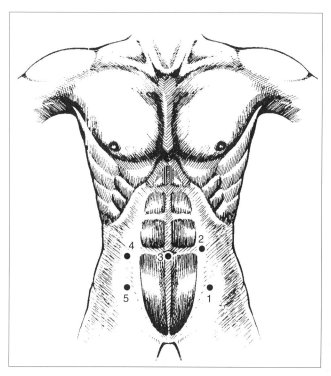

Fig. 2. Trocar placement for resection of the right colon and transverse colon. Ports 1, 2 and 3 are the only ports utilized for an assisted procedure. Ports 4 and 5 added only if vascular division and anastomosis are to be intracorporeally accomplished

resection, whereas a previous open cholecystectomy through a Kocher incision may render the mobilization of the hepatic flexure and exposure of the middle colic vessels very difficult and contraindicate laparoscopy if the surgeon's experience is limited. Preoperative evaluation and preparation of the patient do not differ from those utilized prior to conventional colonic resections (see Preoperative Work-up). The surgeon initially stands on the left side of the patient with a monitor on the right side. Another monitor is placed near the head of the patient on the left side to be viewed by all other personnel (Fig.1). The first assistant stands on the right side of the patient and a second assistant is usually located between the patient's legs (Fig.1). After establishment of pneumoperitoneum, a 10/12-mm port is placed through a 1-cm transumbilical incision. This incision can be made vertically rather than horizontally, so that it can be subsequently incorporated into the 2- to 4-cm transumbilical incision needed to exteriorize the specimen, thus enhancing the cosmetic result. Three additional ports are usually required for right colectomy or transverse resection. One port is placed in the suprapubic region to the right of the rectus muscle (Fig. 2) and another is placed midway between the umbilicus and xiphoid to the left of the rectus muscle (Fig. 2). This latter position avoids the falciform ligament [103]. The fourth trocar may be placed in the left lower quadrant lateral to the rectus muscle (Fig. 2) [103]. Positioning these ports lateral to the rectus muscle obviates epigastric vessel injury. Secondly, such a position is ergonomically superior for lateral mobilization and vascular control. Before starting the dissection, the laparoscopic surgical field must be prepared. The small bowel is gently retracted using a clamp or a retractor. Retraction is facilitated by rotating the table to the left. A steep Trendelenburg position is also helpful for this purpose. The cecum

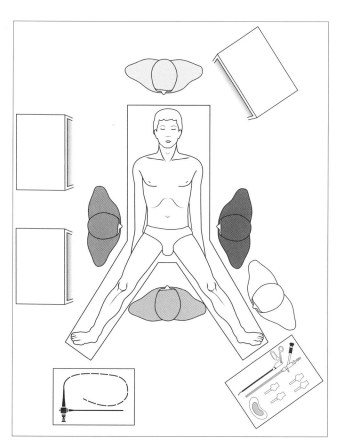

Fig. 1. Position of patient, personnel and equipment in the operating room for a laparoscopic resection of a right-sided lesion. The surgeon stands opposite the target organ

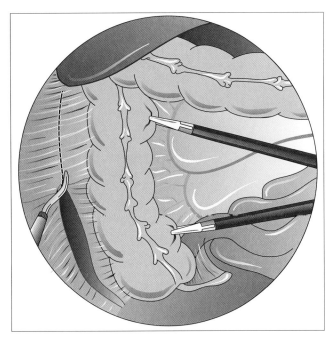

Fig. 3. The colon is retracted anteriorly and medially by two 10 mm diameter atraumatic endoforceps. The colon is mobilized from the retroperitoneum by means of a 10 mm diameter electrocautery scissors

must be mobilized first if resection of the right colon is planned. The terminal ileum and the cecum are gently grasped with a forceps to provide traction and countertraction while the surgeon divides the retroperitoneal attachments with a 10-mm-diameter monopolar electrocautery scissors. Retraction is facilitated by using one grasper through the left-sided port, and the scissors through the other left-sided port. Thus, the surgeon is "two-handed." After the cecum has been mobilized, the right colon is grasped proximally and distally and retracted medially (Fig. 3) thereby exposing the white line of Toldt. This avacular plane is then divided. During mobilization of the right colon from the retroperitoneum, the anatomic position of the right ureter, spermatic and iliac vessels, and duodenum are always verified. As in open surgery, peristalsis

helps to identify the ureter. In cases of severe pelvic inflammation, intraoperative cystoscopic positioning of the ureteric stents may be helpful. Such indications include recurrent ileocolonic Crohn's disease with a large right retroperitoneal phlegmon.

Next, the hepatic flexure is mobilized. This maneuver is probably the most difficult during right colonic resection because of the risk of duodenal injury. Reverse Trendelenburg position and tilting the table to the left can help in this phase to achieve a better view. The camera can also be moved from the umbilical port to a right sided port. The hepatocolic ligament is divided beyond the point of resection of the transverse colon. If necessary, clips or loops are applied at vessels around the flexure. If resection of the transverse colon is the proposed operation, the omentum is detached from the transverse colon dissecting through the avascular plane between these two structures. The dissection is then extended beyond the splenic flexure. After the entire segment of bowel to be resected has been mobilized, the mesenteric vascular supply is divided. If an extracorporeal anastomosis is planned (a lapar-

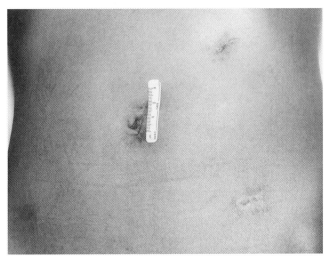

Fig. 5. Postoperative appearance of a patient after laparoscopic-assisted right colon resection

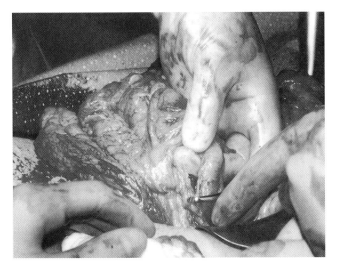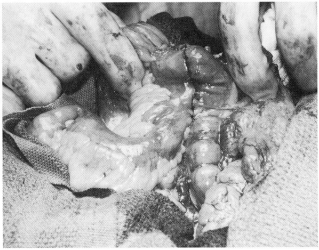

Figs. 4 A, B. **A.** The abdominal colon is eviscerated through a small incision. **B.** The anastomosis has been created

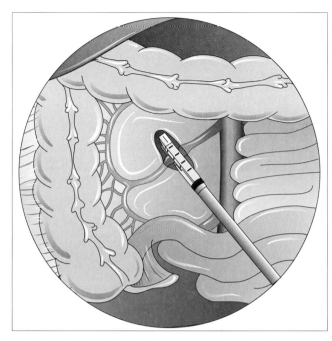

Fig. 6. The ileocolic artery is divided at its origin using an endoscopic linear-cutter stapler

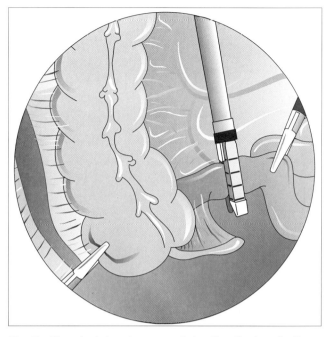

Fig. 7. Two stapled ends are created cutting the bowel with an endoscopic stapler

oscopic-assisted resection), the segment of bowel along with its vascular supply is eviscerated through an incision as small as 2–3 cm (Figs. 4A and B). The incision can easily be made by enlarging the incision for the transumbilical port. Others [43] use an incision made in the right upper quadrant or in the midline. We prefer to enlarge the transumbilical incision to achieve a better cosmesis (Fig. 5). Once the colonic segment has been eviscerated, vascular ligation, resection, and anastomosis can be done quickly, safely, and in a cost-effective extracorporeal manner. Once the anastomosis and mesenteric defect repair have been performed, the bowel is returned into the abdomen. The incision is sutured and pneumoperitoneum is reestablished. The abdomen is inspected for hemostasis and for anastomotic position.

If the mesentery is too short to be extracted, vascular ligation and resection must be accomplished intracorporeally. Such additional laparoscopic work requires two additional 10–12 mm ports. These extra ports are placed on the patient's left side in a mirror-image configuration to the two rigth-sided ports (Fig. 2). As in open surgery, vascular ligation is facilitated by skeletonization of the vessels in the mesenteric fat. For this purpose the mesentery is divided carefully by the electrocautery scissors. Some authors [97] suggest the use of a second laparoscope behind the colon to transilluminate the mesentery and identify the vessels. However, the cost and need for an extra port seem unjustifiable. The ileocolic artery is usually easily recognized, and it is doubly clipped or doubly ligated. The right colic artery and the right branch of the middle colic artery are also ligated by clips or endoloops. If the entire transverse colon must be transected, the middle colic artery must be divided at its origin. The veins are usually ligated separately. Sometimes, it is helpful to divide the vessels with an endostapler containing a vascular cartridge (Fig. 6). In case of potentially malignant neoplasm, these major vessels must be ligated at their origins. Once the vessels are divided and the lines of resection are free of vascular attachments, the bowel can be transected.

If a completely intracorporeal procedure is desired, the bowel is then transected distally and proximally by the 60-mm endoscopic stapler (Fig. 7), thus creating two stapled ends of bowel. Two to three ports are inserted to facilitate suction irrigation, and additional clamps to limit contamination during bowel manipulation. The bowel ends are then grasped with Babcock clamps and the antimesenteric corners of each staple line are excised. The two ends of the bowel are aligned and a side-to-side (functional end-to-end) anastomosis is then created with a third application of the 60-mm stapler. The cartridge side of the stapler is placed in the colonic lumen and the anvil blade is placed into the small bowel lumen (Fig. 8A). Using a 60-mm stapler, a single application usually adequate. The cut edges of the bowel are then grasped with Babcock clamps and the anastomosis is inspected for hemostasis. The lumen can be irrigated with saline, providone iodine, or both. The opposing cut edges of the bowels are held with Babcock clamps and the enterotomy is closed with another firing of the endoscopic stapler (Fig. 8B). Closure of the mesenteric defect can be done by suture or by the application of hernia clips [14]. The resected specimen is placed in a bag and removed through a large port (33 mm) or through a small incision. The abdomen is inspected and the hemostasis is assured. The anastomosis must be free of tension and well vascularized. The pneumoperitoneum is released and the incisions are closed.

The laparoscopic-assisted right colectomy with extracorporeal anastomosis is a relatively safe procedure with only a few complications reported in the literature, which include bleeding [101], anastomotic leaks [34, 55] and deep venous thrombosis [34]. This technique is obviously faster and more cost-effective than is the completely laparoscopic procedure with intracorporeal anastomosis. The laparoscopic-assisted approach is also helpful when the resection is performed in patients with Crohn's disease. In such a case intracorporeally handling the fragile mesentery can be very difficult, if not haz-

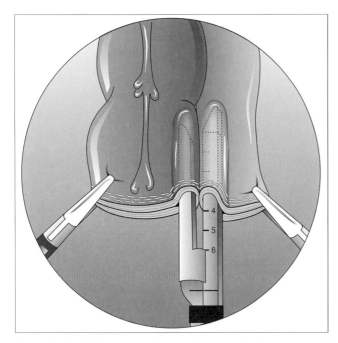 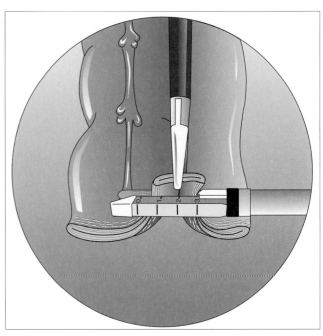

Figs. 8 A, B.   A. The stapler is introduced into the ends of the bowel and is then fired. **B.** Closure of the enterotomy is accomplished by means of a stapler

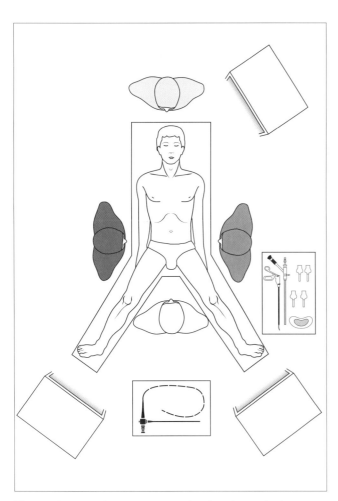

Fig. 9.   Position of patient, personnel, and equipment in the operating room for laparoscopic resection of a left-sided lesion

ardous, and also if one or more strictureplasties are required, they can be best accomplished extracorporeally. Operative time is only slightly increased in most series of extracorporeal anastomosis [33, 102, 109]. Because of technical difficulty, time commitment, cost, potential for contamination, and the ultimate need for an incision for specimen retraction, intracorporeal anastomoses are rarely performed. One surgeon showed a "beautiful" video in which 8 ports and 10 stapler applications had been spent performing a completely intracorporeal resection and anastomosis. At the conclusion of this Herculean feat, an incision was made through which the specimen was delivered. After specimen removal, the entire anastomosis was extracorporealized for "inspection." This lapse in judgement represents a triumph of technology over common sense. Such wanton operations are not to be condoned, because they offer more benefit to the surgeon's ego than to the patient's pathology.

Left Hemicolectomy, Sigmoid Colectomy, and Anterior Resection of the Rectum

Laparoscopic resections of the left colonic or rectal lesions should not differ from traditional resections. Because of the technical difficulties in mobilizing the splenic flexure and in dissecting the rectum, left resections are more challenging than right resections. Conversely, the possibility of using a conventional circular stapler for anastomosis renders left colonic resections well suited for a completely laparoscopic approach. Left hemicolectomy, sigmoid colectomy and anterior resection of the rectum have been reported for a large variety of diseases including malignancy [34, 109], diverticulitis [69, 71, 109], and other benign diseases [71, 73].

The patient is prepared as described previously and placed in the supine modified lithotomy position in Allen Stirrups to allow transanal access for both the colonoscope and the sta-

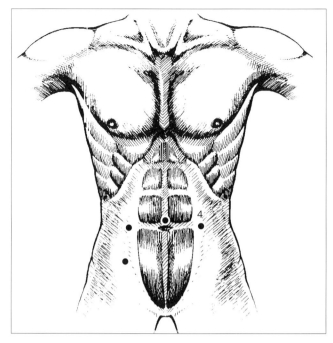

Fig. 10. Trocar placement for a laparoscopic resection of a left-sided lesion Trocar 4 is an optional fourth port used only during anterior resection

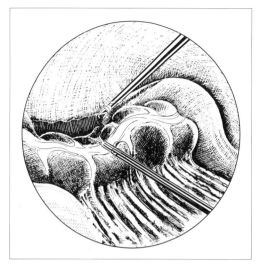

Fig. 12. The sigmoid colon and the rectum are retracted medially and the colon is mobilized from the retroperitoneum using a 10 mm diameter Babcock clamp and a 10 mm diameter electrocautery scissors

pling device. A steep Trendelenburg position and rotation of the table to the right are also used. The surgeon stands to the right side of the patient (Fig. 9). The monitors are placed at the foot of the table at 45 ° angles (Fig. 9). During splenic mobilization the surgeon stands between the patient's legs just in front of the target organ. Port placement varies depending on the type of procedure. The first port (10/12 mm in size) is placed transumbilically, and after inspection of the abdominal cavity, the other two or three ports are placed as follows: for left hemicolectomy or segmental sigmoid resection, a second port is usually placed in the suprapubic region in the right lower quadrant (Fig. 10). The third port is usually placed in the right upper quadrant lateral to the rectus. In case of anterior resection of the rectum, the fourth port is placed on the right

side (Fig. 10). The procedure starts with the mobilization of the left colon from the retroperitoneum (Fig. 11). The position of the table (Trendelenburg and rotation to the right) helps to keep the loops of small bowel away from the operating field. The colon is grasped through the rightsided port with an atraumatic forceps and retracted medially to expose the line of Toldt. The division of the peritoneal attachments is accomplished with the 10 mm diameter electrocautery or scissors, starting in the pelvis and then along the left paracolic gutter (Fig. 12). During this maneuver identification of the ureter is crucial. Once the descending and sigmoid colon have been mobilized, the colon is retracted laterally and toward the abdominal wall to expose the mesentery and allow vascular dissection (Figs. 13 and 14). The left colonic mesentery is separated from Gerota's fascia. After splenic flexure mobilization, the origin of the inferior mesenteric vein at the duodenum should be clear. The mesentery is then scored and the ves-

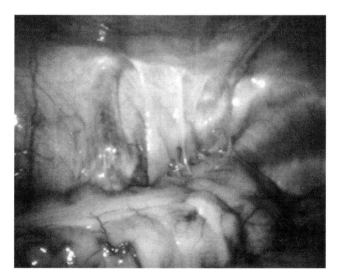

Fig. 11. Peritoneal attachments of the left colon

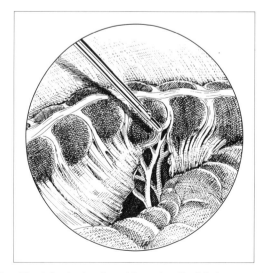

Fig. 13. After lateral retraction of the colon, the inferior mesenteric artery and vein are dissected

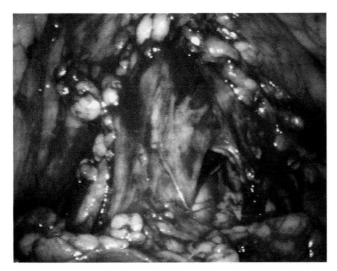

Fig. 14. The vascular pedicle is isolated and prepared for transsection

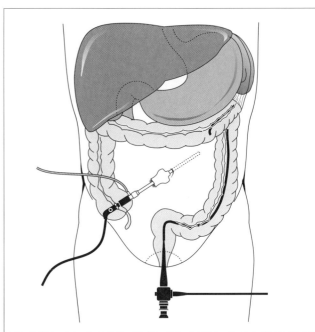

Fig. 16. The splenic flexure is retracted using the tip of the colonoscope

sels are ligated by endoloops or a 30-mm vascular stapling device (Fig. 15). The extent of the dissection and vascular ligation depends on the proposed operation. In case of resection of a potentially malignant neoplasm, the inferior mesenteric artery is ligated at the aorta. The inferior mesenteric vein is also ligated at the same level. During anterior resection of the rectum, the splenic flexure is always mobilized to achieve a tension-free anastomosis. Mobilization of the splenic flexure can be difficult due to a short mesocolon and to the attachment of this portion of the colon to the spleen. The splenic flexure is gently retracted medially to achieve good exposure of the splenic ligament. To avoid splenic tear it is important that the splenic flexure itself is not pulled upon. Excellent splenic flexure retraction can be achieved using a colonoscope [78]. Using a separate video monitor, the colonoscope is advanced beyond the flexure. The tip of the colonoscope is then retroflexed in a wide angle and, while watching the intraperitoneal video monitor, the surgeon controlling the colonoscope gently retracts it in the caudal direction (Fig. 16). The

ligament and the peritoneal attachments are now well exposed and can be safely divided. The dissection can be extended to the transverse colon. Dissection of the rectum to a point distally to the lesion is accomplished by retracting the rectum laterally, anteriorly, and cephalad (Fig. 17). The plane between the mesorectum and the Waldeyer's fascia is divided with the 10-mm cautery scissors providing total mesorectal excision (Fig. 17). Wide lateral margin excision is also necessary during anterior resection of the rectum for neoplasia. As

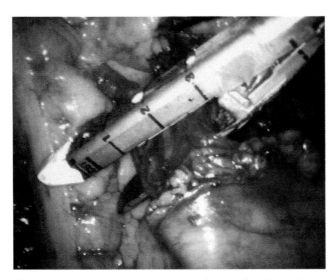

Fig. 15. Transsection of the mesenteric vessels with a 30-mm Endo-GIA (vascular cartridge)

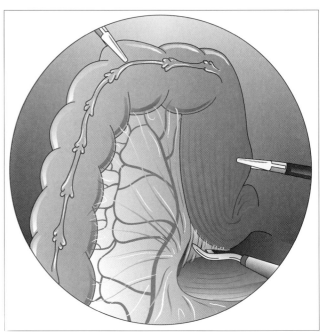

Fig. 17. The rectum is pulled upward and Waldeyer's fascia is divided

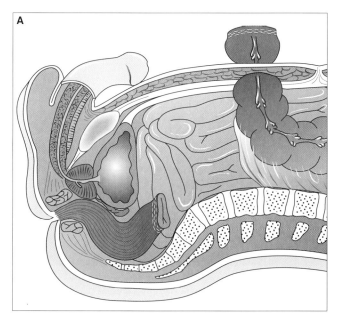
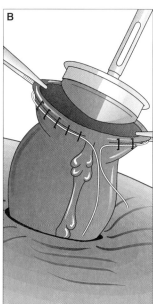
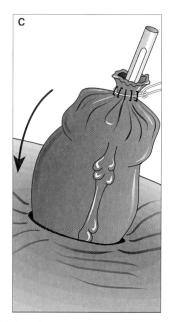

Figs. 18 A, B, C.   A. The proximal end of the bowel is delivered through the abdominal wall. **B.** The anvil is introduced into the bowel lumen and **C.** secured with a purse-string suture

in standard anterior resection, all pelvic dissection is undertaken with electrocautery. It is seldom necessary to use suture ligatures or clips in either setting if an oncologically appropriate total mesorectal and wide lateral excision is routinely performed [37, 38, 63]. During this phase the laparoscope provides an excellent view: the sympathetic nerves are clearly visible at the sacral promontory while anteriorly the seminal vessels can be identified to guide the dissection.

In case of sigmoid colectomy or anterior resection of the rectum an end-to-end anastomosis can be performed using several techniques. The fastest and easiest way is presently the double-stapled anastomosis with the extracorporeal purse string. The right iliac fossa 10-mm port is exchanged for an 18-mm port. The rectum is then transected using a 60-mm endoscopic linear-cutter stapler. Verification of the stapler position can be done by a proctoscope or a sigmoidoscope. Rectal wash-out prior to stapler application can be performed. After distal division of the rectum, the left upper 10-mm port is exchanged for a 33-mm port through which the left colon is then easily delivered (Fig. 18 A). The left colon is then transected and a proximal purse-string suture is created to secure the anvil of the circular stapler into the lumen (Figs. 18 B and C). The

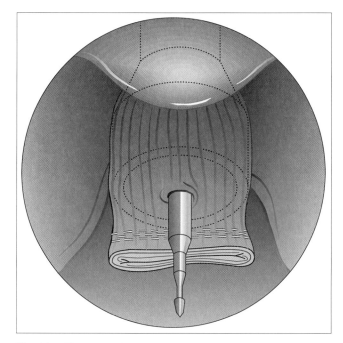

Fig. 19.   The trocar of the circular stapler pierces the rectal stapled stump

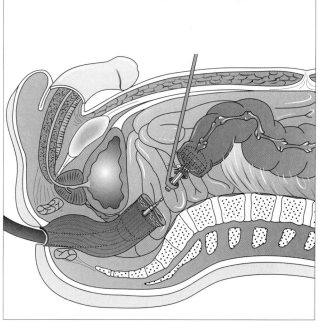

Fig. 20.   The anvil of the stapler is connected with the shaft of the circular stapler under laparoscopic guidance

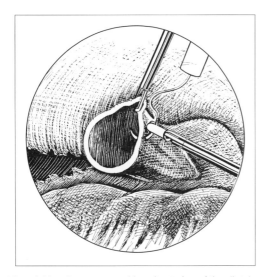
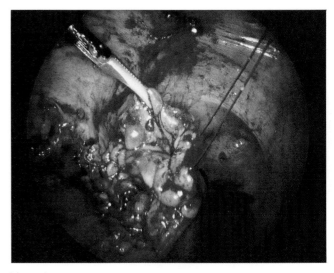

Figs. 21 and 22.   Intracorporeal hand-suturing of the distal purse-string suture.

colon is returned into the abdominal cavity and pneumoperitoneum is reestablished. The circular stapler is transanally introduced and the trocar is used to pierce the stapled rectal
stump (Fig. 19). Under laparoscopic guidance, the anvil of the
stapler is connected with the shaft of the circular stapler that
has pierced the rectal stump. The special Allis anvil grasping
clamp (Ethicon Endosurgery Inc. Cincinnati, Ohio) is very
helpful for this maneuver (Fig. 20). The stapler is fired and the
integrity of the resulting anastomosis is verified by both inspection of the donuts and air insufflation. The advantage of this
technique is the avoidance of the hand-sewn distal purse-
string suture, a process that is extremely difficult, time-consuming, and has the potential for pelvic contamination.

Other techniques of intracorporeal anastomosis have been
reported. The distal or proximal purse string can be intracorporeally fashioned with a hand-sewn technique (Figs. 21 and 22)
or by endoscopic loop purse strings. Transanal introduction of
the circular stapler is carried out with the anvil placed on the instrument (Fig. 23). The anvil is positioned in the proximal colon
stump (Fig. 24). For easier tying of the purse-string sutures,

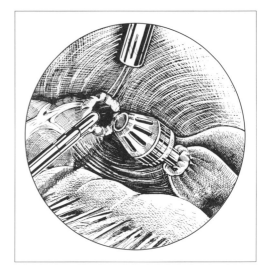

Fig. 24.   The anvil is positioned in the descending colon

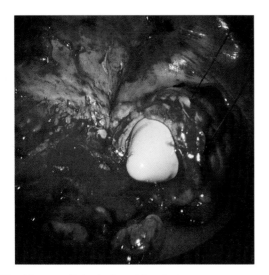

Fig. 23.   Transanal introduction of the stapler

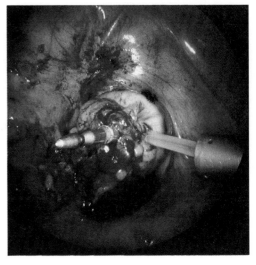

Fig. 25.   Extracorporeal tying of the hand-sewn monofilament
purse-string suture

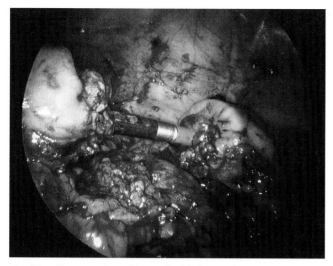

Fig. 26. Reconnection of the anvil with the stapler

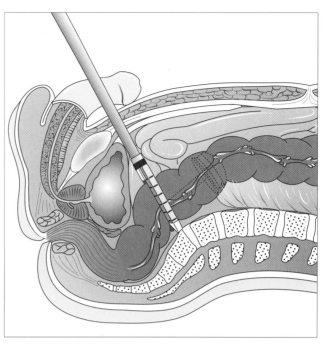

Fig. 28. The bowel is transected proximally; the anvil of the circular stapler is proximal to the line of resection

the instrument can be disconnected (Fig. 25). The anvil is reconnected with the stapler (Fig. 26) and the instrument is fired (Fig. 27). However, in a series reported by Phillips [69] of 51 laparoscopic colectomies in which an intracorporeal hand-sewn purse string or endoscopic loop was used for both ends of the resected bowel, the circular stapled anastomosis was incomplete in 18 % of cases. This high rate of incomplete anastomosis has not been reported in series in which an extracorporeal purse string was utilized [34, 102, 109].

Thus, intracorporeal endoloop purse-string placement is ill-advised unless one desires experience at repair of anastomotic defects [14]. In order to obviate the need for a distal purse string and then an incision to exteriorize the bowel, a triple-stapling technique has been described [27]. In this variation the anvil of the stapler is transanally introduced and, under colonoscopic guidance, is brought to a level proximal to the proximal line of resection. The bowel is then transected distally and proximally by a stapling device (Fig. 28). The anvil of the circular stapler is delivered through the proximal stapled end of the bowel and docked with the shaft of the circular

stapler, which has been introduced transanally to pierce the rectal stump. The anastomosis is certainly not easy to do, and pushing the anvil beyond a neoplasm seems ill-advised.

Complications reported for resections of the left colon include ureteric injuries [34], anastomotic leaks [34, 102], occult bleeding [71, 102], and intra-abdominal abscess [102]. However, complications can be related to the "learning curve," and it can be predicted that with more experience, the rate of complications decreases. In our opinion, the double-stapled technique with extracorporeal fashioning of the proximal purse string is the technique preferred for rectosigmoid or anterior resection. Transanal circular stapler introduction is a procedure already familiar to all surgeons, and the need for an intracorporeal hand-sewn anastomosis is avoided.

Total Abdominal Colectomy

Total abdominal colectomy is a procedure rarely performed laparoscopically. Indications include mucosal ulcerative colitis, Crohn's disease, familial adenomatous polyposis, and colonic inertia [105]. Removing the entire colon requires mobilization of the large intestine in all the abdominal quadrants, thus increasing the length of surgery.

The patient is prepared as for other laparoscopic procedures. After introduction of the camera through a transumbilical port, three additional ports are inserted as shown in Figure 29. The position of the surgeon and personnel varies depending on the segment of colon being mobilized. The entire colon is mobilized as described for other right and left colectomy. If the rectum is to be spared, mobilization is undertaken to the level of the sacral promontory. If proctocolectomy must be undertaken, the upper two thirds of the rectum are also mobilized as described for anterior resection. If rectal dissection is not easily accomplished, the remainder of the dissection can

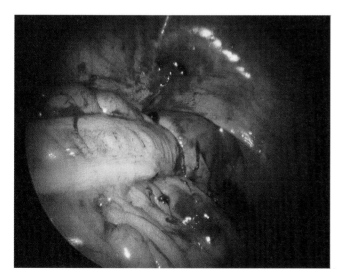

Fig. 27. Stapled anastomosis

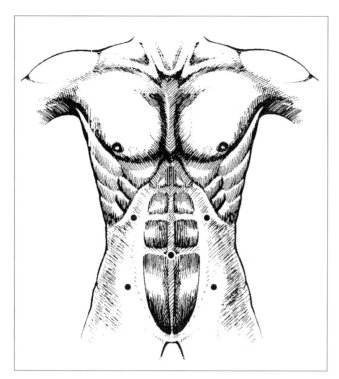

Fig. 29. Trocar placement for laparoscopic-assisted total abdominal colectomy

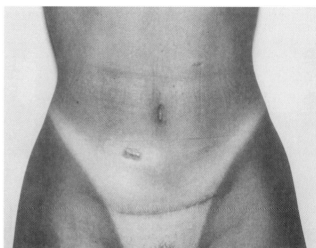

Fig. 31. Scars several months after closure of a laparoscopically created loop ileostomy

be completed during the extracorporeal phase. After full mobilization of the intra-abdominal portion of the colon and rectum, the entire segment is eviscerated through a small infraumbilical midline or Pfannenstiel incision (Fig. 30A). The mesentery is transected and the vessels are ligated in standard fashion. Completion of rectal dissection, transection of the bowel, creation of the ileoanal reservoir and anastomosis are performed according to conventional technique [104]. The advantages of a laparoscopic approach for total colectomy must be sought in the reduction of the length of incision (Fig. 30B). This cosmetic improvement is usually requested by patients with familial adenomatous polyposis, mucosal ulcerative colitis, and colonic in-

ertia, who tend to be relatively young (Fig. 31). However, no other advantages are currently offered by laparoscopic total colectomy [11]. Moreover, one more recent series [77] compared laparoscopic total colectomy to other laparoscopic colorectal procedures. It was found that total abdominal colectomy was associated with significantly more complications than were segmental laparoscopic resections [13]. Likewise, laparoscopic total abdominal colectomy has a higher complication rate than open total abdominal colectomy [82].

Ileostomy and Colostomy

Fecal diversion can be laparoscopically accomplished by the creation of a loop or an end ileostomy or an end colostomy [30, 48]. A technique of laparoscopic cecostomy has also been described [22] in a patient with cecal dilatation due to colonic pseudo-obstruction. However, cecostomy, whether performed laparoscopically or through a standard incision, is mentioned only to be condemned.

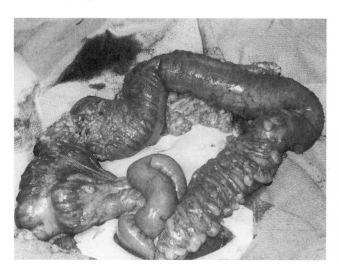

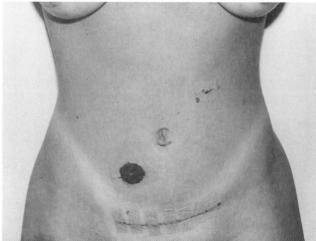

Figs. 30A, B. **A.** Abdominal colon and terminal ileum lying on the abdomen after being laparoscopically mobilized and delivered through a Pfannenstiel's incision. **B.** Scars and Brook ileostomy after laparoscopic-assisted total abdominal colectomy

Creation of a loop ileostomy is ideally suited for a laparoscopic approach. For the creation of a loop ileostomy, two ports are usually required. The first port is 10/12 mm in size and is introduced in the upper midline, midway between the umbilicus and the xiphoid. Another 10-mm port is usually placed in the intended stoma site. An optional third 10/12-mm port can be placed at the contralateral position if adhesiolysis is required. If adhesions are present, they can be lysed to render the small bowel completely mobile. An atraumatic forceps is inserted and the small intestine is gently manipulated. The most distal portion of ileum that reaches the anterior abdominal wall without tension is chosen for creation of the stoma. If a third port has been used, this loop is marked as to proximal and distal direction by placing either staples or clips on the mesentery close to the bowel wall. This maneuver helps to appropriately orientate the bowel before maturation. The bowel is then gently grasped with a laparoscopic Babcock clamp. The stoma port site, Babcock clamp, and the bowel are now withdrawn as a unit (Fig. 32). To facilitate the passage of the loop of ileum, the fascia can be stretched [45] or, as in our experience [95], incised. The fascia is exposed with the skin retractors and incised under direct vision using the electrocautery against the insulated shaft of the Babcock clamp as it is angled upward. Incision of the fascia helps to prevent fascial outlet obstruction that can ensue from normal postoperative stomal swelling [95]. Once the ileum is exteriorized, the pneumoperitoneum is reestablished and, through the laparoscope, hemostasis and anatomic orientation are verified. This verification of nonrotation is especially important if the two-port technique was utilized without bowel marking. If desired, the bowel can be divided and an end ileostomy created. The two other ports are removed, the pneumoperitoneum is released, and the stoma is matured. The patient can be discharged within 2–4 days after surgery [45], in most cases, with little postoperative discomfort and better cosmesis as compared with the open technique.

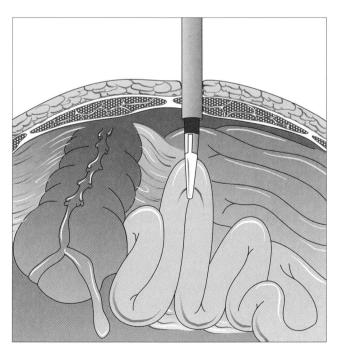

Fig. 32. The small bowel loop is brought out along with the trocar and the Babcock clamp

Subsequent stoma closure can also be effected without a formal laparotomy. A parastomal incision is made and the stoma is circumferentially dissected from the surrounding fascia and abdominal wall. The ileostomy is resected and the anastomosis is created extracorporeally according to traditional technique [107]. Laparoscopic loop ileostomy is a safe and promising alternative to "open" loop ileostomy. Even if not yet proven, laparoscopic creation of a loop ileostomy may result in less adhesions than "open" loop ileostomy.

Laparoscopic creation of a loop colostomy was reported in 1991 by Lange et al. [48]. Later, other reports [30] suggested that this procedure is feasible and carries no increased risk as compared with laparotomy. A laparoscopic colostomy is also created as a part of an abdominal perineal resection [30, 102]. The procedure is similar to that described for ileostomy with mirror-image port placement. The major difference is that, although both an end or a loop ileostomy are acceptable, a loop colostomy is vastly inferior to an end colostomy. Therefore, during colostomy creation intracorporeal vascular and bowel division, as previously described, are performed. The distal end of the proximal bowel is then delivered through the port as for anvil placement. However, instead of anvil placement, the stoma is matured. A circular incision around the trocar, including skin and fascia, helps in the delivery of the bowel [30]. The abdomen is inspected through the laparoscope for torsion, tension, or bleeding prior to stoma maturation.

Hartmann's Procedure

Hartmann's resection is well suited to a laparoscopic approach. The laparoscopic technique is similar to that for sigmoid colectomy or anterior resection of the rectum with the exception of performing an end colostomy instead of an end-to-end anastomosis. However, in a clinical setting the indications to perform a laparoscopic Hartmann's resection are limited to palliative treatment of colorectal cancer and a few other less frequent conditions.

Closure of the Hartmann's pouch can be safely accomplished laparoscopically, the only difficulty being adhesions from previous surgery in an inflamed pelvis. In such a case, however, the patient already has a laparotomy incision, thus negating the cosmetic benefits.

The procedure starts by dissecting the stoma free of the abdominal wall after which the anvil of the circular stapler is introduced into the bowel lumen and secured with a purse-string suture. The bowel is then placed inside the abdomen and an 18- or 33-mm port is secured into the fascial incision. Two other 10/12-mm ports can be placed in the abdomen under direct vision. Accurate dissection of the rectal stump is necessary for a safe end-to-end anastomosis. The continuity of the intestine is restored with a double-stapled technique as previously described for anterior resection of the rectum.

Other Laparoscopic Colorectal Procedures

Other laparoscopic colorectal procedures have been reported, but their practice is still confined to anecdotal reports or experimental studies in a laboratory setting. Laparoscopic repair of traumatic injury to the bowel is another possible application. Recurrent episodes of intestinal obstruction have been treated successfully by laparoscopic adhesiolysis [75].

Another potential use of the laparoscope is polypectomy [8]. In this case the laparoscope can guide the colonoscopic resection of polyps in difficult cases, or a colotomy and polyp excision can be performed by laparoscopic or assisted technique.

Cleveland Clinic Florida Experience

Between August 1991 and March 1996, 193 laparoscopic colorectal procedures were performed in the Department of Colorectal Surgery at the Cleveland Clinic Florida. After a training period, including practice in an animal model and cholecystectomy in humans, clinical experience commenced. A prospective registry included information pertaining to diagnosis, indication for surgery, age, gender, surgical procedure performed, length of surgery, and length of hospitalization. Indications for surgery are listed in Table 3. The mean age of patients was 48.5 years (range 12–88 years) with 81 males and 112 females. The procedures performed included 38 total abdominal colectomies (TAC), 80 segmental colonic or bowel resections, 34 stoma creations, and 41 others including abdominoperineal resection, Hartmann's creation or closure, anterior resection or rectopexy (Table 4). All procedures were per-

Table 3. Laparoscopic colorectal surgery: Indications at Cleveland Clinic Florida

Inflammatory Bowel disease (n = 79)

Crohn's disease	37
Mucosal ulcerative colitis	23
Diverticulitis	19

Neoplasia of Colon and Rectum (n = 68)

Colonic polyps	27
Colonic carcinoma	13
Rectal carcinoma	12
Familial adenomatous polyposis	9
Anal carcinoma	3
Anal melanoma	2
Kaposi's sarcoma	1
Small bowel lymphoma	1

Functional Bowel Disorders (n = 30)

Fecal incontinence	15
Constipation	12
Rectal prolapse	3

Other Forms of Colitis, Proctitis, Ulceration and Colorectal disease (n = 16)

Irradiation proctitis	3
Ischemic colitis	2
Sigmoid volvulus	2
Severe anal stenosis	2
Chronic abdominal pain	2
Colonic tuberculosis	1
Rectal tuberculosis	1
Arterio-venous malformations	1
Anal ulcer (AIDS)	1
Small bowel laceration	1
Total	193

Table 4. Laparoscopic colorectal procedures at Cleveland Clinic Florida

Total abdominal colectomy (n = 38)

Ileoanal reservoir (J pouch)	28
Ileorectal anastomosis	8
End ileostomy	2

Segmental resection (n = 80)

Right hemicolectomy	50
Left hemicolectomy	4
Sigmoid colectomy	24
Small bowel resection	2

Diverting procedures (n = 34)

Diverting ileostomy	27
Diverting colostomy	7

Other minor procedures (n = 41)

Hartmann's creation or closure	12
Rectopexy	4
Adhesiolysis	8
Abdominoperineal resection	7
Low anterior resection	6
Ileorectal anastomosis with ileostomy closure	4
Total	193

Table 5. Location of tumors and procedures

	Right colon	Sigmoid or left colon	Rectum	Anus	Total (n)
Segmental Resection	11	3	–	–	14
Diverting procedures	–	1	5	1	7
Low anterior resection	–	–	3	–	3
Abdominoperineal resection	–	–	4	3	7
Hartmann's procedure	–	1	–	–	1
Diagnostic laparoscopy and biopsy	–	–	1	1	2
Total	11	5	13	5	34

formed according to the surgical principles adopted in open surgery. All patients underwent standard preoperative management as previously described. For right colectomies the segment of bowel to be resected was laparoscopically mobilized. A 2- to 4-cm vertical transumbilical incision was then made and vessel ligation, resection, and anastomosis were extracorporeally performed. For left-sided lesions the intracorporeal division of the distal bowel was accomplished with a 60-mm linear-cutting stapler. All specimens were retrieved through a 33-mm laparoscopic port. The anastomosis was performed with the double-stapled technique after extracorporeally securing the anvil of the circular stapler to the proximal bowel. A total of 34 patients had resection for malignancy (Table 5). A curative resection was undertaken in 24 patients including careful dissection of the mesorectum along with excision of a wide lateral margin. The high ligation of the mesen-

Table 6. Complications after laparoscopic colorectal surgery: Cleveland Clinic Experience

Intraoperative Complications (n = 30; 15.5 %)

Recognized enterotomy or colotomy	11
Major bleeding	6
Anastomotic leak	4
Minor bleeding	4
Adjacent organ injury	2
Abdominal wall hematoma	1
Cardiac arrhythmia	1
Intubation difficulty	1
Total	30 (15.5 %)
None	163 (84.5 %)

Postoperative complications (n = 55; 28.5 %)

Prolonged ileus	11
Wound infection*	9
Stoma related problems	5
Pelvic abscess or peritonitis*	4
Anastomotic leak*	3
Bleeding	1
Port site hematoma	1
Port site hernia	2
Atelectasis	4
Cardiac arrythmia	3
Pneumonia	3
I. V. Fluid overload	2
Catheter sepsis	2
Urinary tract infection	1
Anemia	1
Renal failure	1
Mallory-Weiss tear	1
Myocardid infarction	1

*All patients were receiving high doses of steroids for inflammatory bowel disease

teric vessels provided a large excision of the lymph-node-bearing tissue. 15 patients were operated for curative intent and pathology revealed 5 Dukes' A, 8 Dukes' B, and 2 Dukes' C tumors with a mean of 19 lymph nodes per specimen. 9 patients with anal carcinoma or leiomyosarcoma and malignant melanomana were excluded from this study.

There was no mortality; 41 patients (21 %) required conversion to open surgery, due to bleeding or adhesions. The overall complication rate was 31 % including 15.5 % intraoperative and 28.5 % postoperative complications (Table 6). In a period of 4 years, for the purpose of analysis, 175 patients were chronologically divided into 5 consecutive groups. Procedures were classified as either basic or complex. Complex procedures were those in which there was either a fixed tumor, an abscess or fistula, or extensive intraabdominal adhesions prior to surgery. Complex procedures performed each year ranged from 37 % to 66 %. As well, the percentage of patients with adhesions increased from 17 % in 1991 to 29 % in 1995. Despite increased difficulty, intraoperative complication rate fell significantly from 29 % in 1991 to 8 % in 1995 (p<0.005). Additionally, operative length decreased from a mean of 201 minutes in 1991 to a mean of 141 minutes in 1995 (p<0.05). The most significant variable affecting the intraoperative laparoscopic complication rate was surgical ex-

perience measured as the time interval during which surgery was performed (p=0.02). The total complication rate decreased from 29 % during the first period to 11 % by the second period (p<0.04) and 7 % during the third period (p<0.005). Thus, the "learning curve" appeared to have required more than 50 cases to achieve. Moreover, even after the performance of 94 cases, procedures in the total abdominal colectomy and the other procedure groups, were associated with higher intraoperative laparoscopic complication rates than those in the segmental resections and deviating procedure groups (p=0.04). The mean length of hospital stay was 7.1 days (range 2–84 days). No local, locoregional, or port-site tumor recurrence have been observed at a follow-up of 56 months.

These data are consistent with other data reported in the literature, and suggest that laparoscopic colorectal surgery has a steep learning curve. The morbidity was related to the type of surgery, laparoscopic total abdominal colectomy being associated with more complications than other procedures.

Controversies In Laparoscopic Colorectal Surgery

Presently, there are no published results of any prospective randomized clinical trials comparing laparoscopy with open surgery. The only unanimously accepted advantages of laparoscopy in colorectal surgery as compared with laparotomy is improved cosmesis [34, 102, 107]. After appropriate training, laparoscopic colonic resections can be undertaken with an acceptable morbidity and mortality. During laparoscopic surgery all the structures such as ureters, mesentertic vessels, rectal vessels and mesorectum can be easily identified. However, complications related to iatrogenic injuries of the ureters [34], major vessels [102], and other structures [34, 69, 109] have been reported. These complications are probably related to the loss of tactile sensation through the laparoscope and to the learning curve. In our early experience we had an injury to the iliac artery that required rapid conversion to laparotomy. Other complications reported [69] include a rate of intraoperative incomplete anastomosis as high as 18 %. This high rate of intraoperative failure compares poorly with open surgery.

Another concern is the rate of removal of the wrong segment of bowel. Corbitt [18] converted 3 of 18 procedures due to the inability to identify the colonic lesion. Numerous others [11, 15, 25, 49, 61] have also reported removal of the wrong segment of bowel. A higher rate of thromboembolic complications has also been reported in some series [34], and is probably related to the increased operative time and pneumoperitoneum.

One of the parameters used to assess the efficacy and safety of a procedure is the length of hospitalization and return to work. However, hospital discharge and return to previous activity are difficult to objectively assess, and when laparoscopy is compared with laparotomy in colorectal surgery, the two techniques do not show significant differences [79].

Shorter postoperative ileus can contribute to shorter hospital stay. It has been hypothesized that laparoscopic colorectal surgery, because of less trauma and manipulation of the bowel, results in earlier recovery of bowel function. Jacobs et al. [43] in a series of 20 patients, noted that 18 patients tolerated oral fluids on day 1, and 14 patients were discharged within 4 days after surgery. Other authors [66, 86] reported that their patients regained bowel function significantly earlier, assumed regular diet earlier, and, hence, had a markedly shorter hospitalization than patients who underwent laparotomy. However, early oral intake is not unique to laparoscopy. In a prospective randomized trial [76], 161 consecutive patients who underwent elective laparotomy for colonic resection randomly received, in the postoperative period, either an early oral feeding (clear liquids on day 1) or the traditional regimen (clear liquids only after resolution of ileus).

In this study there was no significant difference between the early and regular feeding groups in terms of nasogastric tube reinsertion (11 vs 10 %, respectively), length of hospital stay (6.2 vs 6.8 days, respectively), and overall complication rates (1.4 vs 3.1 %, respectively). Many laparoscopic enthusiasts claim "marked reduction" in hospital stay after laparoscopic as compared with "standard" surgery. However, these surgeons tend to use historic controls [65] or to feed the former patients immediately and discharge them prior to bowel movement. The latter group are kept NPO until resolution of ileus and are discharged only after resumption of full bowel activity.

Another issue surrounding laparoscopic colorectal surgery, and by far the most important, is the adequacy of this technique in the treatment of colorectal cancer [101]. Several concerns arise regarding adequate laparoscopic excision of a neoplasm, especially for rectal cancer where the surgical technique plays an important role in the prevention of local recurrence. It has been demonstrated that an incomplete surgical excision of the mesorectum and an inadequate lateral margin clearance [11, 37, 42, 72] are both associated with locoregional failure and poor prognosis. An improved 5-year survival rate of 78 % and local recurrence of 3–5 % has been achieved by Heald et al. [38] by routine total mesorectal excision. Quirke et al. [72] reported an incidence of recurrence of 85 % in patients with lateral resection margins involved with the tumor. Conversely, the rate of local recurrence if the lateral resection margins were free of tumor was under 5 %. Tate et al compared 11 patients with lesions located at a mean height of 20 cm who underwent laparoscopic resection with 14 patients with tumors at a mean height of 15 cm [93] who underwent laparotomy. Despite the sigmoid location in the former group, the distal margins were as small as 5 mm, clearly an unacceptable margin for cure. Conversely, the smallest margin in the laparotomy group was 2.0 cm, a universally accepted distal margin. In our experience and that of others [34], complete mesorectal excision with wide lateral margins is easily done [34]. The rectum, after full mobilization, can be pulled cephalad, thus facilitating the dissection in the avascular presacral space. Any advantage of radical abdominopelvic lymphadenectomy for rectal cancer, as advocated by several authors [23, 46], still needs to be determined [35], and there are only a few experimental reports in the literature of such a lymphatic excision by laparoscopy [19, 44].

Other controversies that are still under debate relative to laparotomy can be applied to laparoscopy. High ligation of inferior mesenteric artery and harvesting of a large number of lymph nodes are considered to be a part of a curative resection for colonic neoplasms. Several authors [7, 92] have suggested that high ligation of the inferior mesenteric artery and wide mesenteric resection allow a larger and more complete removal of node-bearing tissue, thus improving the survival rate. Unfortunately, other studies [33, 68] have failed to demonstrate any advantages in terms of improved survival for patients treated by high ligation of the inferior mesenteric artery. Moreover, the reports of a 32 % incidence of skip metastases [88], the microscopic deposit of tumor cells in bone marrow [50], the identification of occult hepatic metastases [26], and the detection by radioimmunoassay of extra-anatomic distal nodal involvement [6] seem to support the concept that colorectal cancer has often spread beyond the scope of surgical therapy at the time of diagnosis. In such a case no advantages can be achieved with high ligation of the inferior mesenteric artery and removal of a large number of lymph nodes. A recent study [24] demonstrated that there was no significant difference between the number of lymph nodes removed with laparoscopy or laparotomy. In other series the lymph nodes harvested were very few, with zero [49, 99] to two nodes [93] being retrieved, thus making adequate staging impossible. However, even if the number of lymph nodes removed laparoscopically was "adequate", it cannot be taken as a criterion for the effectiveness of a surgical excision. The number of lymph nodes collected depends not only on the surgeon, but also on the pathologist, and there is a great variability among different pathologists [16].

Other issues also demand a more cautious appraisal of this procedure for colorectal cancer. The CO_2 pressure of 15 mmHg can reduce the venous blood flow and surpass the capillary venous pressure potentially forcing tumor cells to enter the blood stream. The tumor cells theoretically may be forced into lymphatics and veins, then disseminate to the liver and other sites, increasing the rate of distant recurrence. This potential problem may be obviated by the routine use of the "no-touch" technique. This technique, described by Turnbull et al. in 1967 [96], consists of ligation of the lymphovascular pedicle prior to mobilization and removal of the involved colonic segment. However, during laparoscopic surgery the pneumoperitoneum must be well established prior to any dissection. New techniques, such as the gasless procedure [44, 60], may eliminate the concern of tumor cell embolization.

Possibly related to this problem is port-site tumor recurrence. Since Alexander et al. [3] first reported a 67-year-old female patient with a wound recurrence after laparoscopic-assisted right hemicolectomy for a Dukes' A carcinoma, many port-site recurrences following laparoscopic procedures for cure of malignancy have been described. Two recent surveys [59, 105] reported at least 40 cases of port-site recurrences ranging from isolated tumor at the site of port placement to disseminated peritoneal carcinomatosis and port-site recurrence [10, 12, 20, 21, 28, 29, 31, 40, 47, 65, 67, 80, 87, 91]. This complication does not occur only in the port-site through which the specimen is delivered, but can involve any port-site, and more importantly, is not only confined to advanced neoplasia, but has been noted to occur following laparoscopic cholecystectomy for an unsuspected or occult gall bladder carcinoma [12, 59] and after laparoscopic appendectomy performed for acute appendicitis in the case of an unrecognized cecal carcinoma. There has also been a cutaneous tumor seeding from a previous undiagnosed pancreatic carcinoma after laparoscopic cholecystectomy [86] and there have been port implants of gastric [10] and ovarian carcinoma [32, 40, 54]. No explanation for this phenomenon has been given. Port sites seem to be a very favorable place for tumor cell growth, and it is interesting to note that the continuity of the peritoneal layer is disrupted at the port site. There are experimental data suggesting that surgical wounds are fertile sites for neoplastic growth [57, 58], but this complication is virtually absent after standard open procedures [41]. Other factors specifically related to laparoscopy seem to play a role. Firstly, during laparoscopic surgery an increased exfoliation of malignant cells may occur, due to the manipulation of the tumor with the laparoscopic instruments. The pneumoperitoneum may represent a means for these cells to reach the trocar wound. Secondly, the frequent changes of the instruments from one trocar to another and the contact between the specimen and the skin can explain tumor recurrence observed at virtually any port site. Thirdly, during dissection of an organ with an occult carcinoma, the electrocautery may inadvertently cut deeper than realized. This mechanism can explain some cases of tumor recurrence at port site after laparoscopic cholecystectomy for gallstones in patients with an occult carcinoma [21, 59]. Lastly, squeezing of tumor cells from the tumor to port sites [34] or a suction mechanism during withdrawal of the ports may represent other factors responsible for the pathophysiology of this alarming and mysterious complication.

Finally, one question is of paramount importance in considering the appropriateness of this technique in treating colorectal cancer: Laparoscopic resections of colorectal cancer have a short period of follow-up (up to 5 years), and there have already been many locoregional recurrences reported [34]. Some of these fears were borne out in a recent survey of the members of the American Society of Colon and Rectal Surgeons [15]. Basically, although approximately 31 % of surgeons perform laparoscopic colectomy for cure of carcinoma, only 6 % would have their own rectal carcinoma laparoscopically resected. This double standard is very distressing. Laparoscopic "curative" resection of colorectal cancer should not have a higher rate of locoregional recurrence compared with open procedures, because total mesorectal excision, wide lateral margin resection, and wide lymph node excision can be accomplished. However, logic and fact are different entities, and a longer follow-up period is needed to prove this theory.

Conclusion

Laparoscopic colorectal surgery can be undertaken with an acceptable morbidity and mortality. The only currently proven advantage is cosmesis. Adequate training is required before clinical experience, and a steep learning curve must be expected. In the near future new technology will hopefully render laparoscopic colorectal surgery easier. Definitions (Table 7) need to be accepted to facilitate communication among surgeons and between surgeons and patients. For benign disease laparoscopy is a reasonable alternative.

When performed by appropriately trained surgeons in appropriately selected patients, it undoubtedly has advantages.

For malignant disease prospective randomized trials are needed to determine the safety and efficacy of this procedure. The increasing number of port-site recurrences and the lack of long-term follow-up are the major issues that need to be addressed. Presently, curative resection of malignancy should only be performed within the confines of a prospective randomized trial. However, palliative resection of widely disseminated carcinoma remains an excellent laparoscopic procedure.

Table 7. Definitions

Laparoscopic resection

All phases performed intracorporeally and/or through ports
No incision:
Vascular ligation
Bowel transection
Anastomosis
Mesenteric defect repair (right side)*
Anastomosis verification (left side)*

Laparoscopic-assisted resection

One or more of the above phases performed through an incision

Converted

Any incision made sooner than planned *or* larger than planned *or* any incision ≧ 5 cm

*If applicable

References

1. ADIS DG, SHAFFER N, FOWLER BS ET AL.: The epidemiology of appendicitis and appendectomy in the U.S. Am J Epidemiol 143 (1990) 910–925.
2. ALEXANDER JW, ALTEMEIR WA: Susceptibility of injured tissue to hematogenous metastases: an experimental study. Ann Surg 159 (1964) 933–944.
3. ALEXANDER RJY, JACQUES BC ET AL.: Laparoscopically-assisted colectomy and wound recurrence (letter). Lancet 341 (1993) 249–250.
4. AMERICAN SOCIETY OF COLON AND RECTAL SURGEONS: Policy Statement. Dis Colon Rectum 34 (1991) 5a.
5. AMERICAN SOCIETY OF COLON AND RECTAL SURGEONS: Policy Statement on Laparoscopic Colectomy. Dis Colon Rectum (1994).
6. ARNOLD MN, SHNEEBAURS J ET AL.: Intraoperative detection of colorectal cancer with radioimmunoguided surgery and cc 49, a second generation monoclonal antibody. Ann Surg 216 (1992) 627–632.
7. BACON HE, KHUBCHANDANI IT: The rationale of aortoileopelvic and high ligation of the inferior mesenteric artery for carcinoma of the left half of the colon and rectum. Surg Gynecol Obstet 119 (1964) 503–508.
8. BALLANTYNE GH: Polypectomy. IN: Ballantyne GH, Leahy FP, Modlin IM (eds.). Laparoscopic sugery. W.B. Saunders, Philadelphia (1994): 508–521
9. BARTOLO DCC: Ureteric injury in laparoscopic surgery. Presented at the International Society of University of Colon and Rectal Surgeons 15th Biennial Congress. Singapore, July 2–6, 1994.
10. CAVA A, ROMAN J ET AL.: Subcutaneous metastases following laparoscopy in gastric carcinoma. Eur J Surg Oncol 16 (1990) 63–67.
11. CAWTHORN SJ, PARUMS DV ET AL.: Extent of mesorectal spread and involvement of lateral resection margin as a prognostic factor after surgery for rectal cancer. Lancet 335 (1990) 1055–1059.
12. CLAIR DG, LAUTZ DB ET AL.: Rapid development of umbilical metastases after laparoscopic cholecystectomy for unsuspected gallbladder carcinoma. Surgery 113 (1993) 355–358.
13. COHEN SM, NOGUERAS JJ, WEXNER SD: Laparoscopic colorectal surgery: ascending the learning curve. World J Surg 20 (1996): 277-282.
14. COHEN SM, CLEM MS, WEXNER SD, JAGELMAN DG: An initial comparative study of two techniques of laparoscopic colonic anastomosis and mesentery defect closure. Surg Endosc 8 (1994) 130–134.
15. COHEN SM, WEXNER SD: Laparoscopic colorectal surgery: Are we being honest with our patients? Dis Colon Rectum 38 (1995): 723–727.

16. COHEN SM, WEXNER SD, SCHMITT SL, NOGUERAS JJ, LUCAS FV: Effect of xylene clearance of mesentric fat on harvest of lymph nodes after colonic resection. Eur J Surg 160 (1994) 693–697.

17. COOPERMAN A, KATZ V ET AL.: Laparoscopic colon resection: a case report. Surg Lap Endosc 2 (1) (1991) 79–81.

18. CORBIT JD: Preliminary experience with laparoscopic-guided colectomy. Surg Laparosc Endosc 2 (1) (1992) 79–81.

19. DECAINI C, MILSOM JW, BOHM B, FAZIO VW: Laparoscopic oncologic abdominoperineal resection. Dis Colon Rectum 37 (1994) 552–558.

20. DOBRONTE Z, WITTMANN T ET AL.: Rapid development of malignant metastases in the abdominal wall after laparoscopy. Endoscopy 10 (1978)127–130.

21. DROUARD F, DELAMARRE J ET AL.: Cutaneous seeding of gallbladder cancer after laparoscopic cholecystectomy (letter). N Engl J Med 31 (1991) 1316.

22. DUH QY, WAY IW: Diagnostic laparoscopy and laparoscopic cecostomy for colonic pseudo-obstruction. Dis Colon Rectum 36 (1993) 65–70.

23. ENKER W, URBAN L ET AL.: Enhanced survival of patients with colon and rectal cancer is based upon wide anatomic resection. Ann Surg 190 (1979) 350–360.

24. FALK PM, BEART RW, WEXNER SD: Laparoscopic colectomy: a critical appraisal. Dis Colon Rectum 36 (1) (1993) 28–34.

25. FINGERHUT A: Laparoscopic assisted colonic resection: The French experience. In: Jagar R, Wexner SD. Laparoscopic colorectal Surgery. Churchill-Livingstone, New York (1996) 253–257. Presented at the 4th World Congress of Endoscopic Surgery. Kyoto, Japan, June 16–19, 1994.

26. FINLAY IG: Occult hepatic metastases: Has the die been cast prior to surgery? Presented at the Post-graduate Course, Principles of Colon and Rectal Surgery, University of Minnesota Medical School, September 24–26, 1992.

27. FLESHMAN JW, BRUNT ML, FREY RD, BIRNABAUM E, SIMMANG CL ET AL.: Laparoscopic anterior resection of the rectum using a triple stapled intracorporeal anastomosis in the pig. Surg Laparosc Endosc 3 (2) (1993) 119–126.

28. FLIGELSTONE I, RHODES M, FLOOK D, PUNTIS M, CROBSY D: Tumour innoculation during laparoscopy (letter). Lancet 342 (8862) (1993) 59.

29. FONG Y, BRENNAN MF ET AL.: Gall bladder cancer discovered during laparoscopic surgery. Potential for iatrogenic tumor dissemination. Arch Surg 128 (1993)1054–1056.

30. FURHMAN G, OTA DM: Laparoscopic intestinal stomas. Dis Colon Rectum 37 (5) (1994) 444–449.

31. FUSCO MA, PALUZZI MW: Abdominal wall recurrence after laparoscopic-assisted colectomy for adenocarcinoma of the colon. Dis Colon Rectum 36 (1993) 858–861.

32. GLEESON NC, NICOSIA SV ET AL.: Abdominal wall metastases from ovarian cancer after laparoscopy. Am J Obstet Gynecol 169 (1993) 522–523.

33. GRINNELL RS: Results of ligation of inferior mesenteric artery at the aorta in resections of carcinoma of the descending sigmoid and colon and rectum. Surg Gynecol Obstet 120 (1965) 1031–1036.

34. GUILLOU PJ, DARZI A ET AL.: Experience with laparoscopic colorectal surgery for malignant disease. J Surg Oncol 2 (Suppl 1) (1993) 43–49.

35. HARNSBERGER JR, VERNAVA AM ET AL.: Radical abdominopelvic lymphadenectomy: historic perspective and current role in the surgical management of rectal cancer. Dis Colon Rectum 37 (1994) 73–87.

36. HASSON HM: A modified instrument and method for laparoscopy. Am J Obstet Gynecol 110 (1971) 886–887.

37. HEALD RJ, HUSBAND E ET AL.: The mesorectum in rectal cancer surgery: the clue to pelvic recurrence. Br J Surg 69 (1982) 613–616.

38. HEALD RJ, RYALL RDH: Recurrence and survival after total mesorectal excision for rectal cancer. Lancet 1 (1986) 1479–1482.

39. HORGAN PC, O'CONNELL PR, SHINKAIN LA, KIRWAN WO: Effect of anterior resection on anal sphincter function. Br J Surg 76 (1989) 783–786.

40. HSIU J, FRED T ET AL.: Tumor implantation after diagnostic laparoscopic biopsy of serous ovarian tumors of low malignant potential. Obstet Gynecol 68 (1986) 90.

41. HUGHES ESR, McDERMOTT FT, POLGLASE AL, JOHNSON WR: Tumor recurrence in the abdominal scar tissue after large-bowel surgery. Dis Colon Rectum 26 (1983) 571–572.

42. IRENE O, LUK IS ET AL.: Surgical lateral clearance in resected rectal carcinomas: a multivariate analysis of clinopathologic features. Cancer 71 (6) (1993) 1972–1976.

43. JACOBS M, VERDEJA JC, GOLDSTEIN HS: Minimally invasive colon resection (laparoscopic colectomy). Surg Laparosc Endosc 1 (3) (1991) 144–150.

44. KARAMURA YJ, SAVADA T, MUTO T, NAGAI H: Laparoscopic assisted colectomy and lymphadenectomy with abdominal wall lifting method. Dis Colon Rectum 37 (1994) 16.

45. KHOO RE, MONTREY J, COHEN MM: Laparoscopic loop ileostomy for temporary fecal diversion. Dis Colon Rectum 36 (10) (1993) 966–968.

46. KOYAMA Y, MORIYA Y ET AL.: Effects of extended systemic lymphadenectomy for adenocarcinoma of the rectum: significant improvement of survival rate and decrease of local recurrence. Jpn J Clin Oncol 14 (1984) 623–632.

47. LANDEN SM: Laparoscopic surgery and tumor seeding. Surgery 144 (1993) 131–132.

48. LANGE V, MEYER G, SHARDEY M, SCHILDBERG FW: Laparoscopic creation of a loop ileostomy. J Laparoendosc Surg 1 (3) (1991) 307–312.

49. LARACH SW, SALOMON MC ET AL.: Laparoscopic-assisted abdominoperineal resection. Surg Laparosc Endosc 3 (1993) 115–118.

50. MADOFF RD: Laparoscopic colectomy: Should we do it for cancer just because we can? 5th Annual Colorectal Disease Symposium. Fort Lauderdale, Florida, February 24–26, 1994: 382–383.

51. McDERMOTT JP, DEVEREAUX DA, CAUSHAJ PF: Pitfall of laparoscopic colectomy: an unrecognized synchronous cancer. Dis Colon Rectum 37 (6) (1994) 602–603.

52. MILSOM JW, LAVERY IC, BOHM B, FAZIO VW: Laparoscopically assisted ileocolectomy in Crohn's disease. Surg Laparosc Endosc 3 (2) (1993) 77–80.

53. MILSOM JW: Current status of treatment of rectal prolapse using laparoscopic technique. 5th Annual Colorectal Disease Symposium in Fort Lauderdale, Florida (1994). 391–392.

54. MIRALLES RM, PETIT J ET AL.: Metastatic cancer spread at the laparoscopic puncture site. Report of a case in a patient with carcinoma of the ovary. Eur J Gynecol Oncol 6 (1989) 442–444.

55. MONSON RT, DARZI A, DECLAN-CARRY P, GUILLOU P: Prospective evaluation of laparoscopic-assisted colectomy in an unselected group of patients. Lancet 340 (1992) 831–833.

56. MUNRO W, AVRAMOVIC J, RONEY W: Laparoscopic rectopexy. J Laparosc Surg 3 (1) (1993) 55–58.

57. MURTHY GM, GOLDSCHMIDT RA ET AL.: The influence of surgical trauma on experimental metastases. Cancer 64 (1989) 2035–2044.

58. MURTHY SM, SUMMARIA JL ET AL.: Experimental metastases at sites of surgical trauma (abstract). Proc Ann Meet Am Assoc Cancer Res 31 (1990) A393.

59. NDUKA CC, MONSON JRT, MENZIES-GOW, DARZI A: Abdominal wall metastases following laparoscopy. Br J Surg 81 (1994) 648–652.

60. NEWMAN L, LUKE JP ET AL.: Laparoscopic herniorrhaphy without pneumoperitoneum. Surg Laparosc Endosc 3 (1993) 213–215.

61. NGOI SS, KUM CK, GOH PMY ET AL.: Laparoscopic colon resection: the Singapore experience. Poster presentation at the Tripartate Colorectal Surgery Meeting, Sydney, Australia, October 17–20, 1994.

62. NOGUERAS JJ, JAGELMAN DG: Principles of surgical resection: influence of surgical techniques on treatment outcome. Surg Clin North Am 73 (1) (1993) 103–116.

63. ORKIN BA: RECTAL CARCINOMA: treatment. In: Beck DE, Wexner SD (eds.) Fundamentals of anorectal surgery. McGraw-Hill, New York (1992) 260–369.

64. O'ROURKE N, HEALD RJ: Laparoscopic surgery for colorectal cancer. Br J Surg 80 (10) (1993) 1229–1230.

65. ORTEGA A, BEART R, ANTHONE G, SCHLINKERT R: Laparoscopic bowel resection: a consecutive series (abstract). Dis Colon Rectum 37 (1994) 22.

66. PETERS WR, BARTELS TL: Minimally invasive colectomy: Are the potential benefits realized? Dis Colon Rectum 36 (1993) 751–756.
67. PEZET D, FONDRINIER E ET AL.: Parietal seeding of carcinoma of the gallbladder after laparoscopic cholecystectomy. Br J Surg 79 (1992) 230.
68. PEZIM ME, NICHOLLS RJ: Survival after high or low ligation of the inferior mesenteric artery during curative surgery for rectal cancer. Ann Surg 200 (1984) 729–733.
69. PHILLIPS EH, FRANKLIN M ET AL.: Laparoscopic colectomy. Ann Surg 216 (1993) 703–742.
70. PIER A, GÖTZ F, BACHER C: Laparoscopic appendectomy in 625 cases: from innovation to routine. Surg Laparosc Endosc 1 (1) (1991) 8–13.
71. QUATTLEBAUM JK JR, FLANDERS HD, USHER CH: Laparoscopically assisted colectomy. Surg Laparosc Endosc 3 (2) (1993) 81– 87.
72. QUIRKE P, DIXON MF ET AL.: Local recurrence of rectal adenocarcinoma due to inadequate surgical resection. Lancet 1 (1986) 1996–1998.
73. REDWINE DB, SHARPE DR: Laparoscopic sequential resection of the sigmoid colon for endometriosis. J Laparoendosc Surg 1 (1) (1991) 217–220.
74. REICH H, MCGLYNN F ET AL.: Laparoscopic repair of full thickness bowel injury. J Laparoendosc Surg 12 (1991) 119–122.
75. REISSMAN P, LIGUMSKY M, BLOOM A, DURST AL: Laparoscopic adhesiolysis: a treatment for recurrent obstruction due to adhesions. Min Invas Ther 3 (1994) 103–104.
76. REISSMAN P, TEOH TA, COHEN SM, WEISS EG, NOGUERAS JJ, WEXNER SD: Is early oral feeding safe after elective colorectal surgery? Dis Colon Rectum 37 (4) (1994) 14–15.
77. REISSMAN P, WEXNER SD, NOGUERAS JJ, JAGELMAN DG: Complications of laparoscopic colorectal surgery. 4th World Congress of Endoscopic Surgery (abstract). Kyoto, Japan, June 16–19, (1994) 94.
78. REISSMAN P, TEOH TA, PICCIRILLO M, NOGUERAS JJ, WEXNER SD: Colonoscopic-assisted laparoscopic colectomy. Surg Endosc 8 (1994) 1352–1353.
79. REIVER D, KMIOT WA, COHEN SM, WEISS EG, NOGUERAS JJ, WEXNER SD: A prospective comparison of laparoscopic procedures in colorectal surgery (abstract). Dis Colon Rectum 37 (4) (1994) 22.
80. RUSSI EG, PERGOLIZZI S ET AL.: Unusual relapse of hepatocellular carcinoma. Cancer 70 (•) 1483–1487.
81. SAYE WB, RIVES DA, COCHRAN EB: Laparoscopic appendectomy: three years experience. Surg Laparosc Endosc 1 (2) (1991) 109–115
82. SCHMITT SL, COHEN SM, WEXNER SD ET AL.: Does laparoscopic assisted ileal pouch anal anastomosis reduce the length of hospitalization? Int J Colorectal Dis 9 (1994) 134–137.
83. SCOGGIN SD, FRAZEE R: Laparoscopic-assisted resection of a colonic lipoma. J Laparoendosc Surg 2 (1992) 185–189.
84. SCOGGIN SD, FRAZEE RC, SNYDER SK, HENDRICKS JC, ROBERTS JW, SYMMONDS RE, SMITH RW: Laparoscopic-assisted bowel surgery. Dis Colon Rectum 36 (1993) 747–750.
85. SEMM K: Endoscopic appendectomy. Endoscopy 15 (1983) 59–64.
86. SENAGORE AJ, LUCHTEFELD MA ET AL.: Open colectomy versus laparoscopic colectomy: Are there differences? Am J Surg 59 (8) (1993) 549–554.
87. SIRIWARDENA A, SAMARJI WN: Cutaneous tumor seeding from a previous undiagnosed pancreatic carcinoma after laparoscopic cholecystectomy. Ann R Coll Surg Engl 75 (1993) 199–200.
88. SHIDA H, BAN K ET AL.: Prognostic significance of location of lymph node metastases in colorectal cancer. Dis Colon Rectum 351 (1992) 1046–1050.
89. SOCIETY OF AMERICAN GASTROINTESTINAL ENDOSCOPIC SURGEONS (SAGES) 1990. Granting of privileges for laparoscopic general surgery. Los Angeles, May 1990.
90. SOCIETY OF AMERICAN GASTROINTESTINAL SURGEONS (SAGES): Guidelines for General Surgery Resident Education in Gastrointestinal Endoscopy 1993. Surg Endosc 7 (1993) 144–145.
91. STOCKDALE AD, POCOCK TJ: Abdominal wall metastases following laparoscopy: a case report. Eur J Surg Oncol 11(1985) 373–375.
92. SUGARBAKER PH, CORLEW S ET AL.: Influence of surgical technique on survival in patients with colorectal cancer: a review. Dis Colon Rectum 25 (1982) 545–557.
93. TATE JJ, KWOK S ET AL: Prospective comparison of laparoscopic and conventional anterior resection. Br J Surg 80 (1993) 1396–1398.
94. TEOH TA, REISSMAN P, WEISS EG, VERZARO R, WEXNER SD: Enhancing cosmesis in laparoscopic colon and rectal surgery. Dis Colon Rectum 38 (1995) 213–214.
95. TEOH TA, REISSMAN P, COHEN SM, WEISS EG, WEXNER SD: Laparoscopic loop ileostomy (letter). Dis Colon Rectum 37 (6) 514.
96. TURNBULL RB, KYLE K ET AL.: The influence of the no-touch isolation technique on survival rate. Ann Surg 166 (1967) 420–425.
97. UDDO JF: Right hemicolectomy with intracorporeal anastomosis. In: Ballantyne GH, Leahy PF, Modlin EM (eds.): Laparoscopic surgery. W.B. Saunders Philadelphia (1994).
98. VALLA JS, LIMONNE B, VALLA V, MONTUPET P, DAOUD N, GRINDA A, CHAVRIER Y: Laparoscopic appendectomy in children: report of 465 cases. Surg Laparosc Endosc 1 (3) (1991) 166–172.
99. VAN YE TM, CATTERY RP ET AL.: Laparoscopically assisted colon resections compare favorably with open technique. Surg Laparosc Endosc 4 (1994) 25–31.
100. VERNAVA AM, DEAN P: Preoperative and postoperative management. In: Beck DE, Wexner SD (eds.): Fundamentals of anorectal surgery. McGraw-Hill, New York (1992) 50–56.
101. VERZARO R, TEOH TA, WEXNER SD: Laparoscopic colorectal surgery: risk factors for local recurrences. Reg Cancer Treat 7 (1994) 183–187.
102. WEXNER SD, COHEN SM ET AL.: Laparoscopic colorectal surgery: a prospective assessment and current perspective. Br J Surg 80 (1993) 1602–1605
103. WEXNER SD, JOHANSEN OB: Laparoscopic bowel resection: advantages and limitations. Ann Med 24 (1992) 105–110.
104. WEXNER SD, JAMES K, JAGELMAN DG: The double stapled ileal reservoir and ileoanal anastomosis: a prospective review of sphincter function and clinical outcome. Dis Colon Rectum 34 (1991) 105–110.
105. WEXNER SD, COHEN SM: Port site metastases after laparoscopic surgery for cure of malignancy: a plea for caution. Br J Surg 82 (1995): 295–298.
106. WEXNER SD, JOHANSEN OB, NOGUERAS JJ, JAGELMAN DG: Laparoscopic total abdominal colectomy. A prospective trial. Dis Colon Rectum 35 (1992) 651–655.
107. WEXNER SD, TARANOW DA, JOHANSEN OB ET AL: Loop ileostomy is a safe diversion for fecal incontinence. Dis Colon Rectum 36 (4) (1993) 349–354.
108. WILLIAMS NS, DIXON MF ET AL.: Reappraisal of the 5 cm rule of distal excision for carcinoma of the rectum: a study of distal intramural spread and of patient's survival. Br J Surg 70 (1983) 150–154.
109. ZUCKER KA, PITCHER DE ET AL.: Laparoscopic-assisted colon resection. Surg Endosc 8 (1994) 12–18.
110. WEXNER SD, WEISS EG: Laparoscopic Resection of Colorectal Carcinoma: Is it safe? Presented at the annual meeting of the Society of Gastrointestinal Endoscopic Surgeons. Philadelphia, Pennsylvania, March 13–16, 1996.

17. | Transanal Endoscopic Microsurgery

L. E. SMITH

Introduction

Colorectal cancer is the most lethal gastrointestinal cancer in the Western world. In the United States there are approximately 60,000 cases of rectal cancer each year, and about half of these result in death. The precursors to carcinoma are a large number of adenomas, both tubular and tubulovillous types.

The removal of benign lesions transanally has been practiced using standard instruments for decades; however, only lesions in the distal half of the rectum are readily accessible. Rectal cancers that are small and meet certain clinical criteria have been successfully removed from the distal half of the rectum. The removal or destruction has taken the form of excision, cryotherapy, contact radiation therapy, laser therapy, or electrocoagulation. Needless to say, removal or destruction of all the cancer cells results in cure. The criteria for removal is the same in all cases when deciding which small cancers are amenable to local management.

Only in the past 10 years has it been possible to work effectively on neoplasms in the proximal half of the rectum. The difficulty has been adequate exposure and instruments that would reach to the proximal half of the anorectum. On average the rectum is 15 cm long, and working above the 8-cm level is extremely difficult with standard operating equipment. Fortunately, Gerhard Buess designed equipment that included large diameter operating proctoscopes and long instruments with miniature working tips for use in the upper rectum [2-6].

Prior to the advent of this equipment, most of these operations required an abdominal approach for either benign or small malignant lesions. Unfortunately, this often meant colostomy, either permanent if an abdominal perineal resection was performed, or temporary if a low anterior resection was performed. The morbidity that accompanied this pelvic surgery was great in that bladder dysfunction and sexual dysfunction were frequent.

Another approach to the upper rectum required a parasacral incision usually with removal of the coccyx, but which frequently resulted in fistula formation [8]. A trans-sphincteric approach as per York-Mason entails cutting the sphincter and reapproximating it after surgery [11].

Unfortunately, an incised sphincter may not work as well as it did prior to being incised. Hence, the stage was set for a treatment that could avoid the aforementioned difficulties.

Indications

Transanal endoscopic microsurgery (TEM) may be applied to all benign lesions found within the rectum. These should of course be verified by biopsy, and the proximal margins of the lesions should be scrutinized in order to be assured that the site can be removed with a margin and be sutured closed. Even large villous tumors may be removed in this fashion. Circumferential villous tumors can be removed, but the patient must be repositioned frequently. Needless to say, this is a formidable technical feat.

Small carcinomas may also be removed by this technique. A small carcinoma measures 3 cm in size or less. Specifically, small cancers can be excised locally with a high probability of cure. Tumors that are polypoid are more easily cured than those that are ulcerated. If the lesion is confined to the mucosa and submucosa, a cure rate above 90 % can be expected. If the carcinoma invades into the muscularis propria, the cure rate is decreased. Any carcinoma penetrating full thickness through the wall as a T3-staged lesion should not be treated by local means.

Clinically, the small carcinoma should be carefully assessed digitally for mobility. If the cancer is mobile, i.e., it is not tethered, the clinical criteria of full-thickness penetration, it is a suitable lesion for local removal.

In the past 10 years, with the advent of endoluminal ultrasound, our clinical impression for depth of invasion could be checked [1, 7]. Using the ultrasound, the layers of the bowel wall, which are displayed as rings on the ultrasound image, and hence, the tumor depth, can be plotted. (Figs. 1A and B). In addition to the direct examination of the local invasion, lymph nodes may be identified in the surrounding pararectal tissue. An opportunity is afforded to go back clinically to find if nodes can be reached with the finger and to see what their size and consistency is. Lymph nodes over 5 mm in size may direct the surgeon to perform a more radical surgery. After local excision, any lymph node that is noted should be followed in the postoperative period for progressive enlargement suggesting lymph node metastasis. Prior to embarking upon local excision for carcinoma, a computerized tomography of the abdomen and pelvis is warranted to see that there are no sites that are consistent with metastasis.

An incurable cancer of the rectum may be palliated by local TEM. Tumor may be resected or electrocoagulated to maintain an open lumen, to avoid the symptoms of obstruction. Hemorrhage can also be stopped with these techniques.

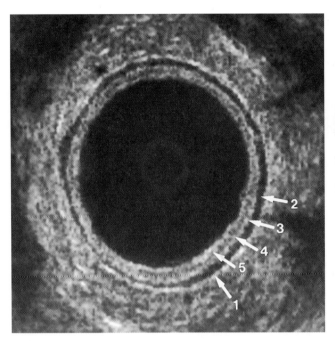 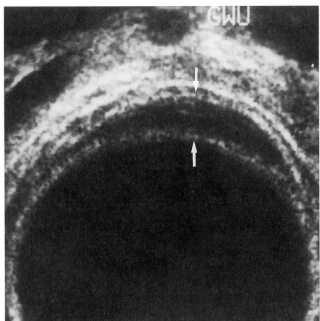

Figs. 1A, B. **A.** Rectal ultrasound. Normal „rings" seen. (1) Hypoechoic interface between muscularis propria and perirectal fat; (2) hyperechoic muscularis propria; (3) hypoechoic interface between submucosa and muscularis propria; (4) hyperechoic mucosa/submucosa layer; (5) hypoechoic interface between the balloon and mucosa. **B.** Abnormal rectal ultrasound. Between the arrows is a thickened hyperechoic ring consistent with the mucosal layer. This may represent a T1 carcinoma or a benign neoplasm

Contraindications are few. Lesions that extend out of the area where direct visualization is possible are of course not amenable to this treatment. If there is a stricture from other disease or surgery, performing a TEM is not possible. Carcinomas overlying the vagina are not good choices for TEM, because a rectovaginal fistula may ensue. Those overlying the cul-de-sac of the peritoneal cavity should be approached cautiously, but this is not an absolute contraindication. A hole from a full-thickness excision can be repaired. The most difficult decision is deciding whether the operating proctoscope will reach high enough to allow adequate excision of the lesion and closure of the wound. Those extending into the sigmoid colon are particularly problematic, because the proximal margin is out of view.

Instruments

An insufflation machine that allows 6 l/min insufflation of carbon dioxide is required. A pressure limit is chosen so that the rectum can be held open for good exposure, and 15 mmHg are not exceeded. A vacuum pump is built into the system so that suction can be applied at a lower pressure than that which is used to maintain exposure. Therefore, the rectal walls do not collapse during the procedure inadvertently. An electrocautery machine is needed, which provides both a cutting and a coagulation current. High-frequency electrocoagulation allows fine cutting for dissection of the tumor. The coagulation current is the primary source for hemostasis.

Large bore operating proctoscopes have been designed for reaching into the rectum (Fig. 2). These are 15 and 20 cm long, and the diameter is 4 cm. They come equipped with a face plate, which locks in providing a gas-tight fit. Plastic

sleeves snap onto the ports in the face plate. Onto these sleeves are fitted caps with holes through which instruments are inserted. These caps fit tightly around the instruments preventing gas leakage (Fig. 2). A microscope for the surgeon is introduced through another port in the face plate (Fig. 3). There is a smaller port through the microscope for a monocular attachment for an assistant. A video camera can be coupled to the monocular attachment so that others in the room and the assistants can see.

Long instruments include the following: an electric knife, a needle holder, a clip applier, two forceps, angled both right and left, scissors, angled both right and left, a water-suction probe, and a needle for injection (Fig. 4). The clip applier is particularly valuable, because these clips attached to a suture take the place of knots. Knot tying is extremely difficult with small instruments in a small space; therefore, these clips are a tremendous advantage.

Operative Technique

The patient is prepared in the usual fashion for a colorectal procedure including both a mechanical and antibiotic bowel preparation [9, 10]. The patient should be admonished to work very hard to be absolutely free of solid stool. Informed consent should include the possibility of laparotomy and ostomy should serious complications be encountered that necessitate closure of a perforation or access to control hemorrhage. If a cancer is detected, it may be reasonable to go ahead with a cancer operation at that time if it is felt that the extent of invasion is greater than that acknowledged in the preoperative evaluation. Anesthesia can be regional, but is usually general anesthesia with an endotracheal tube. The

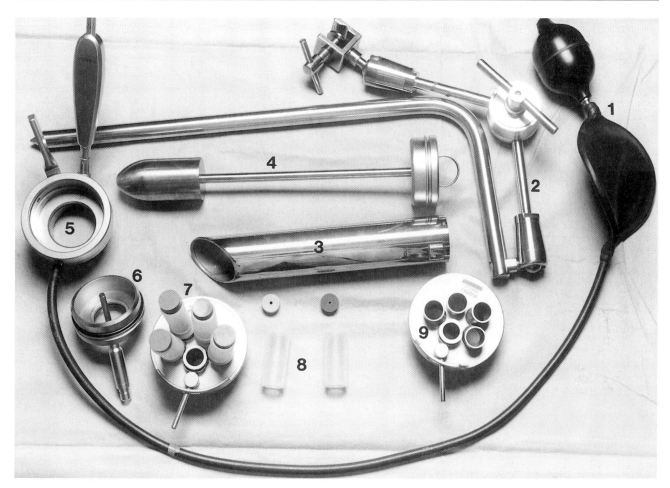

Fig. 2. Operating proctoscopy system. (1) Insufflation bulb connected to the face plate with a clear window ; (2) Martin arm for attachment of the proctoscope to the operating table; (3) a 20-cm operating proctoscope; (4) obturator for insertion; (5) face plate with clear window for positioning; (6) face plate, opposite side; (7) working face plate with silastic sleeves and caps attached; (8) silastic sleeves and caps not attached; (9) working face plate without sleeves

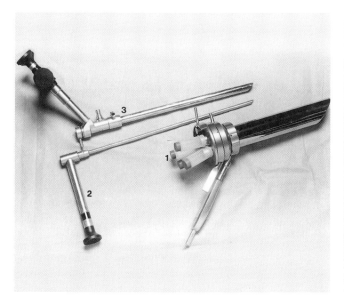

Fig. 3. Optic system with proctoscope. (1) Proctoscope with face plate and sleeves mounted; (2) camera probe which passes through the port in the binocular optic; (3) binocular optic, which passes through the uppermost part in the proctoscope face plate

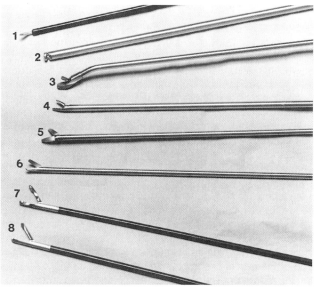

Fig. 4. Transanal endoscopic surgical instruments. (1) Electric knife; (2) clip applier; (3) angled needle holder; (4) straight needle holder; (5) (6) scissors, both right and left angled; (7) (8) forceps, both right and left angled

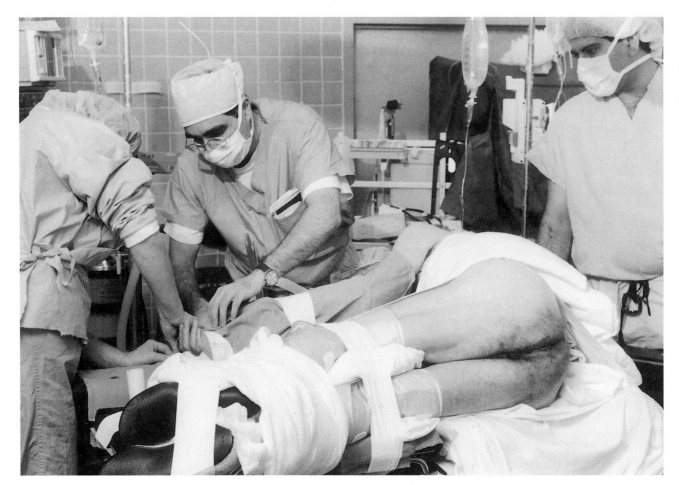

Fig. 5. The patient is positioned with the hips flexed and the anus over the end of the operating table. Note that this can be achieved in a knee/chest position or a supine position using support stirrups

patient must be placed on the operating table with the center of the tumor directly down. The hips must be acutely flexed in order to allow direct access to the anus (Fig. 5). In the supine position the stirrups may be placed such that the legs are pulled up over the abdomen. In the lateral position the knees must be flexed and extended out onto an adjoining support. In the prone position, the table must be acutely flexed in order to permit the hips and knees to be drawn down tight and spread apart for access to the anus. It sometimes requires ingenuity to find means to support the feet in this position. A catheter is inserted into the bladder and the rectum is irrigated. A rigid sigmoidoscopy is used to verify the position of the tumor and empty residual fluid out of the rectum. Sterile drapes are placed over the patient, leaving the anal area exposed.

A clear glass face plate is locked onto the operating proctoscope for the initial insertion. The operating proctoscope has an obturator that is tapered and allows easier introduction while well lubricated. Once the scope tip is placed over the tumor, a Martin fixation arm is applied to the table and the other end of the arm is fixed to the scope to keep it rigidly in place for the operator. Then the operating face plate and microscope are mounted. The face plate is fitted with sleeves and initially with caps with no holes in them to maintain gas tightness. The tubing for insufflation, irrigation, suction, and gas-pressure monitoring line are attached (Fig. 6).

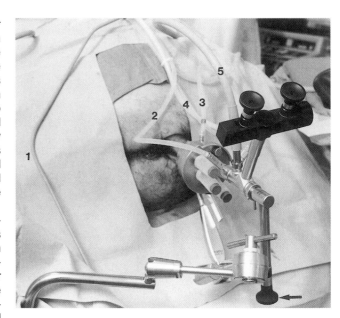

Fig. 6. Lines attached to scope. (1) A line is attached to the suction probe; (2) carbon dioxide insufflation; (3) carbon dioxide flow monitor line; (4) water infusion line; (5) light source cable. The arrow points to the television coupler

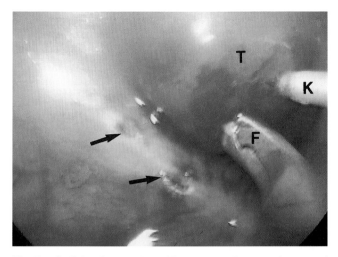

Fig. 7. Outlining the neoplasm. The arrows point to marks created by the electric knife 1 cm from the tumor (T); knife (K); forceps (F)

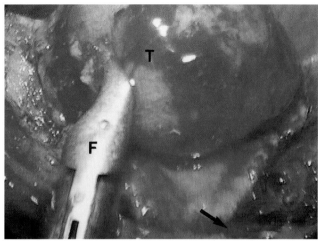

Fig. 9. Full-thickness incision. The marking dots are connected by an incision through the rectal wall to the perirectal fat, tumor (T); forceps (F). The arrow points to the incision

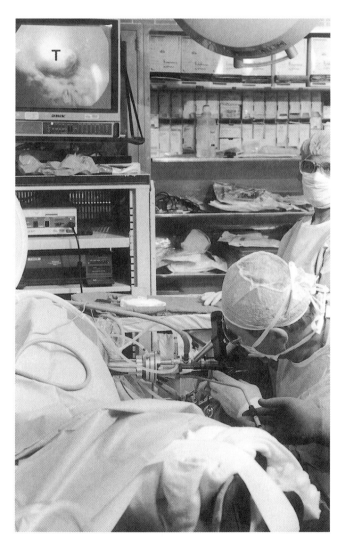

Fig. 8. Transanal endoscopic microsurgery unit in use. The binocular scope provides a three-dimensional field at work. The tumor (T) and instrument tips are seen on the monitor

The scope tip is generally best tilted away from the tumor lifting the opposite wall off of the operating site. This allows the operator to lift his head and straighten his neck for comfort. As the tip of the scope is lifted away from the tumor, a wider field can be seen. The operation is conducted from the right side of the field toward the left. This approach is taken during excision and closure.

The initial step may be to inject an epinephrine solution around the tumor, being careful not to penetrate it. The electrocautery knife is used to provide small dots 1 cm from the tumor margin, which will serve as a guide as to where to make an incision (Fig. 7). At this time the microscope is most helpful in trying to separate the margin of a flat, benign villous tumor and the normal mucosa (Fig. 8). A 1-cm margin is generally desirable especially in a malignant lesion. It is advisable to make the margin on the right side slightly wider in order to create a clear site that can be grasped and pulled without causing direct laceration of the tumor. The previously marked dots are then connected using the high-frequency cutting current. The incision is usually extended through the entire bowel wall until fat is seen. If the operator feels certain that the lesion is benign, it may be removed in the submucosal plane. At this point the mucosa at the right side of the tumor is lifted and undercut using the electric knife (Fig. 9). Whenever bleeders are encountered, they are clamped and electrocoagulated. The knife may be used for direct application of cautery current, but both the suction device and the forceps are also equipped to deliver electrocoagulation. The tumor is resected and carefully inspected to see that the margins appear to be clear of tumor. The wound is again inspected for hemostasis.

Closure of the wound is conducted using 3-0 polydiaxanone (PDS) suture (Fig. 10). This suture is selected because it holds the silver clip readily. Suturing is performed by directing the needle through normal mucosa into the wound at the right lateral end of the excision site (Fig. 11). A simple, running, over and over suture technique is used (Fig. 12). At the end of the suture line another silver clip is applied to secure the closure. Because of the small operating area, the suture material is cut in only 6-cm lengths (Fig. 10). Therefore, a long suture line usually requires more than one 6-cm suture, and

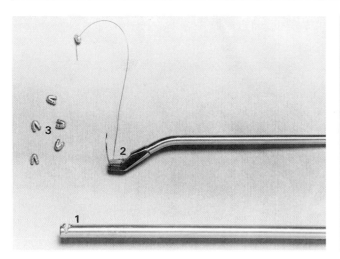

Fig. 10. Clip application system. (1) The clip applier with a split clip mounted; (2) a needle holder with a needle and suture with the clip applied to the tip of the 6-cm suture; (3) five silver split clips

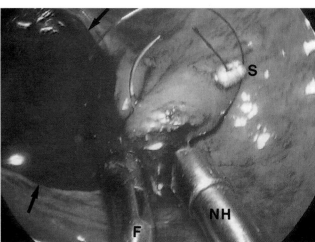

Fig. 12. Continuous suturing. The arrows mark the wound margins. With tissue fixed by the forceps, the needle holder (NH) drives the needle through the upper wound margin. The silver clip (S) is already pulled into and engaged in the end of the wound after the first pass of the needle and suture

hence, the use of more than two silver clips as knots (Figs. 13 and 14).

After removal of the scope, the tumor is pinned flat on a cork board for better pathological examination. Better slides can be created by having better perpendicular cuts.

The patient is usually admitted for observation overnight, but if the lesion is small and the operation went smoothly, some patients may be sent home and followed as an out-patient.

Complications

During introduction of the scope, at times it has been necessary to abort the procedure because the lesion could not be completely seen, due to angulation at the rectosigmoid junction, stricture secondary to previous surgical procedures, or inability to completely visualize the proximal margin of the lesion. The finding of an invasive cancer in what was believed to be a benign lesion might alter the approach. If a perforation into the peritoneum occurs, it may be repaired transanally. If the closure is felt to be tenuous, the abdomen may need to be opened for better closure. In difficult situations where closure is uncertain, a proximal ostomy is appropriate. If a rectovaginal fistula occurs, this must be carefully closed in layers.

The operating proctoscopes have a 4-cm diameter, and there is a significant stretch of the anal sphincter. There may be a laxity of the sphincter while it regains tone. Injection of bupivicaine with epinephrine around the sphincter mechanism may help it relax prior to beginning. On occasion a patient does have a partial loss of continence. In our hands this has been minor and only exhibited as minor soiling episodically. Local infection is manifest by a fever in the postoperative period. These respond well to antibiotics. Interestingly, infection is a rare complication.

Follow-up

The patient is carefully inspected at monthly intervals to see that the wounds heal. Subsequently, the site of excision is carefully inspected for recurrence. On one occasion we have found a hard lump, which we felt obligated to operate upon to define its character. It turned out to be the silver clip, which had been buried under the mucosa during healing. This should be carefully watched for and an operation might be avoided. Large villous tumors are multicentric in origin and may recur on one side or the other of the excision. Small foci can be electrocoagulated should they recur. If a carcinoma recurs, it may be re-resected if it is felt to be superficial, but it may require a radical surgery to obtain the best chance of cure. Certainly, if lymph nodes are discovered by follow-up ultrasound, then a formal, more radical surgery should be recommended. When incurable cancer is the original diagnosis, recurrence may be expected, and this simply must be reexcised to keep the lumen open.

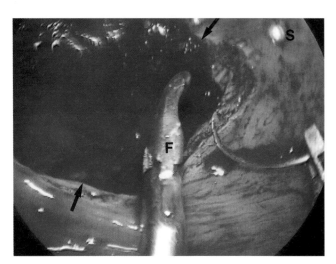

Fig. 11. Closing the wound. The arrows point out the margins of the defect. The forceps (F) and the needle holder are in the foreground. The silver clip (S) is attached to the suture

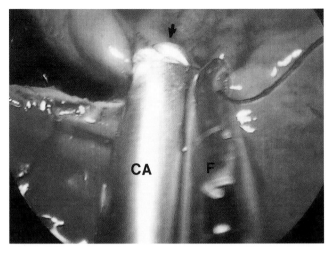

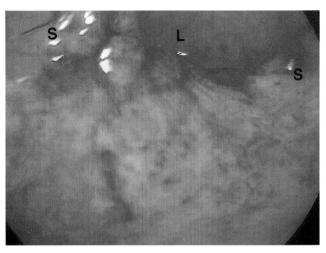

Fig. 13. Clip application. The arrow points to the split silver clip in the tip of the clip applier (CA). The forceps (F) holds the suture taut as the clip is clamped onto the suture

Fig. 14. Closed wound. The silver clips (S) denote the two ends of the incision. The proximal lumen (L) is seen

George Washington University Medical Center Experience

In 3 years 50 patients were treated by transanal endoscopic microsurgery. There were 15 carcinomas, 31 adenomas, and 4 other pathologies including a prolapse, a solitary rectal ulcer, and 2 carcinoids. In the adenoma group there were 14 males and 17 females. In the carcinoma group there were 11 males and 4 females. The dominant number of patients were in the 50-69 years age group.

The tumors were located at levels ranging from 4 to 15 cm. The critical level, above 8 cm, at which the use of standard operating instruments for anal and low rectal lesions is extremely difficult included 25 of the 50 patients. This critical measurement is taken at the lowest margin of the lesion. Of the lesions, 25 were above the 8 cm level, and 3 were at the 15-cm level. Of the carcinomas, 7 were located in the distal half of the rectum and 8 were found in the proximal half of the rectum. Two T-2 lesions were located in the distal half of the rectum. A T-3 lesion and a recurrent carcinoma were excised from the proximal half of the rectum. The T-2, T-3, and the recurrent carcinomas recurred. It is our policy to recommend a proctectomy or low anterior resection for T-2 or greater carcinomas, poorly differentiated carcinomas, and when carcinoma is found within the local lymphatics.

As might be expected, the diameter of the adenomas was larger. By clinical selection, 13 of the carcinomas were 3 cm or less. A 4- and 5-cm adenoma was found to contain a carcinoma. At surgery there was minimal blood loss. There was less than 200 cc of blood loss per patient in 48 patients. One patient had a 300-cc blood loss and another had a 400-cc blood loss. The operating room time averaged 1.9 h. Patients were hospitalized only 0.9 days. In fact, 8 of the patients were sent home immediately after surgery. Early complications included only 2 patients with a temperature, which responded to antibiotics. There was no late hemorrhage or death.

Conclusion

The local excision of benign rectal neoplasms and selected carcinomas has been enhanced by the development of special instruments. Transanal endoscopic microsurgery now permits removal of all such neoplasms including those in the proximal rectum. Cost-effectiveness for a short hospitalization is assured as compared with low anterior resection or abdomino-perineal resection.

References

1. BEYNON J, FOY DMA, ROE AM et al.: Endoluminal ultrasound in the assessment of local invasion in rectal cancer. Br J Surg 73 (1986) 474.
2. BUESS G, THIESS R, GUNTHER M et al.: Endoscopic operative procedure for the removal of rectal polyps. Coloprotology 6 (1984) 254.
3. BUESS G, THIESS R, GUNTHER M et al.: Endoscopic surgery in the rectum. Endoscopy 17 (1985).
4. BUESS G, KIPFMÜLLER K, HACK D et al.: Technique of transanal endoscopic microsurgery. Surg Endosc 2 (1988) 71.
5. BUESS G, KIPFMÜLLER K, HACK D et al.: Clinical results of transanal endoscopic microsurgery. Surg Endosc 2 (1988) 245.
6. BUESS G, MENTGES B, MANNCKE K et al.: Minimal invasive surgery in the local treatment of rectal cancer. Int J Colorect Dis 6 (1991) 77.
7. HILDEBRANDT V, FIEFEL G, SCHWARTZ HP et al.: Endorectal ultrasounds instrumentation and clinical aspects. Int J Colorectal Dis 1 (1986) 203.
8. KRASKE P: Zur Exstirpation des hochsitzenden Mastdarm Krebs. Verh Dtsch Ges Chir 14 (1885) 464.
9. SACLARIDES TJ, SMITH L, KO ST et al.: Transanal endoscopic microsurgery. Dis Colon Rectum 35 (1992) 1183–1191.
10. SMITH L: Transanal endoscopic microsurgery for rectal neoplasms. Gastro Intest Endosc Clin North Am 3 (1993) 329–341.
11. YORK-MASON A: Surgical access to the rectum – a transsphincter exposure. Proc R Soc Med 63 (1970) 91.

18. Laparoscopic Abdomino-Perineal Excision of the Rectum

F. KÖCKERLING, I. GASTINGER, T. RECK, AND F. P. GALL

Introduction

Within a short space of time the combination of reduced surgical trauma, less need for painkillers and early postoperative rehabilitation of the patient prompted the widespread adoption of the minimally invasive clinical procedures of laparoscopic cholecystectomy and appendectomy.

In extensive animal experiments we tested the suitability of the laparoscopic technique for use in clinical colorectal procedures. Three major technical problems were identified and needed to be resolved:

1. Development of a laparoscopic technique for extended lymph node dissection with division of the main vascular structures close to their point of origin
2. Development of safe laparoscopic anastomotic techniques for the colon and rectum
3. Establishment of an oncologically acceptable technique of retrieving specimens without the need for a laparotomy

The results of our experimental studies showed that with the instruments and techniques presently available, extended lymph node dissection with division of the inferior mesenteric artery close to its origin from the aorta is the best candidate for a purely laparoscopic approach. The triple-stapling technique developed by us to perform a laparoscopic anastomosis in the region of the sigmoid colon makes it possible to create such an anastomosis with an acceptable level of risk. The limiting factor is now more likely to be the retrieval of the specimen without a laparotomy.

On the basis of these experimental findings, it seemed logical to assume that their most likely translation to the clinical situation would be laparoscopic abdomino-perineal excision of the rectum with division of the inferior mesenteric artery close to its origin, because with this operation a colostomy is easy to create, and retrieval of the specimen can readily be performed by the perineal surgeon [5, 7, 8, 10, 11].

On August 1, 1992, we carried out the first laparoscopic abdomino-perineal excision of the rectum with ligation of the inferior mesenteric artery close to the aorta. By the middle of 1994, we had used this technique, which is described herein, to treat 18 patients with a low rectal carcinoma, with no serious complications thus far.

Indications

With the increasing use of stapling devices and transanal anastomotic techniques, the indication for sphincter-preserving resection of the rectum for carcinoma has been expanded.

Rectal carcinomas at a distance from the anal verge of 7-8 cm in men and 6-7 cm in women can be removed by means of a low anterior rectal resection followed by a stapled anastomosis. In the borderline area between 4 and 8 cm from the anal verge, the sphincter muscle may also be preserved by performing inter-sphincteric resection with subsequent colo-anal anastomosis. The indication for this procedure is determined by the distance of the tumour from the anal verge and its clinical stage.

With regard to the latter, T2 lesions less than 4 cm and T3 lesions less than 5 cm from the anal verge, as well as all tumors infiltrating the external sphincter, must be resected abdomino-perineally. This also applies to patients with a flaccid sphincter shown by manometry to be insufficient. In the case of T1 tumors, a transanal local sphincter-preserving full-thickness excision of the rectal wall is performed.

Advanced low rectal carcinomas infiltrating neighbouring structures (T4 tumors), e. g. the posterior wall of the vagina, bladder, prostate and/or the seminal vesicles, require an extended rectal excision, and are thus not to be treated by laparoscopy. Thus, the indication for laparoscopic excision of the rectum is a low rectal carcinoma located between 0 and a maximum of 5 cm from the anal verge, and infiltrating the muscularis propria (T2) or, at most, just invading the perirectal fat tissue (T3).

If the perirectal fatty tissue has been widely infiltrated, or if there are extensive lymph node metastases around the tumor, a conventional open surgical technique should be employed. Extended lymph node dissection with ligation of the inferior mesenteric artery close to its origin complies with the oncological principles of radicality. Among curatively operated rectal carcinomas (anterior and low anterior resection and rectal excision), we found metastases in the lymph nodes along the trunk of the inferior mesenteric artery in 3 % of all patients, and in 6.5 % of those with lymph node metastases.

Since 1980 in all anterior and low anterior resections and abdomino-perineal amputations, we have extended the dissection by adding a high, "central" ligation of the inferior mesenteric artery.

The 5-year survival rate observed after curative resection of rectal carcinoma has improved from 53.4 ± 4.7 % in the period 1969-1977 to 69.3 ± 4.6 % in the period 1978-1983, and to 79 ± 7.7 % in the period between 1984 and 1988. According to the results published by the "Deutsche Studiengruppe Kolorektales Karzinom" (German Colorectal Carcinoma Study Group), the percentage of abdomino-perineal rectal resections for carcinoma in 1986 was about 30 %. Presently, the figure is estimated to be about 10-15 %.

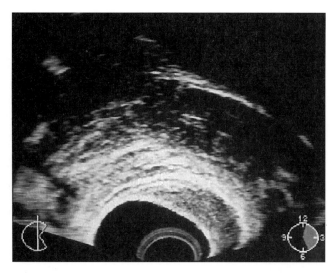

Fig. 1. Preoperative endosonography in a patient with carcinoma of the rectum 3 cm from the anal verge (T3). Curative laparoscopic amputation of the rectum

Preoperative Work-up

In addition to the physical and rectoscopic examinations aimed at determining the height of the tumor from the anal verge, and a histological work-up, we routinely carry out a preoperative endosonography of the rectum (Fig. 1) and a computed tomography (CT) scan of the abdomen. Endosonography has proved capable of providing an accurate assessment of the extent of a rectal carcinoma in 90 % of cases. A further advantage of endosonography is that the surrounding structures, such as the bladder, seminal vesicles, prostate gland, vagina and sacrum, are well visualized. Any infiltration of these structures by the tumor can be detected with a high degree of certainty.

If the carcinoma has reduced the remaining lumen to less than the 2 cm necessary for the endosonographic examination, a CT scan must be done to exclude an infiltration of neighbouring structures. As already mentioned, enlarged lymph nodes do not contraindicate the laparoscopic technique, because they are dissected in the same way as in conventional excision of the rectum, and are thus removed together with the specimen.

To prepare the bowel for the procedure, preoperative lavage using isotonic solution (4-5 l oral) has proved expedient. By adding 50 g high molecular weight dextran/l , absorption of the fluid, which may otherwise be as much as 2 l, can largely be avoided [3]. Prior to the operation, the optimal site for the terminal colostomy is determined by the stoma therapist and marked on the patient's abdomen.

Operative Technique

The patient is first placed in the lithotomy position, with hips somewhat flexed, and is then tilted into a 45-50 % Trendelenburg position to allow the small bowel to move up against the diaphragm out of the operating field. The bladder is catheterized and the catheter is led to one side across the thigh, to which it is then taped. In similar fashion the male genitals are also moved to one side and taped out of harm's way.

After digital examination, the anus is closed with a double purse-string suture to prevent exit of tumour cells. To facilitate the perineal part of the operation, the buttocks are spread apart maximally with the aid of adhesive tape. The patient is draped as for conventional surgery, leaving the abdomen free from the xiphoid to the pubic symphysis and for a considerable distance to either side.

Laparoscopic abdomino-perineal excision of the rectum requires the combined efforts of an experienced team comprising two surgeons of about equal skill and experience, an experienced assistant to operate the camera, and additional assistant for the surgeons and a scrub nurse with experience with laparoscopic surgery.

The two surgeons are positioned on the left and right of the patient. With the latter in the lithotomy position, there is no space next to the surgeons for the cameraman, who therefore takes up his position at the patient's head. The patient's left arm remains at his side, while the right arm is angled away from the body to allow convenient placement of, and access to, arterial and venous lines. The head of the patient is covered on the left side by a drape placed over a stout bar fixed across the operating table, thus enabling the cameraman to work comfortably and unimpaired for the duration of the lengthy laparoscopic colorectal procedure. The video unit, together with the monitor and light source, is placed between the patient's legs. The equipment needed for electrosurgery is situated on the patient's right, and the instrument table and endoirrigator on his left – an arrangement we have found to be most convenient.

The five trocars are positioned in a U-configuration around the umbilicus, with the open part of the U directed towards the pelvis (Fig. 2). The Veress needle and the camera trocar are inserted above the umbilicus somewhat to the left of the midline, with the aim of preserving an adequate distance to the

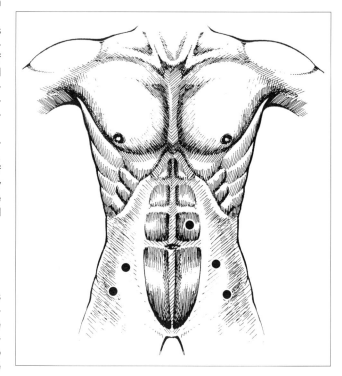

Fig. 2. Placement of ports

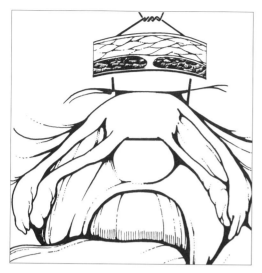
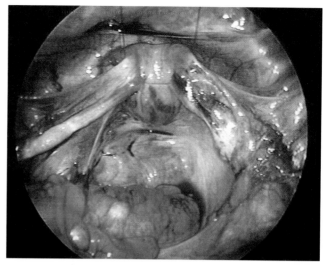

Figs. 3 A, B. Fixation of the uterus and adnexa to the anterior abdominal wall

pelvis while at the same time avoiding insufflation into the liga-mentum teres hepatis.

Two 12-mm working trocars are placed in the left, and two in the right, lower abdomen. The use of 12-mm ports is necessary, because the linear stapler can only be used via a trocar of at least this size, and the optimal angle of approach of the linear stapler changes during the course of the operation. The left upper trocar is inserted at the site pre-selected for the subsequent colostomy.

Prior to the start of the operation, the 30 ° telescope is used to inspect the abdominal cavity and small pelvis. With the aid of cotton applicators the small bowel is moved into the upper part of the abdominal cavity. If necessary, the Trendelenburg position may be increased to ensure that the small bowel remains out of the way. Even the steepest Trendelenburg position has not impeded the operation in any way. The small pelvis is then inspected.

In female patients the uterus and adnexa need to be elevated to facilitate the subsequent manipulations deep within the

pelvis. For this purpose a suture with a straight needle is first introduced through the abdominal wall, and the needle is then passed through the ligamentum latum uteri below the adnexa on the right. The needle is then turned 180 °, passed through the ligamentum latum to the left of the uterus behind the ad-nexa and out again through the abdominal wall. The uterus and adnexa are then drawn up to the abdominal wall and se-cured in place by tying the suture outside the body (Figs. 3A and B). With this technique a good view of the female pelvis is obtained and dissection is facilitated.

For dissection and other preparatory work, the use of cotton applicators is indispensable. They can readily be used to apply tension to the tissue so that dissection can be carried out with-out risk of injury particularly to the wall of the colon or rectum. Dissection is begun by dividing the embryonic attachments of the sigmoid colon to the lateral wall of the abdomen using co-agulation (Figs. 4A and B). The sigmoid and descending parts of the colon are mobilized towards the splenic flexure for a length sufficient to allow subsequent tension-free colostomy.

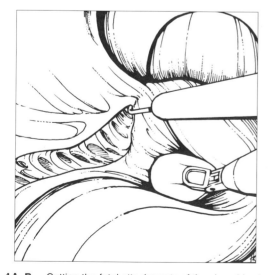
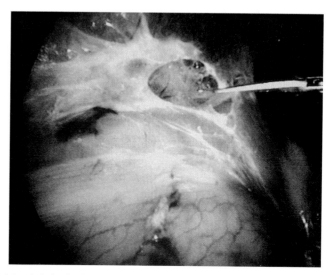

Figs. 4 A, B. Cutting the fetal attachments of the sigmoid colon to the lateral abdominal wall using electro-coagulation

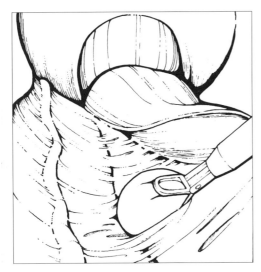 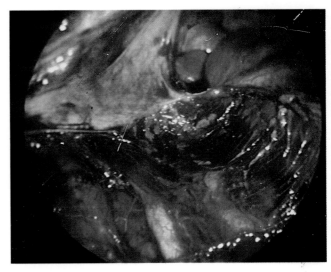

Figs. 5A, B. Dissection of the left ureter where it crosses the left common iliac artery

After dividing the peritoneum in the plane of the fascia of Gerota, the mesosigmoid and descending mesocolon can be freed with a cotton applicator - from the fascia of Gerota to the aorta. Particular care must be taken to identify and expose the left ureter where it crosses the left common iliac artery (Figs. 5A and B). When the mesosigmoid has been adequately mobilized to the aorta, the sigmoid is moved aside to the left with cotton applicators and, approaching from the right, the peritoneum is divided above the aorta, below the plane of the inferior mesenteric artery or superior rectal artery (Figs. 6A and B). While doing this a gap opens up in the mesosigmoid between the plane of the aorta and the longitudinal axis of the superior rectal artery. Into this gap a cotton applicator is now inserted from the left (Figs. 7A and B) to lift the sigmoid, together with the mesosigmoid, towards the abdominal wall.

During this procedure the dorsal fascial space opens up between Waldeyer's fascia and the mesorectum, and the lateral peritoneum of the rectum is put under tension. The delicate connective tissue fibres between the leaves of the dorsal fascial space can now be divided in steps using the coagulation scissors (Figs. 8A and B) so that the dorsal fascial space opens up and further dissection can be performed down to the floor of the pelvis.

The pelvic dissection is continued only for as long as it is easy to do. Finally, dissection is continued cephalad towards the trunk of the inferior mesenteric artery. Dissection in the plane between the aorta and the major mesosigmoid blood vessels presents no problem, because this mesosigmoid attachment contains very few vessels. When the trunk of the inferior mesenteric artery is exposed (Fig. 9), the artery is picked up with an endodissector (Figs. 10A and B).

Because transection of the inferior mesenteric artery at its origin is best accomplished with the linear stapler, the thickness of the tissue of the vessel must first be measured with the aid of a gauge (Fig. 11). The scale on the device usually

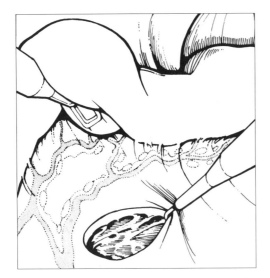 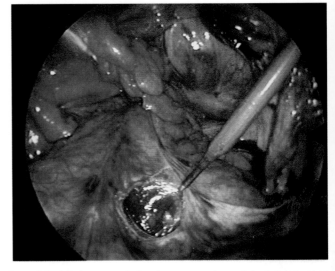

Figs. 6A, B. The peritoneum above the aorta and below the vascular plane of the inferior mesenteric artery or superior rectal artery is incised from the right side

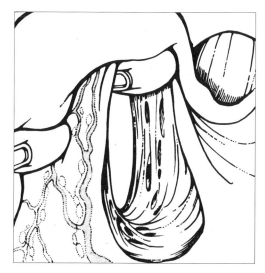
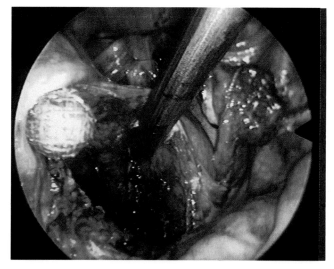

Figs. 7 A, B. Insertion of a cotton applicator into the gap between the aorta and plane of the long axis of the superior rectal artery in the mesosigmoid

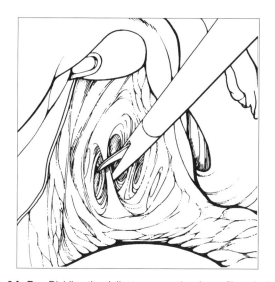
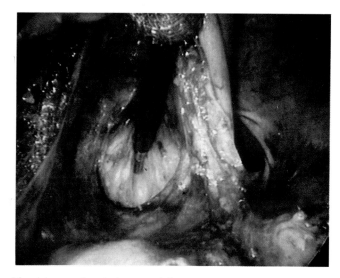

Figs. 8 A, B. Dividing the delicate connective tissue fibres in the dorsal fascial gap using electro-coagulation

indicates the need for a white vessel cartridge. A 30-mm Endo-GIA with the white vessel cartridge in place is then introduced via a 12-mm port, and the inferior mesenteric artery is divided close to the aorta (Figs. 12 A and B). Each of the two ends of the transected vessel is reliably closed with three rows of staples (Fig. 13). Alternatively, the inferior mesenteric artery can be divided using PDS clips (Fig. 12 A). After dividing the inferior mesenteric artery at the trunk, the cranial boundary of the lymph node dissection is established. The colon is then divided stepwise with the Endo-GIA at the junction between the descending/sigmoid colon and the mesocolon. Here also the thickness of the tissue is measured with the gauge before each application of the stapler (Fig. 14).

For transection of the colon a blue cartridge, and for dividing the mesenterium a white vessel cartridge, is usually required. Transection of the colon at the transition of the descending to sigmoid with the stapler leaves the proximal and distal ends of the bowel safely closed with three rows of staples each (Figs. 15 A and B and 16 A and B). The distal end of the bowel is now grasped with a colon forceps and pulled

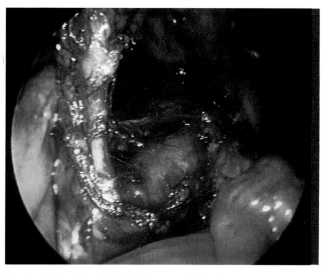

Fig. 9. Dissection of the inferior mesenteric artery

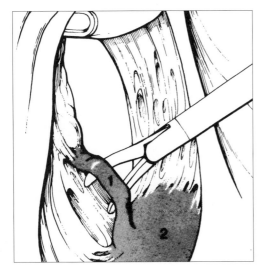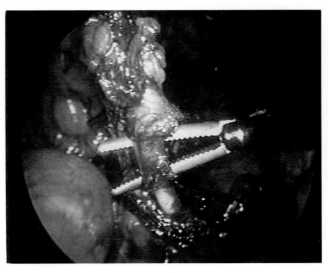

Figs. 10A, B.   Picking up the inferior mesenteric artery with an endo-dissector (1 inferior mesenteric artery; 2 aorta)

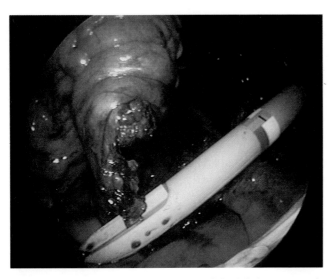

Fig. 11.   Measurement of the thickness of the inferior mesenteric artery with a gauge

cephalad (Fig. 17), and the pelvic dissection is continued. A U-shaped incision placed medially and somewhat caudal to the ureter is then made in the pelvic peritoneum around the rectum (Figs. 18A and B).

As in conventional surgery, dorsal mobilization of the rectum is performed. The mesorectum is pushed aside ventrally using cotton applicators, and the dorsal fascial gap is opened up with coagulation scissors or a coagulation hook down to the floor of the pelvis (Fig. 19).

Anterior mobilization of the rectum is accomplished in the male in the recess of Dennonvilliers' fascia, and in the female in the obliterated fascial gap dorsal to the vagina. For this purpose the bladder or vagina are moved aside ventrally with two cotton applicators. Traction is applied to the rectum using the colon forceps, and dissection is continued into the fascial gap using the coagulation scissors or hook (Fig. 20). Here also dissection should be performed as far as possible towards the pelvic floor.

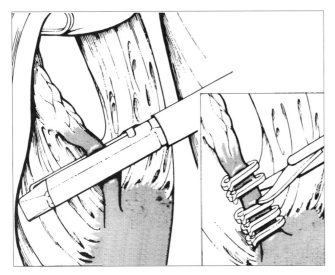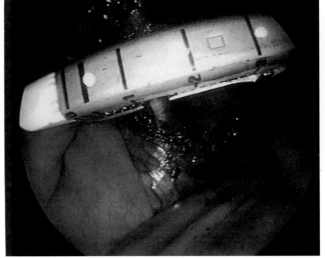

Figs. 12A, B.   Dividing the inferior mesenteric artery at its point of origin using the linear stapler or eventually between absorbable clips

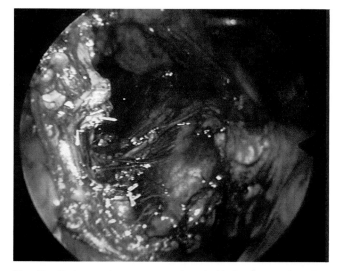

Fig. 13. Both vascular stumps are closed with three rows of staples

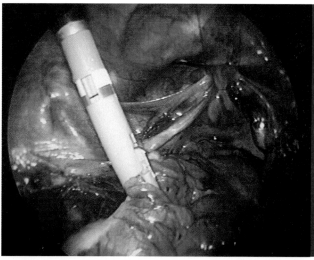

Fig. 14. Gauging the thickness of the tissue at the descending colon/sigmoid junction

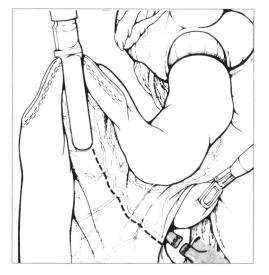

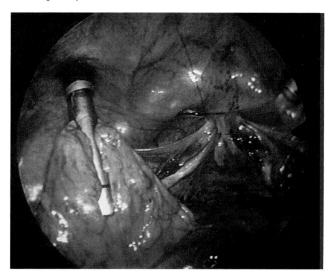

Figs. 15 A, B. Transecting the colon at the descending colon/sigmoid junction with the linear stapler

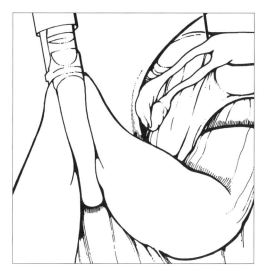

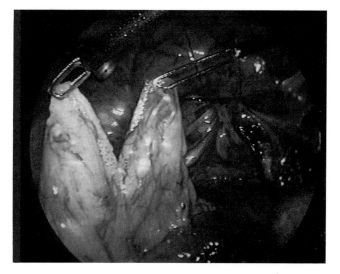

Figs. 16 A, B. Each end of the transected colon is safely closed with three rows of staples

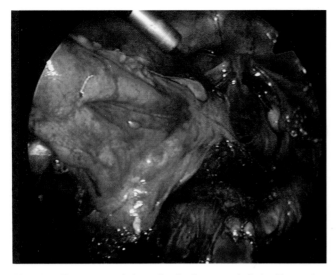

Fig. 17. The stump of the colon is drawn cephalad with a colon forceps

Following dorsal and ventral dissection in the fascial gaps in front of and behind the rectum, it only remains to divide the paraproctia and the middle rectal artery. A cotton applicator is placed first in the anterior, and then in the posterior fascial gap, and the rectum is moved towards the respective opposite wall of the pelvis. In the paraproctia, which are thus put under tension, the middle rectal artery can be dissected, picked up with an instrument and then clipped (Figs. 21 A and B). After dividing the middle rectal artery on the left and right, mobilization of the rectum in the small pelvis is completed by dividing the paraproctia with the coagulation hook.

The abdominal part of the operation is then finished by constructing the terminal stoma. For this purpose the 12-mm port at the colostomy site, selected preoperatively, has to be replaced by a 20-mm or 33-mm "retrieval" port. To do this the skin is first excised around the 12-mm trocar, and a crosswise incision is made in the fascia. After introducing the trocar, the proximal end of the colon is grasped with a strong grasping forceps and drawn up into the port (Figs. 22 A and B). By releasing the pneumoperitoneum, the proximal end of the colon,

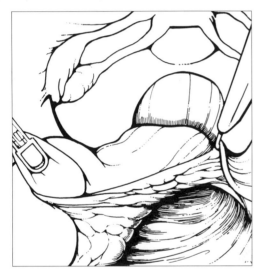
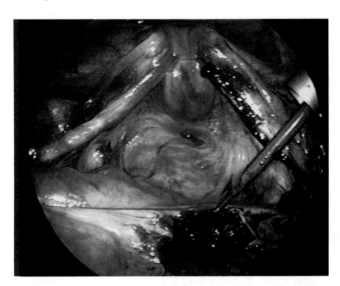

Figs. 18 A, B. The peritoneum is incised in U-shaped fashion around the rectum

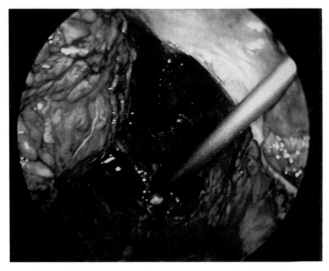

Fig. 19. Mobilization of the rectum in the dorsal fascial space down to the floor of the pelvis

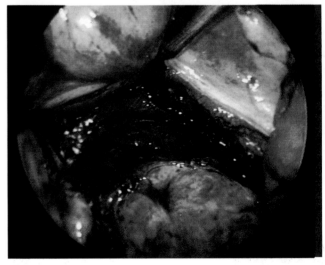

Fig. 20. Mobilization of the rectum in the ventral fascial space

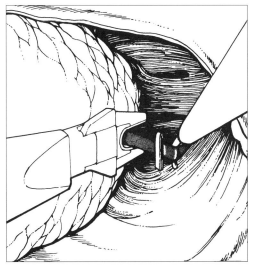 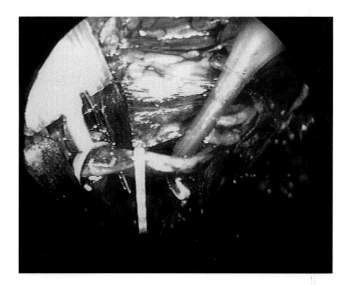

Figs. 21 A, B.   Dividing the middle rectal artery between clips

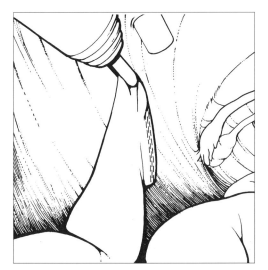 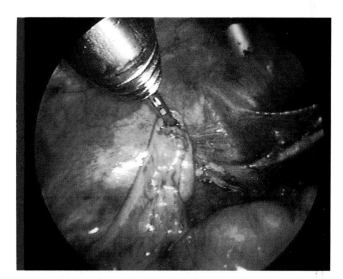

Figs. 22 A, B. The proximal end of the colon is grasped and drawn up into the 20-mm retrieval port

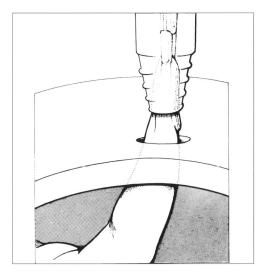 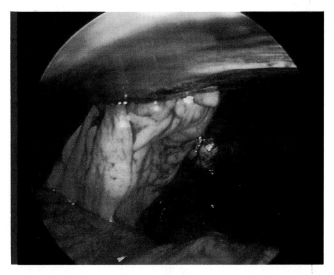

Figs. 23 A, B.   On releasing the pneumoperitoneum, the end of the colon moves tension-free through the abdominal wall

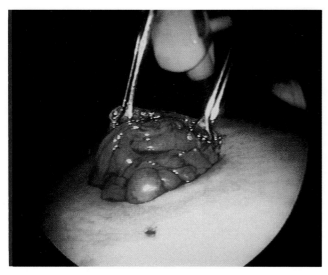

Fig. 24. The exteriorized proximal end of the colon showing the row of staples

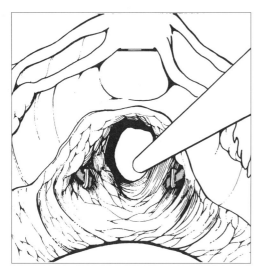
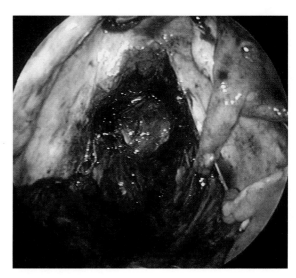

Figs. 25 A, B. View of the small pelvis after laparoscopic amputation of the rectum and hemostasis

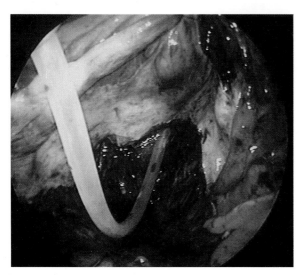

Fig. 26. Robinson drain placed in the small pelvis

together with the port, can readily be delivered through the abdominal wall (Figs. 23 A and B and 24). The row of staples is then opened with a diathermy instrument, and the end of the descending colon is sutured to the skin using single sutures.

Finally, the tension-free position of the descending colon can be inspected via the telescope (Fig. 23 B), excluding any torsion. Although the pneumoperitoneum has been released, the trocars remain in situ so that upon conclusion of the perineal part of the operation, the pelvis can again be inspected for residual bleeding.

The sacral part of the operation is performed using the technique described by Gall [3]. As greater facility is gained, laparoscopic mobilization of the rectum can be effected right down to the floor of the pelvis so that via the perineal wound, merely the levator ani muscles on either side of the rectum need to be divided, which is done in steps.

After the management of the sacral wound cavity, a mild pneumoperitoneum is re-established, and the sacral hollow is inspected intra-abdominally for residual bleeding. If necessary, hemostasis can be carried out either with the coagulation forceps or with the endoclip device (Figs. 25 A and B).

Upon completion of the operation, a Robinson drain is placed in the small pelvis via the left or right lower port (Fig. 26). The specimen retrieved via the perineal wound (Fig. 27) shows the high ligation of the inferior mesenteric artery and the en bloc lymph node dissection. Otherwise, our specimens differ in no way from those obtained after conventional amputation of the rectum. The number of lymph nodes dissected together with the specimen vary between 6 and 45, a range that corresponds to that normally found with conventional excision.

Results

By the middle of 1994, 18 patients had been operated on using the technique described herein. In an additional patient the operation had to be converted, because diverticulosis noted preoperatively at colonoscopy turned out to be severe diverticulitis and, in addition, aneurysms of both common iliac arteries displacing the ureters were found.

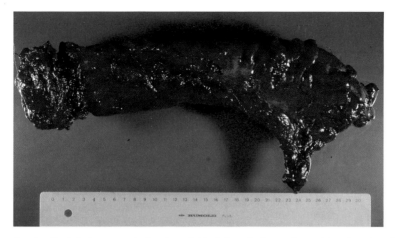

Fig. 27.   Surgical specimen showing the inferior mesenteric artery divided close to the aorta, and lymph nodes dissected en bloc

With the exception of three poorly healing perineal wounds, the postoperative course following laparoscopic amputation of the rectum was free from complications. With growing experience operating time had decreased to 4.5 h. With further improvements in instruments and additional experience, the operation may be expected to take about 4 h.

In all our patients the location of the tumor, clinical staging and the endosonographic findings were such that amputation of the rectum had to be the treatment of choice. A sphincter-preserving operation could not possibly have been considered in any of them.

In two patients with stenosing low rectal carcinoma and pulmonary and/or hepatic metastases, the excision was palliative. In all others the laparoscopic procedure was performed with curative intention. In an additional patient a solitary metastasis in the liver was resected in a second operation.

After laparoscopic excision of the rectum, the postoperative course is appreciably more favourable both for the patient and the nursing staff. Patients rarely complain of abdominal pain, merely pain associated with the perineal wound. More rapid mobilization of the patient is possible.

As a rule the colostomy is active on the second or third post-operative day. Also, the patient experiences hunger earlier, so that uptake of oral alimentation might even have to be restrained. Because of the absence of a laparotomy wound, management of the colostomy is considerably facilitated (Fig. 28).

Discussion

Laparoscopic colorectal surgery for carcinoma requires strict compliance with oncological principles of radicality, with the systematic dissection of lymph nodes and assurance of an adequate margin of clearance [1-4, 6-10, 12].

An important prerequisite for the clinical introduction of laparoscopic abdomino-perineal excision of the rectum was the development in animal experiments of laparoscopic techniques for lymph node dissection in the small pelvis and along the large vessel trunks. This provided the necessary basis for the clinical implementation of laparoscopic colorectal surgery to treat carcinomas.

Thanks mainly to the high ligation of the inferior mesenteric artery close to its origin from the aorta, and the ability to per-

form pelvic dissection, the abdominal part of the abdomino-perineal procedure of rectal amputation makes it possible to clear out the lymph nodes completely. Retrieval of the specimen is effected via the perineal wound. The indication for laparoscopic abdomino-perineal excision of the rectum is established on the basis of the physical examination, rectoscopic determination of the height of the tumor and the results of endosonography or CT.

If a rectal carcinoma is higher than 4-5 cm from the anal verge, a deep anterior rectal resection with a stapled anastomosis or an inter-sphincteric rectal resection with a trans-anal hand-sewn anastomosis and a protective loop ileostomy

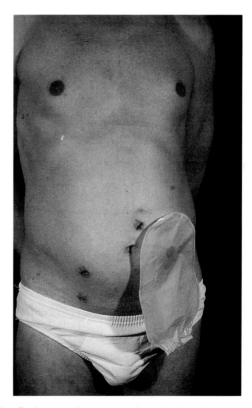

Fig. 28.   Patient wearing a stoma bag 10 days after laparoscopic excision of the rectum

has now become possible. If the carcinoma is lower than 4-5 cm from the anal verge, and if the carcinoma is limited to the mucosa and sub-mucosa (T1 tumor), it can be removed with adequate radicality by means of a transanal full-thickness excision provided that inspection of the specimen reveals no lymph node invasion.

If the lesion is an advanced low carcinoma infiltrating neighbouring structures, such as the posterior wall of the vagina, bladder, prostate or seminal vesicles (T4 tumors), an extended conventional procedure must be carried out, eventually including intraoperative radiation therapy. Thus, the indication for laparoscopic amputation of the rectum is T2 and T3 tumors located less than 4-5 cm from the anal verge; suspected lymph node metastasis is not considered a contraindication. Because clearance of the lymph nodes is effected as in conventional rectal amputation, any involved lymph nodes can be removed laparoscopically.

The histopathological workup of the specimens revealed no peculiarities as compared with conventional specimens. The number of lymph nodes removed together with the specimen was between 6 and 45, and thus corresponded to the normal range removed during a conventional excision of the rectum. No tearing of our specimens or tumors was observed. With the exception of two palliative procedures in patients with hepatic and pulmonary metastases. All the other procedures were assessed by the pathologist to be curative. Thus, there are no technical objections against the use of this minimally invasive procedure for treatment of low rectal carcinoma. A greater number of patients in prospective randomized trials [1, 3, 4, 5, 12] are needed to compare local recurrence rates and long-term results of laparoscopy with open colorectal procedures.

In our patients the postoperative course can only be described as very good. They recovered from the operation more quickly, and they hardly ever complained of abdominal pain. As a result, they could be mobilized earlier. Over the long term, preservation of the integrity of the abdominal wall may result in a reduction in the incidence of scar and stomal hernias in such patients.

The prerequisites for laparoscopic colorectal operations are considerable experience and skill in laparoscopic surgery and conventional colorectal surgery, and an appropriately well-trained team. Experimental training as a team seems advisable. The precise role of laparoscopic colorectal surgery in curative treatment of colorectal cancer still needs to be determined.

Until laparoscopic surgery for curative procedures for colorectal cancer has proven to be oncologically sound, it should be performed only in the context of prospective trials [5].

References

1. BEART RW JR: Laparoscopic colectomy: status of the art. Dis Colon Rectum 37 (1994) 47-49.
2. BLEDAY R, BABINEAU T, FORSE RA: Laparoscopic surgery for colon and rectal cancer. Sem Surg Oncol 9 (1993) 59-64.
3. COHEN SM, WEXNER SD: Laparoscopic colorectal resection for cancer: the Cleveland Clinic Florida experience. Surg Oncol 2 (1993) 35-42.
4. FRANKLIN ME JR., RAMOS R, ROSENTHAL D: Laparoscopic colonic procedures. World J Surg 17 (1993) 51-56.
5. GUILLOU PJ: Laparoscopic surgery for diseases of the colon and rectum - quo vadis? Surg Endosc 8 (1994) 669-671.
6. JACOBS M, VERDEJA JC, GOLDSTEIN HS: Minimally invasive colon resection (laparoscopic colectomy) Surg Laparosc Endosc 1 (1991) 144-150.
7. KÖCKERLING F, GASTINGER I, SCHNEIDER B, KRAUSE W, GALL FP: Laparoscopic abdominoperineal excision of the rectum with high ligation of the inferior mesenteric artery in the management of rectal carcinoma. Endosc Surg 1 (1993) 16-19.
8. KÖCKERLING F: Laparoscopic abdominoperineal excision with high transection of the inferior mesenteric artery. Surg Oncol Clin North Am 3 (1994) 731-743.
9. PHILLIPS EH, FRANKLIN M, CARROLL BJ, FALLAS MJ, RAMOS D, ROSENTHAL R: Laparoscopic colectomy. Ann Surg 216 (1992) 703-707.
10. O'ROURKE NA, HEALD RJ: Laparoscopic surgery for colorectal cancer. Br J Surg 80 (1993) 1229-1230.
11. SACKIER JM, BERCI G, HIATT JR, HARTUNIAN S: Laparoscopic abdominoperineal resection of the rectum. Br J Surg 79 (1992) 1207-1208.
12. WEXNER SD, COHEN SM, JOHANSEN OB, NOGUERAS JJ, JAGELMAN DG: Laparoscopic colorectal surgery: a prospective assessment and current perspective. Br J Surg 80 (1993) 1602-1605.

19. | Laparoscopic Rectopexy

F. KÖCKERLING, I. GASTINGER, T. RECK, AND F. P. GALL

Introduction

On account of its low morbidity and recurrence rates, recto-pexy using Wells' procedure is the most commonly employed surgical approach to rectal prolapse. Collective statistics show a mortality rate of 1.2 %, and a recurrence rate of 3 % for this operation [3]. These good results illustrate the super-iority of the transabdominal techniques over extra-abdominal procedures [5, 6, 8]. In our experience also, the Wells' proce-dure for rectopexy has been used with success for more than 2 decades, initially employing an Ivalon sponge, and later a Marlex or Prolene mesh. Nevertheless, despite the simplicity and good results of transabdominal correction of rectal pro-lapse, a less invasive operative procedure for the treatment of this benign condition would be most desirable.

On the basis of laparoscopic colorectal experimental stud-ies performed in the animal model and our clinical experience with laparoscopic abdomino-perineal excision of the rectum with high transection of the inferior mesenteric artery we have developed a laparoscopic version of Wells' procedure for rec-topexy [4]. In terms of the intra-abdominal manipulations in-volved, there is no fundamental difference between the lapar-oscopic and the conventional approach, but the absence of a laparotomy makes surgery less stressful for the patient.

Indications and Contraindications

The indication for laparoscopic rectopexy is the same as for an open Wells' procedure through a laparotomy. A relative contraindication may be seen in previously operated upon pa-tients, in whom the indication for the laparoscopic procedure must be assessed on the basis of existing scars and of ex-pected adhesions. Also, in patients with severe cardiac and/or pulmonary or other risk factors we reject the abdominal ap-proach in favour of an extra-abdominal procedure.

Preoperative Work-up

In addition to the usual routine examinations, pre-operative evaluation of anal sphincter pressure is obtained. A defeco-gram and rectoscopy are routinely performed. Further patho-logical findings in the colon are excluded by colonoscopy or a barium enema. If the rectal prolapse is associated with an elon-gated sigmoid colon, laparoscopic resection of the sigmoid colon can also be performed together with rectopexy (Fryk-man-Goldberg operation).

Operative Technique

To minimize the risks of peritonitis in the event of intra-opera-tive injury to the bowel, we consider pre-operative lavage of the colon to be of great importance. The patient is placed on the operating table in the lithotomy position with the hips somewhat flexed, and then moved into a steep (30-40 °) Tren-delenburg position. This ensures that the small bowel moves into the upper part of the abdomen, thus permitting a better view of the pelvis. The patient is draped in the usual manner, leaving the abdomen free from the xiphoid to the pubic sym-physis and for a considerable distance to either side. Two sur-geons of equal skill and experience take up their position to the left and right of the patient, and the assistant responsible for the camera stands near the head of the patient, whose left arm is placed along his/her side. The patient's right arm is angled away from the trunk for anaesthesiological manage-ment. The video "tower" comprising monitor, light source, etc. is placed between the patient's legs.

The Veress needle is inserted cranial to the umbilicus and somewhat to one side of the midline to ensure that the came-

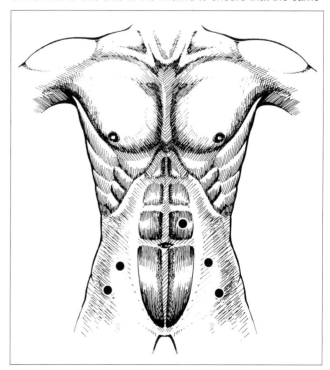

Fig. 1. Placement of ports for laparoscopic rectopexy

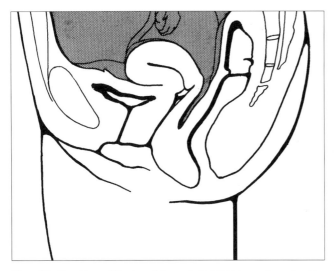 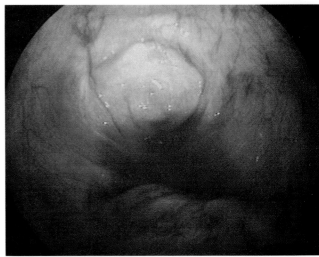

Figs. 2A, B.   View of the hernial sac during laparoscopic exploration of the small pelvis

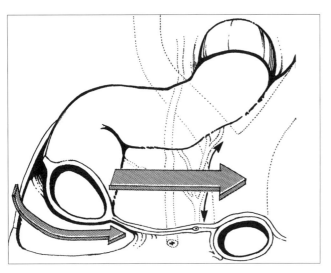 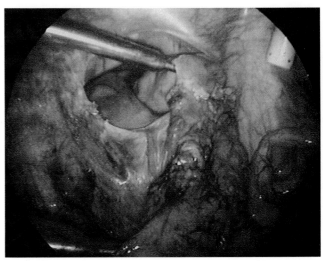

Figs. 3A, B.   **A.** Mobilization of the mesosigmoid along Gerota's fascia   **B.** Laparoscopic view from cephalad

ra port is at a sufficient distance from the pelvis and also from the working ports on the left and right. The pneumoperitoneum is created in the usual way, the maximum pressure employed being limited to 12 mmHg. The four working trocars are placed in a semi-circular configuration, i. e. two in the left and two in the right lower abdomen (Fig. 1).

In female patients the uterus and adnexa are fixed to the abdominal wall with a suture (see Fig. 3, Chap. 18). This ensures that the uterus does not impair the view when the rectum is being mobilized. The pelvis can readily be inspected, and the herniation of the bowel can typically be recognized by an enlarged Douglas pouch (Figs. 2A and B).

The first step is to mobilize the sigmoid colon. For this purpose the congenital adhesions to the lateral wall of the abdomen must be divided using coagulation while traction is applied by pushing the colon to the right. Only gentle traction is applied to the colon using cotton applicators. The procedure is continued, again with the aid of cotton applicators, by dissecting, from the left, the sigmoid mesocolon from Gerota's fascia down to the aorta (Figs. 3A and B). Particular care must

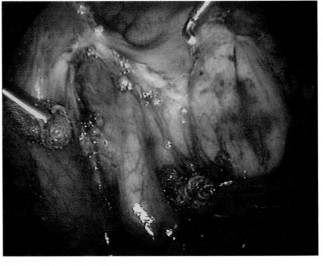

Fig. 4.   Dissection of left ureter

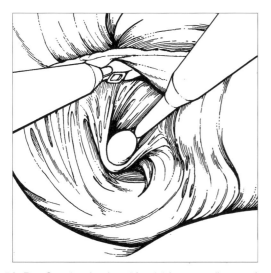
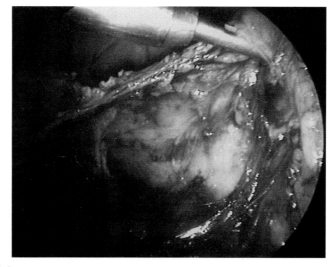

Figs. 5A, B.   Opening the dorsal fascial (retrorectal) space from the left

be taken to identify the ureter where it crosses the common iliac artery medially to the spermatic or ovarian vein (Fig. 4).

Dorsal mobilization of the rectum is the same as in conventional surgery. The mesorectum is lifted up with a cotton applicator, thus permitting access to the dorsal fascial gap (Figs. 5A and B). The delicate fibre attachments between the leaves of the retrorectal space are then divided as far as possible down to the floor of the pelvis (Fig. 6). When further opening of the dorsal retrorectal space is no longer possible, the sigmoid is moved to the left and the lateral peritoneum at the entrance to the pelvis is incised (Figs. 7A and B). The mesenterium is lifted up to the abdominal wall with a cotton applicator (Figs. 8A and B).

In order to mobilize the rectum right down to the floor of the pelvis, the paraproctia on either side must be divided stepwise using electro-coagulation (Fig. 9). Larger vessels are closed with titanium clips and transected. Because the herniated bowel causes an enlargement of the Douglas pouch between the posterior wall of the vagina and the anterior wall of the rectum, dissection in the anterior fascial gap is largely

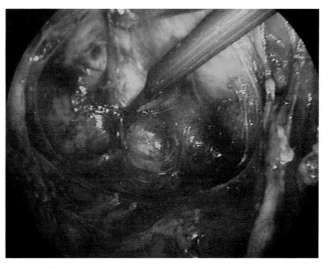

Fig. 6.   Dissection down to the floor of the pelvis in the dorsal retrorectal space

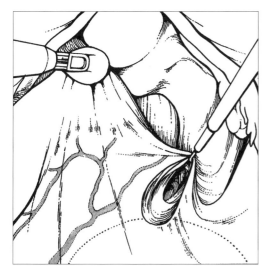
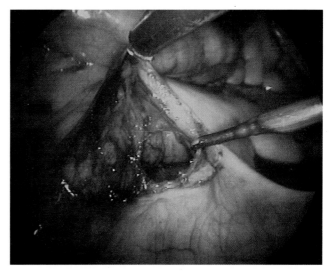

Figs. 7A, B.   **A.** Incision of the lateral peritoneum at the level of the promontorium.   **B.** The sigmoid colon has been moved aside to the left

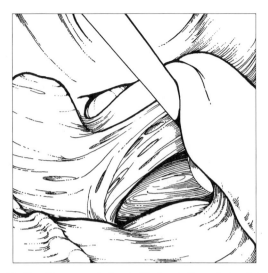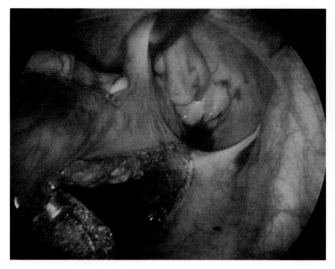

Figs. 8A, B. The mesenterium is lifted up to the anterior abdominal wall with a cotton applicator

unnecessary. Moreover, extensive dissection here can result in damage to autonomous nerve fibres. Adequate mobilization of the rectum can be achieved by extensive dorsal dissection in the pre-sacral space and division of the paraproctia on both sides (Figs.10A and B).

A strip of non-absorbable mesh (Marlex, Prolene, Surgipro) is cut to size (Figs. 11A and B) outside of the patient. In order to facilitate its reliable fixation to Waldeyer's fascia with sutures or staples, three openings are cut in the mesh. The latter is now rolled up, introduced into the abdomen via one of the working ports (Figs. 12A and B) and unrolled in front of the sacrum (Fig. 13).

Several methods are available for securing the mesh to Waldeyer's fascia: the use of the hernia stapler (Figs. 14A and B) or intra or extra-abdominally knotted single sutures (Figs. 15A, B and C). A conventional knotting technique is used, and the extracorporeal knots are introduced through the port with the aid of a knot pusher. Besides the staples, some single sutures suffice to provide secure fixation of the mesh. The windows previously cut in the mesh enable fixation to be per-

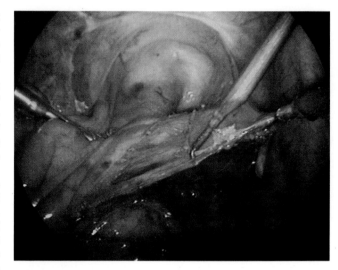

Fig. 9. Further incision of the lateral rectal peritoneum towards the small pelvis. The paraproctia on both sides are divided with a coagulation instrument and blood vessels are clipped

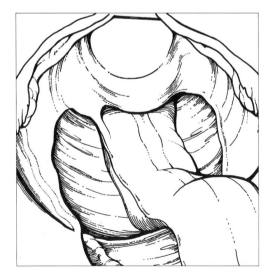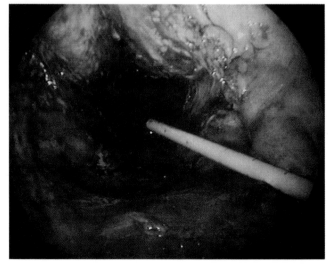

Figs. 10A, B. Complete mobilization of the rectum after dissection in the dorsal retrorectal space and division of the paraproctia on both sides

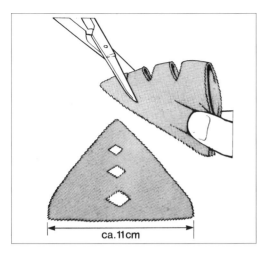 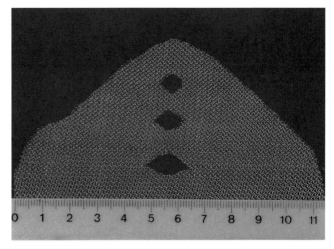

Figs. 11A, B. Cut-to-shape non-absorbable mesh with three central "windows" for reliable fixation to Waldeyer's fascia under direct vision

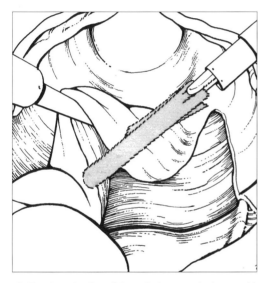

Figs. 12A, B. Introduction of the rolled-up mesh via a working port

formed under direct vision, thus helping to prevent damage to the pre-sacral venous plexus. After establishing a firm connection between mesh and Waldeyer's fascia, the rectum is placed in the mesh "cradle" and, using cotton applicators, cephalad traction is applied. At this point the two ends of the mesh can be trimmed as required; care must be taken to wrap no more than three-quarters of the circumference of the rectum in the mesh to avoid development of a stenosis. The rectum, under traction in the cranial direction, is then fixed to the lateral ends of the mesh using 6-8 single sutures knotted extracorporeally (Figs. 16A and B). Care should be taken to ensure that the needle passes only through the muscular layer of the rectal wall and does not penetrate the lumen; otherwise, contamination of the mesh may occur. When the tensioned rectum has been adequately fixed, the Douglas pouch is seen to be appreciably reduced in size (Figs. 17A–C). After irrigating the pelvis and performing meticulous hemostasis where needed, a silicone drain is placed in the pelvis and exteriorized via one of the trocars. The other trocars are removed under direct vision and the defects are closed in layers.

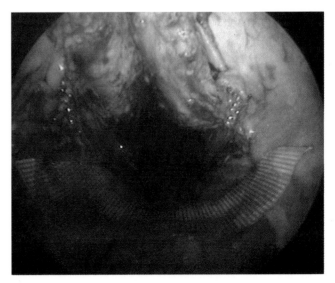

Fig. 13. The mesh positioned in front of Waldeyer's fascia

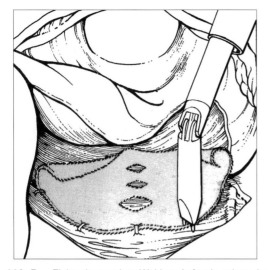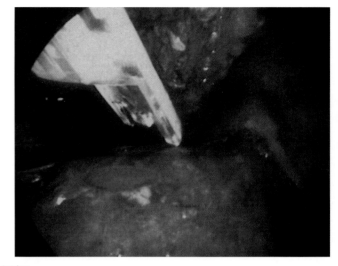

Figs. 14A, B.   Fixing the mesh to Waldeyer's fascia using a hernia stapler

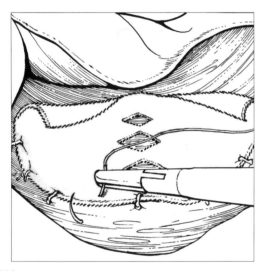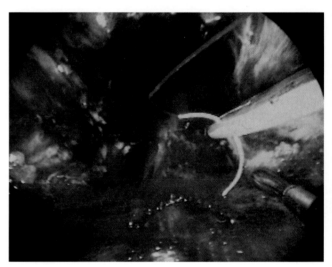

Fig. 15A.   **Fig. 15C.**

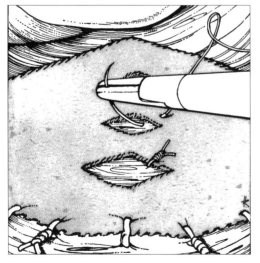

Because foreign material has been introduced into the body, the course of prophylactic antibiotics begun during the operation (see Chap. 5) is continued for another 5 days. When normal bowel function is resumed (usually from the third day onward), a light diet is permitted. Because straining during defecation should be avoided, a mild laxative may be prescribed where necessary.

Results

Between April 13th, 1992, and the middle of 1994, we performed a Wells' rectopexy procedure using the laparoscopic approach in 15 patients. The first two procedures took about 4.5 h, but the operating time was finally reduced to 3 h. In all 15 patients the entire operation was carried out laparoscopically; conversion to a conventional procedure was never required. In all patients both the intra-operative, and in particular the post-operative, course was free of complications. As observed in the case of laparoscopic cholecystectomy, the

Figs. 15A, B, C.   Additional fixation of the mesh to Waldeyer's fascia using single sutures

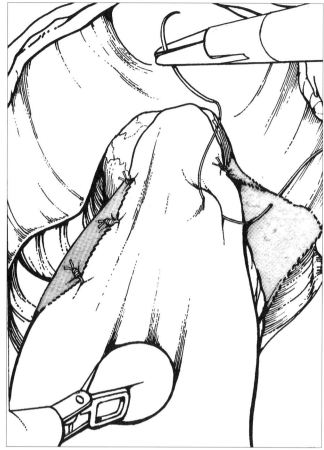

16A.

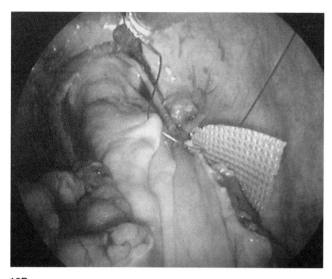

16B.

Figs. 16A, B. The mobilized rectum under mild cephalad traction is cradled in the mesh, each end of which is fixed to the rectum with 3-4 single sutures

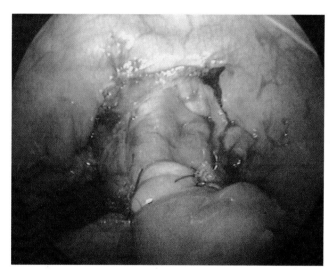

17B.

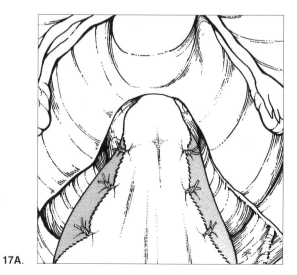

17A.

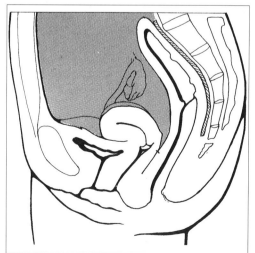

17C.

Figs. 17A, B, C. Rectopexy has been completed. The mobilized rectum is under cephalad traction and the Douglas pouch is now smaller

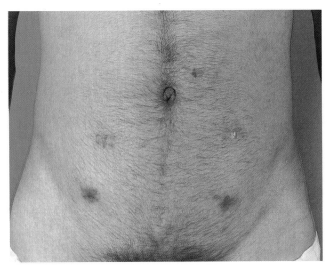

Fig. 18.　The patient 4 weeks after laparoscopic rectopexy

The non-absorbable mesh used for securing the rectum to Waldeyer's fascia can be fixed using either the hernia stapler or single sutures, or both techniques. The knots are made outside the body and then introduced and tightened with the aid of the knot pusher. This obviates any need for a specific laparoscopic knotting technique, which, however, depending on personal preference, can also be employed. Which of the mesh materials used by us will prove the most suitable over the long term has not yet been determined. Presently, no mesh-related infection has been observed. There is little difference between the various materials used in terms of handling, but there may be individual preferences. Securing of the rectum to the mesh for three-quarters of its circumference can also be accomplished by using single sutures. This way, as in the conventional procedure, reliable fixation of the mobilized rectum, under traction, to Waldeyer's fascia can be accomplished.

The principles of rectopexy using Wells' operation have thus now been adapted for laparoscopic approach. An open method for the correction of rectal prolapse that has been used successfully for decades can now be offered as a minimally invasive procedure. This is to the benefit of the patient, who profits greatly from the reduction in stress associated with the laparoscopic procedure. We consider it important that further advances in laparoscopic colorectal surgery should aim at modifying proven conventional methods as little as possible by developing suitable laparoscopic instruments. This, however, requires not only knowledge of the laparoscopic technique and appropriate training, but also mastery of conventional surgical methods.

patients were virtually pain-free in the post-operative phase, and were rapidly mobilized.

Presently, one recurrence of rectal prolapse has been observed, caused by initial use of absorbable suture material. Because, however, the operative method is in principle no different from that of conventional surgery involving laparotomy, the recurrence rate may be expected to be low. In our patients the mean hospital stay was 7 days. However, if circumstances require, or if the patient so wishes, the duration of hospitalization may be shortened even further (Fig. 18).

Discussion

In view of the low rate of complications and recurrence, abdominal procedures are the ones mainly recommended for the surgical treatment of rectal prolapse. However, the fact that numerous extra-abdominal procedures have also been tried is a reflection of a desire to offer the patient a less invasive way of treating this benign condition. However, the extra-abdominal procedures are associated with a high recurrence rate [3]. We are of the opinion that abdominal rectopexy using laparoscopic techniques represents an ideal compromise that provides effective treatment while causing only minimal stress to the patient [1, 2, 4, 7].

On the basis of the results of preliminary extensive experiments in animals, we were able to develop a laparoscopic version of Wells' procedure for rectopexy to be used in the clinical setting. Except for the route of access, it basically does not differ from the conventional approach. The mobilization of the rectum down to the floor of the pelvis, as already practiced in abdomino-perineal excision of the rectum, is done in the same way in the case of rectal prolapse by entering the dorsal retrorectal space and dividing the paraproctia. This approach enables complete mobilization of the rectum down to the floor of the pelvis.

References

1. BERMANN IR: Sutureless laparoscopic rectopexy for procidentia. Dis Colon Rectum (1992) 689-693.
2. CUSCHIERI A, SHIMI SM, VANDER-VELPEN G, BANTING S, WOOD RAB: Laparoscopic prosthesis fixation rectopexy for complete rectal prolapse. Br J Surg 81 (1994) 138-139.
3. ENCKE A, DOERTENBACH JG: Der Rektum- und Analprolaps. In: Bünte H, Junginger TH (eds.): Jahrbuch der Chirurgie 3, Biermann Verlag (1990) 115-129.
4. KÖCKERLING F, GASTINGER I, RECK T, SCHNEIDER B: Laparoskopische Eingriffe am Rektum. Langenbecks Arch Chir (1993) (Suppl) 111-116.
5. KRUYT RH, DELEMARRE JBVM, GOOSZEN HG, VOGEL HJ: Selection of patients with internal intussusception of the rectum for posterior rectopexy. Br J Surg 77 (1990) 1183-1184.
6. MADDEN MV, KAMM MA, NICHOLLS RJ, SANTHANAM AN, CABOT R, SPEAKMAN CTM: Abdominal rectopexy for complete prolapse: prospective study evaluating changes in symptoms and anorectal function. Dis Colon Rectum 35 (1992) 48-55.
7. MUNRO W, AVRAMOVIC J, RONEY W: Laparoscopic rectopexy. J Laparoendosc Surg 3 (1993) 55-58.
8. SAYFAN J, PINHO M, ALEXANDER-WILLIAMS J, KEIGHLEY MRB: Sutured posterior abdominal rectopexy with sigmoidectomy compared with Marlex rectopexy for rectal prolapse. Br J Surg 77 (1990) 143-145.

Other Abdominal Operations

20. Laparoscopic Appendectomy

K. A. Zucker and R. Josloff

Introduction

Although laparoscopic biliary tract surgery was clearly the procedure that heralded the recent revolution in endoscopic surgery, the appendix was actually the first gastrointestinal organ to be removed with the idea of performing a minimally invasive surgical procedure. In 1975 Dekok, in the Netherlands, described a technique that could be best described as laparoscopic-assisted appendectomy. In this procedure the diagnosis was confirmed and the appendix mobilized as much as possible under laparoscopic guidance. Then, a small fascial opening was made in the right lower quadrant of the abdomen allowing the appendix and mesoappendix to be ligated using conventional instruments [3]. In 1982 Kurt Semm, in Kiel, Germany, was the first surgeon to report a successful case of appendectomy performed completely under laparoscopic guidance [13]. Semm, an experienced laparoscopic gynecologist, was operating on a young woman with lower abdominal pain and discovered an endometrial implant at the appendiceal-cecal junction. He then mobilized the cecum from the surrounding tissues and ligated the base of the appendix with pre-tied laparoscopic ligatures. He removed the appendix through the umbilical cannula site. Interestingly, Semm at that time cautioned that laparoscopic surgery was probably not advised in the setting of acute appendicitis because of the possibility of intra-abdominal infection or fecal fistula. Within a few years, however, Schreiber, another German gynecological surgeon with extensive laparoscopic experience, reported a small series of successful appendectomies in women with acute inflammation [11]. Unfortunately, for several years most general surgeons shunned the concept of laparoscopic gastrointestinal surgery and this operation was initially adopted by only a handful of innovative surgeons in Europe and North America.

By 1991 Pier (Germany) and associates had performed over 625 consecutive laparoscopic appendectomy procedures with superb results [6]. Their need for conversion from laparoscopic to open laparotomy was less than 2 % with an overall morbidity rate of less than 1%. Pier also reported that in their institution laparoscopic appendectomy could be completed in most cases in 20 min or less. This large series demonstrated for the first time that minimally invasive surgical techniques could be successfully used not only in early appendicitis, but also in complex patients with advanced inflammation, perforation, and even in those individuals with periappendiceal abscesses. Pier and coworkers, along with many other surgeons in Europe and North America, now firmly believe that laparoscopic appendectomy offers several advantages over conventional open surgery. These advantages include diminished postoperative pain, a more rapid return to normal activities, decreased incidence of wound infection, and the ability to examine the entire abdominal cavity without the need for enlarging any abdominal incisions. The latter is a particular advantage when operating on patients with systemic signs of inflammation and peritoneal findings and yet the appendix is found to be normal (the so-called false-negative or innocent appendix). The laparoscopist may easily examine the other abdominal and pelvic organs without the need for extending any of the abdominal incisions and, in most cases, deal successfully with any other disorders that may mimic acute appendicitis.

Two small prospective randomized trials comparing laparoscopic and conventional appendectomy appear to support these premises [9, 1]. McKenna et al. [9] from Ireland reported their results with 65 patients randomized to either group. Two patients in the laparoscopic group (2/30; 0.6 %) required conversion to open laparotomy because of intraoperative findings. The time required to complete appendectomy was nearly the same for both groups (61 min vs 51 min). Patients in the laparoscopic group were discharged a mean of 2 days (range 1–7) after surgery as compared with 3 days (range 1–7) in the open group. Postoperative complications in the two groups were also similar. A comparable prospective randomized study was also published by Atwood et al. in 1992. Their findings were almost identical to those of McKenna et al. [9]. Although no objective data was presented, both groups also felt that the amount of postoperative discomfort was less with the laparoscopic group of patients.

Indications and Contraindications

Presently, there would appear to be very few contraindications for attempting laparoscopic surgery in any patient with suspected appendicitis. The most common, in our opinion, would be surgeon inexperience with the technique. Other relative contraindications include history of prior lower abdominal or pelvic surgery, evidence of diffuse peritonitis, strong suspicion of an underlying malignancy (i. e., perforating cecal carcinoma), and uncorrectable coagulopathies. Another possible contraindication would be seen in the patient with severe comorbid illnesses (congestive heart failure, COPD, etc.) where a regional anesthetic may be indicated. Although a small number of surgeons have reported successful therapeutic laparoscopic surgery with regional and even local anesthesia, little is known regarding the pulmonary and hemodynamic effects of a pneumoperitoneum in the awake patient. Another potential contraindication is the pregnant patient with suspected acute appendicitis. Little is known regarding the risk of carbon dioxide pneumoperitoneum to the fetus, although many surgeons have recently reported performing successful laparoscopic surgery in the first and second trimesters without maternal or fetal compromise [2,12].

It is essential in any proposed laparoscopic procedure that the patient (and if appropriate, the family) be made aware of the possible need to convert to an open laparotomy based on operative findings. It should be emphasized that such a decision does not indicate that a complication has occurred, but instead represents sound clinical judgment based on operative findings.

Preoperative Work-up

The decision to perform laparoscopic appendectomy should be based on the exact criteria used for conventional open surgery: A detailed history and physical examination is performed, appropriate blood work, routine urinalysis, and plain radiographic films of the abdomen and chest should all be obtained. In selected individuals a preoperative ultrasound or CT scan may also be requested if there is some question regarding the possible cause of the patient's discomfort and physical findings. In our practice we administer a broad-spectrum antibiotic intravenously 30–60 min prior to the operative procedure.

Operative Technique

Patients are usually placed in the supine position with both arms tucked along the side. The surgeon stands on the left side of the patient with the first assistant positioned directly across. Some surgeons prefer a modified lithotomy position

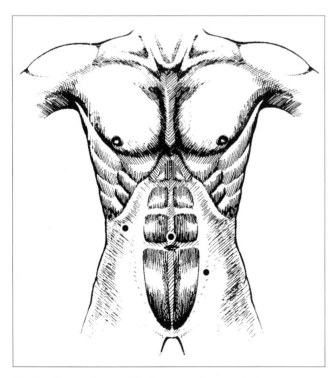

Fig. 1. Trocar placement for laparoscopic appendectomy

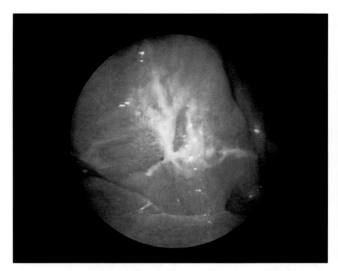

Fig. 2. Large inflammatory phlegmon surrounding appendiceal abscess

when operating on younger women because it allows for the use of a blunt, transvaginal probe for manipulation of the uterus and adnexa. Video monitors are usually placed at the foot of the operating table so as to be in direct view of the entire surgical team. The patient should be securely strapped to the operating table if the surgeon has requested extreme movements of the table in order to expose the right lower quadrant of the abdomen and pelvis (Trendelenburg position with a left tilt). Both a bladder and nasogastric catheter are routinely inserted, because decompression of these organs will minimize their risk of injury as well as facilitate exposure of the upper and lower abdomen.

A pneumoperitoneum may be established using either the percutaneous (Veress needle) or open (Hasson) techniques. We prefer the open method because there may be an accompanying ileus in many patients with acute appendicitis, which increases the risk of blind needle or trocar injury to the underlying viscera. This modified cannula is usually placed just above the umbilicus (Fig. 1). The abdominal cavity is then insufflated to a maximal pressure of 14–15 mmHg and the video laparoscope is inserted. We prefer an angled (30–45 °) over a forward (0 °)-viewing laparoscope because of its greater versatility in viewing intra-abdominal structures. Two additional cannulas (10- to 12-mm diameter) are also inserted into the abdominal cavity. Occasionally, a fourth trocar (10/12 mm) may be placed in the right mid- to upper abdomen to assist with retraction and/or dissection in more difficult cases. The abdominal cavity is then explored to confirm the diagnosis and assess the feasibility of continuing the laparoscopic approach.

Atraumatic Babcock-like forceps are then inserted into the suprapubic trocar and the cannula placed in the left lower quadrant of the abdomen and used to identify the cecum and appendix. Often, the inflamed appendix will be readily exposed with minimal manipulation. If the appendix is not visible by simple retraction of the cecum, we begin by bluntly dissecting along the lateral peritoneal attachments of the ascending colon. The cecum is then mobilized medial and cephalad in order to expose the juncture with the appendix. For a right-handed surgeon the cecum is grasped with a Babcock clamp inserted through the suprapubic port and pulled gently toward the midline. A curved Metzenbaum scissors guided through

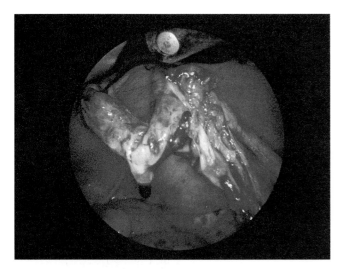

Fig. 3. Inflamed appendix may be grasped with atraumatic or Babcock forceps

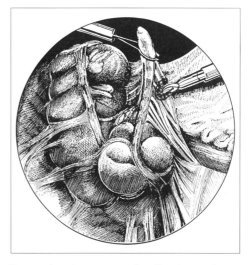

Fig. 5. Transection of mesoappendix with scissors after coagulation

the left abdominal cannula is then used to divide the lateral and posterior attachments of the cecum. This maneuver allows the terminal ileum and cecum to be rotated toward the patient's left thereby exposing its posterior surface. In nearly all cases this maneuver will allow the surgeon to expose and dissect free either a retrocecal or pelvic appendix. In some cases the entire right lower quadrant of the abdomen may be filled with a large inflammatory phlegmon (Fig. 2). Loops of small and large bowel are then freed from the inflammatory phlegmon wall until an appropriate anatomical landmark is identified. The use of a cylindrical gauze inserted through one of the cannulas and grasped with a forceps can help break up these inflammatory adhesions and facilitate blunt dissection down to the cecum. This type of gauze will also absorb any blood in the region and help prevent subsequent tissue staining, which may hinder identification of the ileocecal junction.

After identifying the appendix, it should be freed from any adhesive attachments to other loops of bowel or peritoneum so that its juncture with the cecum is readily visible. This is usually accomplished with a combination of blunt and sharp dissection. The tip of the appendix can usually be grasped safely with an atraumatic forceps (Fig. 3) or pre-tied endoscopic ligature without fear of crushing or perforating it. If the tip of the appendix is already perforated, a similar loop ligature can be used to minimize further peritoneal contamination.

Two methods of ligating and dividing the appendix are in common use. Until recently, the most common method of controlling the appendiceal stump was with the use of multiple pre-tied endoscopic ligatures. The mesoappendix is first divided along the length of the appendix. In North America this is usually accomplished by placing surgical clips on each branch of the appendiceal artery, whereas in Europe many surgeons routinely cauterize these small vessels with bipolar electrical energy (Figs. 4 and 5). After exposing the base of the appendix a series of pre-tied loop ligatures are used to ligate the cecal stump. Two ligatures are placed on the cecal side

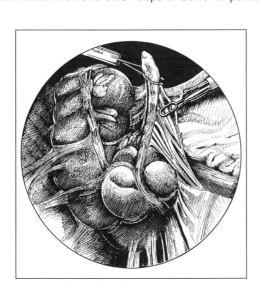

Fig. 4. Mesoappendicular vessels are cauterized using bipolar electrocoagulation

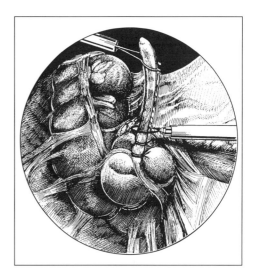

Fig. 6. The appendicular basis may be secured with pre-tied endoscopic ligatures, placing two ligatures on the cecal stump and one on the specimen side

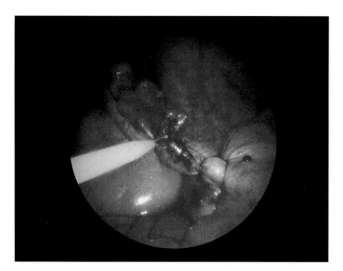

Fig. 7. The pre-tied ligatures are tightened with a knot-pusher

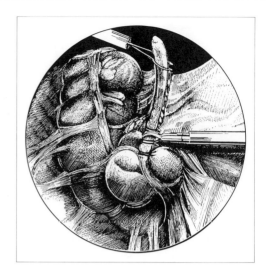

Fig. 8. The appendix is divided sharply with scissors between ligatures

and one on the specimen side (Figs. 6 and 7). The appendix is then divided sharply with scissors (Fig. 8) or with an electrical cautery device. Another method of controlling both the appendix and mesoappendix involves using the endoscopic linear stapler (Endo-GIA). These instruments place three rows of hemostatic staples on each side and simultaneously advance a cutting blade, which divides any tissue within the jaws of the device between the staple lines. Staple cartridges are available in lengths of 30 or 60 mm and accept multiple staple configurations designed for different thicknesses of tissue (see Chap. 4). After completely mobilizing the appendix, a small window is made in the mesoappendix near the base of the cecum. The stapler is usually introduced through the suprapubic cannula and the jaws are placed around the window in the mesentery enclosing the mesoappendix. The instrument is fired and the staple line is checked for hemostasis. The stapler cartridge is replaced, positioned across the base of the appendix, and then fired once again (Figs. 9 and 10). Although endoscopic linear staplers are relatively expensive (and dis-

posable), they are much faster than placing individual ligatures. Most surgeons feel that the savings in operating room costs at least partially make up for the extra expense of the disposable staplers.

With either the ligature or stapled technique the result is an everted appendiceal stump. Most contemporary surgeons, however, were trained to invert the remnant into the wall of the cecum, despite the fact that a large prospective randomized trial comparing everted vs inverted appendiceal stump closure showed no difference in clinical outcome [4]. A method of inverting the appendiceal stump into the wall of the cecum, however, has been described using laparoscopic suturing techniques [10]. Fortunately, such maneuvers appear to be unnecessary because there have been no problems reported to date with leaving an everted appendiceal remnant.

After separating the appendix from the cecum, the next step is removal of the specimen from the abdominal cavity. As mentioned previously, one apparent advantage of laparos-

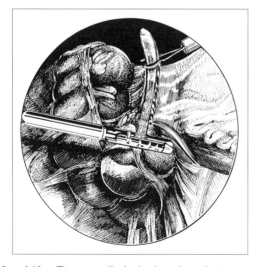

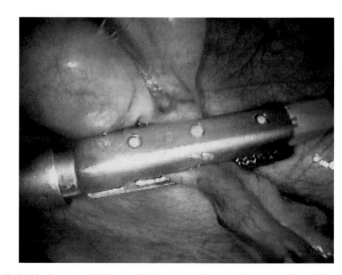

Figs. 9 and 10. The appendicular basis and cecal stump are controlled with three staple lines each by the application of a 30-mm Endo-GIA

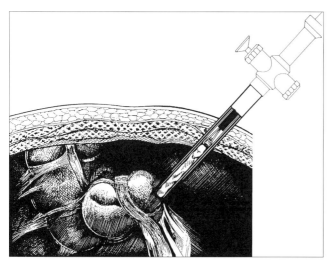
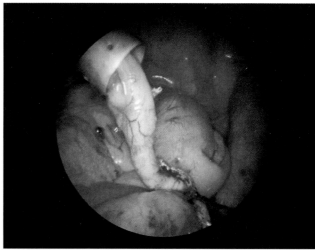

Figs. 11 and 12. The appendix is grasped by the stump and extracted from the abdominal cavity through one of the cannulas without contamination of the abdominal wall

copic appendectomy is the ability to remove any infected or contaminated tissues without coming in contact with the tissues of the abdominal wall thereby resulting in a much lower incidence of wound infections. If the appendix is small, it can often be removed simply through one of the laparoscopic cannulas (Figs. 11 and 12). In most cases, however, the inflamed appendix is too edematous and inflamed to pull through even a 12-mm laparoscopic cannula. In these cases most surgeons choose to place the appendix within an impermeable specimen bag. Initially, surgeons used gas-sterilized condoms or portions of a sterile operating room glove, which were then pushed through one of the cannulas and into the abdomen. Recently, however, commercially produced specimen bags have become available, which are easier to use and stronger. The appendix is placed inside the bag (Fig. 13) and extracted through one of the cannula sites, usually the suprapubic site. If necessary, the fascial opening can be enlarged with right-angled retractors until the appendix can be removed.

The next important step is to copiously irrigate the abdomen and pelvis with saline. Many of the irrigation devices in current use are gas powered and can quickly flood the peritoneal cavity with several liters of fluid. Larger (10 mm) pool-tipped suction probes are also available, which can remove most purulent débris. Drainage catheters are used only if a localized or contained abscess cavity is identified. A 10-mm or larger closed suction drain can be inserted through one of the laparoscopic cannulas and positioned within the abscess cavity. The external portion of the catheter can be pulled out through one of the lower port sites (usually the supraumbilical) as the cannula is removed. Finally, all trocar sites larger than 5 mm should be closed at the fascial level. In nearly all cases we also close the skin (sutures or staples), even in advanced cases of appendicitis with abscess formation.

Complications Associated with Laparoscopic Appendectomy

For the most part any complication associated with open appendectomy can also occur during laparoscopy. These complications include postoperative abscess formation, appendiceal stump leak/blowout, wound infection, and early or late intestinal obstruction. Both methods of securing the appendiceal stump (pre-tied suture ligation and stapled closure) appear to be equally effective with no greater incidence of leakage when compared with conventional methods of closure in open surgery. As mentioned previously a number of large retrospective clinical series have supported the premise that laparoscopic appendectomy is associated with fewer wound infection problems than open surgery. Unfortunately, the small number of published prospective randomized trials thus far published have not included enough patients to confirm this observation. No information is yet available concerning the incidence of postoperative abscess formation. Although some early critics of this procedure proposed that the laparoscopic approach to the perforated appendix would not be adequate in terms of infection control, no such observation has been made in any of the papers published to date.

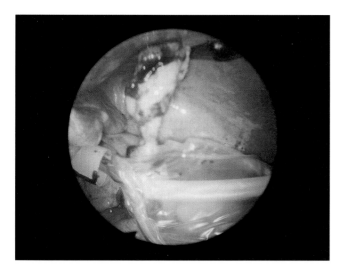

Fig. 13. A large, inflamed appendix can be extracted within a specimen bag to avoid contamination of the abdominal wall

Problems associated solely with laparoscopic appendectomy are, for the most part, related to the establishment of the pneumoperitoneum and placement of the various trocars. As mentioned previously, many surgeons prefer an open or Hasson technique over blind insertion of a Veress needle, because many individuals with acute appendicitis will also present with some ileus and intestinal distension. Use of a Hasson cannula, however, does not eliminate the possibility of a visceral injury, because enterotomies and other visceral injuries may still occur when attempting to enter the peritoneal cavity through a very small (1.5–2.0 cm) incision [5]. Another possible type of injury that may occur more frequently with laparoscopic surgery is iatrogenic lesion of the small bowel or colon from the use of endoscopic instruments. With laparoscopic surgery the surgeon is unable to directly palpate the tissues and instead uses specially designed instruments that are 30–35 cm long. The length of these devices as well as the fact that the abdominal wall and cannulas further dampen the "feel" of the tissues makes it difficult for the surgeon to judge how much traction/retraction or crushing force is being applied to the tissues. In addition, the rigid abdominal wall also acts as a fulcrum that can magnify such forces without the full appreciation of the surgeon. This problem is further compounded by the fact that the surrounding large and small bowel are often inflamed, which may render them more susceptible to such injuries. Therefore, enterotomies from instrumentation may occur more frequently than in open surgery. If such an injury should occur, conversion to open laparotomy for repair is usually indicated. In some cases very experienced endoscopic surgeons may feel comfortable with laparoscopic repair of such injuries.

Discussion

Although laparoscopic appendectomy appears to have several advantages over open surgery, many surgeons remain reluctant to adopt this approach. Inexperience with laparoscopic bowel surgery is certainly one reason for this hesitancy, but other valid concerns, such as increased cost, have also been proposed. As with most new laparoscopic procedures the true cost relative to conventional surgery has not been adequately addressed. Operating room charges are usually greater, especially when disposable instruments are used, but whether this is offset by decreased time in the hospital and shorter convalescence is unknown.

Presently, many surgeons have adopted a policy of selectively offering laparoscopic intervention to their patients, such as performing open surgery in young males, where there is little doubt of the diagnosis. Laparoscopic surgery would then be reserved for individuals where there was a greater likelihood of nonappendiceal problems such as younger women and older patients with atypical presentations. The increasing use of diagnostic laparoscopy in this latter group of patients has raised some questions regarding the most appropriate management when the appendix appears normal on endoscopic examination. In some series as many as 20 % of patients taken to the operating room are found to have a normal appendix especially if the patient population includes women of child-bearing age [8]. Some surgeons have advocated leaving the appendix in place in such situations in an attempt to reduce the incidence of "false-negative appendectomies." Most contemporary laparoscopic surgeons, however, would

disagree with this premise and still remove a normal-appearing appendix in this situation for two reasons [7]: Firstly, in a small percentage of patients the appendix may appear grossly normal, but subsequent histological examinations reveal early or mucosal appendicitis. Secondly, failure to remove the appendix may result in confusion if the pain and other signs of localized right lower quadrant peritonitis return. In addition, the patient may relate a history of undergoing a previous appendicitis, although it may have been left in situ. Most surgeons have adopted a policy of removing even a normal-appearing appendix in order to avoid any such confusion that could potentially result in a delay of appropriate treatment. The only exception to this policy would be in a situation where the cecum was extensively involved in an acute inflammatory process from another pathological source. Removal of the appendix in such a circumstance could result in a fecal fistula and/or intra-abdominal abscess.

In conclusion, laparoscopic appendectomy has become a valuable alternative to the open procedure in most patients. The greatest benefit, however, seems to be the possibility of inspecting the whole abdominal cavity and especially the pelvic region in young women in which the diagnosis is still uncertain. Therefore, the laparoscopic procedure offers the advantage of performing a diagnostic laparoscopy at the same time, which can never be done through the usually small incisions in open surgery.

References

1. ATTWOOD SE, HILL AD, MURPHY PG, THORNTON J, STEPHENS RB: A Prospective Randomized Trial of Laparoscopic versus Open Appendectomy. Surgery 112 (1992) 497–501.
2. CURET MJ, ZUCKER KA: Laparoscopy during Pregnancy. In Press: Archives Surg. 1996.
3. DE KOK, HJM: Laparoscopic Appendectomy: A New Opportunity for Curing Appendicopathy. Surg. Laparosc. Endosc. Vol. 2 (4) (1992) 297–302.
4. ENGSTROM L, FENYO G: Appendectomy: An Assessment of Stump Invagination: A Prospective Trial. Br. J. Surg. 72 (1985) 971–972.
5. FITZGIBBONS RJ, SALERNO GM, FILIPI CJ: Open Laparoscopy. In "Surgical laparoscopy" (eds) ZUCKER KA, BAILEY RW, REDDICK EJ. Quality Medical Publishing, St. Louis, pp. (1991) 87–99.
6. GÖTZ A, PIER A, BACHER C: Laparoscopic Appendectomy in 625 cases: From Innovation to Routine. Surg. Laparosc. Endosc. 1 (1) (1991) 8–13.
7. HOFFMANN J, RASMUSSEN OO: Aids in the Diagnosis of Acute Appendicitis. Br. J. Surg. 76 (1989) 774–779.
8. JESS P: Acute Appendicitis: Epidemiology, Diagnostic Accuracy and Complications. Scand. J. Gastroenterol. 18 (1983) 161–163.
9. MCKENNA OJ, AUSTIN O, O CONNELL PR, HEDERMAN WP, GOREY TF, FITZPATRICK J: Laparoscopic versus open Appendectomy: A Prospective Evaluation. Br. J., Surg. 79 (1992) 818–820.
10. O'REILLY MJ, REDDICK EJ, MILLER WD, SAYE W: Laparoscopic Appendectomy. In "Surgical laparoscopy: Update" (eds) ZUCKER KA, BAILEY RW, REDDICK EJ. Quality Medical Publishing. St. Louis, MO. pp. (1993) 301–326.
11. SCHREIBER J: Experience with Laparoscopic Appendectomy in Women. Surg. Endosc. 1 (1987) 211–216.
12. SCHREIBER J: Laparoscopic Appendectomy in Pregnancy. Surg. Endosc. 4 (1990) 100–102.
13. SEMM K: Endoscopic Appendectomy. Endoscopy 15 (1983) 59–64.
14. WELCH NT, HINDER RA, FITZGIBBONS RJ: Laparoscopic Incidental Appendectomy. Surg. Laparosc. Endosc. Vol. 1 (2) (1991) 116–118.

21. | Laparoscopic Splenectomy

R. J. ROSENTHAL AND E. H. PHILLIPS

Introduction

The importance of the spleen has been debated since the ancient Greeks. From a historical point of view, its immunologic role has only recently been established. For the past 25 years, surgical extirpation for the slightest reason has been replaced by efforts to save all or some of the splenic mass especially in children. Nevertheless, occasionally the entire spleen must be removed because of intrinsic disease, hypersplenism, or for diagnosis. The operative technique for total splenectomy is well known, and until 4 years ago had not significantly changed since the first splenectomy was performed in 1826.

A generous vertical or subcostal incision has been the accepted approach for splenectomy, and the results have been excellent. However, critically ill patients are often considered for splenectomy. Increasingly, elderly patients with advanced lymphoma and severe pancytopenia are referred for urgent splenectomy. Of course, the risks of surgical intervention must balance the potential advantages. "Open" splenectomy in patients with splenomegaly greater than 1,000 g has a 30 % morbidity and a 10–15 % mortality [1].

The laparoscopic revolution has shown that upper abdominal surgery, such as cholecystectomy and antireflux surgery performed without large abdominal wall incisions, significantly shortens hospital stay and decreases morbidity. Subsequently, laparoscopic techniques have been applied to splenectomy in the hope that morbidity and mortality would decrease as well as postoperative discomfort and hospital stay.

The complex vasculature and the many peritoneal attachments of the spleen seem to defy the laparoscopic approach. In fact, just over 15 years ago it was common to routinely remove the spleen for even minor tears of the splenic capsule. But surgical experience with splenic salvage and partial splenectomy has increased familiarity with the vascular supply to the spleen. Application of this knowledge and the basic principles of surgery (exposure, tension, countertension, precise dissection, and vessel ligation) under the magnification of the laparoscope have led to the successful removal of the spleen by endoscopic techniques.

Indications

At its present stage of development laparoscopic splenectomy is best suited to the removal of normal-sized spleens in the elective setting [7]. Slightly enlarged spleens can be re-

moved as the surgeon gains experience, the patient is thin, and the body habitus permits. Only the most experienced surgeons can approach spleens greater than 1,000 g and deal with the special technical problems involved. Most surgeries have been performed for idiopathic thrombocytopenic purpura. Other diseases that require splenectomy, but are associated with normal-sized spleens, such as those seen in patients undergoing staging for Hodgkin's disease and some cases of acquired hemolytic anemia, are good candidates for laparoscopic splenectomy. Certain cases of myeloid metaplasia, lymphoma, and leukemia that have normal or slightly enlarged spleens may also be considered for laparoscopic splenectomy when indicated to decrease transfusion requirements. The early results of laparoscopic splenectomy on enlarged spleens suggest that as experience is gained and technology advances the more fragile patients (often on steroids) will benefit with the lower morbidity and mortality that results from the lack of an upper abdominal incision and the concomitant early ambulation it affords.

Preoperative Work-up

Autologous blood is obtained for all elective cases. Patients should receive preoperative immunization with Pneumovax, hemophilus influenza, and meningococcus vaccines. All operations are performed under general endotracheal anesthesia. Preoperative splenic artery embolization is considered in obese patients, patients with AIDS, or patients with splenomegaly.

Operative Technique

Patients are positioned on an electric operating table on a bean bag for easier position change during surgery – left side up. This becomes an important aid when dissecting the splenorenal and the splenophrenic ligaments in obese patients or patients with enlarged spleens. A 30 ° viewing angled laparoscope is important for visualization.

Following creation of the pneumoperitoneum with a Veress needle or open Hasson technique, a 10/11-mm trocar is placed in the umbilical area or supraumbilical area in the tall patient. A general inspection of the abdomen is performed with special attention to possible accessory spleens. A 5- or 10-mm trocar is placed in the subxiphoid area (Fig. 1), and a 10/11-mm trocar (the operating trocar) is placed halfway

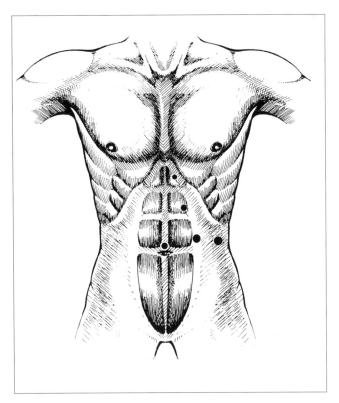

Fig. 1. Position of trocars for laparoscopic splenectomy

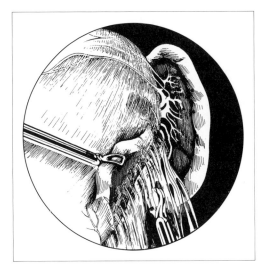

Fig. 3. Widening of the incision in the gastrocolic ligament using scissors

between the subxiphoid and the umbilical trocar. A 10/11-mm trocar (the lateral trocar) is placed in the left axillary line half-way between the costal margin and the iliac crest. A 12-mm trocar (the stapler trocar) is placed halfway between the um-bilicus and the lateral trocar. In a very tall patient, when the trocar for the laparoscope is placed above the umbilicus, the left lateral trocars are moved up correspondingly.

The operation is begun by ligating the splenic artery in the lesser sac. The stomach is reflected anteriorly and the colon is retracted inferiorly with Babcock or atraumatic graspers

placed via the two lateral trocars. A window in the gastrocolic omentum is opened with electrocautery (Fig. 2) and enlarged with scissors (Fig. 3). The pancreas is retracted posteriorly and inferiorly with a fan retractor. The tortuous splenic artery is usually pushed up into view by this maneuver. The perito-neum is lifted with a grasper placed via the subxiphoid trocar and is divided using scissors placed via the operating trocar (Fig. 4). The splenic artery is then grasped, elevated, and oc-cluded with a large endoclip or ligature (Figs. 5 and 6). In some cases a stapler may be used for transsections of the hilar vessels (Fig. 7). The surgeon performs these tasks using a two-handed technique: The left hand operates through the subxiphoid trocar and the right hand through the midline (op-erating) trocar.

In normal or slightly enlarged spleens, attention is paid to the colosplenic attachments. They are divided sharply or with electrocautery. The spleen is grasped with a ring forceps grasper or lung clamp and elevated anteriorly and medially (with the patient positioned left side up) via the lateral trocar.

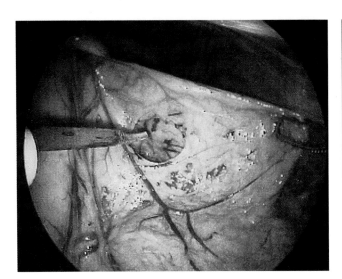

Fig. 2. Opening of a window in the gastrocolic ligament with electro-cautery

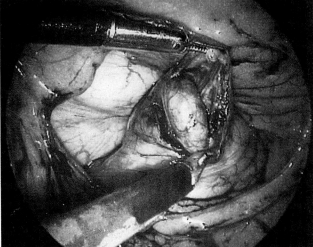

Fig. 4. Incision of the peritoneum for dissection of the splenic artery

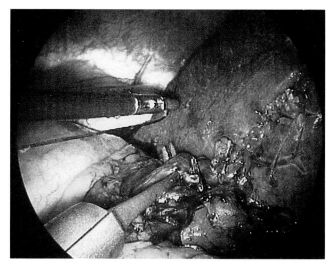

Fig. 5. An extracorporeal tie is brought around the splenic artery

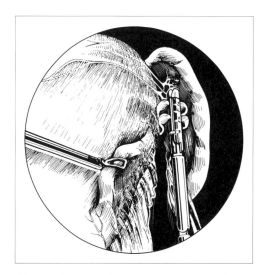

Fig. 7. Transsection of the hilar vessels with the stapler

The splenorenal ligament is divided with scissors and/or electrocautery hook. An electrocautery hook device with suction and irrigation facilitates this dissection and is critical when bleeding is encountered.

The dissection is taken cephalad as far as possible. Division of the splenophrenic attachments allows the spleen to be completely elevated exposing the hilar vessels. If splenomegaly prevents extensive mobilization, the operation is more difficult and more dangerous, because the hilar vessels need to be divided first. In the normal-sized spleen the inferior hilar vessels are divided until more of the retrosplenic, splenorenal and/or splenophrenic attachments can be reached. Although some authors divide the hilar vessels first, this approach leaves one with fewer options if bleeding is encountered when dissecting the hilar vessels, because it is much more difficult to control the bleeding if the spleen is not already mobilized. This is especially true in the more difficult laparoscopic splenectomy. In the truly massive spleen this type of mobilization is impossible.

After division of as much of the posterior peritoneal attachments as possible, the inferior pole vessels are dissected (Fig. 8) and divided (Fig. 9). The central vessels and the superior pole vessels are then sequentially ligated and divided. Finally, the short gastric vessels are divided. The techniques of vessel ligation include endoscopic loops, clips, intra- and extracorporeal ties, and Endo GIA staplers. Ties and Endo GIA staplers are less likely to be disrupted by retractors than clips, and are therefore preferred. The Endo-GIA staplers are excellent, but still require proper dissection of the vessels and adequate-sized windows to allow safe insertion of their "jaws". Adequate dissection of the vessels should be performed in case there is bleeding from the staple lines. It is dangerous to blindly insert the Endo GIA stapler on the hilar vessels and "fire" it blindly, because the device may only be cutting halfway across a splenic vein or artery. It needs to be stressed that proper dissection of hilar "windows" and application of the staplers is critical. The stapler is especially useful when dividing the short gastric vessels, be-

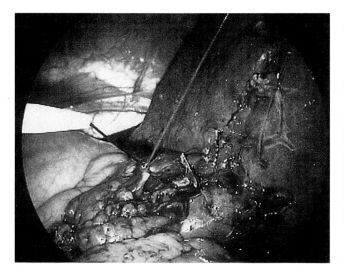

Fig. 6. The splenic artery is ligated after the vein has been closed with a clip and transsected

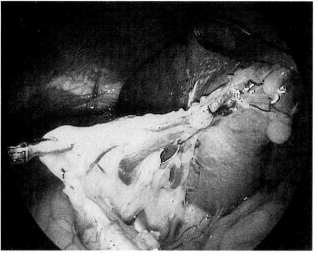

Fig. 8. Dissection of the inferior pole vessels

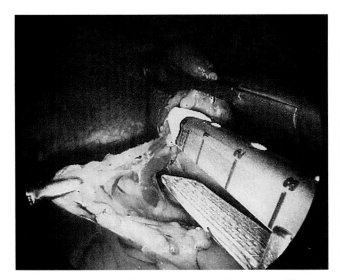

Fig. 9.   Division of the inferior pole vessels with the Endo-GIA

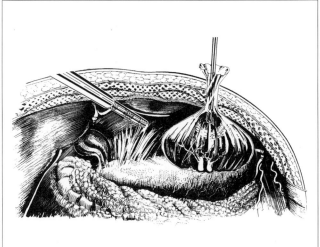

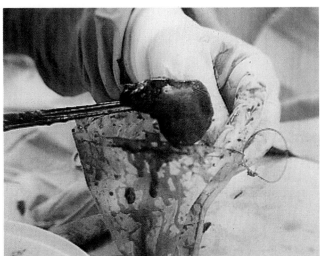

Figs. 11 and 12.   Extraction of the morcellated spleen without contamination of the abdominal wall

cause the staple lines are secure even when the stomach distends.

If the spleen has already been mobilized when bleeding is encountered during the dissection of the hilar vessels, the rapid application of the endovascular stapler can quickly and securely stop the bleeding in most cases. Even a grasper can apply pressure until the field has been suctioned and a plan for ligation of the vessel is agreed upon. If the spleen has not been mobilized, control of hemorrhage is much more difficult.

After the spleen is detached, it is placed in a Cook Urologic specimen bag, which is presently the strongest and safest bag (Fig. 10). If pathologic analysis is not crucial, the spleen can be morcellated manually with a ring forceps or mechanically with a tissue morcellator (Cook Urologic, USA) at the site of the 12-mm trocar (Figs. 11 and 12). If the procedure is performed for Hodgkin's disease, lymphoma, or other tumors that require careful pathologic analysis, the specimen can be removed intact via a lower abdominal incision or enlargement of the umbilical trocar site. Before CO_2 is removed, Bupivacaine is injected at each trocar site. Then the fascia is closed at each 10- to 12-mm trocar site with a suture.

Results

Reports of successful laparoscopic splenectomy have been published and presented at surgical meetings in recent months, but no large series have been accumulated. Our group first attempted laparoscopic splenectomy in January 1992 in a patient with Hodgkin's disease. Presently, we have performed successful laparoscopic splenectomy in 33 patients, and failed in 3 other patients. Laparoscopic splenectomy was performed/attempted in 16 patients with idiopathic thrombocytopenic purpura, 8 patients with lymphoma, 4 patients with Hodgkin's disease, 3 AIDS ITP, and 2 patients with multiple splenic abscesses. The reasons for conversion to "open" surgery were intraoperative bleeding (n = 2) and obesity preventing adequate exposure (n = 1). Eleven patients had successful preoperative splenic artery embolization and laparoscopic splenectomy. All others had successful laparoscopically guided splenic artery ligation in the lesser sac. Nine patients (27 %) had accessory spleens (one patient had two). Significantly, patients who were attempted laparoscopically and were converted were not harmed by the attempt.

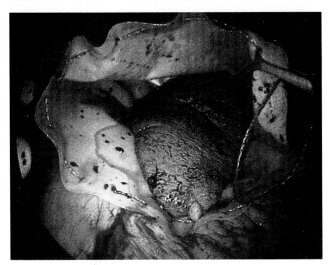

Fig. 10.   The spleen is placed in a retrieval bag

The average blood loss was 300 cc (range 25–800 cc), and 2 patients required transfusion of autologous blood. The average length of surgery was 161 min (range 120–225 min), and the average postsurgical stay was 3.6 days compared with 9.3 days for 8 patients who underwent "open" splenectomy because of massive splenomegaly during the same period. There were four minor complications, one major complication, and no deaths in the laparoscopic or converted group. Complications included minor wound infections, pleural effusion, atelectasis, and 1 patient had a 1-cm incision in his diaphragm sutured laparoscopically. Table 1 shows the comparison between successful laparoscopic splenectomies, converted splenectomies, and open splenectomies.

Table 1. Average results comparing laparoscopic splenectomy (LS), open splenectomy (OS), and converted splenectomy (CS)

	n	Stay (SD)	Operation time (SD) min	Complications (minor)	Complications (major)	Deaths
LS	33	3.6 (2)	161 (76)	4 (12 %)	1 (3 %)	0
OS	7	9.3 (4)	123 (37)	2 (29 %)	1 (14 %)	1
CS	3	7.7 (5)	173 (21)	1	0	0
p-value		< 0.0005	< 0.01	0.18	0.32	0.32

Stay = postsurgical stay in days; SD = standard deviation
Laparoscopic splenectomies (LS), converted splenectomies (CS), open splenectomies (OS).

The results varied with spleen size. The postsurgery stay for patients with massively enlarged spleens did not quite reach statistical significance, because they had predominantly lymphoma, myeloproliferative disease, or other serious hematologic conditions requiring hospitalization for treatment, although the patients technically could have gone home after recovering from their splenectomy. Table 2 compares results with spleen size. The hospital stay was also affected by age and shortened by the laparoscopic technique (Table 3). Other surgeons have also had excellent results. Table 4 summarizes their experiences.

Table 2. Relation between length of hospital stay and spleen weight

	< 200 g*	200-1,000 g*	> 1,000 g*
	n Stay (SD)	n Stay (SD)	n Stay (SD)
LS	21 (95 %) 3.1 (1)	8 (80 %) 3.4 (1)	4 (36 %) 7.7 (4)
OS + CS	1 (5 %) 5.0 (0)	2 (20 %) 8.5 (6)	7 (64 %) 9.5 (4)
p-value	< 0.05	< 0.005	0.1

* All values approximate

Table 3. Relationship between age and hospital stay

Operation	Patient age (years)	
	< 65 SD	> 65 SD
LS	3.0 (33) 1	5.2 (9) 3
OS + CS	7.6 (7) 4	13.0 (3) 2

Table 4. Experience overview of other centers with laparoscopic splenectomy

Surgeon	Attempted	Completed	Complications	Deaths
Cuschieri	17	16	2	0
Mulvihill	25	21	2	1
Lefor/Flowers	31	24	3	1
Delaitre	18	15	1	0
Schlinkert	8	7	0	0
Ou	10	10	2	0
Poulin	17	17	4	0
Phillips/Carroll	36	33	5	0
Total	162	143	19	2

Discussion

As surgeons gain greater familiarity with laparoscopic techniques, more surgeons will seek to apply those skills to procedures that clearly benefit the patient. However, not all operations will be performed as safely or with demonstrable advantage to the patient. Nevertheless, laparoscopic splenectomy is one of the advanced laparoscopic procedures that clearly has a place in the surgical armamentarium. It is accompanied by less postoperative pain and shorter postsurgical stay than traditional splenectomy. Although relatively few cases have been performed, the results are as dramatic as were the early results of laparoscopic cholecystectomy. Early ambulation, early recovery of bowel function, and earlier hospital discharge are evident with a successful laparoscopic splenectomy. A significant number of patients admitted for splenectomy also receive steroid treatment, thus being exposed to a higher rate of wound complications. These patients may expect special benefit from the small trocar incisions. As in the early days of laparoscopic cholecystectomy, selected patients were chosen for the first cases. Subsequently, more challenging cases were performed.

In the future the technical problems associated with splenomegaly will be resolved, and these cases will be able to be performed laparoscopically. Splenic salvage in trauma may be feasible in experienced hands, but presents considerable challenges of exposure and retraction. Initially, patients selected for laparoscopic splenectomy should have normal-sized spleens. Obese patients should be avoided until experience is gained, and these patients should have preoperative splenic artery embolization. As in any surgery, open or Laparoscopic, proper training and an appreciation of one's own limits is the difference between dangerous and safe surgery. Although the laparoscopic approach benefits our patients, it does so only if it is performed safely.

References

1. CARROLL BJ, PHILLIPS EH, SEMEL CJ, FALLAS M, MORGENSTERN L: Laparoscopic splenectomy. Surg Endosc 6 (1992) 183–185.
2. CUSHIERI A, SHIMI S, BANTING S, VANDER-VELPEN G: Technical aspects of laparoscopic splenectomy: hilar segmental devascularization and instrumentation. J Roy Coll Surg Edin 37 (6) (1992) 414–416.
3. DELAITRE B, PHILLIPS EH: Laparoskopische Splenektomie. In: Brune, I. B., K. Schoenleben (eds.): Laparo-Endoskopische Chirurgie. Hans Marseille Verlag, Munich (1993) 273–280.
4. HIATT JR, GOMES AS, MACHLEDER HI: Massive splenomegaly. Arch Surg 125 (1990) 1363–1367.
5. KITANO, KOBAYASHI SM, SUGIMACHO K: Laparoscopic surgery for pancreatic and splenic disorders. Surg Endosc (abstract) 8 (5) (1994) 449.
6. LEFOR, AT, MELVIN WS, BAILEY RW, FLOWERS JL: Laparoscopic splenectomy in the management of immune thrombocytopenia purpura. Surgery 114 (3) (1993) 613–618.
7. PHILLIPS EH: Laparoscopic splenectomy. In: Hunter, JG., JM. Sackier (eds.): Minimally invasive surgery. McGraw-Hill, New York (1993) 309–313.
8. PHILLIPS EH, CARROLL BJ, FALLAS MJ: Laparoscopic splenectomy. Surg Endosc (in press).
9. TULMAN, DELAITRE SB, CADIÈRE CB: Laparoscopic splenectomy. Surg Endosc (abstract) 8 (5) (1994) 449.

22. | Laparoscopy in the Acute Abdomen

I. B. BRUNE

Introduction

The use of laparoscopy for diagnostic purposes dates back to the beginning of the 20th century (see Chap. 2). As an alternative to exploratory laparotomy, laparoscopy has been proposed from time to time within the past decades [1, 5, 8, 9], but never really became established because there were no therapeutic possibilities.

With the evolution of other non-invasive diagnostic tools, such as ultrasonography, CT scan, MRI and other radiological techniques, diagnostic laparoscopy, which had mainly been performed under local anesthesia, almost completely disappeared.

Since 1989 laparoscopic surgery has rapidly become very popular. Many operative techniques have been developed so that presently most surgeons are able to perform minor therapeutic laparoscopic operations for acute abdominal problems [3, 7, 10]. Thus, a new form of laparoscopy in the acute abdomen, performed under general anesthesia and presenting therapeutic options, has evolved.

Laparoscopy should not replace preoperative workup. It should be performed with the aim of verifying or correcting the diagnosis established by the usual investigative techniques [6]. As with any surgical intervention, there are certain risks, although laparoscopic complications are rare in the hands of well-trained surgeons. Therefore, the indications for laparoscopy in the acute abdomen must be carefully evaluated.

After laparoscopic verification of diagnosis, there are several options:

1. No surgical therapy is necessary
2. The surgical procedure can be performed laparoscopically
3. Operative therapy requires laparotomy

The decision whether to finish the operation laparoscopically or convert to laparotomy depends not only on the pathology, but also on the experience and laparoscopic training of the surgeon. In no case should laparoscopy be performed if it presents an added risk to the patient.

The four main steps in laparoscopy for acute abdominal diseases are:

1. Insufflation of the peritoneal cavity
2. Systematic exploration of the whole abdominal cavity
3. Surgical treatment, laparoscopically or via laparotomy
4. Peritoneal lavage

Establishment of a Pneumoperitoneum

The patient is placed in a supine position well secured to the table, because exploration of the four quadrants of the abdominal cavity often requires steep Trendelenburg or reverse Trendelenburg positions combined with significant side-to-side rotation. The stomach is emptied with a nasogastric tube and the bladder catheterized.

Insufflation of the abdomen with carbon dioxide in a patient with an acute abdomen may be accompanied by higher risks than in the more common elective procedure. The bowel may often be very distended because of intestinal obstruction or paralytic ileus, and is therefore more prone to injury during placement of the Veress needle or introduction of the first trocar. Also, many patients with an acute abdomen have previously been operated upon and as a result may have intra-abdominal adhesions.

Puncture of the abdominal cavity with the Veress needle is best performed in the left upper quadrant of the abdomen, because the likelihood of encountering adhesions is least in this area. Before starting insufflation, the correct position of the needle must be established using the standard tests. Once the pneumoperitoneum has been established, the first trocar is placed near the umbilicus. Before introduction of the first trocar, it may be advisable to puncture the abdomen in the region of the umbilicus with a syringe containing saline. If gas bubbles appear upon aspiration, adhesions are unlikely. If there is any doubt, open access using the Hasson trocar should be performed. Trocars allowing incision and perforation of the abdominal wall under visual control are available (see Chap. 4). Because the danger of intestinal lesion is higher in an acute abdomen, disposable trocars equipped with safety shields or retractable tips should be used. These additional safety precautions may be helpful, but should not prevent the surgeon from exercising extreme care when introducing the first trocar. The secondary trocars must be placed under direct vision and positioned according to the pathology identified by laparoscopic inspection. Trocars of 5 or 10 mm may be used: For most surgical instruments 5 mm are sufficient. However, another 10-mm port may be useful to introduce the laparoscope from another angle.

It is important to place the trocars so that the instruments will be at right angles to one another, because manipulation with parallel instruments can be extremely difficult. Also, the distance of the trocars from the operating field must be sufficient to permit free movement of instruments or the use of a stapler, the jaws of which must be completely within the abdominal cavity to permit full opening of the instrument.

Exploration of the Four Quadrants of the Abdomen

To confirm or exclude a diagnosis, the abdominal cavity must be systematically explored. Following a standard routine of exploration helps in making a correct diagnosis. Very often the procedure is difficult because of the presence of dilated bowel loops and/or adhesions.

The exploration begins with the inspection of the pelvis. The table is tilted in the Trendelenburg position so that the bowel loops and omentum fall into the upper abdominal region. If ascites is present, it is aspirated and a specimen sent for bacteriological examination. In young women with pelvic pain of unknown aetiology, thorough gynaecological inspection is crucial. The uterus and tubes are lifted up and inspected for the presence of endometriosis or other lesions. Adhesions to the ovaries are transected to permit complete inspection and exclusion of cysts or tumours.

To explore the caecum and the right lower quadrant of the abdomen the Trendelenburg position is maintained with rotation of the table to the left. Inspection of the appendix, caecum and ileum sometimes requires division of adhesions in this region. Starting at the ileo-caecal valve, the small bowel is inspected loop by loop, carefully handling the bowel wall with atraumatic forceps. Inflammatory diseases can be excluded as well as a Meckel´s diverticulum. The small bowel is followed up to the ligament of Treitz, which is exposed by rotating the table to the right.

Examination of the large bowel begins with the rectum behind the urinary bladder, which must be lifted towards the abdominal wall. The large bowel is followed along the sigmoid and descending colon. Adhesions between the bowel and the abdominal wall may have to be divided to safely exclude a perforated diverticulitis or pericolic abscess. Further inspection is carried out along the splenic flexure, transverse colon, hepatic flexure and ascending colon ending up at the caecum.

After complete exploration of the infra-colic area, the upper quadrants of the abdomen are examined. Systematic inspection of the liver is performed. To adequately examine the diaphragmatic surface of the liver, a 30° angled optic must be used. Laparoscopic ultrasonography of the liver should be routinely performed when the equipment is available. The ultrasound probes are 10 mm in diameter and have rigid or flexible tips. Biopsies are taken from lesions either under direct vision or under ultrasonographic control.

The gallbladder and hepato-duodenal ligament are inspected as are the pylorus, proximal duodenum and anterior surface of the stomach. The best view of the hiatus can be obtained by introducing a 30° laparoscope through a trocar placed in the midline between the xyphoid and the umbilicus.

The retro-gastric space is only explored when a pancreatic lesion or posterior gastric ulcer are suspected. Access to the lesser sac may be gained either by opening the lesser omentum through the avascular area along the lesser curve or through an incision in the gastro-colic ligament.

Pathological Findings and Therapeutic Consequences

Whether therapy is performed laparoscopically or via a laparotomy depends on the experience of the surgeon with the laparoscopic technique.

The most frequent causes of acute upper abdominal pain are acute cholecystitis and ulcer perforation. Cholecystectomy for acute cholecystitis can usually be managed laparoscopically, and rarely requires a laparotomy (see Chap. 6).

A perforated ulcer can easily be sutured laparoscopically if it is located on the anterior surface of the stomach or duodenum [7]. In case of a duodenal ulcer, débridement of the edges and closure of the defect with full-thickness interrupted sutures is sufficient. A gastric ulcer must be excised for histological exclusion of malignancy prior to suturing. Although peritoneal lavage is possible laparoscopically, it is preferable to perform laparotomy in patients with a significant generalized peritonitis.

In young women with right pelvic pain, laparoscopy is the preferred method for distinguishing between gynaecological disorders and appendicitis [11, 12]. If an acute appendicitis is found, appendectomy can be carried out laparoscopically (see Chap. 20). If appendicitis is not encountered, the small bowel is inspected to rule out an inflamed Meckel's diverticulum, which can be removed laparoscopically (see Chap. 25). In most situations the patient can be spared an unnecessary laparotomy [4].

An obstruction caused by a single adhesion can be treated laparoscopically [3], but creation of a pneumoperitoneum carries a high risk of intestinal injury because of the dilated small bowel.

Mesenteric ischaemia may be difficult to prove or exclude laparoscopically [2], because it is impossible to palpate the mesenteric vessels. The laparoscopic use of Doppler ultrasonography may help to compensate for this deficiency. If intestinal ischaemia is found, the decision whether to perform a resection laparoscopically or via a laparotomy depends on the local extent of the ischaemia and its anatomical distribution, as well as on the individual laparoscopic experience of the surgeon.

In the case of abdominal trauma, laparoscopy allows a complete exploration of the abdomen [13]. The inspection must be carried out systematically and starts with examination of the parietal peritoneum. If there is no injury to the parietal peritoneum, there can be no penetrating injury to the intraperitoneal contents. Blunt trauma however must be thoroughly excluded by following the routine examination described above.

If a perforation of the parietal peritoneum is found, it is lined up with the skin incision to determine the direction of the stab, and an extensive exploration along this line is carried out. In patients with a low thoracic stab wound, the diaphragm must be examined carefully with a laparoscope introduced through a trocar placed in the midline between the xyphoid and the umbilicus. Retroperitoneal lesions are only occasionally identified laparoscopically.

Peritoneal Lavage

Extensive irrigation of all four quadrants of the peritoneal cavity with saline warmed up to 37 °C requires a highly performant irrigation-suction device. The loss of pneumoperitoneum must be compensated for by high rates of insufflation. Irrigation is continued until the aspirated liquid is clear. Fibrinous exudate is carefully removed and aspirated. Postoperative management is determined by diagnosis and the type of operation performed.

Discussion

Laparoscopy in the patient with acute abdomen may presently be an alternative to laparotomy. It offers the advantage of confirming the diagnosis via a less invasive access with small incisions, reduced pain and better cosmesis for the patient. In an increasing number of cases therapy can also be achieved laparoscopically. These aspects justify a laparoscopic trial, even in those patients in whom conversion to laparotomy becomes necessary and who are therefore subject to a longer operative time.

The inability to palpate intra-abdominal structures, such as the mesenteric vessels, is still a problem limiting the applicability of laparoscopy, but may be progressively compensated for by the laparoscopic use of Doppler ultrasonography for vascular structures and laparoscopic ultrasonography for examination of parenchymal organs.

One of the main dangers of laparoscopy in the diagnosis and treatment of patients with acute abdomen is to overlook a pathological finding that may be hidden in localizations that are not readily accessible for inspection. For this reason the surgeon must make sure he has performed a complete systematic inspection of the whole abdominal cavity before drawing the conclusion that no pathology requiring surgical treatment is to be found.

References

1. BAERLOCHER C, ENGELHART G, FAHRLÄNDER H: Die Notfall-Laparoskopie. Leber-Magen-Darm 3 (1973) 11–14.
2. BRUNE IB, SCHÖNLEBEN K: Laparoskopische Sigmaresektion. Chirurg 63 (1992) 342–344.
3. CLOTTEAU JE, PREMONT M: Occlusion sur bride traitée par section sous coelioscopie. Presse Méd. 19 (1990) 1196.
4. DUNN EL, MOORE EE, ELERDING SC: The unnecessary laparotomy for appendicitis – can it be decreased? Am Surg 48 (1982) 320.
5. IBERTI TJ, SALKY BA, ONOFREY D: Use of bedside laparoscopy to identify intestinal ischemia in postoperative cases of aortic reconstruction. Surgery 105 (1989) 686–689.
6. LINDNER H, HENNING H: Die Laparoskopie als diagnostische Methode. Internist 17 (1976) 214–219.
7. MOURET P et al.: Laparoscopic treatment of perforated ulcer. Br J Surg 77 (1990) 1006.
8. PATERSON-BROWN S, ECKERSLEY RT, SIM AJ: Laparoscopy as an adjunct to decision making in the acute abdomen. Br J Surg 73 (1986) 1022–1024.
9. REIERTSEN O et al.: Laparoscopy in patients admitted for acute abdominal pain. Acta Chir Scand 151 (1985) 521–524.
10. SEMM K: Laparoscopic appendicectomy. Endoscopy 15 (1983) 59–64.
11. SPIRTOS NM, EISENKOP SM, SPIRTOS TW: Laparoscopy – a diagnostic aid in cases of suspected appendicitis. Am J Obstet Gynecol (1987) 90–94.
12. WHITWORTH CM, WHITWORTH PW, SANFILLIPO J: Value of diagnostic laparoscopy in young women with possible appendicitis. Surg Gynecol Obstet 167 (1988) 187–190.
13. WOOD D, BERCI G, MORGENSTERN L: Mini-laparoscopy in blunt abdominal trauma. Surg Endosc 2 (1988) 184–189.

23. | Diagnostic Staging Laparoscopy

H. Feussner

Introduction

The aim of diagnostic laparoscopy is to detect pathological conditions and their degree within the abdominal cavity. This examination should be as minimally invasive as possible, but should nevertheless warrant a comprehensive exploration of the whole abdomen.

Direct visual exploration of the abdominal cavity has a long tradition in modern medicine. The first published report on the technique of laparoscopy in humans was from Jacobaeus (Fig. 1) [10]. Kalk further pioneered the use of laparoscopy for the investigation of patients with diseases of the liver [11]. For several decades laparoscopy became an established technique among gastroenterologists, mainly for diseases of the liver. Gradually, however, the increased sophistication of modern imaging procedures, such as ultrasound, computed tomography (CT), and magnetic resonance imaging, put it into oblivion. With the exception of the few authors who still did recommend it for the diagnostic work-up of chronic and acute abdominal pain [15, 21, 22], staging of malignancies [13, 19], in trauma [1, 2, 8], or under emergency conditions [4, 9], the majority of gastroenterologists and surgeons renounced its use. The introduction of laparoscopy in the hands of surgeons starting in 1989 with laparoscopic cholecystectomy induced a revival of diagnostic laparoscopy. The diagnostic value of laparoscopy was further augmented by the fact that now an exploration of the whole abdominal cavity became possible,

and that the third dimension of parenchymatous organs could be assessed by laparoscopic ultrasound. As a result, diagnostic laparoscopy has regained an important place in the preoperative diagnostic workup.

Indications and Contraindications for Diagnostic Laparoscopy

Surgical laparoscopy (or so-called extended diagnostic laparoscopy; EDL) is indicated if neither laboratory findings nor modern imaging techniques clinically provide a clear diagnosis, or if the use of imaging techniques is impossible because of logistic reasons, or if the necessary time is not available.

In particular, EDL can be indicated in the staging of malignant gastrointestinal tumors mainly for esophageal, gastric, and pancreatic cancer. Diagnostic laparoscopy should not be performed in the cases of severe cardiopulmonary decompensation, coagulopathy, and extended abdominal adhesions.

Operative Risk

Extended diagnostic laparoscopy can be considered a relatively safe examination, mortality being below 0.05 %; the overall morbidity rate is between 1 and 5 %. The patient has to be preoperatively informed about usual general risks of abdominal operations (i. e., thrombosis, embolism, impaired wound healing) and particularly about the following:
1. Major bleeding
2. Perforation of stomach as well as small and large bowel
3. Laceration of parenchymatous organs (liver, kidneys, pancreas)
4. Biliary fistula (particularly after liver biopsies)
5. Gas embolism
6. Subcutaneous emphysema

Principally, it must always be emphasized that intraoperatively conversion to an open procedure may be required.

Preoperative Work-up

Patients are prepared and evaluated preoperatively as for other surgical procedures. The day before the operation a peroral laxative is given. All patients receive gastric and urinary decompression by the appropriate catheters. The abdo-

Aus dem westlichen Krankenhause der Allgemeinen Fürsorgeanstalt in Stockholm (Oberarzt: Dr. G. Wilkens).

Ueber die Möglichkeit die Zystoskopie bei Untersuchung seröser Höhlungen anzuwenden.

Vorläufige Mitteilung.

Von H. C. Jacobaeus, Privatdozent in Stockholm.

Die mit der äusseren Körperfläche durch natürliche Oeffnungen in Verbindung stehenden Hohlräume des Organismus, war man seit langem instand gesetzt, mit verschiedenen Licht- und Spiegelanordnungen zu beleuchten und infolgedessen auch mit dem Auge zu untersuchen.

In erster Linie gilt dies von den Harnwegen, wo krankhafte Veränderungen, besonders durch Nitzes Arbeiten, in grosser Ausdehnung diagnostiziert und lokalisiert werden können.

Fig. 1. First published report on laparoscopy by Jacobaeus entitled "About the possibility to use cystoscopy for the examination of serosal cavities" (Münch Med Wochenschr, October 4, 1910)

men is prepared and draped widely. Should laparotomy become necessary during the procedure, the field need not be changed.

Anesthesia

In most cases general anesthesia is required. In elective situations, laparoscopy under local anesthesia with sedation is possible as well. However, in these cases CO_2 should be replaced either by nitrogenous oxygen or by helium. Carbon dioxide causes abdominal pain, and is thus not suitable for laparoscopy under local anesthesia. As soon as any intra-abdominal manipulation is considered, however, general anesthesia is mandatory.

Operative Technique

Modern diagnostic laparoscopy permits not only a visual exploration of the peritoneum and the surface of intra-abdominal organs, but also a surgical exploration of otherwise inaccessible areas such as the lesser sac, the hiatus, or the structures of the hepatoduodenal ligament. Laparoscopic ultrasonography and guided biopsy are also frequently performed (Table 1). Accordingly, modern surgical laparoscopy is no longer comparable to laparoscopy as performed by gastroenterologists in previous decades; therefore, we prefer the term *extended diagnostic laparoscopy* (EDL).

Table 1. Extended diagnostic laparoscopy

Pneumoperitoneum
    Insertion of ports

Anti-Trendelenburg position
    Exploration of upper abdomen

Trendelenburg position
    Exploration of lower abdomen

Surgical dissection of lesser sac, etc.

Laparoscopic ultrasonography

Biopsies

Position of the Patient

Because in EDL the patient's position has to be changed intraoperatively, care has to be taken to strap the patient safely to the table. The operation begins in the reverse Trendelenburg position for the inspection of the upper abdomen. For a systematic inspection of the lower abdomen, it has to be changed to the Trendelenburg position. The video monitor has to be placed depending on which pathological condition is suspected. If the main findings are expected within the upper abdominal cavity, the screen should be located at the left shoulder of the patient. The surgeon is positioned on the right side (Fig. 2). Thus, an inspection of the lower abdomen is feasible as well.

If, however, more demanding manipulations in the lower abdomen are required, the position of the screen has to be adequately changed.

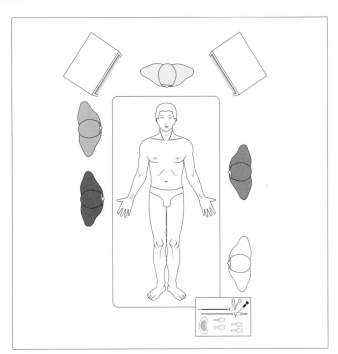

Fig. 2. Positioning of surgical team and laparoscopic equipment for extended diagnostic laparoscopy (EDL).

Trocar Sites

The number and sites of trocars depends on the indication and the suspected findings. In most cases the periumbilical area is selected for the site of insertion of the Veress needle and placement of the first trocar. For staging of gastrointestinal tumors, five trocars are required (Fig. 3).

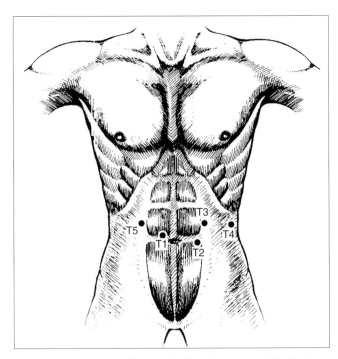

Fig. 3. Trocar sites in EDL. T1, T4, T5: 10-mm ports; T2, T3: 5-mm ports

The examination begins with the patient being in the reverse Trendelenburg position. After having established the pneumoperitoneum, the first 10-mm trocar is inserted in the periumbilical area. In case of doubt, the so-called Hasson technique should be preferred. The 30 ° telescope is passed through the trocar and the peritoneal cavity is inspected. The subsequent trocars are inserted under visual control. The systematic inspection of the abdominal cavity starts in the left upper quadrant. The peritoneum of the abdominal wall is explored first, the laparoscope being directed ventrally in order to identify early manifestations of peritoneal spread. The view is then directed toward the visceral peritoneum, left lobe of the liver, anterior aspect of the stomach, lesser and greater omentum, and the spleen. The left lobe of the liver is elevated and its posterior surface as well as the cardia and lesser curvature of the stomach are inspected.

The telescope is then passed beneath the falciform ligament to the right side of the abdomen. Again, the inspection of the right upper quadrant is started with the exploration of the parietal peritoneum, which is followed by a systematic inspection of the right lobe of the liver including the falciform ligament and the lower margin of the liver. The right lobe of the liver is elevated in order to explore the hepatoduodenal ligament and gallbladder. Subsequently, the patient is brought into a Trendelenburg position. The right colon, caecum, right iliac vessels, and pelvis are explored. The examination is continued by a close inspection of the left middle and lower abdomen including the sigmoid and pouch of Douglas. In female patients this is facilitated by elevating the uterus using a grasping forceps. Systematic inspection of the abdominal cavity is always completed by a dissection and visual exploration of the retrogastric space including the dorsal aspect of the stomach and pancreas.

The greater curvature of the stomach is lifted up with a grasping forceps to extend the gastrocolic ligament. A window is opened in the avascular area below the left gastroepiploic artery. This opening has to be widened sufficiently in order to allow insertion of the laparoscope through trocar T1 or T3. The posterior gastric wall in the fundic area and the body of the pancreas are inspected from T1 (Fig. 4). In a second step

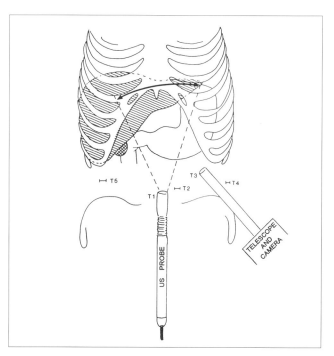

Fig. 5. The ultrasound probe is inserted via incision T1. Probe position is controlled by the telescope in incision T3

the position of the endoscope is changed to trocar T3, which facilitates exploration of the posterior aspect of the antrum and head of the pancreas.

This step is followed by laparoscopic ultrasonography. We use a flexible tipped probe with a diameter of 10 mm. Best results are obtained with a linear scanner of 7.5 Mhz. The telescope remains in T3. The ultrasound probe is inserted via incision T1. Thus, the whole upper abdomen can be examined (Fig. 5). The left lobe of the liver is examined in parallel segments giving a view to the lesser curvature of the stomach as well. After sonography of the left lobe of the liver, the stomach is filled with 200 ml saline and the ultrasound probe is directly applied to the anterior wall of the stomach. The examination of the stomach and pancreas is performed in multiple transverse and parallel cuts. Although it is frequently possible to examine the right liver lobe as well from this position, it may be more convenient to change the probe's position to T5.

The final step is to take biopsies from all suspicious areas. For parenchymatous organs, puncture with a biopsy needle is very easy. Superficial tissue is obtained with a biopsy forceps. Lymph nodes are sampled for pathohistological examination after having been localized by ultrasound. It is of the utmost importance to document localizations of the biopsies in a schematic drawing of the abdomen.

Indications

Staging of Abdominal Malignancies

Despite progress in modern imaging procedures, the selection of patients with gastrointestinal malignancies for curative or palliative treatment still remains a challenge to the surgeon. The need for proper preoperative staging is augmented by the

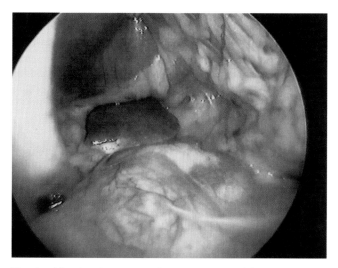

Fig. 4. View into lesser sac. Center: pancreas; right upper corner: posterior gastric wall. Note lymph node beside the body of the pancreas

possibilities of alternative forms of treatment such as neoadjuvant chemotherapy and radiation therapy. The aim of EDL should be to avoid those cases in whom patients had to undergo laparotomy only to reveal unsuspected incurable disease. Laparoscopy is used for diagnosis and biopsy of a primary tumor, assessment of operability, evaluation of metastatic disease, and in a few cases the search for an unknown primary tumor. Despite modern imaging techniques, such as sonography, endosonography, CT, and magnetic resonance imaging, four conditions still cannot be assessed reliably in many cases:

1. Infiltration of neighboring organs
2. Early manifestations of peritoneal spread
3. Lymph node infliction
4. The presence of small metastases of a size smaller than 1 cm

This obvious diagnostic gap can be closed by laparoscopy.

Esophageal Cancer
Although at first glance laparoscopy seems to be of little help in the diagnostic workup of esophageal carcinoma, several studies emphasize its use: Dagnini and Caldironi studied 369 patients with esophageal cancer [6]. Laparoscopy showed intra-abdominal metastases in 52 patients (14 %) in the liver, peritoneum, omentum, gastric wall, and lymph nodes. In another 36 (9.7 %) patients metastases of the gastric wall and lymph nodes could be demonstrated. Additionally, important information could be given concerning the general operative risk for the patient. For instance, 53 patients (14.3 %) suffered from cirrhosis of the liver, which precluded radical surgical therapy. The rate of false-negative findings, as confirmed by surgical exploration, was only 4.4 %.

A more recent study by Watt et al. [20] compares the sensitivity, specificity, and accuracy of laparoscopy, ultrasound, and CT in detecting intra-abdominal metastases of carcinoma of the esophagus and cardia. The evaluation of 90 patients demonstrated clearly that laparoscopy is more sensitive and accurate concerning hepatic metastases, and is by far the most reliable method to detect peritoneal spread. In this series no morbidity or mortality was associated with laparoscopy. The authors consider laparoscopy a safe and reliable method to determine the intra-abdominal status obviating the need for surgery in patients with malignant dysphagia.

Not infrequently it is argued that the quality of new CT scanners and ultrasound devices have made this comparison obsolete. This does not hold true. Even presently the detection of peritoneal spread is problematic, and the involvement of lymph nodes and small metastases is still very difficult to prove or to exclude even by well-advanced imaging procedures. On the other hand, the technique of modern diagnostic laparoscopy makes it possible to expose formerly inaccessible regions such as the hiatus and the diaphragmatic crura, and to sample important lymph nodes, particularly of the celiac axis. Moreover, it has to be taken into account that laparoscopic ultrasound further enhances the diagnostic precision. In our own patients we became more and more inclined to use preoperative laparoscopy prior to esophagectomy. This was stimulated by the fact that we perform transthoracic esophagectomy first and then use the transabdominal route for gastric interposition. If after transthoracic esophagectomy unsuspected intra-abdominal findings, such as peritoneal spread or cirrhosis, are detected, the operation will have to be completed, but will only be palliative. Preoperative laparoscopy helps to avoid these cases. We examined 28 patients with esophageal carcinoma. In 9 of them the tumor was located above the tracheal bifurcation, and in 19 it was located beneath. All of them were either staged T3 or T4 by endosonography and/or CT. Laparoscopy was indicated because of suspicion of liver metastases in 9 cases, peritoneal spread in 8 cases, infiltration of the diaphragmatic crura in 8 cases, and liver cirrhosis in 3 cases. Liver metastases could be ruled out in 3 and confirmed in 6 cases, peritoneal spread was found in 5 of 8 patients, and infiltration of the diaphragm in 4 of 8 patients. Cirrhosis of the liver was found in all of the patients in whom it had been suspected.

Accordingly, 10 of 28 patients were operated upon. Laparoscopic findings proved to be correct in 8 instances, whereas laparoscopy turned out to be falsely negative in 2 cases. In one case a liver metastasis had not been detected, and in another case infiltration of the diaphragmatic crura had been overlooked. On the whole, laparoscopy helped to clear the diagnosis in as many as 26 of 28 cases if it is considered that positive findings were accepted only if they could be proven by biopsy. Accordingly, we are convinced that laparoscopy should be performed in any instance of esophageal cancer in which abdominal manifestations are suspected or cannot be ruled out reliably.

Gastric Cancer
Progress in multimodality treatment has increased the management options in patients with gastric cancer. Exact evaluation of each new treatment depends on accurate staging of the tumor, associated lymph nodes, and distant metastases. The aim of EDL is to identify reliably the group of patients that is fit for primary surgery, and to find out those who will have potential benefit from preoperative chemotherapy. Last, but not least, diagnostic laparotomy should become unnecessary.

The results of conventional laparoscopy (i. e., without laparoscopic ultrasound) have been described in the literature. In one study [13] laparoscopy was performed in 40 patients whose gastric cancer appeared to be resectable according to the prelaparoscopic work-up. During laparoscopy formerly unrecognized distant metastases were found in 5 patients (12.5 %) and locally advanced, unresectable cancer in 11 patients (27.5 %). Thus, unnecessary laparotomy could be avoided in 40 % of patients.

In another study the sensitivity, specificity, and predictive value of laparoscopy for the staging of gastric cancer and for the detection of liver metastases were evaluated [16]. A total of 369 patients were examined. The following parameters were assessed:
1. Serosal infiltration
2. Tumor fixation
3. Metastases to lymph nodes
4. Peritoneal spread
5. Liver metastases

For the detection of liver metastases subgroups were also submitted to liver scintigraphy, sonography, and determination of alkaline phosphatase levels. Peritoneal dissemination and liver metastases were most accurately detected by laparoscopy (efficiency 89.4 % and 96.5 %, respectively). Up to now it has been argued that laparoscopy is still relatively poor for establishing resectability, because posterior fixation of a gastric tumor was hard to establish or exclude. This can be easily achieved, however, by dissection of the retrogastric space as described previously.

In our own prospective study we investigated to what extent EDL is able to influence treatment strategies in this type of cancer. A diagnosis of peritoneal secondary spread into adjacent structures was only accepted when confirmed histologically. The information gained by laparoscopy was classified as follows:

1. No additional information gained; findings of prelaparoscopic staging confirmed.
2. No alteration of tumor stage, but important additional findings influencing patient management discovered.
3. The tumor was downgraded to a more favorable stage.
4. The tumor was upgraded to a less favorable stage.

In those patients undergoing primary resection after laparoscopy, the results of laparoscopy were compared with the findings at the operation and pathological examination.

Laparoscopy was performed in 111 consecutive patients: 81 males (72 %) and 30 females (28 %); median age was 55 years (range 28–80 years) with advanced gastric cancer (T3 and T4). All had been considered suitable for chemotherapy treatment prior to surgical therapy. Patients with a T3 or T4 tumor, but without secondary spread, were considered for initial chemotherapy followed by gastrectomy. Those found to have peritoneal carcinomatosis, regardless of the "T" grade of tumor, were offered appropriate palliative treatment only.

Pretherapeutic staging in all patients was obtained by endoscopy and biopsy, endosonography, conventional ultrasound scanning, and CT. Patients with a T1 or T2 tumor were not entered in the study because the frequency of peritoneal carcinomatosis was considered to be too low to justify routine laparoscopy. The tumor was predominantly located in the upper third of the stomach in 47 patients (42.3 %), in the middle third in 51 patients (46 %), and in the distal third in 13 patients (11.7 %). Using Lauren's classification [8], the tumor was of intestinal type in 51 patients (46 %) and of nonintestinal type in 60 patients (54 %). The overall results of laparoscopy are shown in Fig. 6. In 56 of 111 patients (50.4 %) the findings of laparoscopy and preoperative staging were identical. In 6 of 111 patients (5.4 %) laparoscopy revealed additional findings not connected with the gastric cancer, but important enough to alter therapeutic management. Five patients were found to have cirrhosis of the liver as confirmed by biopsy and one patient an ovarian carcinoma.

Laparoscopy and biopsy downgraded the tumor in 17 of 111 patients (15.3 %). Prior to this test it was suspected that there was infiltration of the liver in 10 patients, pancreas in 6, diaphragm in 2, and peritoneal spread in 4.

The tumor was upgraded in 28 patients (25.3 %). Peritoneal secondaries were found in 26 patients, infiltration of adjacent organs in 3, and distant metastases in 4 (3 hepatic and 1 colonic). Overall, detailed laparoscopy with laparoscopic ultrasound altered the preoperative diagnosis in 51 of 111 patients (46 %) with advanced gastric cancer leading to changes in management in 45 of them (40.5 %).

In those patients in whom laparoscopy showed a lower tumor stage, infiltration of adjacent organs was excluded in 16 patients. This resulted in a change from T4 to T2 classification in 9 patients, all of whom underwent primary resection according to our protocol. In all 9 patients the findings at operation and pathological assessment confirmed the results of laparoscopy. Four patients in whom peritoneal spread could be excluded by laparoscopy were treated by preoperative chemotherapy. Chemotherapy could be avoided in 26 patients found to have suspected peritoneal secondaries. Overall, the planned management had to be changed in 45 of 51 patients in whom the diagnosis was altered by laparoscopy (including the 6 patients with additional laparoscopic findings) or 40.5 % of the group of 111 patients.

These data convincingly show that diagnostic laparoscopy has the potential to improve significantly the precision of preoperative staging in gastric carcinoma.

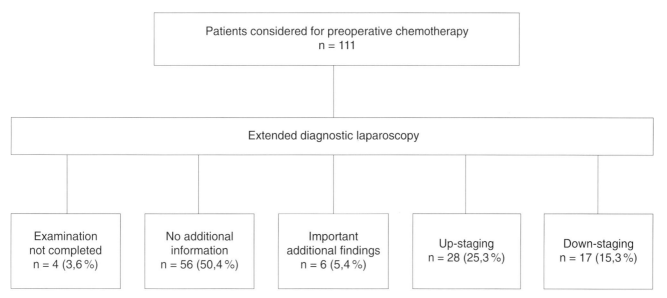

Fig. 6. Outcome of EDL in the staging of gastric carcinoma. According to endoscopy, endosonography, and CT, 111 patients appeared to be candidates for preoperative chemotherapy. Prelaparoscopic staging was confirmed in 50.4 % of patients, but therapeutic strategy was changed by EDL in 40.5 % of them

Pancreatic Carcinoma

According to the literature, approximately 10,000 patients/year are subjected to laparotomy in the U. S. in whom a pancreatic tumor finally turns out to be unresectable. It is likely that a more liberal use of laparoscopy could clearly be of benefit, because it is less invasive and abbreviates the time of hospitalization for the patient who only has a limited life expectancy.

Even with the less sophisticated technique as used a couple of years ago by Warshaw et al. (without laparoscopic ultrasonography) [18], laparoscopy brought significant additional information after CT and angiography primarily by the detection of small peritoneal metastases. On the whole, additional findings could be assessed by visual exploration alone in as much as 30% of cases.

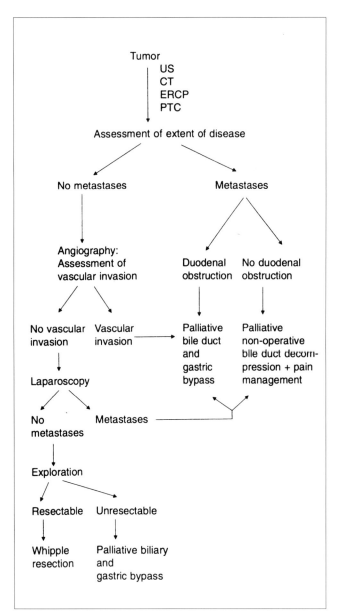

Fig. 7. The place of EDL in the diagnostic workup of pancreatic carcinoma. If laparoscopy is negative, curative resection is considered. (According to [12])

In a more recent study by Murughia et al. [14] laparoscopic ultrasound was included. A total of 12 patients appeared to have a resectable carcinoma of the pancreas according to preoperative imaging techniques. By visual inspection during laparoscopy, resectability had to be excluded in 4 of these patients. By the additional use of laparoscopic ultrasound, another 2 patients turned out to be inoperable. Accordingly, inappropriate laparotomy could be avoided in 6 of 12 patients. Laparoscopy, however, turned out to be falsely negative in one of the remaining 6 patients who was operated upon for cure.

Conclusively, EDL is helpful in identifying the patients in whom laparotomy will not lead to curative resection. In our own practice laparoscopy is therefore integrated into the regular preoperative work-up as suggested by Karl and Carey [12]. It is performed regularly after CT and angiography prior to considering a curative resection (Fig. 7). There is no doubt that growing experience and more widespread use of laparoscopy will further emphasize its diagnostic potential.

Conclusion

The diagnostic value of direct visual inspection of the abdominal cavity by laparoscopy has been proven historically. As an investigation, it went out of favor temporarily because of the introduction of modern imaging procedures; however, the benefits of diagnostic laparoscopy have been rediscovered. This new trend has been brought about by two facts:
1. The ever-increasing requirements of a precise preoperative work-up not provided by the shortcomings of sophisticated procedures, such as CT, sonography, nuclear magnetic resonance, etc., but can be provided by EDL.
2. Laparoscopy has been established as a useful diagnostic and therapeutic tool for the surgeon. Because it provides valuable and comprehensive information with minimal disturbance to the patient, EDL can be recommended as an easily available, reliable, and safe procedure.

References

1. BERCI G, DUNKELMAN D, MICHEL SL et al.: Emergency minilaparoscopy in abdominal trauma: an update. Am J Surg 146 (1983) 261–265.
2. CARNEVALE N, BARON N, DELANEY HM: Peritoneoscopy as an aid in the diagnosis of abdominal trauma: a preliminary report. J Trauma 17 (1977) 634–641.
3. CLARKE PJ, HENDS LJ, GOUGH MH, KETTLEWELL MGW: The use of laparoscopy in the management of right iliac fossa pain. Ann R Coll Surg Engl 68 (1986) 68–69.
4. CORTESI N, ZAMBARDA E, MANENTI A et al.: Laparoscopy in routine and emergency surgery. Am J Surg 137 (1979) 647–649.
5. CUSHIERI A, HENESSY TPJ, STEPHENS RB, BERCI G: Diagnosis of significant abdominal trauma after road traffic accidents. Preliminary results of a multicentre clinical trial comparing minilaparoscopy with peritoneal lavage. Ann R Coll Surg Engl 70 (1988) 153–155.
6. DAGNINI G, CALDIRONI MW: Laparoscopy in abdominal staging of esophageal carcinoma. Gastrointest Endosc 32 (1986) 400–402.
7. FEUSSNER H, KRAEMER SJ, SIEWERT JR: Technik der laparoskopischen Ultraschalluntersuchung bei der diagnostischen Laparoskopie. Langenbecks Arch Chir 379 (1994) 248–254.
8. GAZZANIGA AB, SLANTON WEW, BARTLETT R: Laparoscopy in the diagnosis of blunt and penetrating injuries to the abdomen. Am J Surg 131 (1976) 315–318.

9. IBERTI TJ, SALKY BA, ONOFREY D: Use of bedside laparoscopy to identify intestinal ischemia in postoperative cases of aortic reconstruction. Surgery 105 (1989) 686–689.

10. JACOBAEUS HC: Über die Möglichkeit, die Zystoskopie bei Untersuchung seröser Höhlen anzuwenden. Münch Med Wochenschr 57 (1911) 2090–2092.

11. KALK H: Die Bedeutung der Laparoskopie und Leberpunktion für die Praxis der Leberkrankheiten. Dtsch Med J 13 (14) (1953) 338–341

12. KARL RC, CAREY LC: Impact of staging on treatment of pancreatic and ampullary carcinoma. Endoscopy 25 (1993) 69–74.

13. KRIPLANI AK, KAPUR BML: Laparoscopy for preoperative staging and assessment of operability in gastric carcinoma. Gastrointest Endosc 37 (1991) 441–443.

14. MURUGHIA M, PATERSON-BROWN S, WINDSOR JA, MILES WFA, GARDIN OJ: Early experience of Laparoscopic ultrasonography in the management of pancreatic carcinoma. Surg Endosc 7 (3) (1993) 177.

15. PATERSON-BROWN S, ECKERSLEY JRT, SIM AJW, DUDLEY HFA: Laparoscopy as an adjunct to decision making in the "acute abdomen". Br J Surg 73 (1986) 1022–1024.

16. POSSIK PA, FRANCO EL, PIRES DR., WOHNRATH DR, FERREIRA EB: Sensitivity, specificity and predictive value of laparoscopy for the staging of gastric cancer and for the detection of liver metastases. Cancer 58 (1986) 1–6.

17. SACKIER JM, BERCI G, PAZ-PARTLOW M: Elective diagnostic laparoscopy. Am J Surg 161 (1991) 326-331.

18. WARSHAW AL, GUN ZY, WETTENBERG J, WALTMAN C: Preoperative staging and assessment of resectability of pancreatic cancer. Arch Surg 125 (1990) 230–233.

19. WARSHAW AL, TEPPER JE, SHIPLEY WU: Laparoscopy in the staging and planning of therapy for pancreatic cancer. Am J Surg 151 (1986) 776–780.

20. WATT J, STEWART J, ANDERSON J: Laparoscopy, ultrasound and computed tomography in cancer of the oesophagus and gastric cardia: a prospective comparison for detecting intra-abdominal metastases. Br J Surg 76 (1989) 1036–1039.

21. WHITWORTH CM, WHITWORTH PW, SANFILLIPO J, POLK HC JR.: Value of diagnostic laparoscopy in young women with possible appendicitis. Surg Gynecol Obstet 167 (1988) 187–190.

22. WOOD RAB, CUSCHIERI A: Laparoscopy for chronic abdominal pain. Br J Surg 60 (1979) 900.

Pediatric Surgery

Critical Comments

S. RUBIN

Laparoscopic and thoracoscopic procedures in adults have been described since 1910 [3]. It is only since the publication of Gans and Berci [2] and the successful European [1, 4] and American [5, 6] pediatric clinical experience that endoscopic surgical treatment has been accepted as an alternate choice to the standard open procedure.

Medical management includes diagnosis and treatment. The sick child with a surgically treatable condition often has a single pathology. Diagnosis is clinical and verification may require a simple test. For example, the palpation of the pyloric "tumor" confirms the diagnosis of pyloric stenosis. If we are unable to feel the "tumor", then an ultrasound will be diagnostic. Treatment is usually standard. In our example, we correct the fluid and electrolyte imbalance and then perform a quick, safe pyloromyotomy under general anesthesia. Oral feedings are resumed within hours of the operative procedure and no further treatment is required. Even in complex pathologies, the results of surgery are excellent. Nevertheless, pediatric surgeons are always striving to improve the surgical care.

In adult surgery in addition to gynecology, endoscopic surgery is recommended for cholecystectomy, pleural empyema and spontaneous pneumothorax. It is the accepted alternative to standard open procedures such as splenectomy, fundoplication, appendectomy, inguinal hernia, intestinal resection and resection of the kidney and adrenal. Laparoscopy is used extensively as a diagnostic tool.

The advantage of endoscopic surgery to the patient are that the surgery is less extensive with no cutting of muscles. The postoperative course is less painful with a rapid return to normal physical activitiy.The smaller operative incisions are cosmetically more acceptable.

The disadvantages are technical and operator-dependant. They include a longer operative time, and possible damage to structures caused by the instrumentation, e.g. puncture by the trocar, or cautery burn and electrical sparking, especially if monopolar cautery is used. Insufflation may cause air embolism, adversely ventilation, oxygenation, and acid-base balance or produce a pneumothorax. Implantation of malignant tumors especially sarcomas in the trocar tracts may occur. The operative cost for most procedures is increased. The endoscopic surgical method of treatment is new, and long-term statistical comparison to standard open procedures in many procedures is not yet available.

Whereas genito-urinary, gastro-intestinal and respiratory endoscopy in children are routine procedures, the role of endosugery requires careful assessment. Although the advantages in the individual patient are similar to those in an adult, the technical difficulties are potentially greater. There is at present no standard laparoscopically performed operation such as cholecystectomy. Infrequent use of the technique has a negative impact on the expertise of the pediatric surgeon and the operating room staff.

Until recently, the small pediatric market restricted development of appropriate instrumentation. In the small patient, the available operative field is not only confined, but the distance between the ports is limited and the crowding of instruments hampers their use. There is an increased potential for complications including tissue injury, anesthetic difficulties and inordinately lengthy procedures.

Despite the above, pediatric surgical ingenuity has convinced the industry that smaller instruments are useful not only for children but for adults as well. Consequently, a close liaison had developed between pediatric endosurgeons and the endoscopic instrument manufacturing industry [2]. Today, improved illumination and optics have sporned a wide array of smaller laparoscopes and better cameras. Small specialized ports and fine atraumatic instrumentation have permitted a similar range of procedures to be safely performed in children, infants and neonates as in adults.

The limiting factor in laparoscopy must reside with each individual operating room and endosurgical team. Although economic considerations are important, the selection of mode of surgical treatment must be ethically dictated. Thus the patient should receive the best treatment that the pediatric surgeon can offer.

The indications for laparoscopy as of June, 1996 are both diagnostic and therapeutic and may be listed as follows:

Diagnostic

Definitive:	Debilitating unresolved abdominal pain
	Impalpable undescended testis
	Intersex
Possible:	Staging of tumors
	Biopsy
Questionable:	Inguinal hernia diagnosis
	Jaundice in neonates and infants
	Abdominal trauma

Therapeutic

Definitive:	Cholecystectomy
	Fundoplication
	Adnexal pathology
	Lung biopsy
	Spontaneous pneumothorax
	Thoracic empyema
Possible:	Appendectomy
	Abdominoperineal pullthrough for Hirschsprung's disease
	Meckel's diverticulum
	Adhesive intestinal obstruction
	Renal surgery
	Adrenal resection
	Peritoneal dialysis
	Ventriculo-peritoneal shunts
	Mediastinal masses
	Thymectomy
	Pulmonary resection
	Pericardiectomy
	Diaphragmatic plication
Questionable:	Pyloromyotomy
	Inguinal hernia repair
	Orchiopexy
	Gastric and intestinal stomas
	Intestinal volvulus
	Obstructive uropathy
	Heller myotomy
	Patent ductus arteriosus closure

In addition combined open and laparoscopic procedures for many of the above conditions, especially those involving intestinal resections, may limit the operative trauma and improve the postoperative course.

The pace of the technical development of endosurgery and its increasing acceptance by both the public and pediatric practitioners is resulting in continued improvement and wider application. Specifically, insufflation may be avoided by the use of special parietal retractors; small, fine and ergonomic instruments are replacing the large cumbersome adult instrumentation; increased safety and lower cost of lasers and ultrasonic devices are improving hemostasis while decreasing tissue injury; the inherent problem of loss of palpation in endosurgery is being partly overcome by the introduction of endoscopic ultrasonography; correction of anatomical fetal abnormalities is a future possibility.

In our enthusiasm, we as pediatric surgeons must continue to upgrade our knowledge and skills, whilst maintaining the highest standard of ethics.

References

1. CORTESI N: Laparoscopy in routine and emergency surgery. Am Surg 137 (1979) 647.
2. GANS SL, BERCI G: Advances in endoscopy of infants and children. J Pediatr Surg 6 (1971) 199.
3. JACOBAEUS HC: Kurze Übersicht über meine Erfahrungen mit der Laparoskopie. Münch Med Wochenschr 58 (1911) 2017
4. KARAMEHMEDOVOC O, DANGEL P, HIRSING J et al.: Laparoscopy in childhood. J Pediatr Surg 12 (1977) 929.
5. RODGERS BM, TALBERT JL: Thoracoscopy for diagnosis of intrathoracic lesions in children. J Pediatr Surg 11 (1976) 703.

24. Extramucosal Pylorotomy by Laparoscopy

J. L. ALAIN AND D. GROUSSEAU

Introduction

Laparoscopy was most probably described for the first time by Jacobaeus [5]. The first publications on this method performed on adult patients were written by Kalk and Brühl [6]. It is worth noting that for as long as half a century, laparoscopy had never been attempted in children. During the 1960s some pediatric surgeons started using the technique for biopsy and abdominal exploration [4]. With increasing indications for laparoscopic procedures, these were extended to operations in very young children always taking into consideration the necessary precautionary measures.

Extramucosal pylorotomy may now be performed through the laparoscopic approach in young infants presenting with congenital hypertrophic pyloric stenosis. In conventional surgery this operation had first been described by Ramstedt [8] and Fredet [3] at the beginning of the century. It has scarcely been modified since.

In May 1990 we performed our first laparoscopic extramucosal pylorotomies in infants presenting with hypertrophic pyloric stenosis [1].

Precautions in Anesthesia and Contraindications

Before considering laparoscopy in young children, it is necessary to bear in mind all the ventilatory and hemodynamic problems related to celioscopy in infants. At this young age alveolar ventilation is proportionally much greater as compared with adults. Consequently, any variation in inspired gas concentration will considerably bear its effects on alveolar and arterial gas concentration. Moreover, hypercapnia may be aggravated by abdominal hyperpression, aspiration, the Trendelenburg position or, by inadequate airway control.

In young infants definitive closure of shunts is achieved several weeks after birth. Until then, any increase in pulmonary arterial pressure secondary to hypoxia, hypercapnia, acidosis, or hypovolemia could result in a return to fetal circulation. It is thus vital to exclude the presence of any preexisting disorder that might be a contraindication to the procedure. It is also necessary to assure the absence of congenital heart disease, respiratory problems, or a relative hypovolemia, which must be corrected beforehand.

Peroperative Anesthesiologic Monitoring

The parameters considered are of two types:

1. Those routinely surveyed in all infants, i. e., the recording of arterial blood pressure, oxyhemoglobin saturation, and the branching of an electrocardioscope
2. Additional parameters must be continuously monitored, due to the creation of the pneumoperitoneum: The quantity of gas insufflated and the intraperitoneal pressure (IAP) must be permanently measured

The insufflation itself must be very slow and progressive so as not to exceed an IAP of 6–8 cm H_2O. Capnometry is mandatory and allows the following:

1. An instantaneous measure of expired CO_2 pressure (PE CO_2), which immediately reflects the arterial CO_2 pressure (Pa CO_2)
2. A rapid regulation of ventilatory parameters so as to maintain an optimal $PaCO_2$
3. Early detection of complications such as gas embolus or acute hypovolemia

Anesthesia

After premedication with an anticholinergic agent, general anesthesia with endotracheal intubation and controlled ventilation are necessary. Halothane should be avoided because of its deleterious effects to the heart.

Operative Technique

Position of the Infant

The infant is placed at the end of a mattress or of a warmed operating table with his lower limbs slightly abducted and his feet facing the surgeon. The size of the trocars is selected according to the height and weight of the infant whose abdominal cavity is very small. The endoscope allows direct vision at an angle of $0°$. It has a caliber of 3.5 mm. The grasping and spreading forceps, spatula, and scalpel are introduced through 4-mm trocars. The scalpel has been specially developed for pylorotomy in infants (K. Storz, Tuttlingen, Germany).

Introduction of the Instruments

The sites are chosen in accordance with the position of the umbilicus, the midline, and the costal margin, as well as the presumably most common location of the pyloric olive (Fig. 1).

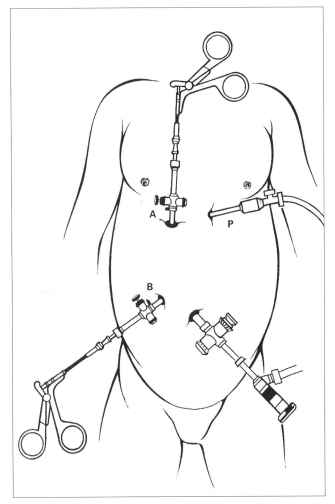

Creation of the Pneumoperitoneum

After manual bladder evacuation using external pressure, according to Créde's maneuver, a Veress needle is introduced below the left costal margin 1 cm from the midline. Syringe testing verifies its intraperitoneal placement. The needle is left in place to lift the left hepatic border throughout the operation. Carbon dioxide gas is slowly insufflated. Very close survey of intra-abdominal volume and pressure, as well as insufflated gas quantity are mandatory so as not to exceed a pressure of 6–8 cm H_2O in the young infant. Any abnormal rise in capnometry makes an immediate exsufflation absolutely necessary.

Placing the Laparoscope

The umbilicus is carefully desinfected. Through a short incision in its right inferior quadrant, a trocar is placed and the 4-mm endoscope is introduced at a 0° inclination through the trocar. To avoid accidental exteriorization of the trocar during the operation, it is advisable to secure the rubber collar of the trocar to the abdominal wall with a suture. The pyloric olive is now located using the laparoscope. Accordingly, the sites of introduction of the other trocars are decided upon.

Placing Trocars A and B of 3.5-mm Diameter (Figs. 1 and 2)

Trocar A is placed on the right 3 or 4 cm below the hepatic border and lateral to the midline. Through this trocar an atraumatic grasping forceps is introduced to hold the duodenum a few millimeters distal to the pyloric olive. Trocar B is placed at a right angle above the pyloric olive. It allows the successive introduction of the scalpel, spatula, and spreading forceps.

Incision of the Pylorus

Incision of the pylorus is carried out along the avascular area (Fig. 3). A scalpel with a retractable blade is used through trocar B (Fig. 4). The incision is started at the thickest point of the pyloric olive and extended laterally along the pylorus. Two dangerous manoeuvres must be avoided:

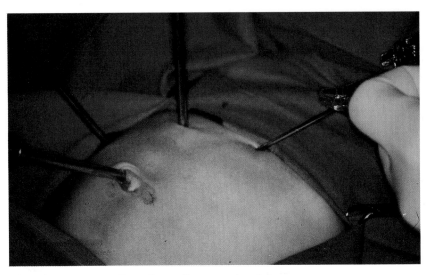

Fig. 1 and 2.   Position of the trocars (schematic illustration and intraoperative site)

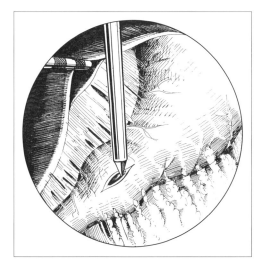 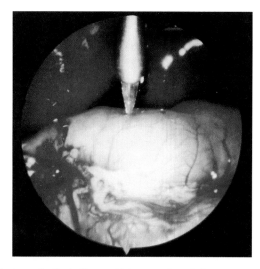

Figs. 3 and 4.   Incision of the pylorus in the avascular area with the scalpel (schematic illustration and intraoperative site)

1. Pushing the scalpel in too deeply. For this purpose a special scalpel is chosen, the blade of which is of a precisely limited length. Because the gastric mucosa may be easily injured, the incision is extended only just to permit the introduction of the spatula followed by the spreading forceps
2. Moving up too far toward the stomach: At the oral side of the hypertrophic pylorus, the stomach wall is very thin, sometimes creating a pseudodiverticulum (Fig. 5). Here the danger of perforating the mucosa is very high

Divulsion of the Pylorus

After incision of the surface of the pyloric olive, the scalpel is withdrawn. In its place a blunt spatula is introduced and rotated 90° between the edges of the incision. This maneuver facilitates the introduction of the spreading forceps. The closed tip of the spreading forceps is placed in the incision. The divulsion is obtained by spreading out the arms of the forceps, which possess small spurs protecting them from sliding over the muscular edges (Fig. 6). The retraction must be performed very slowly and very gradually by repeatedly opening

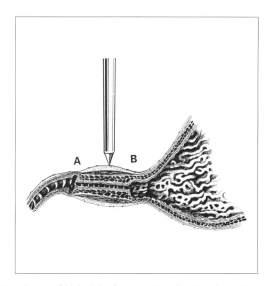

Fig. 5.   Areas of high risk of mucosal perforation (pseudodiverticulum) on each side of the pylorotomy (A and B)

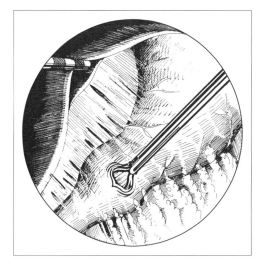 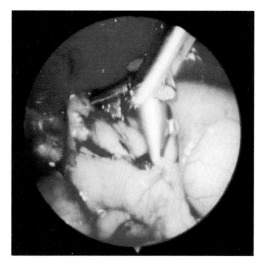

Figs. 6 and 7.   Divulsion of the transected muscular layer with a forceps (schematic illustration and intraoperative site)

the forceps in the direction of the two extremities of the olive (Fig. 7).

If a fibrous bridge persists, it is advisable to withdraw the forceps and reintroduce the spatula, not the scalpel, in order to transect the fibrosis. After complete pylorotomy, the gastric mucosa protrudes through the incision of the muscular layer. Usually, no bleeding results from this intervention. In case of any mishap, very fine electrocoagulation may be applied; in fact, we have never had to use it.

Verification of Gastric Mucosal Integrity

To exclude mucosal injury, air is injected through a nasogastric tube using a syringe. Normally, no bubbles are seen at the bottom of the incision. At the slightest doubt of gastric mucosal injury, a laparotomy becomes mandatory in order to verify or exclude it, and to suture any accidental mucosal break. Before trocar withdrawal, complete CO_2 exsufflation must be carried out at the end of the procedure. The skin incisions at trocar sites A and B are closed with sutures.

Postoperative Course

Analgetics are recommended during the first postoperative hours. Oral feeding may start on the evening of the same day; it is difficult to evaluate the degree of postoperative discomfort in the young infant related to the absence parietal incision. According to our pediatric anesthesiologist, an improvement was observed compared with open surgery.

Personal Experience and Results

Since May 1990, 83 infants (19 girls and 64 boys) have undergone laparoscopic pylorotomy in our hospital. No consequent mortalities were observed. None of the pylorotomies were found to be insufficient necessitating a complementary act or reintervention. However, two complications were observed, leading to a change of technique and a modification of the instruments. In both cases the surgeon did not perform laparotomy, although at air insufflation through the nasogastric tube there seemed to be a slight doubt about mucosal integrity.

The following day, laparotomy was decided upon for these two infants. Gastric mucosal perforation was confirmed. The perforation was found toward the gastric end of the incision and probably caused by the scalpel blade. This avoidable complication justifies the need for the utmost care and vigilance while verifying the absence of gastric mucosal perforation using the air injection test through the nasogastric tube. It also implicates the necessity for a conversion to laparotomy on the least shadow of doubt.

Ever since technique modification, no further remorse over accidental perforation has haunted the success of the procedure. This applies to the past 50 cases. The modifications consist of:

1. Use of a new scalpel, the blade of which has a standard depth and ridged borders attempting only one incision with the blade and never applying the second, even if the pylorotomy appears to be incomplete
2. Systematic use of a spatula after the incision is made and before the introduction of the spreading forceps so as to facilitate the process of spreading out the edges

Conclusion

Laparoscopic extramucosal pylorotomy is easily applicable in young infants. Laparoscopic myotomy is as safe and effective as conventional surgery, and offers the potential benefits of shortened hospital stay and minimum cosmetic deformity [9]. Prerequisites for a successful laparoscopy include extensive laparoscopic experience on the part of the surgeon, the use of specially adapted instruments, and the respect of all precautions concerning anesthesia. This approach must be left open to discussion as one of the options of surgical intervention, not forgetting the simplicity and low morbidity subsequent to classic conventional laparotomy.

Strict precision and great care are mandatory. It is up to the surgeon to choose the method he or she considers safe in his or her hands. The future outcome of this new surgical approach depends on the rigorous restriction of its practice to surgeons highly trained in laparoscopy within the domain of pediatrics.

Acknowledgments

The author thanks D. Grousseau, B. Longis, G. Terrier, and A. Longis of the Department of Pediatric Surgery, Dupuytren University Hospital, Dupuytren, France. He also thanks K. Storz GmbH, P. O. Box 230, D-78503 Tuttlingen, Germany.

References

1. ALAIN JL, GROUSSEAU D, TERRIER G: Extramucosal pylorotomy by laparoscopy. J Pediatr Surg 26 (1991) 1191–1192.
2. ALAIN JL, GROUSSEAU D, TERRIER G: Extramucosal pyloromyotomy by laparoscopy. Surg Endosc 5 (1991) 174–175.
3. FREDET P, LESNE E: Sténose du pylore chez le nourrisson, résultat anatomique de la pylorotomie sur un cas traité et guéri depuis 3 mois. Bull Mém Soc Nat Chir 54 (1908) 1050.
4. GANS SL, BERCI G: Advances in endoscopy of infants and children. J Pediatr Surg 6 (1971) 199–233.
5. JACOBAEUS HC: Über die Möglichkeit die Zystoskopie bei Untersuchung Seröser Höhlungen anzuwenden. Münch Med Wochenschr 57 (1910) 2090–2092.
6. KALK H, BRUHL W: Leitfaden der Laparoskopie und Gastroskopie. Thieme, Stuttgart (1951).
7. LOBE TE, SCHROPP KP (EDS.): Pyloromyotomy. In: Pediatric laparoscopy and thoracoscopy. W. B. Saunders Company, Philadelphia (1994).
8. RAMSTEDT C: Zur Operation der angeborenen Pylorusstenose. Med Klin 8 (1912) 1702.
9. TAN HL: Pylorotomy by laparoscopy in children. In: Graber (ed.): Abdominal laparoscopy surgery. McGraw-Hill, New York.

25. Meckel's Diverticulum and other Embryonic Vestiges of the Umbilical Duct

J. WALDSCHMIDT AND F. SCHIER

Introduction

Meckel's diverticulum is an embryonic vestige of the umbilical duct. It occurs in 1.5–2 % of the general population. There are other even rarer intra-abdominal remnants of the embryonic umbilical duct (persistent umbilical duct, Roser cyst, vitelline duct cyst, enteral filament, and terminal filament) and the umbilical vessels (ligamentary vestiges of the vitelline artery and vein) [9, 12, 13].

Meckel's diverticulum as well as the intra-abdominal ligaments can be the cause of chronic abdominal pain and an acute abdomen (Figs. 1–3) [11, 12]. The most frequent complications are listed in Table 1.

Indications and Contraindications

In cases of detected Meckel's diverticulum or a ligamentary vestige of embryonic umbilical duct structures, resection is indicated due to the complications that may be involved with these conditions. Meckel's diverticulum can be detected radiologically, scintigraphically or incidentally during laparos-

copic appendectomy or other laparoscopic interventions (Table 2). Looking for Meckel's diverticulum and other embryonic ligamentary vestiges should be an integral part of every diagnostic and surgical laparoscopy.

Table 1. Complications of embryonic umbilical duct vestiges

Gastrointestinal bleeding

Diverticulitis

Perforation

Intussusception

Strangulation ileus due to torsion of the diverticulum, volvulus of the diverticulum-carrying or ligament-fixed ileum segment, adherence in a hernia (Littré's hernia), knotting

Bowel obstruction by inversion and eversion in an open umbilical duct

Compression ileus due to diverticular tumor, overdistension, parasites, bezoars, foreign bodies

Kinking due to traction

Ileum stricture in chronic diverticulitis

Hemorrhagic ascites

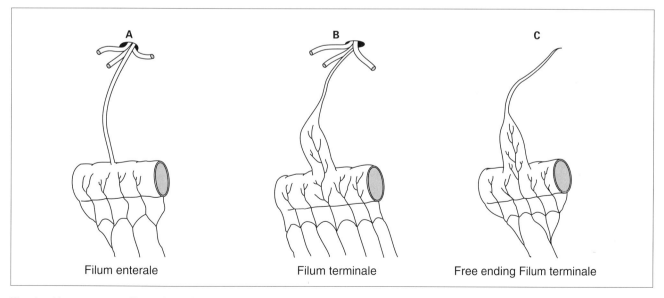

Filum enterale   Filum terminale   Free ending Filum terminale

Fig. 1. Ligamentous malformations of the omphaloenteric duct. **A.** Complete obstruction of the vitelline duct forming an enteral filament. **B.** A terminal filament results in the case of an existing Meckel's diverticulum. **C.** The terminal filament can tear at the omphalus and adhere with its free end to another site or float freely

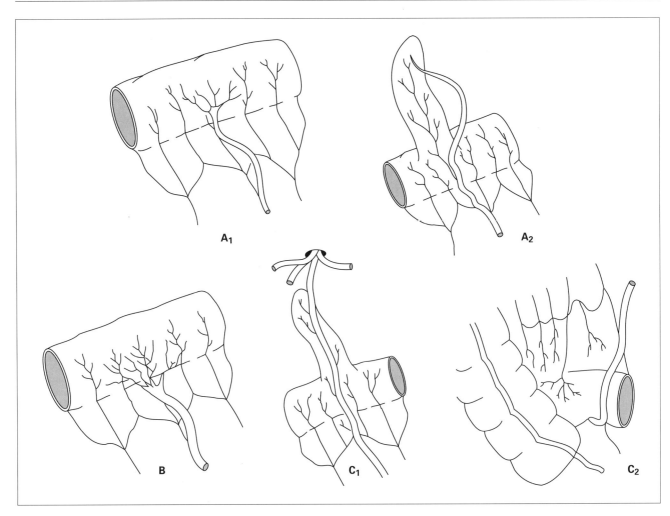

Fig. 2. Remnants of the umbilical arteries. **A₁.** Lig. mesoenterale. **A₂.** Mesodiverticular ligament. **B.** Radiculomesenteric ligament. **C₁.** Omphalomesenteric ligament of the right vitelline artery. **C₂.** Omphalomesenteric ligament of the left vitelline artery

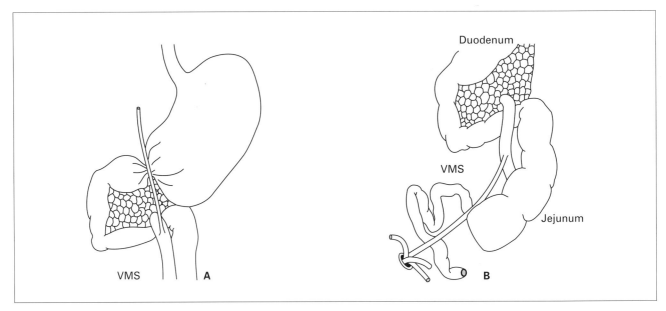

Fig. 3. Ligaments arising from a persistent left umbilical vein. **A.** Persistence of the central segment with compression of the duodenal bulb or pylorus. **B.** Persistence of the peripheral segment with a fibrous ligament between the omphalus and the transverse mesocolon

The contraindications are limited to exceptions, such as a diverticulum discovered by chance in premature and neonates during diagnostic laparoscopy. Further contraindications include a delayed ileus with gangrene of the diverticulum-carrying loop of the small intestine, peritonitis, and diverticulum perforation with advanced inflammation of the surrounding area, which seriously interferes with the visualization of the diverticulum. Furthermore, the general contraindications of anesthesia must be considered in neonates and infants.

Preoperative Work-up

Diagnostic laparoscopy is indicated if there is adequate clinical suspicion of Meckel's diverticulum (umbilical abnormalities; see Table 2). In recurring subileus, gastrointestinal bleeding and in cases of chronic pain, other causes must be excluded such as chronically recurring intestinal inflammation and mesenteric lymphadenitis (yersinia infection, toxoplasmosis, verminosis, campylobacter, etc.), inflammatory/ulcerative diseases of the gastrointestinal tract (Crohn's disease, duodenal ulcer), renal malformation, biliary tract diseases, diseases of the uterine appendages, nutritional intolerance, metabolic disorders (diabetes mellitus, lipid metabolism), and immunovasculitis associated with Schönlein-Henoch purpura. An active search for these causes should be undertaken (stool specimens, serological tests, X-rays).

Table 2. Indications for laparoscopic diverticulum resection

Incidental detection

Clinical detection of a diverticulum (radiologically, scintigraphically)

Clinical suspicion of Meckel's diverticulum
    In umbilical abnormalities: umbilical hernia, fistula, polyp, sinus, cysts, tissue heterotopy
    Recurring abdominal pain
    Recurring subileus conditions
    Recurring intestinal bleeding

Acute abdomen by ileus or gastrointestinal bleeding

Meckel's diverticulum must be taken into consideration for each case of intestinal bleeding in small children, possibly even in infants, but more rarely in older children. Technological and radiological detection by endoscopy, sonography, contrast-enhanced imaging of the gastrointestinal passage, or by other imaging procedures (CT, NMR) is only very rarely successful. These diagnostic procedures are very stressful and time-consuming, and therefore should be avoided in cases of massive intestinal bleeding.

The preoperative detection of a hemorrhaging Meckel's diverticulum is carried out most reliably and rapidly with scintigraphy. Scintigraphic detection is based on the frequent existence of heterotopic gastric mucosa in the diverticulum (Fig. 4). This is enhanced with sodium pertechnetate ^{99m}Tc. In cases of hemorrhaging Meckel's diverticulum, heterotopic gastric mucosa is encountered in 90 % and very reliably demonstrated with previous thyroid suppression and pentagastrin stimulation. False-positive findings can be simulated in intussusception, AV fistulas, angiomas, aneurysms, hydronephrosis, duplications, Peutz-Jeghers syndrome, and urinary stasis [5, 8, 10, 13].

A Meckel's diverticulum or a ligament can also cause intestinal obstruction. Infants and small children generally present with strangulation through torsion, volvulus, or ligamentary obstruction, with intussusception in older children. Mesenteric ischemia is accompanied by extremely severe pain, vomiting and circulatory shock; bloody stools and signs of peritonitis occur later, and speed is required. An X-ray of the abdomen in an upright or lateral recumbent position confirms the diagnosis and should be the impetus for immediate laparoscopy.

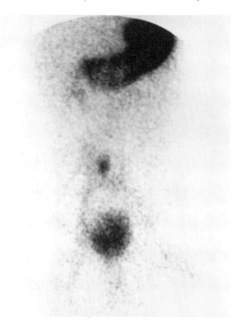

Fig. 4. Scintigraphic detection of a hemorrhaging Meckel's diverticulum 30 min after ^{99m}Tc pertechnetate administration, previous thyroid suppression, and pentagastrin stimulation in a 2½-year-old boy

Operative Technique

Positioning, arrangement of the instruments, and the position of the surgeon and nurse are as in an appendectomy. The surgeon and the scrub nurse sit or stand on the left side of the child, with the assistant on the right. In school children the position of the trocar can be selected as in adults (Fig. 5) [14].

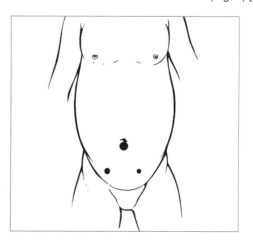

Fig. 5. Trocar placement for laparoscopic resection of Meckel's diverticulum

The Veress cannula and the 10-mm optical trocar are inserted at the lower edge of the omphalus. Under laparoscopic visual control, the first working trocar (5 mm) is inserted in the left suprasymphysic area, lateral to the rectus sheath; the second working trocar (7 mm) on the right, lateral to the rectus sheath. In infants and small children the umbilical region, however, must be avoided, because accompanying umbilical abnormalities can be expected in a large percentage, and injuries could be made due to the high bladder and the still-fragile umbilical arteries in the lateral umbilical folds. The Veress cannula and the optical trocar are thus inserted at the Munro point (Fig. 6).

The Nd:YAG laser is advantageous and preferred especially for infants and small children, due to its precise guidance and good hemostasis. Dissection of Meckel's diverticulum and its removal are performed in the contact mode with 25 W with an impulse duration of 0.5 s and an impulse interval of 0.3 s. Possibly required hemostasis is carried out in the noncontact mode with 35 W. As a light conductor a 0.4-mm bare fiber is used in infants, and a 0.6-mm bare fiber in older children.

A vitelline duct cyst is generally located directly adjacent to the umbilicus. Here, it can be removed with high-frequency diathermy or with the laser (Fig. 7). It should be evacuated before extraction. In case of a connection to the ileum, the connection to the intestinal lumen must be transected between double ligatures.

Embryonic ligaments are resected. Exclusive transection is inadequate. Due to the strong vascularization of these taut, fibrous cords, the ligaments should be ligated at their points of attachment or resected under coagulation with high-frequency diathermy or – preferentially – with the laser (Fig. 8 and 9).

In cases of a narrow-based diverticulum extending from the ileum, resection is performed as in an appendectomy. The tip of the diverticulum is fixed with laparoscopic grasping forceps.

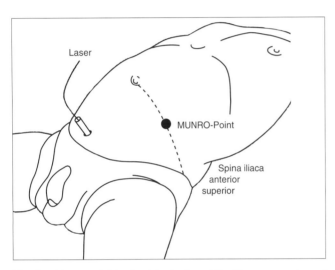

Fig. 6. Munro point for the introduction of the Veress cannula and the optical cannula in neonates and infants

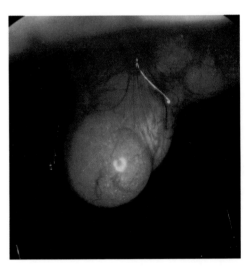

Fig. 7. Embryonic ligament of the umbilical duct at the umbilicus in a 7-year-old boy

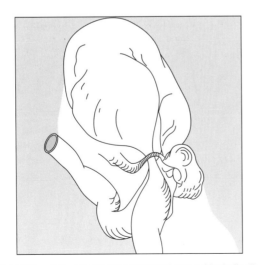

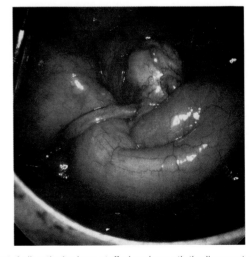

Figs. 8 and 9. A 7-year-old boy presented with a Meckel's diverticular ligament. A diverticular loop stuffed underneath the ligament and was strangulated. Resection of the diverticulum and ligament as well as appendectomy were performed. **8.** Schematic drawing. **9.** Laparoscopic photograph

The vascular pedicle is occluded and divided with high-frequency diathermy or with the laser (Figs. 10–12). The diverticulum is emptied into the intestinal lumen, then the base is ligated with a Roeder loop. A second Roeder loop closes the diverticular sack. The resection of the diverticulum is performed between the two ligatures. The mucous membrane on the diverticular stump is devitalized with high-frequency diathermy or with the laser. The stump is sealed with fibrin. A small platelet of Interceed can also be applied for adhesion prophylaxis [14].

In cases of wide-based attachment the diverticulum is raised after its mobilization with the antimesenteric intestinal wall until it is stretched into a tent shape. In infants and small children further procedures are performed as with a narrow-based diverticulum, whereby the ileum wall is included tangentially in the ligature. In older children the resection follows after placing 6 rows of staples with the Endo-GIA. The sta-

pling device places a triple row of clip sutures in the intestine as well as in the diverticulum, which reliably closes the lumen without endangering perfusion. The Endo-GIA must be applied diagonally in order to avoid stenosis of the intestinal lumen. Care must also be taken not to grasp the mesenteric ileum wall in the staple line. Exteriorization of the diverticulum, as described by Attwood [1] and Ng et al. [6] for adults, is not necessary in children.

Technical Difficulties and Possible Problems

To perform a safe laparoscopy in infants and neonates several technical aspects that differ from laparoscopy in adults must be taken in consideration (Table 3). In those very small patients the distance between the abdominal wall and the intra-abdominal organs is very short resulting in a close work-

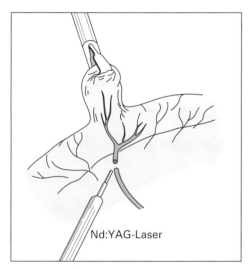

Fig. 10. Grasping the tip of the diverticulum. Separation of the mesenteriolum after previous obliteration of the artery and vein with the Nd:YAG laser

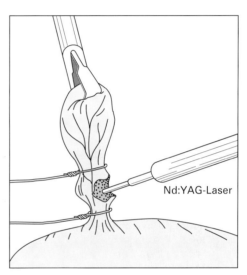

Fig. 12. Second endoloop. Transecting the diverticulum at its base, between the ligatures. Vaporization of the stump mucosa, fibrin sealing

ing distance. Even when using specially developed short instruments the space for manipulations is limited.

In adaptation to the smaller anatomical conditions, 5-mm laparoscopes are used in infants and neonates. The reduced diameter impairs light transmission, and therefore intra-abdominal illumination may not be as good as in the adult.

Table 3. Special aspects of the laparoscopic technique in neonates and infants

Close working distance

Small optics (reduced light transmission)

Individual puncture sites
   In neonates at the Munro point
   In small children in the diagonal contralateral quadrant

Thin abdominal walls (gas losses, unreliable fixation of the cannula)

Thin greater omentum (floating, blurring optics, and obstructing cannula)

Lower insufflation pressure (elevation of diaphragm)

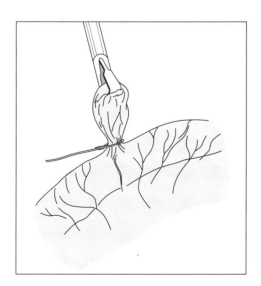

Fig. 11. Ligature at the diverticulum base (endoloop); the antimesenteric intestinal wall is raised in a tent shape

The umbilical region must be avoided for puncture with the Veress needle and the first trocar. In this area the danger of a lesion to the bladder or hemorrhage from the umbilical arteries is highest. Therefore, blind punction with the first trocar should be carried out at the Munro point in neonates. In infants the first trocar can be placed in the diagonal-contralateral quadrant.

The abdominal wall in small children and infants is still very thin and fragile giving the trocars little hold. To prevent accidental extraction of the trocars and gas loss along the outer side of the trocar sheath, additional fixation may be necessary. The greater omentum is also thin and contains less fat than in the adult: It therefore has a tendency to float around and blurr the view or obstruct the cannulas.

When resecting a diverticulum, attention should be paid not to grasp the contralateral ileum wall in the ligature or staple row. Furthermore, careful inspection of the whole abdominal cavity is mandatory to safely exclude other abnormalities (Figs. 1A–C) that might also require laparoscopic treatment.

Precise anesthesiological monitoring is of primary importance, because the pneumoperitoneum can have a severe impact on circulation and blood gas pressure in infants and neonates (see Chap. 24). To minimize these negative effects, it is advisable to keep the intra-abdominal pressure as low as possible.

Discussion

Meckel's diverticulum should be actively looked for in every laparoscopy performed in children. Resection becomes mandatory with the identification of a diverticulum, due to the threat of numerous severe complications. Laparoscopy is possible at every age and with every body size; the special features of laparoscopy in neonates and infants should, however, be considered. The use of the Nd:YAG laser is especially valuable in these cases because of the small cannula.

Valuable information can be obtained from a thorough case history and an exact inspection of the umbilicus. Searching for associated malformations, such as ligamentous vestiges of the umbilical duct and the accompanying embryonic vessels, as well as for alterations at the omphalus and the mesenteric root, should be performed during laparoscopy. These must also be removed; the umbilical hernial orifice should be closed.

The advantage of laparoscopic diverticulum excision versus an open procedure is the better overview of the abdominal cavity without the impaired position of the organs to each other caused by retractors. Thus, the diagnosis of concomitant abnormalities at the omphalus and mesenterium (ligaments, terminal filament, cysts, etc.) is easier and more reliable. In addition, they can be less traumatically treated. Using the laser probably causes fewer adhesions, because there is neither blood nor fibrin extravasation at the cut surface.

The disadvantages of laparoscopy become obvious with a complicated Meckel's diverticulum. Orientation and preparation are especially difficult in perforation with strong reactions in the surrounding area or with torsion; however, these complications are rare. Another possible risk consists of an incomplete resection if ectopic mucosa is not limited to the diverticulum, but extends to the ileum. This situation rarely occurs. It can be avoided by the tent-shaped raising of the antimesenteric intestinal wall and placement of endoligatures.

For excising Meckel's diverticulum a 30-mm Endo-GIA (12-mm trocar) is used in older children, and an endoloop (5-mm trocar) is used in small children and infants. The diverticular stump does not require additional coverage, but the mucosa in the stump should be devitalized so that a smooth scar forms. This can be performed the least traumatically with the laser, because the laser effect can be precisely controlled and thermal damage is limited. There is also a greater sealing effect with the laser than with high-frequency diathermy or Endo-GIA resection [2, 4, 7].

We performed a laparoscopic diverticulum resection in six patients (four endoligatures and two Endo-GIAs) without intraoperative or postoperative complications. The youngest child was 2.5 years old.

Although the previous results are still based on a very small patient population, they are, however, encouraging. Only further experience on a larger patient population will be able to determine the value of laparoscopic diverticulum resection as compared with open surgery.

References

1. ATTWOOD SE, McGRATH J, HILL ADK, STEPHENS RB: Laparoscopic approach to Meckel's diverticulectomy. Br J Surg 79 (1992) 211.
2. GIRONA GCL, FOURNET J, CHAMPETIER J: Les Accidents hémorragiques du Diverticule de Meckel. Place de la Laparoscopie dans leur diagnostic. Rev Med Alp Francaises 4 (1985) 79–83.
3. GÖTZ F: Die endoskopische Appendektomie nach Semm bei der akuten und chronischen Appendicitis. Endoskopie Heute 2 (1988) 5–7.
4. HUANG CS, LIN LH: Laparoscopic Meckel's diverticulotomy in infants: report of 3 cases. J Pediatr Surg 28 (1993) 1486–1489.
5. JEWETT TCD, DUSZYNSKI DO, ALLEN JE: The visualization of Meckel's diverticulum with 99mTc pertechnetate. Surgery 68 (1970) 567-570.
6. NG WT, WONG MK, KONG CK, CHAN YT: Laparoscopic approach to Meckel's diverticulectomy. Br J Surg 79 (1992) 211.
7. PANUEL M, CAMPAN N, DELARUE A, PETIT P, SARLES J, DEVRED P: Ultrasonographic diagnosis and laparoscopic surgical treatment of Meckel's diverticulum. J Pediatr Surg 4 (1994) 344–345.
8. RODGERS BM, YOUSSEF S: "False positive" scan for Meckel's diverticulum. J Pediatr 87 (1975) 239–240.
9. RUTHERFORD RB, AKERS DR: Meckel's diverticulum: a review of 148 pediatric patients with special reference to the pattern of bleeding. Surgery 59 (1966) 618–626.
10. SEITZ W, HOFFMAN S, HAHN K: Ergebnisse der Abdominalszintigraphie mit 99mTechnetiumpertechnetat im Kindesalter. Pädiat Prax 21 (1977/1978) 383–390.
11. SÖDERLUND S: Meckel's diverticulum: clinical and histologic study. Acta Chir Scand 248 (Suppl) (1959) 13–233.
12. WALDSCHMIDT J: Intraabdominelle ligamentäre Relikte des Dottersackganges und der Dottersackgefässe. Mschr Kinderheilk 131 (1990) 222–227.
13. WALDSCHMIDT J: Rückbildungsstörungen des Dottergangs, des Allantoisgangs und des ventralen Mesenteriums. In: Waldschmidt J (ed.): Das akute Abdomen im Kindesalter. VCH edition medizin, Weinheim (1990) S. 327–376.
14. WALDSCHMIDT J, SCHIER F: Laparoskopische Abtragung von Meckel Divertikeln und anderen embryonalen Relikten des D. omphalusentericus. Pädiat Prax 46 (1993/1994) 675–684.

26. Laparoscopic Treatment of Cryptorchidism

G. H. JORDAN

Introduction

Cryptorchidism refers to any testis that resides in an extra-scrotal position. This condition can be further classified into dystopic testes (those unable to descend into the scrotum due to an incomplete cord length) and ectopic testes (those that have descended to a nonscrotal location). Although there remains some controversy regarding the cause of the undescended testicle, whether mechanical or hormonal, it is known that both gross and microscopic abnormalities exist in testicular and ductal development of the undescended testis [17]. The consequences of these abnormalities constitute many of the indications for correction of this condition:

1. Possible improved fertility
2. Possible prevention of a significantly higher incidence of testicular malignancy
3. Correction of associated hernias
4. Prevention of testicular torsion
5. Alleviation of the psychological trauma resulting from an empty scrotum [17].

The goal of treatment, to achieve permanent fixation of the testis in the scrotum, may be achieved in some instances by hormonal therapy, but in virtually all instances is attainable through the use of an appropriately chosen surgical technique. The timing of treatment is important, because some studies have indicated that early correction can decrease the incidence of malignancies and improve fertility in adulthood. When one considers these findings and the occasional natural occurrence of spontaneous descent throughout the first year, correction early in the second year of life appears desirable [17].

Evaluation of Cryptorchidism

An important distinction to be made as part of the evaluation is the location of the undescended testicle. Upon clinical examination undescended testes may be either palpable or impalpable. Furthermore, a palpable undescended testicle is either retractile, ectopic, or truly undescended within the canal, whereas an impalpable testis may be either truly undescended (i.e., high canalicular or intra-abdominal in location) or absent [17].

A true retractile testis will be found along the line of descent, and is most commonly palpated in the groin or upper scrotum. These testes withdraw to an extrascrotal position due to a hyperactive cremasteric reflex. If gentle coaxing draws them back into the scrotum and they remain in position without tension, they are not truly undescended. Although it is worthwhile

to reexamine the patient periodically, no further treatment is usually necessary in these cases, because maturation and fertility are reportedly normal in retractile testes, and the vast majority will ultimately come to lie properly in the scrotum.

An ectopic testis is commonly described as a testis that has emerged from the external inguinal ring, but has then been misdirected along the remaining course of its descent. The superficial inguinal pouch between the external oblique aponeurosis and the subcutaneous tissue is the most common site of ectopia, with perineal ectopia, prepenile ectopia, and transverse scrotal and femoral positions being less common. Because these testes do not generally respond to hormonal treatment, it is believed that mechanical impediment to normal descent is a factor in their displacement [10]. The testicle can also take an abnormal path of descent within the abdomen, with testicles having been found adjacent to the upper pole of the kidneys, beneath the liver, and more frequently, in the pelvis, medial to the respective medial umbilical ligament. We have identified these medial abdominal ectopic testicles as being particularly difficult to address at the time of orchidopexy.

Truly undescended testes are the result of a diminished length and fixation of the spermatic vessels. They may be intra-abdominal, intra-canalicular, or emergent (high canalicular or just exiting the external ring). For the most part, the higher the location of the testis, the more severe the degree of maldevelopment, and the more difficult it is to treat by either hormonal or surgical methods [17].

Absent testes may present as either a unilaterally or bilaterally impalpable organ. Only about 20 % of impalpable testis are actually absent, whereas the remainder are in an undetected intra-abdominal or intra-canalicular position.

Preoperative Work-up

A careful physical examination of the patient is often sufficient to rule out the diagnosis of cryptorchidism. A diagnosis of cryptorchidism is based on the inability to either feel a testis in the scrotum or to manipulate a palpable testis into the scrotum. Relaxation of the patient and warming of the examiner's hands will aid in a successful examination, and a gentle milking action from the superior iliac crest toward the scrotum will often deliver an impalpable testis to a palpable or scrotal position. At times it is desirable to place a vaginal lubricant on the examiner's fingertips. The reduced friction often heightens the ability to palpate the difficult-to-locate testicle. Another useful maneuver is to place the patient in the cross-legged position, leaning slightly forward, to relax the cremasteric muscle.

If a careful physical examination does not reveal the location of either a retractile or undescended palpable testis, further evaluation is necessary. Although surgical exploration might seem to be the most probable means of determining the location of the impalpable undescended testis, less invasive means have also been successful. If anorchidism (bilateral impalpable undescended testicles) is suspected, endocrine testing (basal FSH and LH levels and the response of testosterone secretion to HCG stimulation) provides a relatively reliable prediction for the presence of functioning testicular tissue [1, 19]. HCG stimulation testing can yield a false-negative test, though, as it appears not all "functioning" testicular tissue responds alike to gonadotropin stimulation. The author has, in fact, localized testicular tissue (demonstrated by histology) at laparoscopy that failed to respond to accepted protocols of HCG stimulation. In most cases in which both components of this testing were fulfilled, however, this hormonal testing has proven reliable in predicting bilateral congenital anorchidism. On the other hand, if the results are not absolutely definitive, further diagnostic tests should be employed to aid in location of an occult testis.

Tests that have been used to aid in the diagnosis of impalpable undescended testis include pneumoperitoneography using nitrous oxide gas and direct contrast peritoneography [7, 20, 25], computed tomography [26], aortography, selective gonadal arteriography, gonadal venography [14, 24] and magnetic resonance imaging [16]. Although each method has proven useful in certain circumstances, the information gained from these procedures must be considered in the context of their limited accuracy and, in some instances, invasive nature.

More recently, laparoscopy has been found useful in the diagnosis of the intra-abdominal testicle, in the visualization of spermatic vessels and vas deferens as they enter/approach the internal inguinal ring, and to demonstrate blind-ending spermatic vessels or vasae within the abdomen [23]. A number of reports support the increased accuracy of laparoscopic localization as compared with the other modalities described herein. In fact, studies also suggest that laparoscopic localization is more accurate than exploration, particularly extended inguinal exploration [4, 18].

Indications for Use of Laparoscopic Techniques in Diagnosis and Treatment of Undescended Testicles

The laparoscope's first urological application, reported by Cortesi, was as an aid in the localization of the impalpable undescended testicle [6]. Pediatric laparoscopic surgery demands that certain special considerations be made due to the size of the patients, but instruments currently available for therapeutic pediatric laparoscopy in children are limited. Recent advances in endoscopic and accessory instrumentation, however, are accelerating the evolution of these tools, making this approach more practical.

For purposes of diagnosis, laparoscopy has similar limitations to some of the other procedures described herein in its invasive nature and need for general anesthesia. However, its advantages include that it offers an opportunity for a definitive diagnosis in virtually all cases, and at the least, permits assessment of cord length and testicular mobility, thereby allowing planning of the surgical approach.

There are four surgical approaches to the correction of an undescended testicle: inguinal (extended inguinal), primary open abdominal, staged laparoendoscopic, and primary laparoendoscopic [11]. Laparoendoscopic orchidopexy (either primary or staged) is offered as an alternative to primary abdominal orchidopexy or extended inguinal orchidopexy.

The intra-abdominal testis can be found virtually anywhere in the retroperitoneum, but most commonly it is just inside the inguinal ring. The so-called ovarian location (higher abdominal locations), with short vessels but a long looping vas, allows for endoscopic division of the spermatic vessels. The vast majority of intra-abdominal testicles are not associated with the findings of a looping vas deferens, and the lack of that finding does not preclude the performance of orchidopexy by dividing the spermatic vessel leash. Subsequent to the initial ligation of the spermatic vessels, a 6-month wait is followed by the second-stage procedure that is performed via either open or laparoendoscopic techniques. In cases in which the testicle is above the internal ring with mobile vessels, the precise situation will be discussed with the parents, and orchidopexy/orchiectomy will be accomplished according to the decision of the parents and our recommendations. Many surgeons currently favor, in almost all situations, staging the abdominal orchidopexy with the vessels divided at the initial stage followed at 6 months by the testicle being mobilized on an enhanced blood supply that accompanies the vas deferens [3, 5, 22].

Special Considerations for Laparoscopic Surgery in the Child

Children are not simply small adults, and both their size and emotional immaturity present challenges in terms of medical care. Because children often undergo anesthesia while crying (with concomitant swallowing of air), they are at risk for gastric distention. Gastric distention predisposes to injury from the insufflation needle and/or blind primary access cannula placement. Therefore, unless a child is completely quiescent during induction of anesthesia, and there is absolutely no question of gastric distention, a nasogastric tube should be placed.

Experience with observational laparoscopy in children has shown that children are also especially susceptible to emphysematous complications during insufflation. In the early experience with pediatric laparoscopy, hypercarbia was thought to be related to the development of emphysema, and it was therefore presumed that children were at increased risk and required more intensive monitoring than adults. Recent experience has disproved this fear, however, and it is now known that children tolerate pneumoperitoneum well, with little hypercarbia. The emphysematous phenomenon arise more frequently in children, due to looser attachment of the peritoneum to the extraperitoneal structures.

A child's small size can present both advantages and disadvantages to the laparoscopic surgeon. One advantage to a child's dimensions is that they permit easy identification of landmarks. Palpation of the bifurcation of the great vessels and the sacral promontory are usually effortless, and abdominal or pelvic masses are easily detected in most children. In addition, children tend to have less preperitoneal fat, making the depth of the abdominal wall thinner, with less chance of inappropriate preperitoneal insufflation should a Veress needle approach be elected.

Unfortunately, the smaller size of pediatric patients also puts them at an increased risk for complications. Cannula placement must be approached with care for several reasons. Diminished space between the anterior abdominal wall and the vital organs in the child increases the risk of complications resulting from placement of the Veress needle and primary access cannula. Also, the bladder of a child is more of an intra-abdominal organ, making bladder decompression mandatory to avoid injury with cannula placement. Finally, looser attachments of the peritoneum to the extraperitoneal structures often create problems with access cannula placement.

Due to the risks of blind cannula access and the ease with which open cannula placement can be accomplished in children, at this center we have abandoned both Veress needle insufflation and blind cannula access.

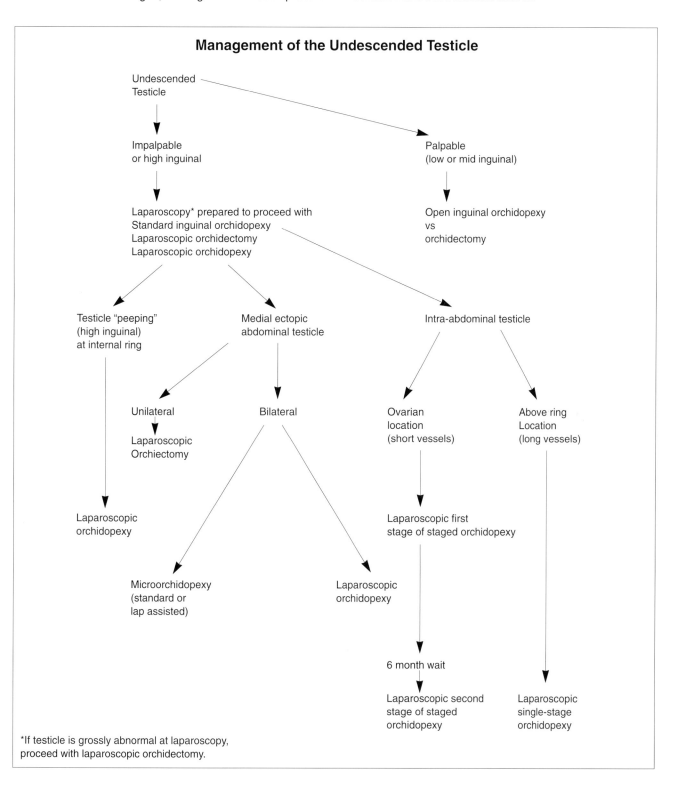

Management of the Undescended Testicle

Undescended Testicle

→ Impalpable or high inguinal

→ Palpable (low or mid inguinal)

Impalpable or high inguinal → Laparoscopy* prepared to proceed with
Standard inguinal orchidopexy
Laparoscopic orchidectomy
Laparoscopic orchidopexy

Palpable (low or mid inguinal) → Open inguinal orchidopexy
vs
orchidectomy

Laparoscopy branches to:
- Testicle "peeping" (high inguinal) at internal ring
- Medial ectopic abdominal testicle
- Intra-abdominal testicle

Testicle "peeping" → Laparoscopic orchidopexy

Medial ectopic abdominal testicle → Unilateral / Bilateral

Unilateral → Laparoscopic Orchiectomy

Bilateral → Microorchidopexy (standard or lap assisted) / Laparoscopic orchidopexy

Intra-abdominal testicle → Ovarian location (short vessels) / Above ring Location (long vessels)

Ovarian location (short vessels) → Laparoscopic first stage of staged orchidopexy → 6 month wait → Laparoscopic second stage of staged orchidopexy

Above ring Location (long vessels) → Laparoscopic single-stage orchidopexy

*If testicle is grossly abnormal at laparoscopy, proceed with laparoscopic orchidectomy.

Instrumentation for Pediatric Laparoendoscopic Surgery

A complete assortment of endoscopic instruments should be available in the room used for a pediatric laparoscopic procedure. These instruments must be varied in application, and can be insulated to be compatible with monopolar cautery. In addition to the endoscopic instruments (endoscopes, cannulas, and trocars), a complete laparotomy set must be in the room and open. A high-intensity light source is essential for pediatric laparoscopy as well.

Reusable trocars (particularly larger access cannulas) become dull with use and push, rather than penetrate, the peritoneum. Due to smaller space tolerances in the child, a dull trocar is a deadly weapon. Disposable cannula systems offer the advantage of sharp trocars, but although adaptable, are designed for adult use, and are far from optimal. However, recent innovations in disposable cannulas have made their use in children easier, and new designs of trocars and shielding mechanisms have made cannula placement far less anxiety-provoking in children.

A valid concern is that many currently available laparoendoscopic instruments are too large for small children. True open access cannulas are not useful for children. Fortunately, experience has shown that standard cannulas with fixation devices can be adapted with few problems for open placement in the child. Some instruments have 10-mm shafts, and the working elements are tapered to 5 mm. For many pediatric applications, 5-mm ports are all that are required. For other cases the need to place a 10-mm or larger cannula rests on whether multiclip appliers or staplers will be used. A 5-mm reusable vascular clip applier is available for use in Europe; however, at the time of this writing, it is not marketed for use in the United States. Most 5-mm laparoscopic lenses provide excellent optics and illumination for laparoscopic surgery in the young child. In the older child (> 5 years old), 10-mm optics are preferable. As instrument manufacturers rise to the cause, more instruments are being downsized to 5 mm (see Chap. 4). In some cases cannula placement can be facilitated by using the laparoscopic instruments from within to help create the peritoneotomy, or by using the laparoendoscopic instruments through the cannula.

Length and diameter of instrumentation are concerns in pediatrics. Long instruments push the surgeon and assistant away from the operative field and, with the size of the child's abdomen already a limiting factor, compound the difficulties. A trend that will benefit pediatric applications is that 5-mm instruments are now being shortened for ease of use in pelvic node dissection. However, shortening the shaft will only solve half the problem. A major shortcoming of currently available laparoscopic instruments is the undue length of the noninsulated working portion of the instrument in the limited confines of the child's peritoneal cavity.

A laparoscopic coagulation device is required, and monopolar cautery devices with isolated ground seem to dominate. The engineering limitations of bipolar devices have slowed their development, but as more aggressive laparoscopic bowel surgeries are developed, some encouraging bipolar devices are becoming available.

Preparation of the Patient

In laparoscopic surgery the patient is placed supine on the operating room table. For intersex evaluation a low lithotomy position is useful, allowing for simultaneous cystoscopy/vaginoscopy and laparoscopy. It is best for the patient to be flat on the operating room table, and the table moved to achieve the extremes of Trendelenburg, reverse Trendelenburg, or rolled positions, if possible. Arms should be tucked at the side, due to the potential risk of brachial plexus injury with extension. As in adult laparoscopic surgery it is essential for the child to be fixed to the table with belts, tape, and/or shoulder fixation devices to prevent sliding or rolling during movement of the table.

The field is prepared so that the position and extent of draping are suitable for an open abdominal procedure, if necessary. The skin preparation is nipple line to mid-thigh, table side to table side. A urethral catheter is inserted, and in most cases the anesthesiologist places a nasogastric/oral gastric tube for decompression of the stomach. Warming blankets are used, because a child can lose body heat during a laparoscopic procedure almost as readily as with an open procedure.

Cannula Placement in the Pediatric Patient

Trocar placement must be modified in the pediatric patient (Fig. 1). The usual primary access cannula for pelvic surgery is periumbilical, but additional suprapubic and McBurney's point ports do not work well for access and pelvic surgery in children. The differences in relationships of the pelvic structures in the child's abdomen as compared with adults can potentially lead to territorial disagreements between the surgeon, camera holder, and assistant. We have learned that displacement of the lateral cannulas in a cephalad direction seems to alleviate these problems while providing excellent access to all areas of the child's pelvis, and specifically to the internal inguinal ring and iliac vessels. Because there are many perforators from the inferior epigastric vessels in the area of the umbilicus, the movement of these lateral cannulas in

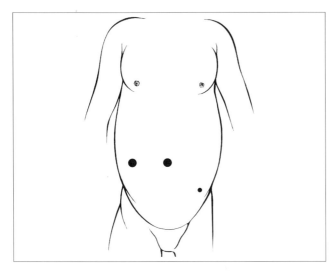

Fig. 1. Typical cannula placement for (R) laparoscopic orchidopexy. For diagnostic laparoscopy, only the subumbilical port is used. Should one require a 10-mm lateral access cannula, that would be placed ipsilateral to the testicle

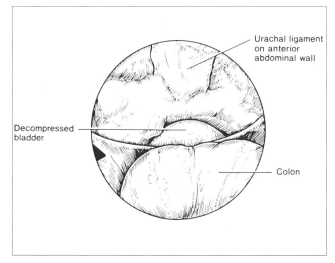

Fig. 2. View of the midline in the child. The transverse vesical fold is easily appreciated. The medial umbilical ligaments are just outside the view of this field. (Used by permission, AUA Update Series, Lesson 34, vol X, 1991, American Urological Association)

a cephalad direction opens the possibility of complications, due to an increased potential for bleeding. Experience with this modification to standard cannula placement schema thus far has not led to problems with abdominal wall bleeding. We place a 5- or 10-mm primary access cannula, depending on the age of the child, through which the appropriate telescope is inserted. Because a displaced lens actually hinders rather than improving vision, due to space limitations in most children, there is no advantage to using a 30 ° lens for pelvic procedures. The lateral access cannulas are 5 mm.

Diagnostic Laparoscopy for the Impalpable Undescended Testicle

The laparoscopic exploration begins with a transverse incision approximately 1 cm in length. Care is taken to place the

incision in a natural periumbilical (either infra or supra) skin crease. The incision is extended to the level of the fascia using blunt dissection. Most children have only a small amount of subcutaneous adipose tissue, and the fascia is readily apparent. The child is then placed in a 15 ° Trendelenburg position. The abdominal wall is grasped and elevated, and two fascial sutures are placed well to the lateral aspects of the incision. The elevation of the abdominal wall during placement of these sutures helps protect against inadvertent suture placement through the peritoneum.

As already mentioned, at our institution we have abandoned blind access and Veress insufflation. After placement of the fascial sutures, the abdominal wall is elevated and the fascia is opened in the midline. Joseph skin hooks are used to elevate the fascial incision. The peritoneum is easily identified and opened. The skin hooks are then repositioned to elevate both the peritoneum and fascia. A blunt-tip trocar and cannula with fixation threads is dilated into the abdominal cavity, and a good gas seal is achieved. The scope is introduced, verifying proper cannula placement, and insufflation is begun directly through the cannula. Again, beginning insufflation pressures should be less than 5 mmHg.

The abdomen is inspected. The bladder and loops of the sigmoid colon are easily identified (Fig. 2). Extending bilaterally from the bladder toward the umbilicus are the obliterated umbilical arteries (medial umbilical folds or ligaments). The urachus (median umbilical ligament) is in the midline between the obliterated umbilical arteries. Viewing the pelvic sidewall, the spermatic vessels course toward the internal inguinal ring. Most children have minimal extraperitoneal pelvic fat, so the iliac vessels are readily seen, as are the deep inferior epigastric vessels (lateral umbilical ligaments). Identification of cord structures can be facilitated by placing slight traction on the spermatic cord and pulling down on the descended testicle (Figs. 3 A and B).

Due to the dimpling of the peritoneum, this maneuver allows the area at the internal ring to be visualized. On the side of a normally descended testicle, the vas deferens is typically obvious as it passes from the internal ring to the retrovesical recess. Any indirect hernias and patent processus vaginalis are noted (Figs. 4A and B).

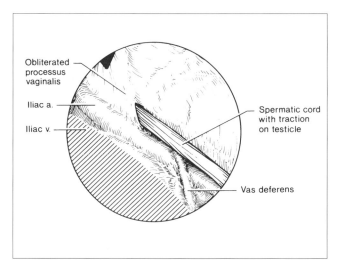

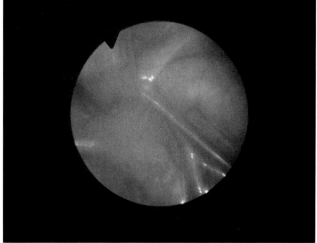

Figs. 3 A, B. Normal right groin with a descended testicle and no evidence of patent processus. **A** Line drawing. **B** Photograph. (Used by permission, AUA Update Series, Lesson 34, vol X, 1991, American Urological Association)

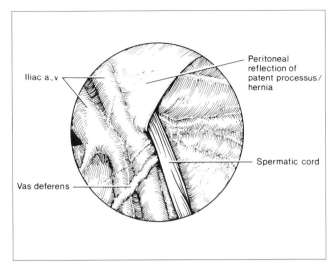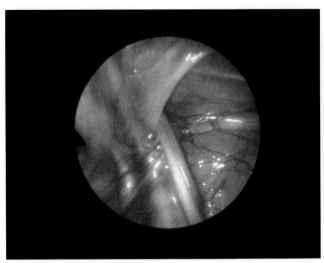

Figs. 4 A, B. Right groin demonstrating a patent processus. **A** Line drawing. **B** Photograph. This could be the appearance of a normally descended testicle with a hernia or an inguinal maldescended testicle with a hernia. (Used by permission, AUA Update Series, Lesson 34, vol X, 1991, American Urological Association)

Attention is next directed to the side of the undescended, impalpable gonad of the patient. The spermatic cord is often seen extending through the inguinal ring, and if a patent processus vaginalis is noted, gonads or remnants are usually present distally. However, absence of a patent processus does not eliminate the possibility of gonadal remnants in the inguinal area. Furthermore, it has been the experience of the author that gonadal remnants may contain viable tubules, and because these remnants may carry the same malignant potential as the undescended gonad itself, removal of the gonadal remnant is recommended.

In the past these remnants were recovered via an inguinal incision. We have found, however, that in about 80 % of cases they may be removed laparoscopically, thus avoiding the additional morbidity of an inguinal incision. In situations where an inguinal incision is required, the laparoscopic dissection allows for the incision to be small. Often no more than 1 cm in length is required.

In many cases the cord structures extend through the ring with a patent processus. If the testicle is not visible in the abdomen, gentle pressure in the external canal will push a canalicular "peeping" testicle/emerging testicle back through the internal ring (Figs. 5A and B). These testicles can be easily managed via primary laparoscopic orchidopexy.

For diagnostic laparoscopy there are a number of retractors that can be placed through 5-mm ports that permit gentle manipulation of bowel loops. With manipulation of the table, and second ports for manipulating instruments, the entire retroperitoneum and sidewall can be examined to the level of the inferior pole of the kidney, as well as the liver, gall bladder, area of the falciform ligament, and stomach.

Direct observation of blind-ending spermatic vessels is proof of testicular absence. The vas may end blindly nearby or at the same site, but it is the termination of the spermatic vessels that is pathognomonic for a nonexistent gonad (Fig. 6). When a blind-ending vas but no blind-ending vessels are

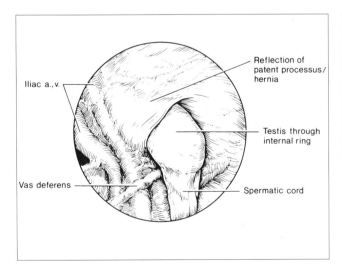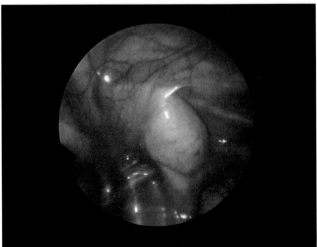

Figs. 5 A, B. Right groin depicting a low abdominal or an emerging testicle, which has been pushed up adjacent to the patent processus. **A** Line drawing. **B** Photograph. (From J Urol 152:1249–1252)

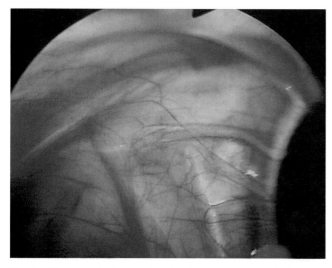

Fig. 6. Photograph showing the classic appearance of blind-ending vessels and a blind-ending vas ending proximate to each other (left groin). (From J Urol 152:1249–1252)

present at the internal ring, it is important to carry the inspection as high up along the sidewall toward the kidney as possible. The testicle and vas/epididymis form from different fetal anlage, and it is possible that the vessels end blindly, or the gonad itself will be at a position higher up in the retroperitoneum, far distant from the paragonadal structures. Occasionally the opposite exists, and blind-ending gonadal vessels are seen on the pelvic sidewall with no obvious blind-ending vas deferens. In this situation the gonadal structures should be immediately caudal to the blind-ending vessels, and the inspection should be adequate to declare testicular absence.

Staged Fowler-Stephens Orchidopexy

Intra-abdominal testicles with short spermatic vessels can be addressed by staged orchidopexy. As early as 1903, Bevan advocated the division of the spermatic vessels "to aid with

orchidopexy" [2]. Fowler and Stephens later described a two-stage approach based on collateralization along a long loop of vas deferens [8, 9]. In recent years this procedure has been modified by division of the spermatic cord vessels with the testicle left in situ at a first stage, and the testicle brought down onto the richer vasal collaterals at a later date.

In the past the disadvantage to this approach lay in the possibility that the child would be subjected to two laparotomies. However, Bloom described a modification in which the first-stage occlusion of the spermatic vessels is accomplished with pelviscopic clipping, and 6 months later the testis is relocated on its enhanced vasal collaterals by open techniques [3]. This two-step procedure has not only been successful in cases of long vasal loops (designated by Stephens as a prerequisite for the Fowler-Stephens orchidopexy) [8, 9], but also in patients who have a high abdominal testis and a nonlooping vas. The "short," nonlooping vas deferens is in fact the most common anatomic pattern in the intraabdominal testis.

Vascular clips may be used to ligate the cord, and in some cases the cord can be clipped without exposing it from its extraperitoneal location. Some centers merely coagulate the spermatic vessels using electrocautery. A more formal approach to the first stage may be required in the larger child, however.

At a number of centers the second stage of the staged orchidopexy has been performed laparoscopically. This is technically a relatively simple procedure, because the extensive dissection of the spermatic cord required for primary orchidopexy is not required, and the broad paravasal peritoneal flap is easily developed and transposed with the vas deferens.

Primary Laparoscopic Orchidopexy for the Abdominal Undescended Testicle

A single-stage orchidopexy can be used for an impalpable testicle that is emerging or proximal to the internal ring and has vessels that permit mobilization (Figs. 7 A and B). Recently, we and others have also extended the applications of primary laparoscopic orchidopexy to high palpable inguinal testicles. This surgery is performed endoscopically with the patient in about 30 ° of Trendelenburg and 20 ° of lateral tilt.

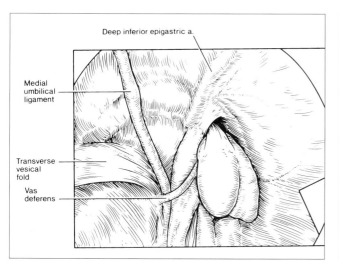
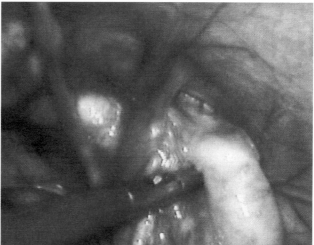

Figs. 7 A, B. Appearance of the right groin with a low abdominal testicle. Laparoscopic orchidopexy to be accomplished on this testicle. **A** Line drawing. **B** Photograph. (From J Urol 152:1249–1252)

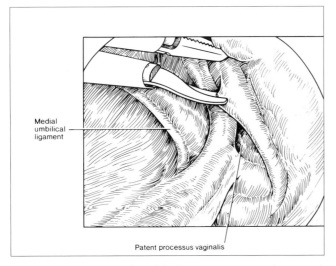

Fig. 8. The perineum adjacent to the patent processus is grasped. An incision is created adjacent to the patent processus. (From J Urol 152:1249–1252)

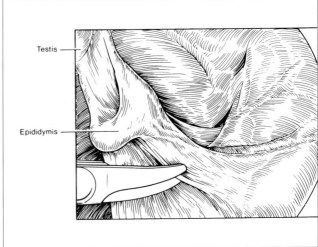

Fig. 10. The testicle is retracted free in the abdomen, and the lateral peritoneotomy is extended allowing for dissection of the tissues adjacent to the spermatic vessel leash and vas deferens. (From J Urol 152:1249–1252)

The procedure requires the use of at least two lateral 5-mm accessory cannulas. Lateral to the spermatic cord at the upper pole of the testicle (in the case of a true abdominal testicle), a peritoneal incision is continued in a cephalad direction (Fig. 8). Using blunt dissection the spermatic cord is rolled medially and elevated from the retroperitoneal tissues. The gubernaculum is opened adjacent to the patent processus vaginalis, and its anterior peritoneum is opened laterally. If a loop of the vas deferens is identified, it is reflected in a cephalad direction. The testicle is retracted with grasping forceps at the point of reflection of the gubernaculum from the lower pole of the testicle, and the remainder of the gubernacular attachments are cauterized and divided (Fig. 9). In the case of the high inguinal testicles an incision is made adjacent to the

patent processus, and the hernia sac is dissected from the spermatic vessel.

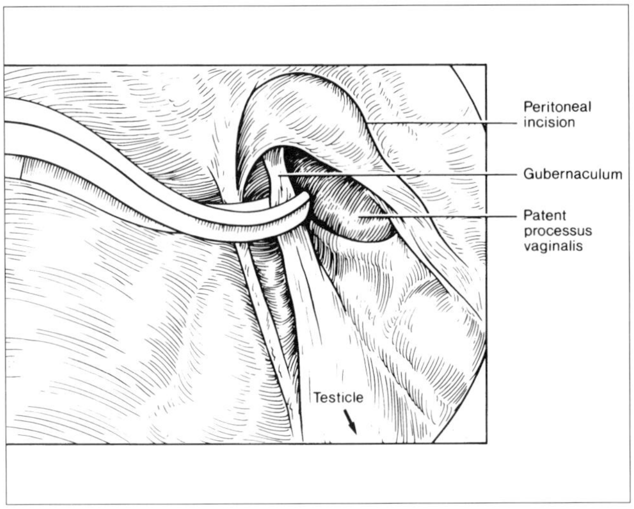

Dissection is then extended to the peritoneum overlying the vas deferens medial to the testicle. The peritoneum is opened medially over the vas deferens, i. e., elevated carefully to preserve its adjacent vessels. The vas is mobilized 2.5–3.0 cm medial to its reflection over the obliterated umbilical artery. The peritoneotomy overlying the vas is continued to join the lateral peritoneotomy (Fig. 10) immediately proximal to the globus major of the testicle. The spermatic cord is then further freed via sharp and blunt dissection, allowing the testicle to be moved extensively within the pelvis.

A small transverse skin incision is made at the base of the involved hemiscrotum and carried to the Dartos fascia. A subdartos pouch is created, and the Dartos is secured with Prolene sutures. A hemostat is used to develop a canal to the level of the pubic tubercle. The fascia, but not the peritoneal cavity, is penetrated with the clamp, and the tip of the clamp is directed to the medial umbilical ligament. The tips of the clamp are both directed by palpation and visualized by the laparoscope as they indent the peritoneum.

A 5-mm blunt rod is introduced along the course of the developed canal. The indentation of the rod is observed, and the cannula is introduced into the peritoneal cavity under direct vision just medial to the obliterated umbilical vessel. A threaded dilator is passed over the rod (Fig. 11) expanding the canal to 10 mm in diameter, allowing for placement of a 10-mm cannula. This 10-mm cannula allows for placement of a grasper into the abdomen to cautiously withdraw the testicle into the scrotum (Fig. 12). A special testicular grasping forceps has been designed allowing the bulk of the testis to be nontraumatically grasped. With gentle manipulation the testicle is placed in the canal. As the spermatic vessels come under tension, the vas and spermatic cord are further freed from the associated attachments, allowing descent into the base of the hemiscrotum without tension. The testicle is secured in the Dartos pouch and the skin is closed as shown in Figures 13 and 14.

Fig. 9. Incision has been continued around the patent processus freeing the testicle and allowing it to be retracted in a rostral direction. The caudal descent of the vas has been identified, and the gubernaculum is divided. (From J Urol 152:1249–1252)

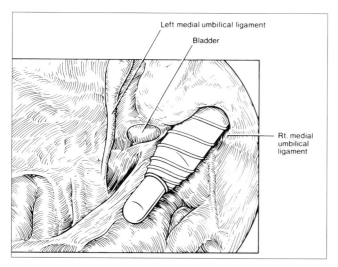

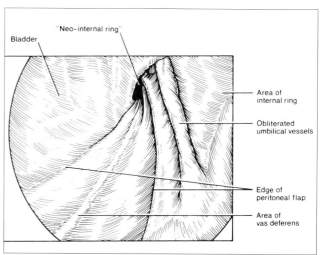

Fig. 11. The intra-abdominal dissection on the spermatic vessel and vas deferens is complete. Dartos pouch has been prepared, and the canal of Nuck has been developed. A 5-mm rod has been passed medial to the right medial umbilical ligament, and a threaded dilator passed over that, expanding the canal to accept a 10-mm cannula. (From J Urol 152:1249–1252)

Fig. 13. The testicle has been fixed to the Dartos pouch. Scrotal incision is closed. The figure shows the typical appearance of the spermatic vessels and "triangle of peritoneum" as they pass through the "neo-internal ring"

After intraperitoneal pressures are lowered, the area of dissection is irrigated and inspected, and the accessory sheaths are removed. The child can be recovered and discharged as an outpatient. Of undescended testicles, 52.5 % are found in the inguinal position [15], with the frequency for the impalpable high inguinal testicle (emergent/"peeping" testicle) not documented. The emergent or "peeping" testicle has been recognized as difficult to manage with inguinal access alone. In a series recently reported by Jordan, Robey and Winslow, the patients had true low intra-abdominal testicles or impalpable, high inguinal testicles [13]. Since October 1991, we have performed 27 laparoendoscopic orchidopexies in 24 patients in which there has been sufficient time to evaluate the surgical results (greater than a 6-month follow-up). Of those, 24 were

singlestage orchidopexies; three were the second stage of a staged Fowler-Stephens orchidopexy in which the first-stage clipping had also been accomplished laparoendoscopically (Figs. 15A and B). In the United States, as of this writing, well in excess of 100 laparoscopic orchidopexies have been performed with excellent results and essentially no morbidity.

Laparoendoscopic Orchidectomy

An adult or child will occasionally present with an impalpable undescended testicle that is grossly abnormal upon endoscopic observation (Fig. 16). Orchidectomy is indicated in these cases, and can be performed endoscopically. The dis-

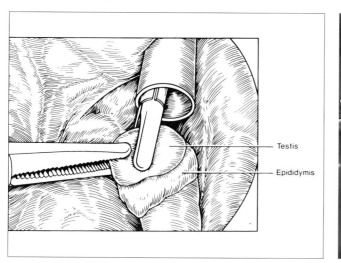

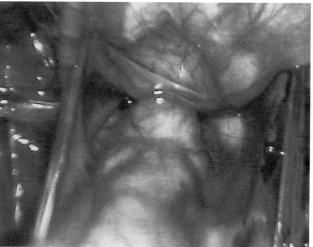

Fig. 12. A 10-mm cannula has been passed, and a grasping forceps (modified spoon grasping forceps) has been used to grab the substance of the testicle and retract the testicle into the scrotum

Fig. 14. Photograph of the pelvis of a child who has just undergone bilateral laparoscopic primary abdominal orchidopexy. Note the spermatic cords passing bilaterally just medial to their respective medial umbilical ligaments

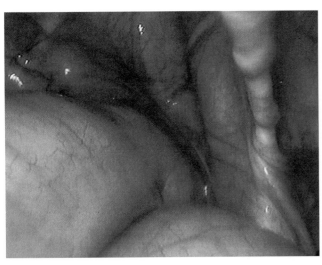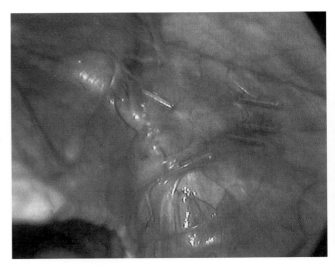

Figs. 15 A, B. Laparoscopic appearance of the right-groin area in a child 6 months following a primary laparoscopic orchidopexy. **A** The appearance of the spermatic cord passing just medial to the medial umbilical ligament. **B** The appearance of the area of the internal ring in the same child with the clips marking the area of the herniorrhaphy

section begins with division of the gubernacular attachments. The testicle can then be dissected in a cephalad direction so that it remains attached by the vas deferens and the short spermatic vessels. Many times there is nearly complete dissociation between the testicle and epididymal/vasal structures. To separate the connections that exist, the vas can be divided with electrocautery, and the spermatic vessels with vascular clips, following ligation (Fig. 17).

In most cases these abnormal testicles can be recovered directly through the cannula. In the case of the adult, in whom the gonad may be larger, the testicle is manipulated into a small endobag, with the bag then brought out through the accessory cannula site. Although the endobag and testicle are larger than the cannula puncture site, dilation of the tract is

accomplished with gentle traction of the bag, and the sac holding the testicle can be popped through.

Discussion

The literature supports diagnostic laparoscopy as the single most accurate modality for the diagnosis and localization of the impalpable undescended gonad. As judged by our experiences and those reported in the literature, laparoendoscopic orchidopexy is also a valid procedure, accomplishing a surgery that is identical to that of open techniques, with diminished surgical morbidity. With experience operative time compares favorably with open techniques, and although there is

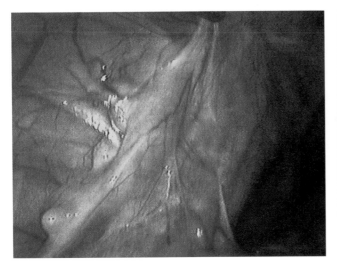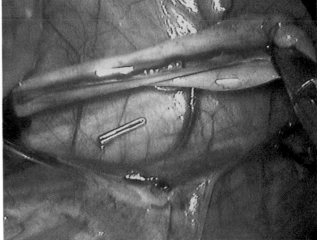

Fig. 16. Laparoscopic appearance of the left groin of a 10-year-old child. Of note is the fact that this patient has had a prior open inguinal exploration with no gonad found. In the mid-upper portion of the figure, marked by the end of a retractor, a stitch can be seen at the site of the prior exploration. At the lower left of the figure, a grossly abnormal gonad is noted

Fig. 17. In the same child as described in Figure 16, the appearance of the gonad as laparoscopic orchidectomy is being performed. The clip is being placed across the spermatic vessel leash. A clip placed in the middle portion of the figure allows estimation of the size of the gonad

no question that the procedure is best suited for the low intra-abdominal testicle found at the internal ring or the high inguinal or emergent testicle, even in children, and even for an inguinal incision/procedure, we believe laparoscopic surgery offers advantages.

Our experience has identified the difficulty of the "medial abdominal ectopic" testicle, and further experience will help to define whether the correct management modality for these difficult cases is orchidopexy or, in situations where there is a contralateral normally descended testicle, orchiectomy. The ability to perform orchiectomy via laparoendoscopic techniques raises some interesting issues. In the past an adult who achieved the age of 32 years with an impalpable undescended testicle was not felt to be a candidate for orchidectomy, in that the laparotomy required for removal of the testicle carried a greater morbidity than the patient's chance of developing an intra-abdominal malignancy. This issue may be re-evaluated as the morbidity of laparoendoscopic techniques is proven to be less than that of laparotomy.

In short, we believe that these procedures have proven their efficacy and validity, and we continue to apply them in our practice. Truly, the management of the impalpable cryptorchid gonad in virtually all cases has become the arena of the laparoscopic surgeon.

References

1. AYNSLEY-GREEN A, ZACHMANN M, ILLIG R ET AL.: Congenital bilateral anorchia in childhood: a clinical, endocrine and therapeutic evaluation of twenty-one cases. Clin Endocrinol 5 (1976) 381.
2. BEVAN AD: The surgical treatment of undescended testicle: a further contribution. JAMA 41 (1903) 718.
3. BLOOM DA: Two-step orchidopexy with pelvioscopic clip ligation of the spermatic vessels. J Urol 145 (1991) 1030.
4. BODDY SA, CORKERY JJ, GORNALL P: The place of laparoscopy in the management of the impalpable testis. Br J Surg 72 (11) (1985) 918–919.
5. CALDAMONE AA, AMARAL JF: Laparoscopic stage 2 Fowler-Stephens orchiopexy. J Urol 152 (1994) 1253–1256.
6. CORTESI N, FERRARI P, ZAMBARDA E ET AL.: Diagnosis of bilateral abdominal cryptorchidism by laparoscopy. Endoscopy 8 (1979) 33.
7. DWOSKIN JY, KUHN JP: Herniagrams in undescended testes and hydroceles. J Urol 109 (1973) 520.
8. FOWLER R, STEPHENS FD: The role of testicular vascular anatomy in the salvage of high undescended testis. Aust N Z J Surg 29 (1959) 92.
9. FOWLER R, STEPHENS FD: The role of testicular vascular anatomy in the salvage of high undescended testis. In: Webster R (ed.): Congenital malformation of the rectum, anus, and genitourinary tracts. Livingstone, London (1963) 306.
10. JONES PG: Undescended testes. Aust Paediatr J 2 (1966) 36.
11. JORDAN GH, BLOOM DA: Laparoscipic genitourinary surgery in children. In: Gomella LG, Kozminski M, Winfield HN (eds.): Laparoscopic urologic surgery. Raven Press, New York (1994) 223.
12. JORDAN GH, ROBEY EL, WINSLOW BH: Laparoendoscopic surgical management of the abdominal/transinguinal undescended testicle. J Endourology 6 (1992) 157.
13. JORDAN GH, WINSLOW BH: Laparoscopic single stage and staged orchiopexy. J Urol 152 (1994) 1249–1252.
14. KHADEMI M, SEEBODE JJ, FALLA A: Selective spermatic arteriography for localization of an impalpable undescended testis. Radiology 136 (1980) 627.
15. KLEINTEICH B, HADZISELIMOVIC F, HESSE V ET AL.: Kongenitale Hodendystopien. Thieme, Stuttgart (1989).
16. KOGAN BA, HRICAK H, TANAGHO EA: Magnetic resonance imaging in genital anomalies. J Urol 138 (1987) 1028–1030.
17. KOGAN SJ: Cryptorchidism. In Kelalis PP, King LR, Belman B (eds.): Clinical pediatric urology, 2nd edn, vol 2. W. B. Saunders Co., Philadelphia (1985) 864.
18. KOYLE MA, PFISTER R, JORDAN GH, WINSLOW BH, EHRLICH R: Laparoscopic surgery in the patient with previous negative inguinal exploration of impalpable testis (in preparation).
19. LEVITT SB, KOGAN SJ, SCHNEIDER KM ET AL.: Endocrine tests in phenotypic children with bilateral impalpable testes can reliably predict "congenital" anorchism. Urology 11 (1978) 11.
20. LUNDERQUIST A, RAFSTEDT S: Roentgenologic diagnosis of cryptorchidism. J Urol 98 (1967) 219.
21. MOORE RG, PETERS CA, BAUER SB, MANDELL J: Laparoscopic evaluation of the nonpalpable testis. J Urol 151 (3) (1994) 728–731.
22. RANSLEY PG, VORDERMARK JS, CALDAMONE AA, BELLINGER MF: Preliminary ligation of the gonadal vessels prior to orchiopexy for the intra-abdominal testicle: a staged Fowler-Stephens procedure. World J Urol 2 (1984) 266.
23. SILBER SJ, COHEN R: Laparoscopy for cryptorchidism. J Urol 124 (1980) 928.
24. WEISS RM, GLICKMAN MG, LYTTON B: Clinical implications of gonadal venography in the management of the nonpalpable undescended testis. J Urol 121 (1979) 745.
25. WHITE JJ, HALLER JA JR, DORST JP: Congenital inguinal hernia and inguinal herniography. Surg Clin North Am 50 (1970) 823.
26. WOLVERSON MK, JAGANNADHARAO B, SUNDARAM M ET AL.: CT in localization of impalpable cryptorchid testes. Am J Roentgenol 134 (1980) 725.

Inguinal Hernia

Critical Comments

R. STOPPA

Hernia repair has awakened public interest in questions such as safety, benignity, postoperative comfort and satisfaction. At the same time, the high rate of hernia repair creates a community problem with respect to socio-economic costs and recurrence. Thus, a sort of "correct policy" has appeared in hernia surgery, which includes the tactical obligation to satisfy minimum and maximum rules, i.e., a minimum of anesthesia, post operative discomfort, hospitalization, iatrogenic complications and disability versus maximum reproducibility of good results. This is because hernia surgery is a form of plastic surgery that has a deontological obligation of providing good results versus simplicity of performance. Moreover, the efficiency of repair is dependent on the quality of surgery and the quality of groin structures. It is therefore necessary to person-alize the repairs and to maintain selective indications of di-versified procedures while taking into account the diversity of groin hernias. Another general remark is related to the fact that coelioscopic hernia surgery which is still in its early stages, appeared at a time when discussions about classification of hernias and selective indications of open techniques were still in progress. Thus, all kinds of hernia repairs have been approached by endoscopy. This does not make it easier to appreciate the complexity of these operations today.

The two chapters on hernia repair were written by very skilled coelioscopic surgeons, namely J. L. Dulucq and R. J. Fitzgibbons, whose work I highly respect. The reported procedures and results are technically sound and highly efficient. I share the reserved general opinion about coelioscopic simple raphies (Ger, Popp), transabdominal plugs (Schultz), and intraperitoneal patches (Spaw), because of apparently poor results, and I shall focus my remarks on coelioscopic prosthetic repairs performed through trans- or preperitoneal approaches.

Convinced as I am of the value of posterior prosthetic repair, I am pleased to observe that the principles that I proposed 30 years ago for the great reinforcement of the visceral sac (GPRVS) are now being praised by coelioscopic surgeons. I agree with the posterior route. The use of mesh is the only way to avoid any tension and prevent limitation of the repair extent provided one uses a large piece of mesh so that intra-abdominal pressure defined by the Pascal Hydrostatic Principle will be limited. I trust that the technique will enhance good long-term results. The wall structures are preserved, and there is an immediate increase in postoperative comfort and patient satifsaction even if the cosmetic result is not regularly satisfactory in thin young women. The technique also bears the benefit of easy exploration of all associacted defects, frequent or rare, and of all associated abdominal pathologies when using the transabdominal approach. A particular advantage of this is the ability to avoid the difficulties of an anterior dissection (and risks of injury to the nerves or the cord) when repairing complex recurrent hernias.

However, we must also present the drawbacks of coelioscopic repair and express the hopes of reducing them. Anesthesia is routinely and almost necessarily general. This somehow restricts the possibility of using ambulatory repair in an out-patient setting, and contraindications arise in patients with respiratory or cardiac troubles. The transperitoneal mode of approach is not really minimally invasive, as it converts a superficial operation in an intra-abdominal one with a potential for serious complications. The systematic use of prosthetic material can also be criticized. Although mesh can be considered a great progress in the cure of hernias with a high risk of recurrence, congenital hernias in young patients do not need mesh repair. Moreover the aspect of safety has not been sufficiently evaluated, even if we know that there are now many skilled laparoscopic surgeons who are highly interested in this problem and who have carried out their own studies or participated in multicentre studies on safety. However, there will be an unavoidable chronological delay as we wait for adequate assessment of these results. Some early and medium-term reports indicate problems related to complications and recurrence.

1. Complications: In a multicentre study of 686 patients reported by Fitzgibbons (1995) 5.4 % of all complications were related to laparoscopy, 6.7 % were related to the patient and 17.1 % were related to herniorrhaphy itself. In another multicentre study of 7340 patients reported by Estour (1995), including the J.L. Dulucq experience, workers observed 0.6 % bleeding, 0.12 % visceral injuries, 8.7 % local complications, and 4.42 % secondary complications. Among the complications were unexpected yet serious complications that are really "new" for a classical hernia surgeon, namely, trocar injury to intra-abdominal viscera and large vessels, complications due to CO_2 insufflation or high frequency current use and caused by postoperative neuralgias mesh stapling.

2. Recurrences: Fitzgibbons (1995) observed 4.5 % within 15-30 months, Estour (1995) observed 0-5.9 % within 3-48 months, and Filipi (personal communication, 1996) observed 0-5.1 % within 1-41 months. Although there is no randomized prospective study that compares open versus laparoscopic procedures, the above results are no better than those obtained via open classical repairs. The success of the laparoscopic repairs will probably and hopefully improve with growing experience, a thorough knowledge and teaching of anatomical details, and critical analysis of failures. Overcoming the "learning curve" should also improve the results. This is illustrated by the great difference in the outcome of surgery performed by highly experienced versus moderately experienced surgeons. Thus, coelioscopic hernia surgery does not seem to be equally reproducible in all hands.

It also seems that coelioscopic hernia surgery is more difficult to teach, and learn, and perform than other minimally invasive procedures. Laparoscopic cholecystectomy and appendectomy consist only in removing a more or less destroyed small organ, while hernia repair aims at constructing a solid barrier against the irregular, lifelong tides of intra-abdominal pressure. It is therefore a much bolder enterprise, which expectedly takes time for maturation.

It should also be noted that coelioscopic hernia surgery does not have a satisfactory cost-to-benefit ratio. Thus, although some of its aspects are very interesting and promising, I cannot consider it yet the standard repair method.

Potential indications for coelioscopic hernia repair should result from the application of a universally accepted classification (e.g. the modified Nyhus classification (1989), which takes aggravating factors into account and agrees with the sub-classification by Campanelli (1995) in the group of recurrent hernias). Types III and IV (recurrent) hernias, bilateral and multiple hernias, or hernias associated with an abdominal lesion should be selected for coelioscopic treatment.

Absolute contraindications include high risk for general anesthesia, bleeding disorders, and major intra-abdominal disease. Other contraindications must be carefully evaluated, e.g., large (scrotal, sliding) hernias, and irreducible hernias, young age, obesity, and previous major abdominal operation.

To secure the future of coelioscopic hernia repair, randomized controlled multicentre trials that compare coelioscopic repair techniques to similar conventional techniques must be performed. These trials should utilize paired groups, follow an adequate classification and specify such endpoints as recurrence rates at a minimum of 5 years with less than 5 % of patients lost to follow-up. Further parameters of study should include complications, postoperative pain, time for resumption of various activities using objective tests such as Kehlet's recovery score, Payne's exercise test, and Christensen's fatigue score. I think that laparoscopy-related complications will progressively decrease. The most important goal for laparoscopic surgeons who perform hernia repair should be to demonstrate that the procedure is of real benefit for the patient. This implies achieving a very low recurrence rate (less than 2 %) a decrease in the amount of postoperative pain, and an early return to work. With this thought in mind, let me close by saying: Long live laparoscopic surgery!

27. Laparoscopic Treatment of Inguinal Hernia – The Extraperitoneal Approach

J.-L. DULUCQ

Introduction

Laparoscopic treatment of inguinal hernia provides the patient with a considerable gain in comfort. The technique described below basically consists in inserting an approximately 6 x 11 cm prolene mesh between the muscles and the peritoneal cavity after a laparoscopy-induced pneumoretroperitoneum has been created. This strictly extraperitoneal technique provides a new method of minimally invasive surgery.

The main advantage of using prosthetic material in the repair of inguinal hernias is its long-term durability. Stoppa [17, 18] proved the efficacy and good tissue tolerance of prosthetic pre- and retroperitoneal hernia repair in his various studies. The now standard retroperitoneal approach has produced excellent results to date.

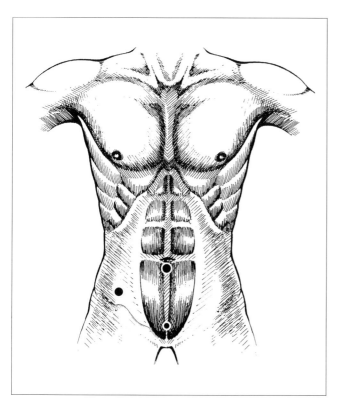

Fig. 1.   Position of trocars in right-sided hernia repair

Indications – Contraindications

In the early stages, we limited use of the method to medium-sized, indirect hernias in male patients. By now, we also perform laparoscopic surgery of indirect hernias occurring with direct hernias, bilateral hernias, medium-sized scrotal hernias, and recurrent hernias. Extremely large scrotal hernias are only sometimes treatable by laparoscopy. Previous sub-umbilical laparotomy is not an absolute contraindication to laparoscopic treatment. However, great caution must be used in positioning the trocars in these patients.

Pneumoretroperitoneum is generally well tolerated, and the contraindications are generally the same as for conventional surgery.

Preoperative Work-up

In addition to a physical examination and the usual laboratory tests, an electrocardiogram and a chest X-ray should be part of preoperative diagnostic studies. A cardiovascular evaluation will be obtained in elderly and sick patients. In some cases, ultrasonography of the abdominal wall may be of help.

Operative Technique

The instrumentation consists of a 0 ° or 30 ° telescope, forceps, a needle holder, and scissors. An applier for the titanium staples is also required for patch fixation. The procedure is usually carried out under general anesthesia. In some patients peridural anesthesia may be chosen. A urinary catheter is inserted. The patient is positioned supine with the legs spread apart. The surgeon stands on the side contralateral to the hernia.

The pneumoretroperitoneum is created with a Veress needle by insufflating one liter of carbon dioxide (CO_2) in Retzius' space via a suprapubic puncture. The tip of the needle must perforate the aponeurosis and will be positioned in Retzius' space. Two 11-mm trocars and one 5-mm trocar are positioned as shown in Figure 1. Soft Teflon™ mandrins for dissection of the retroperitoneal cavity are inserted in the trocars. The first trocar is inserted tangentially via a skin incision in the lower umbilical fossa. From the extraperitoneal position, the trocar is advanced caudally under vision, until it reaches the site of pneumoretroperitoneum. The individual layers are dissected using the Teflon mandrin.

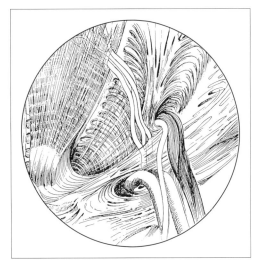

Fig. 2. Topography of the inguinal region from the retroperitoneal aspect

Continuous insufflation of CO_2 is initiated when the first trocar is in place. This induces loosening of peritoneal tissue. The maximum CO_2 pressure must be limited to and maintained at 12 mmHg during the entire procedure.

Another Teflon mandrin inserted via the suprapubic 5-mm trocar is used to displace the peritoneum cranially. Cooper's ligament is the first landmark to be revealed. The epigastric vessels are located by looking up towards the abdominal wall (Fig. 2). The upper border of the hernial sac can then be found. The hernial sac is dissected free along its entire circumference, and it is removed from the iliac fossa (Figs. 3 and 4).

When the hernial sac is visualized from top to bottom, the third trocar is inserted in place in the region of the iliac fossa beside the hernia, and the scissors are inserted.

The hernial sac is mobilized entirely along the hernial ring. Whereas small hernial sacs are placed inside the abdominal cavity, large hernial sacs are exposed down to the base, transsected with an *Endo-GIA* application, and removed.

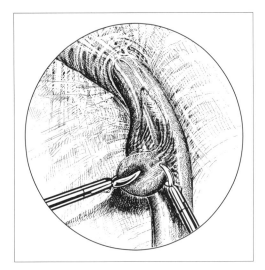
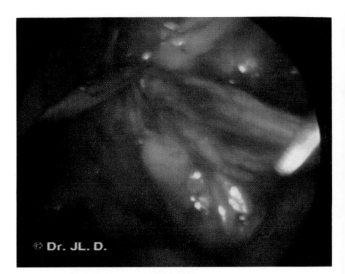

Figs. 3 and 4. The hernial sac is dissected free from the spermatic cord (diagram and intraoperative finding)

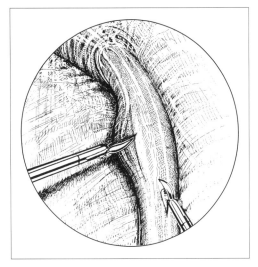
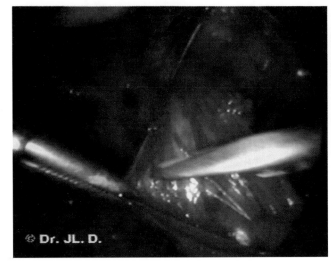

Figs. 5 and 6. Spermatic cord structures can be found under the crevices of the cremaster muscle fibers (diagram and intraoperative finding)

The spermatic cord, testicular artery, pampiniform plexus, and the deferent canal are isolated, freed from the cremaster muscle, and lateralized as far as possible (Figs. 5 and 6). Cooper's ligament and the psoas muscle must be painstakingly demonstrated, because both structures are the main fixation points for the patch.

The prolene mesh is inserted in the iliac fossa via the 11-mm trocar (Figs. 7 and 8).

The lower edge of the mesh is fixed to Cooper's ligament and the psoas muscle using two titanium staples (Figs. 9 and 10).

The mesh thus lies adjacent to the iliac vessels and the lateralized spermatic cord. The mesh can also be fixed in place using single interrupted sutures (Fig. 11).

The patch is positioned over the inner inguinal ring (Fig. 12) and attached to the sides of the epigastric arteries using fibrin glue or two additional titanium staples.

The pneumoretroperitoneum is slowly desufflated at the end of the procedure. Drainage is not necessary.

Complications – Problems

Correct creation of pneumoretroperitoneum is one of the most important steps in the procedure. Insufflation of one liter of CO_2 into the retropubic space makes it possible to loosen infraperitoneal tissue without difficulty. The individual steps for dissecting the hernial sac must be carried out carefully and correctly in order to guarantee reliable results.

In our previous experience, we have observed the following complications:

1. Development of moderate subcutaneous emphysema around the trocar insertion sites. It is important to insert the trocars with great care
2. Development of emphysema in the scrotal region, which can be easily and completely expressed by manual pressure at the end of the procedure
3. Development of postoperative hematoma along the outer inguinal ring, which was completely absorbed after puncture without requiring further treatment

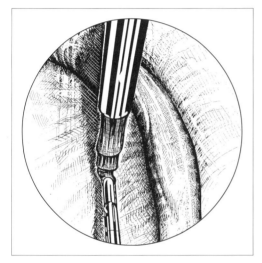
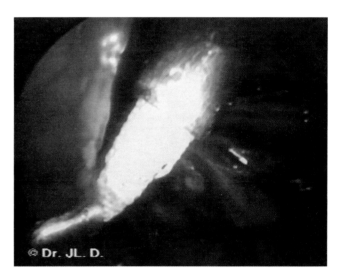

Figs. 7 and 8.   Introduction of the rolled up mesh into the iliac fossa via the 11 mm trocar (diagram and intraoperative finding)

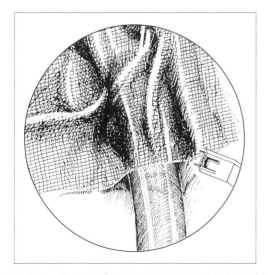
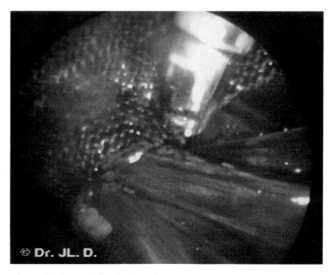

Figs. 9 and 10.   Fixation of the prolene mesh to the sides of the spermatic cord using two titanium staples

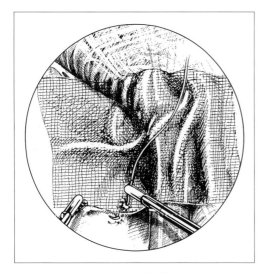

Fig. 11. Fixation of the prolene mesh with single interrupted sutures

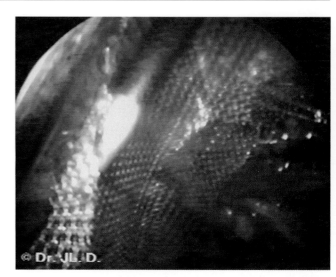

Fig. 12. The prolene mesh is fixed on the hernial gap using fibrin glue

4. Accidental intraoperative penetration of the peritoneum. The laparoscopic technique can still be continued, but equilibrium of intra- and extraperitoneal pressure must be carefully maintained. In small peritoneal lesions, an intra-peritoneal trocar must be inserted to provide a valve

Postoperative Follow-up

Clinical follow-up examinations are performed 1 and 3 months after surgery. Normal physical activity can be resumed from the fourth postoperative day on, and the patient can generally return to work within 10 days.

Results

From June 1990 to June 1995, 864 inguinal hernias were treated according to this method, for 797 patients operated.

There were 462 external oblique inguinal hernias, 272 direct inguinal hernias, 71 direct hernias combined with an external oblique inguinal hernia, 67 bilateral inguinal hernias, and 70 recurrent hernias.

At one month and three months postoperative, all patients were checked. The results were excellent, characterized by extreme robustness and a high degree of reliability. The average hospital stay was 48 to 72 hours.

In the beginning, we had eight conversions to traditional surgery and two conversions to laparoscopic transperitoneal surgery.

Complications – Morbidity

Among those patients, we observed the following complications:
- 26 cases of minor subcutaneous emphysema
- 24 cases of hematoma of the external inguinal orifice, two of which had to be drained surgically.
- 8 immediate reoperations, 7 through laparoscopy, 1 through open surgery.
- 3 immediate recurrences due to inadequate positioning of the mesh, and spontaneous folding of its upper edge.

- 3 laparoscopic reoperations for acute pain in the crural nerve area, demanding immediate removal of the ill-positioned clip fastening the mesh to the psoas muscle.
- 2 immediate laparoscopic reoperation to evacuate a very large hematoma in front of the mesh, not followed by drainage.

These 5 reoperations took place on the 2nd postoperative day. So far, we have not yet observed any recurrence.

Discussion

Laparoscopic treatment of inguinal hernia has many advantages. For example, it is not necessary to dissect broad layers of fascia, as is inevitable in conventional surgery thus reducing tissue trauma to the abdominal wall. The extraperitoneal approach, which has proven its usefulness in conventional surgery for decades, appears a logical alternative.

We have obtained excellent results with the technique since we started using it in June 1990. MacKernan and Phillips [15, 16], as well as Bégin [2, 3, 4, 5] have developed a similar method. Other laparoscopic techniques which make use of a transperitoneal approach have several disadvantages: closure of the peritoneal incision can be problematic [10, 11] and adhesions frequently develop in this region in the later course of healing. Furthermore, pneumoperitoneum is associated with considerably more postoperative problems than pneumoretroperitoneum. Apparently, the least successful results occur when intraperitoneal prosthetic material is stapled in place without a peritoneal covering.

The prolene patch, which is made of inert and relatively stiff material, is well suited for insertion in the preperitoneal space via laparoscopy. Its tissue tolerance is excellent. Fixation is necessary in order to keep the patch from becoming dislocated in the immediate postoperative phase.

When the technique is performed correctly, retroperitoneal repair of inguinal hernias appears to be a new and promising method of minimally invasive surgery. The technique is simple and efficient, and its results are excellent.

References

1. ARREGUI M, DEVIS C, YUCEL O, NAGAN R: Laparoscopic mesh repair of inguinal hernia using a preperitoneal approach: a preliminary report. Surg Laparosc Endosc. 2 (1992) 53–58.
2. BÉGIN G: Surgical Endoscopy 6 (4) (1992).
3. BÉGIN G: Journal de Coelio-Chirurgie 8 (1993).
4. BÉGIN G: Chirurgie Endoscopique 1 (1992).
5. BÉGIN G: Journal of Laparoendoscopic Surgery 1 (1) (1990).
6. CORBITT JD JR.: Laparoscopic herniorrhaphy. Surg Laparosc Endosc. 1 (1991) 23–25.
7. DULUCQ JL: Traitement des hernies de l'aine par mise en place d'un patch prothétique sous-péritonéal en rétropéritonéoscopie. Cahiers de Chirurgie 79 (1991) 15–16.
8. DULUCQ JL: Traitement of Inguinal Hernias by insertions of mesh through retroperitoneoscopy. Post Graduate General Surgery 4 (2) (1992) 173–174.
9. FERZLI G, RABOY A, KLEINERMAN D, ALBERT P: Extraperitoneal endoscopic pelvic lymph node dissections vs. Laparoscopic lymph node dissection in the staging of prostatic and bladder carcinoma. J. of Laparoendosc Surg 2 (1992) 219–222.
10. FITZGIBBONS RJ JR., ANNIBALI R, LITKE BS: Gallbladder and gallstone removal, open versus closed laparoscopy, and pneumoperitoneum. Am J Surg 165 (1993) 497–504.
11. FITZGIBBONS RJ JR.: Laparoscopic hernia repair. In: Proceedings of the Symposium on New Frontiers in Endosurgery. New Brunswick, Ethicon Inc. (1991).
12. HIMPENS J.: Laparoscopic Hernioplasty Using a Self-Expandable (Umbrella-Like) Prothetic Patch. Surg Laparosc & Endosc 2 (4) (1992) 312–316.
13. HIMPENS J: Laparoscopic inguinal hernioplasty: repair with a conventional vs a new self-expandable mesh. Surg Endosc 7 (1993) 315–319.
14. LICHTENSTEIN IL, SHULMAN AJ, AMID PK ET AL.: The tension-free hernioplasty. Am J Surg 157 (1989) 188–193.
15. McKERNAN JB, LAWS HL: Laparoscopic repair of inguinal hernias using a totally extraperitoneal prosthetic approach. Surg Endosc 7 (1993) 26–28.
16. PHILIPS EH, CAROLL BJ, PEARLSTEIN AR, DAYHOVSKY L, FALLAS MJ: Laparoscopic colectomy. Ann. Surg. 216 (1992) 703–707.
17. STOPPA RE, WARLAUMONT CR: The preperitoneal approach and prosthetic repair of groin hernia. In: Nyphus LM, Condon RE (eds): Hernia. Philadelphia (1989) 199–255.
18. STOPPA RE, RIVES JL, WARLAUMONT CR: The use of Dacron in the repair of hernias of the groin. Surg Clin N Am 64 (1984) 269–285.
19. TOY FK, SMOOT RT: Toy Smoot hernioplasty. Surg Laparosc Endosc 1 (1991) 151–155.
20. VERNAY A: La rétropéritonéoscopie: justification anatomique. Expérimentation technique. Expérience clinique. Thèse Med. Grenoble (1980).
21. WEBB DR, REDGRAVEN N; CHAN Y, HAREWOOD LM: Extraperitoneal laparoscopy: early experience and evaluation. Aust N.Z.J. Surg 63 (1993) 554–557.
22. WURTZ A: L'endoscopie de l'espace rétropéritonéal: technique, résultats et indications actuelles. Ann Chir 43 (1989) 475–480.

28. Laparoscopic Inguinal Herniorrhaphy: Transabdominal Preperitoneal Repair

A. A. RYBERG, K. M. ULUALP, D. CORNET, AND R. J. FITZGIBBONS JR.

Introduction

In 1980 in the United States alone, at least 500,000 hernia repairs were performed [24]. This is evidence enough that inguinal hernias remain a common problem. Until recently, modern surgical dictum concerning inguinal hernia repair had been dominated by the principles set forth by Bassini, who developed a technique for inguinal herniorrhaphy that included high ligation of the sac and reinforcement of the inguinal floor [1]. His method for reinforcing the inguinal floor relied on approximating the inguinal ligament to the conjoint tendon. Modifications of Bassini's original technique have been described by many surgeons including Halsted, Shouldice, and McVay [12, 18, 23]. These modifications were an attempt to further reduce recurrence rate and to avoid testicular complications. In expert hands, they have been successful [11]. In routine hospital practice, however, a recurrence rate of 10 % can still be expected [6]. After a failed repair, additional recurrence can be as high as 35 % [2]. The incision used for the classical repair is painful and causes patients to miss approximately 2 weeks of work. An occupation involving physical exertion results in an even more prolonged absence from work. In addition, in those patients who develop complications (approximately 5 %), the total amount of time they are incapacitated may be considerable [14]. These factors have been the stimulus to seek alternative procedures. Laparoscopic inguinal hernia repair represents one alternative.

Lichtenstein popularized the concept of avoiding tension in the closure of hernia defects by suturing polypropylene mesh to Poupart's ligament and the internal oblique muscle [16]. This has been important in the development of laparoscopic hernia repairs because the majority of laparoscopic techniques are also tension-free.

The purpose of this chapter is to describe laparoscopic hernia repair through a transperitoneal access. Indications and contraindications for the laparoscopic technique are also discussed.

Indications and Contraindications

The development of laparoscopic hernia repair stemmed from three key factors: (a) the acceptance of prosthetic materials for herniorrhaphy; (b) the apparent efficacy of the preperitoneal approach; and (c) the development and widespread use of laparoscopy in general surgery. To justify replacement of a safe and effective technique for inguinal hernia repair, such as

classical hernia repair, laparoscopic herniorrhaphy must meet four criteria: (a) reduction of postoperative pain and a shortened time away from work; (b) reduction in recurrence rate; (c) fewer incidences of postoperative neuralgias; and (d) competitive cost for repair [9]. To achieve these goals, laparoscopic inguinal hernia repair, in addition, must be at least as safe as the traditional approach. Adhesive complications related to traversing the peritoneum should not be excessive and the routine use of prosthetic material should not be associated with an increased infection rate. Randomized prospective trials comparing conventional with laparoscopic techniques need to be done to see if these goals have been met.

All adult patients generally felt to be fit for general anesthesia can be considered candidates for laparoscopic inguinal hernia repair. It would seem, however, that patients with recurrent or complicated hernias are particularly suited for a laparoscopic approach because the preperitoneal space has usually not been dissected and previously formed scar tissue can be avoided. There may also be a role for laparoscopy in the pediatric patient, primarily as a tool for evaluation of the opposite side, i. e., placement of a 5-mm telescope through the ipsilateral sac. However, the use of laparoscopic techniques for hernia repair in the pediatric patient has not been well accepted [17]. Using a traditional approach for the repair of an inguinal hernia may be more reasonable in a child with a small indirect inguinal hernia or in an elderly adult with a straightforward hernia who has medical contraindications to general anesthesia.

Those patients who probably should not be considered for laparoscopic inguinal hernia repair may have one or more of the following relative contraindications: uncontrolled coagulopathy, intraabdominal adhesions from previous abdominal surgery, incarceration, severe obesity, or peritonitis. Presently, it is not possible to ascertain absolutely which patients are better suited for laparoscopic herniorrhaphy and which are better suited for the conventional approach. This will be determined with comparative trials when laparoscopic inguinal herniorrhaphy techniques become standardized.

Preoperative Work-up

Verification of a signed investigational consent for laparoscopic inguinal hernia repair should be obtained when the patient arrives in the preoperative area if an intraperitoneal technique is planned. In consultation with the Human Research Committee at Creighton University, we have now abandoned the experimental consent form for the transabdominal preperitoneal and the totally extraperitoneal repairs. In addition to the routine medical and surgical history and physical examination, a chest radiograph and electrocardiogram are obtained if the patient is over 40 years of age and has not had either of the two evaluations within the previous 6 months. Female patients have blood analysis for pregnancy evaluation if they are within the appropriate age range. All patients able to provide a specimen have a urine analysis. Once in the operating room, patients have sequential compression stockings placed and are given 1 g cefazolin intravenously. Should an allergy exist, appropriate antibiotic adjustments are made. Any additional testing would be related to a specific patient and his/her medical history.

Operative Technique

Current laparoscopic herniorrhaphies can be classified as one of three types: (a) transabdominal preperitoneal repair (TAPP); (b) intraperitoneal onlay mesh repair (IPOM); or (c) totally extraperitoneal repair (EXTRA). The TAPP repair is currently the most popular and is the subject of this chapter.

The TAPP laparoscopic inguinal herniorrhaphy is based on the classical preperitoneal repairs popularized by Rives and Stoppa in France and Nyhus and Condon in the United States [19, 26]. It is vital for the surgeon to know the anatomy from a laparoscopic vantage point (Fig. 1). The preperitoneal space can be entered either through a skin incision, as done in conventional repairs, or by making an incision in the peritoneum laparoscopically. Prosthetic material can be placed identically for both procedures.

Entrance into the peritoneal cavity has been an important feature of laparoscopic inguinal herniorrhaphy. Safe entry into the abdominal cavity has been mandatory if complications of laparoscopy, such as major vascular injury, are to be avoided [5]. Most authorities agree that open laparoscopy will prevent the potentially life-threatening complication of major vascular injury [13]. However, the literature does not support the concept that open laparoscopy will prevent injury to solid or hollow organs [4]. Whether an open technique, a Veress needle, or direct trocar insertion is used, the surgeon must use extreme caution when entering the abdominal cavity.

The most efficient operating room setup is depicted in Figure 2. The surgeon will be able to complete the procedure with greater ease if he/she stands on the opposite side of the table from the hernia because the angle for dissection and staple placement will be most appropriate. Once general anesthesia induction has been completed, a Foley catheter should be placed into the patient's bladder to insure continuous decompression. The considerable dissection involved necessitates general anesthesia, although diagnostic laparoscopy can be done under local anesthesia.

Three 10- to 12-mm laparoscopic cannulas are used; one is placed at the umbilicus and the remaining two just lateral to

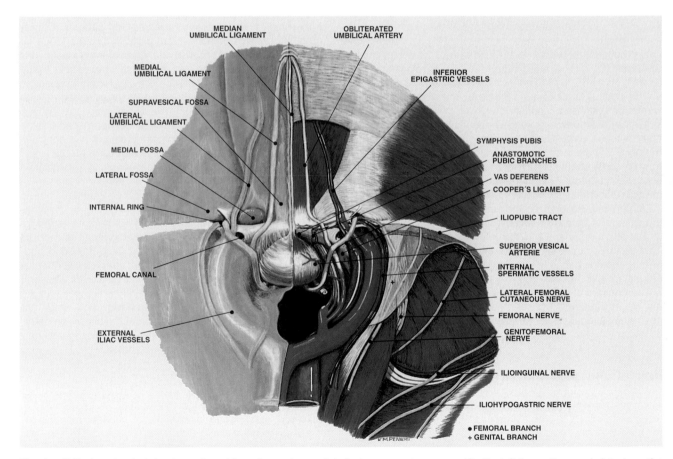

Fig. 1. Critical anatomical structures viewed from the vantage point of a laparoscopic surgeon. On the left the peritoneum is intact; on the right it has been stripped away

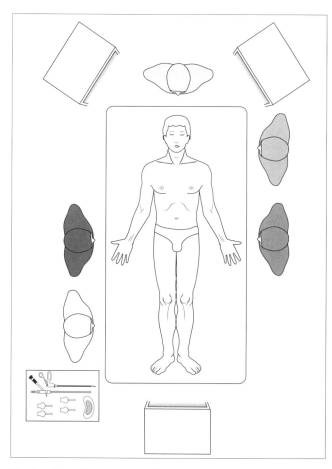

Fig. 2. Operating room setup for a left-sided hernia

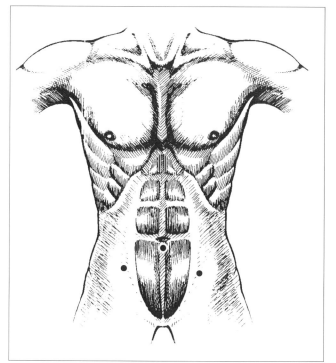

Fig. 3. Port positions for the transabdominal preperitoneal herniorrhaphy of a left-sided hernia

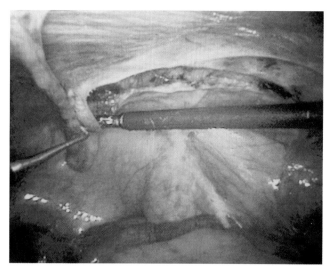

Fig. 4. Complete peritoneal incision

both rectus sheaths (Fig. 3) at the level of the umbilicus. We prefer to use an open technique for placement of the initial cannula. This is accomplished by making a small incision in the skin immediately below the umbilicus and deepening this incision through the subcutaneous fat until a thick raphe is found leading up to the umbilicus. The raphe is grasped at its junction with the fascia with two Kocher clamps placed in line vertically. The fascia is then divided with Mayo scissors. The peritoneum below may be divided in the same action if it is closely adherent to the fascia. Otherwise, the peritoneum can be grasped and divided sharply or opened by blunt finger dissection according to the surgeon's preference. Two sutures are placed on either side of the defect in the fascia and a Hasson cannula is then introduced into the abdominal cavity under direct vision. The Hasson cannula is secured with the previously placed sutures.

Once intra-abdominal access has been established, a CO_2 pneumoperitoneum is created and the laparoscope is introduced through the Hasson cannula, allowing a thorough diag-

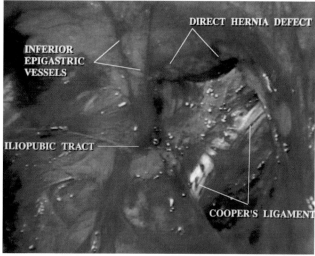

Fig. 5. Peritoneal flap is mobilized downward to display epigastric vessels, iliopubic tract, and Cooper's ligament

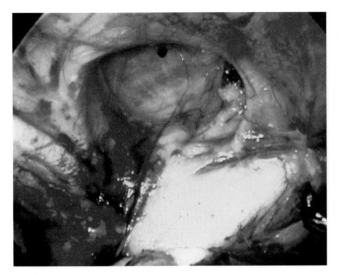

Fig. 6. Cooper's ligament and the iliopubic tract with the pseudosac seen in the defect

nostic laparoscopy. The patient is placed in the Trendelenburg position to let the bowel fall away from the pelvis, permitting good visualization of this area. It is important to examine both myopectineal orifices to confirm the pathology and to examine the contralateral side. The other two cannula, those placed lateral to the rectus sheaths, are then inserted under direct vision. We prefer to use 11- or 12-mm cannulas at both of these sites so that the laparoscope and stapling device can be transferred from cannula to cannula depending on the angle needed to secure the prosthesis. Instruments are placed as follows: A toothed grasper is inserted through the left and a scissors through the right port. The peritoneum is opened by making an incision at the medial umbilical ligament, which may be divided if it appears to compromise exposure. This initial incision into the peritoneum should be made at least 2 cm above the myopectineal defect. As this incision is extended laterally to the anterior superior iliac spine, bleeding from small vessels can be controlled using electrocautery (Fig. 4). The peritoneal flap is mobilized downwardly, away from the overlying abdominal wall, using sharp and blunt dissection.

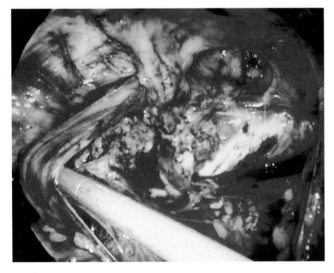

Fig. 7. Dissection of the sac away from the cord structures

The inferior epigastric vessels, Cooper's ligament, and iliopubic tract are exposed (Fig. 5).

The peritoneal flap is mobilized inferiorly, away from the abdominal wall. An important landmark is the inferior epigastric vessels. Cooper's ligament can be visualized inferomedially and the iliopubic tract laterally. If a direct hernia is present, the sac and preperitoneal fat are reduced from the hernia orifice using gentle traction (Fig. 6). The thinned-out transversalis fascia (the "pseudosac"), which lines the defect, is left behind (Fig. 6). The final step to complete the dissection for a direct hernia is done by mobilizing the cord structures away from the peritoneal flap (Fig. 7). Compared with direct hernias, indirect hernias are clearly more difficult to manage [21]. If the hernia sac is small, it can be mobilized from the cord structures and reduced back into the peritoneal cavity. A hook dissector with cautery may be helpful in accomplishing this mobilization and reduction. If the hernia sac is large, extending into the scrotum, complete mobilization of the sac may result in an increased incidence of spermatic cord or testicular complications. Thus, a large hernia is best managed by dividing the sac at the internal ring, leaving the distal part in situ. The proximal portion of the sac should then be dissected away from the cord structures. The spermatic cord must be carefully identified: it is located inferomedially to the internal ring and crosses the origin of the inferior epigastric vessels from the external iliac artery and vein just before it enters the internal ring.

Once the dissection is completed, a tension-free repair is commenced using a mesh prosthesis. Although various types of prosthetic materials can be used, the most popular currently is polypropylene. Earlier recurrences with laparoscopic herniorrhaphy have been felt to be due to inadequate coverage with the prosthesis of all of the potential sites of recurrent groin herniation [22]. Thus, as an absolute minimum, the size of the prosthesis must be no less than 10 x 5 cm [8]. It must be sufficiently large to cover the defect as well as providing extensive overlap so that normal intraabdominal pressure acts on the patch overlying strong healthy tissue keeping the patch in position, rather than allowing it to herniate through the defect.

The cord structures may be encircled with the prosthetic material or simply covered (Fig. 8). There are opponents and proponents of both of these techniques and the literature lacks reliable data with sufficiently long follow-up to settle the controversy. Our preference is the latter to avoid cord-related complications due to more extensive dissection required with the former method. Also, this is a source for the development of recurrence through the mesh.

The appropriately sized mesh should be inserted into the abdominal cavity through either of the two lateral laparoscopic ports. If the decision has been made to slit the mesh to accommodate the cord structures, this should be done prior to inserting the mesh into the abdominal cavity. We have found it helpful for orientation once the mesh is in the abdominal cavity to have rolled one arm of the mesh and to have secured it with a stay suture. Otherwise, one corner of the mesh should be grasped with a 5-mm instrument and quickly placed through one of the 11- or 12-mm lateral cannulas. The instrument should be promptly withdrawn so that excessive CO_2 loss does not occur. The prosthesis is then positioned in place.

Having appropriately positioned the mesh, it should be stapled in place using the following landmarks as observed from the laparoscopic vantage point: symphysis pubis medially, Cooper's ligament inferomedially, iliopubic tract inferolaterally,

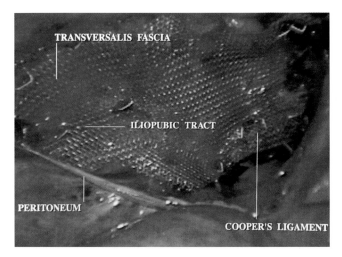

Fig. 8.   Inguinal herniorrhaphy with mesh in place

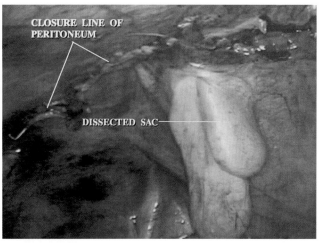

Fig. 10.   Closure of the peritoneum

a point approximately 1 cm medial to the anterior superior iliac spine laterally, and the transversalis fascia superiorly at least 2 cm above the hernia defect (Fig. 8). The currently available hernia stapling devices facilitate the stabilization of the prosthesis and are preferable to suture placement. In order to avoid injury to the lateral femoral cutaneous nerve of the thigh or the femoral branch of the genitofemoral nerve, care must be taken not to staple below the iliopubic tract when lateral to the internal spermatic vessels [10, 15]. A maneuver that is helpful in this situation is the bimanual technique (Fig. 9). Staples should be placed only when the surgeon is able to palpate the head of the stapler. This verifies that the staples are being placed above the iliopubic tract. Staples should be oriented parallel to the nerves, i. e., vertically when stapling

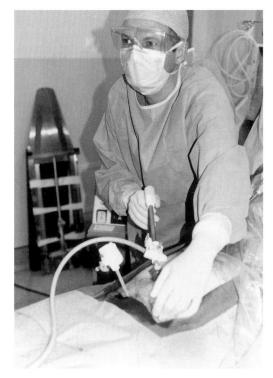

Fig. 9.   Bimanual technique

inferiorly, because the lateral femoral cutaneous nerve of the thigh and the femoral branch of the genitofemoral nerve course in this direction. Superior and lateral placement of staples should be horizontal, corresponding to the direction of the ilioinguinal and iliohypogastric nerves, which lie in a plane superficial to the preperitoneal space but nevertheless can be damaged with too vigorous a bimanual technique. The prosthesis should be tailored to the preperitoneal space during the course of staple placement by trimming the excess in situ and removing it from the abdominal cavity.

The final step is to close the peritoneum over the prosthesis, thus isolating it from the abdominal contents (Fig. 10). It is important not to leave gaps when placing the staples because bowel has been reported to slip between these gaps causing obstruction [11]. This closure may be facilitated by reducing the pneumoperitoneum.

Bilateral hernias are repaired in a similar manner. One long transverse peritoneal incision with a single prosthesis, at least 20 x 60 cm, can be used to cover both defects. However, some authorities prefer two separate pieces of prosthetic material because it is easier to manipulate the smaller prostheses. In addition, this may avoid the theoretical complication that might be encountered if the urachus was patent and an incision was made across it and not recognized.

Personal Experience and Results from the Literature

At Creighton University, we (R. J. F.) have performed 256 laparoscopic hernia repairs in 194 patients (62 bilateral) using the TAPP procedure. The ages of these patients ranged from 15 to 86 years with a mean age of 52 years. As of April 1994, we have follow-up from 2 to 163 weeks. Depending on the complexity and bilaterality of the hernia, operating time averaged 81–127 minutes. A total of 125 hernias were direct, 115 indirect, 11 femoral, and 5 combination. Complications were divided into "general," "laparoscopic," and "local." The most frequent general complication was urinary retention. This occurred in 10 of 194 patients (5.1 %). "Laparoscopic" complications occurred in 8 patients (4.1 %). Minor bleeding occurred during dissection in 3 patients (1.5 %) but none required transfusion. Of those complications that we classified as

Table 1. The three most commonly performed laparoscopic inguinal herniorrhaphies

Name	Critical features	Major advantages	Major disadvantages
TAPP*	Radical preperitoneal space dissection after it is entered through a peritoneal incision	Essentially identical to conventional preperitoneal procedures	Morbidity increased because of radical preperitoneal dissection
	Sac reduced or divided at the internal ring	Prosthesis is covered by peritoneum	Potential for adhesive complications or herniation at sites where peritoneum has been breached
	Large prosthesis placed in the preperitoneal space		
	Peritoneum closed over the prosthesis		
IPOM**	Prosthesis placed intraabdominally with no attempt to cover it	Minimal dissection	Prosthesis potentially in contact with intra-abdominal organs, which may result in erosion or fistula formation
	Landmarks for prosthesis placement are: symphysis pubis medially, anterior abdominal wall at least 2 cm above the defect superiorly, Cooper's ligament inferomedially, the iliopubic tract inferolaterally, and a point medial to the anterior superior iliac spine laterally	Minimal perioperative pain	Potential for adhesive complications or herniation at sites where peritoneum has been breached or prosthetic material has been placed
TEP***	The dissection of the preperitoneal space begins at the umbilicus avoiding the need for a peritoneal incision	Peritoneal cavity is never entered	Technically difficult
	Once the preperitoneal space in the vicinity of the groin is entered, the dissection is identical to the TAPP		Peritoneal breach common especially for the inexperienced

*TAPP transabdominal preperitoneal; **IPOM intraperitoneal onlay mesh; ***TEP totally extraperitoneal

"local," transient groin pain was the most common, occurring in 4 patients (2 %). Persistent groin and leg pain was arbitrarily defined as pain that was present 2 months postoperatively. Groin pain was present in 2 of 194 patients (1 %) at 2 months follow-up, whereas persistent leg pain was present in 3 of 194 patients (1.5 %). All groin and leg pain have subsequently resolved. The hernia recurrence rate after laparoscopic repair using the TAPP approach was 2.3 % (6 of 256).

Similar results are reported in the recent literature [7, 20]. Panton et al. noted a 1 % incidence of chronic pain and no recurrences after 106 repairs using the TAPP approach in 79 patients with a follow-up of 1–2 months [20]. Felix et al. reported no recurrences after 205 hernia repairs in 183 patients with a mean follow-up of 12 months [7]. In rural west-central Minnesota, Brown repaired 84 hernias in 61 patients laparoscopically, 10 of whom had previously had a traditional repair. Of those patients who had the traditional as well as a laparoscopic repair, 100 % would choose to have a laparoscopic hernia repair should they need another hernia repair in the future [3].

In April 1991, a multicenter trial for laparoscopic herniorrhaphy was initiated at Creighton University. The objective was to study the TAPP, IPOM, and EXTRA procedures. Institutions in North America and Europe participated. Data from 869 herniorrhaphies in 686 patients revealed a recurrence rate of 4.5 % with a minimum follow-up of 15 months. Although 61 patients had additional abdominal procedures performed at the time of laparoscopy, these procedures did not adversely affect the herniorrhaphy.

Neuralgias, resulting in transient or persistent leg or groin pain, or numbness, were the most distressing complication. Once surgeons understand the anatomy of the nerves in the region, especially the lateral femoral cutaneous nerve of the thigh and the femoral branch of the genitofemoral nerve, this can be minimized. Six patients (0.87 %) required a secondary abdominal procedure for complications, i. e., painful adhesion, infected mesh, trocar site bleeding, bowel obstruction, bowel perforation, and bladder perforation. Laparotomy was required in two, whereas the other four patients required laparoscopy to correct their complications. Of the patients, 57 % were discharged the day of surgery, 37 % were kept overnight, and 6 % stayed 2 days or more usually as a result of a complication or severe underlying medical illness. There was no significant difference in recurrence rate when comparing the types of laparoscopic inguinal herniorrhaphy. The recurrence rate for individual surgeons was higher in their first ten cases suggesting that the learning curve for this new procedure was significant [10].

The results of a randomized prospective trial involving 75 conventional procedures and 75 laparoscopic procedures have been reported [25]. The laparoscopic repair performed in that investigation was the TAPP. These data suggest that laparoscopic hernia repair causes less pain than conventional hernia repair and enables patients to return to normal activity and work more quickly.

Conclusion

Laparoscopic inguinal herniorrhaphy remains an investigational procedure. The best technique and the exact indications for laparoscopic inguinal herniorrhaphy are presently unclear. The most commonly used inguinal hernia repairs using laparoscopic methods are summarized in Table 1.

Excellent exposure of the preperitoneal space can be obtained with laparoscopy. This can be very useful in repairing many inguinal hernias especially those that are recurrent or otherwise complicated. Laparoscopy should certainly have a place in the armamentarium of general surgeons caring for inguinal hernias although it is unlikely that every inguinal hernia will best be repaired laparoscopically. Preliminary results suggest that further investigation is warranted.

References

1. BASSINI E: Sulla Cura Radicale dell' Ernia Inguinal. Arch Soc Ital Chir 4 (1987) 380.
2. BERLINER, BURSON SL, KATZ P ET AL.: An anterior transversalis fascia repair for adult inguinal hernias. Am J Surg 135 (1978) 633– 636.
3. BROWN RB: Laparoscopic hernia repair: a rural perspective. Surg Laparosc Endosc 4 (1994) 106–109.
4. BYRON JW, MARKENSON G, MIYAZAWA K: A randomized comparison of Veress needle and trocar insertion for laparoscopy. Surg Gynecol Obstet 177 (1993) 259–262.
5. CAMPS, NAGAN JR, ANNIBALI R, QUINN T, ARREGUI M, FITZGIBBONS RJ, JR: Laparoscopic inguinal herniorrhaphy: current techniques. In: Arregui, MR., RJ. Fitzgibbons Jr, JB McKernan, N Kathkouda, H Reich (eds.): Principles of laparoscopic surgery. Springer, New York (1995) 400–408.
6. Conceptualization and measurements of physiological health for adults. Rand, Santa Monica, Calif. (1983) 3–120.
7. FELIX EL, MICHAS CA, MCKNIGHT RL: Laparoscopic herniorrhaphy. Transabdominal preperitoneal floor repair. Surg Endosc 8 (1994) 100–103.
8. FITZGIBBONS RJ JR, VITALE GC, CAMPS J: Laparoscopic inguinal hernia repair. In: Sanfilippo, JS., GC. Vitale, J Périssat (eds.): Laparoscopic Surgery: An Atlas for general surgeons. JB Lippincott, Philadelphia (1995) 207–217.
9. FITZGIBBONS RJ JR, CAMPS J, NGUYEN N: Laparoscopic inguinal herniorrhaphy. In: Cameron, JL (ed.): Current surgical therapy, 5th edn. Mosby Year Book, Philadelphia (1995) 1052–1059.
10. FITZGIBBONS RJ JR, CAMPS J, CORNET D, NGUYEN N, LITKE B ET AL.: Laparoscopic inguinal herniorrhaphy: Results of a multi-center trial. Ann Surg (1994) 21(1): 3–13.
11. GLASSOW F: Short stay surgery (Shouldice technique) for repair of inguinal hernia. Ann R Coll Surg Engl 58 (1976) 133–139.
12. HALSTED WS: The radial cure of inguinal hernia in the male. Bull Johns Hopkins Hosp 4 (1893) 17.
13. HART RO, FITZGIBBONS RJ JR, FILIPI CJ, SALERNO GM: Open laparoscopy for laparoscopic herniorrhaphy. In: Zucker, K, EJ Reddick, BS Bailey (eds.): Surgical laparoscopy. Quality Medical Publishing, St. Louis (1991) 87–97.
14. ILES JDH.: Specialization in elective herniorrhaphy. Lancet i (1965) 751–755.
15. KRAUS MA: Nerve injury during Laparoscopic inguinal hernia repair. Surg Laparosc Endosc 4 (1993) 342–345.
16. LICHTENSTEIN IL, SHULMAN AG, AMID PK, MONTLLOR MM: The tension-free hernioplasty. Am J Surg 157 (1989) 188–193.
17. LOBE TE, SCHROPP KP: Inguinal hernias in pediatrics: initial experience with laparoscopic inguinal exploration of the asymptomatic contralateral side. J Laparoendosc Surg 2 (1992) 135–140.
18. MCVAY CB: Inguinal and femoral hernioplasty: anatomic repair. Arch Surg 57 (1948) 524–530.
19. NYHUS LM: The preperitoneal approach and iliopubic tract repair of inguinal hernia. In: Nyhus, LM, RE Condon (eds.): Hernia. JB Lippincott, Philadelphia (1989) 154–188.
20. PANTON ON, PANTON RJ.: Laparoscopic hernia repair. Am J Surg 167 (1994) 535–537.
21. REDMOND L, SALERNO GM, ANNABALI R, FITZGIBBONS RJ, JR: Laparoscopic herniorrhaphy. In: D Brooks (ed.): Current techniques in laparoscopy. Current Medicine, Philadelphia (1994) 18.1–18.11.
22. SCHULTZ, GRABER LJ, PIETRAFITTA J, HICKOK D: Laser laparoscopic herniorrhaphy: a clinical trial. Preliminary results. J Laparoendosc Surg 1 (1990) 41–45.
23. SHEARBURN EW, MEYERS RT: Shouldice repair of inguinal hernia. Surgery 66 (1969) 450–459
24. Socio-economic Factbook for Surgery. American College of Surgeons (1980).
25. STOKER DL, SPIEGELHALTER DJ, INGH R, WELLWOOD JM: Laparoscopic versus open inguinal hernia repair: randomised prospective trial. Lancet 343 (1994) 1243–1245.
26. STOPPA RE, WARLAUMONT CR: The preperitoneal approach and prosthetic repair of groin hernia. In: Nyhus, LM, RE Condon (eds.): Hernia, 3rd edn J. B. Lippincott, Philadelphia (1989) 199–225.

Thoracoscopic Surgery

Critical Comments

R.J. GINSBERG

In this well-written and beautifully illustrated chapter, the authors have outlined the current status of video-assisted thoracoscopic surgery. One must always keep in mind the goals of these video-assisted techniques lessened postoperative pain, improved cosmetics and shortened hospital stay. There is no doubt that video-assisted surgery has become an accepted approach in the investigation and management of many intrathoracic problems. It is doubtful that all of these goals, however, have been accomplished in other than a few situations.

To my mind, the most important advances that have occured as a result of the video-assisted techniques have been in the development of improved endoscopic instruments and the ability to teach while performing limited access procedures.

The diagnosis and management of most pleural problems can easily be accomplished through a single intercostal incision utilizing operating endoscopes or open instruments such as a mediastinoscope. This includes: diagnosis of indeterminate pleural effusions, pleurodesis of malignant pleural effusion, and localized decortications for empyema. The thoracoscope available with an operating channel allows all of these procedures mentioned to be performed without the necessity of a second port. All of these techniques were well established in thoracic surgical centers prior to the advent of video-assisted techniques. I still continue to use this simplified approach. The value of the newer thoracoscopes is the improved visualization available and the ability to teach while performing the procedure.

On the other hand, video-assisted techniques, with the improved imaging available, have allowed simpler management approaches for specific problems such as chylothorax and sympathectomy to be performed without thoracotomy. Whether or not the video-assisted techniques utilized for spontaneous pneumothorax is an improvement over a small axillary incision with regard to efficacy and postoperative pain is still debatable. There is no doubt, however, that improved visualization and identification of all offending blebs makes thoracoscopic inspection an advantage.

The simplest approach to the diagnosis of an indeterminate nodule remains percutaneous needle aspiration biopsy. This allows for the diagnosis of most malignancies (85 %) without the necessity of general anesthesia, single lung ventilation and the costs incurred in an operating room. As well, the diagnosis of a malignancy prior to operation allows for important preoperative planning. In my own practice, I reserve thoracoscopy for those nodules not diagnosed or diagnosable by percutaneous needle aspiration biopsy.

In the staging of lung cancer, video-assisted thoracoscopic surgery has only a limited place being useful for defining the etiology of pleural effusions and indeterminate second nodules as well as acessing those lymph nodes in the mediastinum unavailable to standard mediastinoscopy techniques. In our own center, it is rare that we find a need for thoracoscopic staging for lung cancer.

As the authors quite rightly indicate, the standard treatment for even peripherally-placed T1N0 lung cancer remains lobectomy. The authors did not stress the importance of lymph node sampling and/or mediastinal lymph node dissection as part of the operative procedure. Certainly, video-assisted techniques can accomplish all of these goals – the question is whether or not there is any advantage at all to these techniques! In the light of current information, there does not appear to be any improvement in postoperative pain or lessened hospital stay utilizing video-assisted thoracoscopic surgery for standard pulmonary resections. Improved pain-relief techniques now available and muscle-sparing incisions appear to be equivalent to video-assisted approaches including postoperative comfort and the ultimate cosmetic effect. Tumor implentation and local recurrence continues to be a concern with minimal access techniques.

Video-assisted techniques have improved the management of posterior mediastinal problems including: small benign tumors, benign esophageal lesions requiring simple excisions, and neurectomies that occaisonally are required for hyperhidrosis, pain relief or acid-suppression. These can all be accomplished with ease using video-assisted approaches. With increasing expertise, it appears inevitable that simple reconstructive esophageal surgery for benign disease (e.g. anti-reflux surgery, myotomies etc.) will be universally performed using limited access techniques.

My major objection to video-assisted thoracic surgery is its misapplication when simpler techniques are available (e.g. thoracentesis and percutaneous needle aspiration biopsy, mediastinoscopy for lung cancer staging, subxyphoid drainage for pericardial effusion, and transcervical thymectomy for myasthenia). A second major concern is the use of minimally invasive approaches in the management of cancer. Primary intrathoracic malignancies require wide, adequate excisions and adequate lymph node staging if not lymph node dissection. Manual palpation to identify metastatic nodules is an important step in the treatment of pulmonary metastases. Limited access ports do not allow this. Of real concern is the temptation for surgeons to do less than adequate dissection and excisions during the conduct of a video-assisted approach. For this reason, great caution should be applied when considering a video-assisted approach in the management of intrathoracic malignancies.

In the future, undoubtedly, further improvement in instrumentation, optical resolution and technical ability will allow surgeons to accomplish virtually everything through minimal access techniques that are now accomplished with open surgery. One always has to be extremely cautious that these techniques are utilized for the benefit of the patient rather than as a "tour de force" for the surgeon and that all oncologic principles are adhered to when using limited access techniques in treating curable malignant disease. Experience has shown us that the first operation should be the definitive goal.

29. Thoracoscopic Surgery

M. J. Mack, R. J. Landreneau, and S. R. Hazelrigg

Introduction

Minimally invasive surgical techniques have been developed and applied to virtually every surgical subspecialty in the past decade. Video-assisted thoracic surgery (VATS) is the term used to describe the application of minimally invasive surgical techniques to perform intrathoracic surgical procedures. VATS is the current thoracic surgical extension of thoracoscopy, which was initially performed in 1910 by Jacobaeus, a Swedish internist who used a cystoscope to perform diagnostic procedures in the pleural space [49]. He proceeded to expand the application of thoracoscopy to lyse pleural adhesions as a therapy for tuberculosis [48, 50, 51]. This collapse therapy became a commonplace bedside procedure performed by thoracic surgeons in tuberculosis sanitoriums worldwide. It remained the mainstay of antituberculosis therapy until the development of effective antimicrobial therapy for tuberculosis late in the 1940s. Subsequently, thoracoscopy became a seldom applied procedure being only occasionally used for diagnosis and management of mainly pleural disease [5, 53]. Significant experience of thoracoscopy in the 1950s and 1960s continued especially in the pediatric-age patient group [106, 107].

During the 1980s significant technological advances resulted in improved video-optical endoscopic equipment. These advances led to the well-known explosion in laparoscopic surgery and prompted interest by surgeons in other fields to explore the use of minimally invasive video-assisted techniques in their specialties [102]. In late 1990 surgeons in a number of medical centers began developing extensive experience with video-assisted techniques for a variety of intrathoracic processes [76].

The primary purpose of the VATS approach is to reduce the postoperative pain and other post-thoracotomy-related morbidity following thoracic surgery without sacrificing the well-established surgical principles of open thoracic surgery [66]. Because the application of minimally invasive surgery has significantly expanded the role of thoracoscopy beyond that of its accepted role as a diagnostic procedure on the pleura, it was felt that a better descriptive term was needed to encompass the wide variety of diagnostic and therapeutic procedures now being performed by thoracoscopic techniques; hence, the term video-assisted thoracic surgery (VATS) [86].

Indications

Whereas virtually every thoracic surgical procedure in the past 4 years has been performed by VATS, current indications

are constantly evolving (Table 1). The main morbidity of traditional open thoracic surgical procedures is the pain and respiratory dysfunction associated with the operative approach. VATS offers a less invasive approach while hopefully allowing the same surgical procedure to be performed as traditionally has been accomplished by open techniques. Although the procedure has been well accepted and its role clearly defined in some disease processes, e. g., spontaneous pneumothorax, its benefit has not been nearly as clearly defined in some other intrathoracic disease entities, e. g., esophageal cancer (see Chap. 9). For the purposes of this discussion we have divided thoracoscopic procedures into diagnostic and therapeutic while attempting to outline where the current indications for the procedures lie.

Table 1. VATS procedures December 1990 – November 1994 ($n = 798$)

Lung resection	($n = 401$)
Nodule	279
Apical blebs/infiltrate	31
Giant bullae	21
Pneumothorax	70
Pleural disease	($n = 165$)
Effusion	90
Chylothorax	3
Empyema	44
Hemothorax	12
Mass	16
Mediastinal disease	($n = 59$)
Biopsy/staging nodules	14
Mass	26
Cyst	10
Thymectomy	9
Pericardial disease	38
Sympathectomy	29
Spine procedures	56
Lobectomy	24
Esophageal procedures	23
Other	3

The current indications for thoracoscopy are listed in Table 2. VATS can be either a diagnostic or a therapeutic procedure, or, as in the case of solitary pulmonary nodules or idiopathic pleural effusions, it can be both diagnostic and therapeutic.

Table 2. Indications for VATS

Location	Diagnostic indications	Therapeutic indications
Pleura	Indeterminate nodule Indeterminate mass	Malignant effusion Empyema Chylothorax Hemothorax
Lung	Indeterminate nodule Diffuse lung disease Metastatectomy	Limited-stage cancer VATS lobectomy ± Metastatectomy Pneumothorax Bullectomy
Mediastinum	Cysts Staging lung cancer Posterior masses Anterior masses	Cysts Thymectomy Posterior masses
Esophagus	Benign tumors	Achalasia ± Esophagectomy Benign tumors
Pericardium	Indeterminate effusions	Effusive pericardial disease
Miscellaneous	Spine disease	Sympathectomy Vagotomy Splanchnicectomy Spine disease

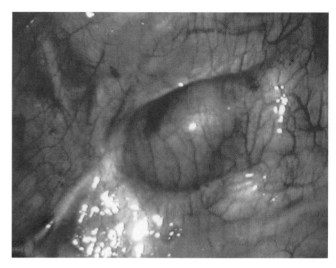

Fig. 1. Thoracoscopic view of an indeterminate pleural-based mass

Pleura

Idiopathic Effusions

Diseases of the pleura were the original indications for thoracoscopy in 1910 and remain a prominent indication for VATS presently [20, 28, 45, 46, 87, 89]. Approximately 25 % of the VATS procedures performed in major centers are for diseases of the pleura [54]. For idiopathic pleural effusions that have eluded less invasive attempts at diagnosis, VATS has been demonstrated to be highly effective [87]. When repeat thoracentesis and needle biopsy of the pleura have not yielded a diagnosis, direct examination of the pleura by video techniques has proven to be virtually 100 % diagnostic for idiopathic effusions. In our experience, the overwhelming majority of idiopathic effusions are revealed to be malignant after direct visual complete examination of the pleural cavity [54]. If a previous history of malignancy exists in the patient with an indeterminate effusion, the likelihood that the current effusion is malignant is virtually 100 %.

Pleural Masses

VATS is also highly effective for the diagnosis of pleural-based masses (Fig. 1). When the differential diagnosis is mesothelioma vs adenocarcinoma or benign disease, directed open biopsy and/or resection of the pleural-based mass is usually successful at yielding a definitive diagnosis [54].

Malignant Effusions

VATS has also been demonstrated to be highly effective as a therapeutic procedure for pleural diseases. In malignant pleural effusions VATS has the ability to completely drain the pleural space, break up areas of loculated fluid, and distribute a sclerosing agent, preferably sterile talc, uniformly through all

visceral and parietal pleural surfaces (Fig. 2). The management of malignant pleural disease is one of the areas in which thoracoscopy has had its greatest impact [1, 19, 37, 72, 112]. In a disease process in which it was previously very difficult to obtain effective palliation, VATS has offered significant palliative management in a minimally invasive manner in these patients who are often terminally ill.

Several sclerosing agents have been instilled by VATS for chemical pleurodesis. Tetracycline and its derivatives, quinacrine, nitrogen mustard, bleomycin, and talc, have all been used [37]. Talc and bleomycin have both resulted in high success rates; however, talc is much less expensive and its success is greater than 90 % in multiple series [72].

Other methods of pleurodesis can be performed by VATS including a mechanical pleurodesis using a gauze sponge, scratch pad, or marlex mesh (Table 3). Similarly, a pleurectomy can be performed if that is the method of choice. These methods of pleurodesis, however, are much more appropriate for the management of benign pleural processes. Patients who

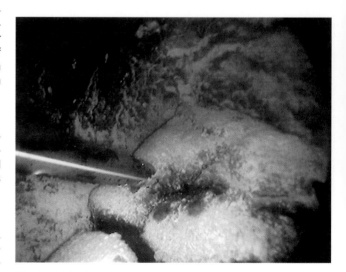

Fig. 2. Talc pleurodesis. Note distribution of talc on all visceral and parietal pleural surfaces

Table 3. Techniques of VATS procedures for pleurodesis

Mechanical
 Gauze abrasion
 Endoscopic kittner

Cautery
 Electrocautery
 Argon beam coagulator
 Laser

Chemical
 Tetracycline derivatives
 Nitrogen mustard
 Bleomycin
 Quinacrine
 Talc

Pleurectomy

have malignant pleural effusions and trapped lung represent an additional problem. The failure of the lung to fully expand after drainage of pleural fluid may be due to tumor encasing the lung, fibrous entrapment of the lung, or endobronchial obstruction. If any of these conditions exist, thoracoscopy will not be effective at palliating the effusion. Malignant entrapment of the lung itself cannot be successfully decorticated (Fig. 3).

Unless complete pleural symphysis can be obtained, reaccumulation of the pleural fluid cannot be prevented. These patients are best treated with either permanent chest-tube palliation or occasional pleural peritoneal shunts [72].

Empyema
Early treatment of pneumonia with antibiotics has resulted in a decreased incidence of empyema. However, empyema remains a relatively frequent problem in thoracic surgery. There are three phases of empyema: firstly, an early acute phase in which the fluid is thin and easily drained by thoracentesis or tube thoracostomy. In the intermediate phases, the fibrinopurulent stage, the fluid is thicker, gelatinous, and a fibrinous peel is present on the visceral pleura. Lastly, empyemas

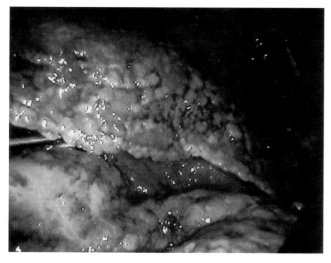

Fig. 3. Entrapment of the lung due to malignant involvement of the visceral pleura

progress to a chronic phase in which a thick fibrous peel exists on the lung, which is difficult to decorticate.

Early empyemas are frequently successfully managed by tube thoracostomy only. However, if the fluid does not immediately and completely drain, VATS has a significant therapeutic role [104]. Similarly, in the fibrinopurulent stage in which the empyema process has been in existence for 3 weeks or less, VATS offers an excellent approach for draining the pleural space and decorticating the fibrinopurulent material from the lung surface. If the empyema has been present for more than 3 weeks, the adherence of the fibrinous peel to the lung may be too dense for adequate decortication to be performed by VATS techniques [25]. If initial attempts at decortication by VATS are unsuccessful, immediate conversion to an open procedure should be performed so that complete reexpansion of the lung can occur.

In patients who are poor candidates for any operative procedure, there has been some success using streptokinase and urokinase in the early fibrinopurulent stages as an alternative to surgical procedure [105]. Thoracic surgeons should always keep this option in mind.

Chylothorax
Chylothorax can be due to either malignant or benign causes. Benign causes are usually traumatic or iatrogenic [24]. There is limited, but successful, experience with the use of VATS for the management of the chylothorax [82]. If conservative measures, such as elemental diets or intravenous hyperalimentation with adequate drainage of the pleural space, have not been successful managing the chylothorax, VATS can be used [47]. By the preoperative oral administration of heavy cream or ice cream, the white milky lymphatic effluent can usually be located in the mediastinum. We have had experience successfully managing chylothoraces after blunt trauma as well as after coronary artery bypass surgery. The leaking thoracic duct can usually be located and successfully ligated.

Hemothorax
There is some experience with VATS for the management of the persistent nonexsanguinating hemothorax as well as the treatment of retained clotted blood [34]. The most common cause of a traumatic hemothorax is laceration of an intercostal vessel. In the stable, nonexsanguinating trauma patient, thoracoscopy has been demonstrated to offer effective management. If simple chest tube drainage does not effect complete evacuation of the thoracic cavity, the subsequent risk of empyema and fibrothorax is increased. Early use of thoracoscopy for continued bleeding after chest tube placement or for evacuation of clots inadequately removed by chest tube drainage is effective management [35]. After removal of the clotted blood, the site of bleeding can usually be identified and controlled. If an intercostal vessel is the source, cautery or endoscopic clips can control the bleeding. Pulmonary parenchymal injuries can be sutured or stapled. Unsuspected diaphragmatic injuries can also be identified [115]. Of course, unstable trauma patients should not be managed by VATS, but rather by an open procedure.

Pulmonary Parenchymal Disease

There are both diagnostic and therapeutic applications of VATS in pulmonary parenchymal disease as listed in Table 2. VATS is a very helpful diagnostic modality for the management of indeterminate solitary pulmonary nodules [78] as well as for obtaining a lung biopsy for the diagnosis of infiltrate of lung disease [26].

VATS can also be therapeutic by offering a less invasive approach for wedge resection of the lung in limited-stage lung cancer in patients who are poor candidates for surgery or have poor pulmonary function [113]. There is also extensive experience with VATS lobectomy for stage I and stage II carcinoma of the lung [35, 57, 58, 84, 110, 123].

Finally, VATS has become the treatment of choice for management of persistent or recurrent spontaneous pneumothorax due to apical bleb disease. Experience with the management of bullous lung disease by both laser ablation and stapled resection of bullous disease via the thoracoscopic approach [10, 41, 43, 46, 93, 95, 119, 121, 126] is also increasing.

Indeterminate Solitary Pulmonary Nodules

Diagnostic modalities available for the management of the indeterminate solitary pulmonary nodule include computerized tomography, sputum cytology, fiberoptic bronchoscopy, and transthoracic fine-needle aspiration biopsy (Table 4) [70, 71, 88, 111].

Table 4. Diagnostic modalities for indeterminate solitary pulmonary nodule

Chest X-ray (serial)
Computerized tomogram
Sputum cytology
Fiberoptic bronchoscopy
Fine-needle aspiration biopsy
Thoracotomy
Thoracoscopy
FDG PET scan
PET (positron emission tomography)

If a peripheral lung nodule cannot be demonstrated to have been present, unchanged in size and configuration for a 2-year period, and cannot be demonstrated to have specific calcification patterns in it, further diagnostic management is mandatory.

Sputum cytology and fiberoptic bronchoscopy have insufficient diagnostic yield to recommend them as routine use in the management algorithm [70]. Standard management of the indeterminate nodule has traditionally included fine-needle aspiration biopsy. However, with the advent of minimally invasive pulmonary resective techniques, VATS has assumed a larger role. The only diagnostic result of a fine-needle aspiration biopsy that avoids operative intervention is a specific benign diagnosis. Data by Calhoun as well as our own indicate that a *specific benign* diagnosis is obtained in less than 5 % of all patients undergoing fine-needle aspiration biopsies for diagnosis in indeterminate nodules [9]. Results using VATS for diagnosis of the indeterminate nodule reveal virtually 100 % sensitivity and 100 % specificity [78]. Although VATS is an operative procedure, its minimally invasive nature, the high diagnostic value, compared with the relatively low yield of fine-needle aspiration biopsy in establishing a *specific benign* diagnosis, all mitigate toward a larger role for thoracoscopy in the management of the indeterminate nodule. Recently, FDG and positron emission tomography (PET) scanning have also been shown to have great diagnostic promise in lung nodules.

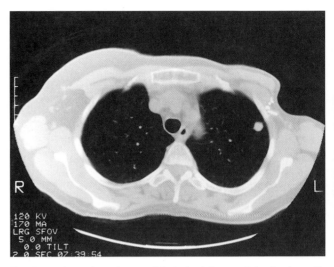

Fig. 4. Indeterminate lung nodule in the left upper lobe that is easily identified and resected by VATS

Candidate nodules for VATS resection include peripheral nodules located in the outer one-third of lung and less than 3 cm in greatest diameter (Fig. 4) [61]. Nodules that are central in location and not adjacent to the visceral pleura or near a fissure present difficulties for VATS resections (Fig. 5). Similarly, nodules less than 1 cm in diameter and not immediately adjacent to a pleural edge also present problems, because the surgeon has lost the ability to palpate the lung, and other sensory input, including visual and instrument tactile input, are necessary for localization. Nodules less than 1 cm in diameter present some difficulty in localization, and unless immediately adjacent to the pleural edge, a preoperative localization technique is preferable [73, 99].

Infiltrative Lung Disease

Development of a new infiltrate that does not resolve spontaneously or on a course of antibiotics mandates further investigation, especially in the cancer patient or in those patients

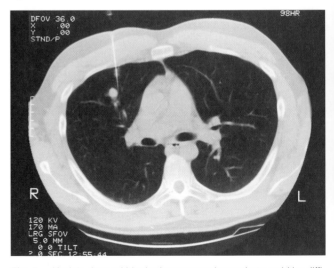

Fig. 5. Nodule deep within the lung parenchyma that would be difficult to identify at VATS. A preoperative localizing wire has been placed

who are immunosuppressed either due to their underlying disease or therapeutic treatment regimens [119, 3]. The differential diagnosis includes the wide gamut of diffuse infiltrative lung processes including sarcoidosis, pulmonary fibrosis, usual interstitial pneumonia (UIP), and if the patient has malignancy or is immunosuppressed, opportunistic infection, chemotherapeutic toxicity, or lymphangitic spread of the patient's malignancy. Determining the etiology is vital in directing future management. Although sputum analysis and transbronchial biopsy with bronchial lavage are initial management steps, surgical biopsy of the lung is frequently required when a definitive diagnostic result is not obtained by less invasive methods.

In this setting the open lung biopsy has been the traditional method for obtaining an adequate sample of lung tissue for diagnostic result. VATS offers a reasonable alternative to open limited thoracotomy for non-ventilator-dependent patients requiring a surgical diagnosis. In our own experience of over 100 patients with diffuse infiltrative lung disease, there has been no operative mortality and no significant morbidity [119].

The postoperative course compares favorably against our early experience with the open lung biopsy in the same clinical setting. Satisfactory tissue for diagnosis of the infiltrative process was obtained in all circumstances. In the ambulatory patient this biopsy can frequently be done as an outpatient procedure or with hospitalization of less than 24 h.

Metastatic Disease

New solitary pulmonary nodules in patients with a previous history of extrathoracic malignancy yields a diagnosis other than the original malignancy in approximately one-third of cases depending on the length of time from the original primary tumor presentation as well as the specific origin of the previous malignancy [55, 108, 109]. When multiple nodules are present and a tissue diagnosis is deemed necessary, fine-needle aspiration biopsy is usually helpful. However, with smaller nodules 1 cm or less, or if a specific diagnosis has not been obtained in fine-needle aspiration biopsy, VATS offers the preferred diagnostic technique for resection of the lung nodule. Whereas surgical resection is effective for the *diagnosis* of a pulmonary metastasis, there is debate as to its therapeutic role. There is potential survival benefit when limited pulmonary disease burden is present in patients with favorable primary tumor histologies [11, 18, 21, 22, 31, 36, 57, 67, 83, 92, 100, 101, 118]. If the primary tumor has been controlled and there is no other site of metastasis, there may be a therapeutic benefit from resection of the pulmonary malignancy in some specific tumors especially sarcoma [101]. There has been concern raised that the restricted ability to palpate the lung with the VATS technique will allow some foci of metastatic disease to be missed, and therefore jeopardize a potential therapeutic result. However, with modern CT scanning techniques, especially the newest generation of "spiral" or "helical" CT scanners, nodules 2 mm in size are consistently identified [62]. Lesions of this size are usually impossible to discriminate, even at the time of open thoracotomy. These nodules can be located by VATS after appropriate preoperative wire-needle localization. Studies have indicated that when more than two or three nodules are found at the time of thoracic exploration, the intervention becomes primarily diagnostic anyway [22]. Therefore, we believe that the VATS approach for metastatic disease is a valid alternative to thoracot-

omy for the resection of limited metastatic disease identified as small peripheral nodules by modern CT scanning techniques as a diagnostic as well as a possibly therapeutic procedure.

In addition, gene therapy is offering promise for oncologic management [12, 81, 90, 114]. VATS offers a good approach for obtaining adequate tumor tissue for cell culture for specific gene therapy including ras and P53 oncogenes. Success of this therapy will depend on the outcome of current ongoing specific oncogene protocols.

Limited Resection for Cancer

When the planned surgical resective procedure for carcinoma of the lung is a nonanatomic wedge resection, the VATS approach offers the preferred method of performing this resection [113]. Standard management of stage I non-small-cell carcinoma of the lung, however, remains lobectomy. Results of the North American Lung Cancer Study Group determine that although there is no survival benefit to lobectomy compared with nonanatomic wedge resection in intraoperatively determined peripheral pathologic stage I non-small-cell carcinoma of the lung, the local recurrence rate was higher following wedge resection or segmentectomy compared with lobectomy [30]. These findings support the continued use of anatomic lobectomy for stage I carcinoma in patients who are able to withstand the procedure.

However, in patients who are at significant risk for a lobectomy due to either age, general medical condition, or impaired pulmonary function, VATS offers the best approach for nonanatomic wedge resection of peripheral primary bronchogenic carcinomas. Shennib et al. have reported their experience in a small number of high-risk elderly patients with significant impairment in cardiopulmonary reserve [113]. The same criteria for resection should be used as those for indeterminate lung nodules, i. e., peripheral lesions less than 3 cm in diameter and located in the outer one-third of the lung, preferably close to a visceral pleural surface or a fissure.

VATS Lobectomy

Significant experience is developing with the use of thoracoscopy for the performance of formal lobectomies and pneumonectomies [57, 58, 84, 110]. The technique involves the use of traditional thoracoscopic ports with the addition of a 5–6 cm "accessory" or "utility" incision for extraction of the specimen at the end of the procedures. At least four large series exist demonstrating that the procedure can be performed safely with no operative mortality (Table 5).
Equivalent lymph node harvesting can be performed by this technique, and generally there appears to be less postoperative pain and reduced hospital stay. However, there is a significant learning curve to the approach and the benefits at this

Table 5. Lobectomy performed by VATS

Center	N	Mortality	Conversion for bleeding	Conversion for technical problems
Roviaro (Milan)	84	0	2	6
McKenna (Los Angeles)	45	0	1	2
Walker (Edinburgh)	50	0	0	5
Kirby (Cleveland)	25	0	1	4

stage are not clear enough to recommend general application of this technique compared with open thoracotomy with limited muscle-sparing incision.

Blebs and Bullous Lung Disease

Spontaneous Pneumothorax
Primary spontaneous pneumothorax occurs in patients without underlying lung disease, and is usually due to the rupture of an apical bleb. Patients are usually young and otherwise healthy. Standard management of the first spontaneous pneumothorax includes observation only if there is minimal collapse or intercostal tube drainage. Successful resolution without subsequent recurrence is the result in 70–75 % of patients [86]. However, in patients who have a recurrent spontaneous pneumothorax or a persistent air leak of greater than 3–4 days' duration, or in patients who are frequent travelers or have hazardous occupations, VATS offers the optimal method of surgically managing the disease.

Multiple series exist now demonstrating the efficacy of VATS and management of primary spontaneous pneumothorax. The largest series is by Yim and colleagues of 100 patients managed over a 3-year period with a 97 % success rate and 2 % recurrence [127].

Secondary pneumothoraces occur in patients with underlying lung disease. The underlying disease is usually bullous emphysema, although it can occur in the face of interstitial lung disease, neoplasms, asthma, or trauma. It is increasingly occurring in patients with acquired immune deficiency syndrome (AIDS) who have pneumocystis pneumonia or tuberculosis [27]. Surgical management of secondary spontaneous pneumothorax in any of these settings is significantly more complicated. In patients with underlying bullous emphysema, surgical intervention frequently means resection of a bullous, which requires advanced stapling techniques, and frequently, laser ablation. Fibrin tissue glue is often required in these circumstances. The thoracoscopic surgeon considering VATS intervention in these patients should be very experienced in VATS operative techniques. The patient with pneumocystis pneumonia in the setting of AIDS has a very short life expectancy (less than 6 months). Conservative management is therefore preferred [23]. Because the lung is very friable, surgical management is much more difficult, and if surgical intervention is necessary, pleurectomy is advised at the time.

Diffuse Bullous Emphysema without Pneumothorax
There is increasing interest in the use of surgery for bullous emphysema either by endoscopic methods or by open techniques [120]. The traditional indication for surgical intervention in bullous emphysema included those patients who had large localized bullae encompassing at least one-third of the hemithorax with evidence of compression of adjacent lung tissue [29]. It was felt that decompression of the bullous would recruit potentially functioning compressed lung tissue and improve breathing capacity in emphysematous patients.

Recently, there have been two developments to renew interest in surgical intervention. Wakabayashi has developed extensive experience using the VATS neodymium:YAG laser bullectomy [122]. By using the laser in a contact mode, Wakabayashi reports a series of 262 patients with subjective improvement in pulmonary function in the majority of patients. There is a mortality rate of 5.3 %, but only a small percentage

of patients had postoperative pulmonary functions evaluated. Lewis et al. reported similar use of VATS using the argon beam coagulator instead of the laser for bullae obliteration [69].

More recently, Cooper et al. have reported on the use of median sternotomy and bilateral stapling to achieve volume reduction of the lung [17]. Respiratory impairment in bullous emphysema is multifactorial. In addition to destruction of lung tissue and compression of adjacent, potentially functioning lung tissue by the emphysematous bullous, a large number of patients with bullous emphysema have hyperinflation of the lung. This causes impairment of the chest wall and diaphragmatic contribution to respiratory function [7]. By reducing the volume of lung tissue by 20–30 %, he has been able to demonstrate improvement in pulmonary function by restoration of diaphragmatic and chest wall function. In 20 patients there was no mortality and the mean improvement in FEV1 was 69 %. Postoperative air leak problems were lessened by the use of bovine pericardium to reinforce staple lines.

A combination of Cooper et al.'s technique [17] and the laser technique is being performed endoscopically by Landreneau (pers. comm.). By the use of the endoscopic stapler as well as the Nd:YAG laser, he is performing volume-reduction surgery with good early results.

Several questions remain unanswered: How are patients best selected for this surgery? Which is the best technique, stapler, laser, argon beam coagulator? Should the procedure be performed unilaterally or bilaterally, endoscopically or open? Although short-term benefits have been demonstrated, will the results be long lasting?

Mediastinal Procedures

The indications for VATS in mediastinal disease include the diagnosis and resection of posterior mediastinal masses [39], excision of mediastinal cysts [42], biopsy of anterior mediastinal masses inaccessible by cervical mediastinal exploration [116], staging of lung cancer [65], and thymectomy for thymoma or myasthenia gravis [79].

Posterior Masses
Posterior mediastinal masses are most frequently benign tumors of neurogenic origin. Preoperative evaluation includes CT scan, and if the tumor is adjacent to the vertebral body, a preoperative CT myelogram is mandatory prior to surgical resection in case tumor extension is present into the epidural space. If this "dumbbell" tumor is present, the resection still can be performed by endoscopic techniques.

Mediastinal Cysts
Mediastinal cysts are approachable and resectable by VATS techniques. However, the mere presence of a mediastinal cyst does not mandate removal. If symptoms exist due to compression of adjacent structures by an enlarged cyst, or if any concern of malignancy exists, VATS offers an ideal approach for surgical removal.

Staging
For staging of lung cancer and biopsy of anterior mediastinal masses, VATS has a definite role. For peritracheal lymphadenopathy or masses, cervical mediastinal exploration (CME) is still the preferred approach. However, for a left-sided lung cancer or for mediastinal masses in the aortopulmonary win-

dow, or in the subcarinal area, VATS offers the optimal approach for biopsy. Left thoracoscopy has replaced the anterior mediastinotomy (Chamberlain procedure) in our practice. A better staging procedure can be performed by the VATS technique because of better visualization and enhanced lighting. The aortopulmonary window, levels 4L, 5, 6, and 7, are all optimally accessed by the VATS approach.

Thymectomy

We have also developed extensive experience with VATS for thymectomy for both limited-stage thymoma and for myasthenia gravis. By the use of the left thoracoscopic approach, we have been able to demonstrate that a total thymectomy can be performed. Although experience is relatively limited (nine patients) and follow-up relatively short (average 2 years), results equal to open techniques for thymectomy have been achieved in myasthenia gravis [79].

Limited-stage thymoma has also been reported to be resected by thoracoscopic techniques [64]. If invasive thymoma is present, however, open techniques should be used.

Pericardium

VATS can be used to diagnose idiopathic pericardial disease as well as for the management of either benign or malignant pericardial disease [38]. For pericardial effusions that remain undiagnosed after less invasive maneuvers, or that are recurrent after catheter drainage, the VATS approach through either the right or left chest can be used [77]. Pericardial effusions that tend to recur after limited pericardial windows, including benign pericardial disease, purulent pericarditis, and radiation-induced pericarditis, are best managed by the VATS technique. Malignant pericardial effusions with a potential for long-term survival (i. e., lymphoma, breast cancer) may also be treated by VATS; however, malignant pericardial disease with a poor prognosis (i. e., secondary to lung cancer) should be managed by a subxiphoid pericardiectomy, which allows a larger pericardial window than by the traditional nonvideo techniques.

Esophagus

A role for VATS has become fairly well established for benign esophageal disease; however, the benefits are less clear in malignant disease. Benign tumors of the esophagus, leiomyomas, can be completely removed by the VATS approach. Because the tumors are intramural in location, they can easily be shelled out and excised completely. Similarly, esophageal duplication cysts are also easily managed by VATS techniques.

Esophageal diverticulum can be excised by VATS techniques. Because pulsion diverticula are usually associated with esophageal motility disorders, a myotomy is usually a necessary part of the procedure.

Pelligrini and associates have developed a significant experience with the use of the VATS approach for managing achalasia [32] (see Chap. 10). By a left thoracoscopic approach, a Heller myotomy can be performed. The technique involves the use of simultaneous esophagoscopy to facilitate the procedure. He has reported good or excellent results in 90 % of the first 28 patients undergoing the procedure.

Although it is possible to perform antireflux procedures through the thoracoscopic approach, it appears presently that reflux disease is best managed surgically by the laparoscopic Nissen procedure (see Chap. 12). The laparoscopic technique has been well defined and results are excellent. The thoracoscopic approach appears to be a much more difficult technique for surgically managing reflux disease.

Although there have been several series of thoracoscopic esophagectomies for cancer, the benefits have not yet been demonstrated [106]. Collard has reported esophagectomy with *en bloc* tumor resection by the thoracoscopic technique [107]. Although it has been amply demonstrated that an esophagectomy with concomitant lymph node dissection can be performed, the technique is cumbersome and the benefits are presently not obvious.

Krasna has demonstrated the use of thoracoscopy for lymph node staging of esophageal cancer [59]. The role of lymph node staging is important for the indication to an adjunctive therapy for positive N-1 disease. Again, however, the benefits of management by this technique have not been demonstrated.

Autonomic Nervous System

Sympathectomy

The indications for dorsal sympathectomy include reflex sympathetic dystrophy (RSD) or causalgia of the upper extremity, hyperhidrosis, and less commonly, vascular disorders [40]. Although experience with endoscopic sympathectomy has been reported for over 50 years, it is only recently that it has been widely used. Large series by Kux [60] and Claes [15] have been reported with sympathectomy. The thoracoscopic approach appears to offer significant advantages over any of the traditional approaches. The lessened morbidity associated with the approach in patients who already have difficult pain-management syndromes appear to mitigate strongly toward VATS.

All patients with reflex sympathetic dystrophy who are potential candidates should have a positive preoperative response to a stellate ganglion block to ensure a positive result from sympathectomy [96].

Thoracic Splanchnicectomy

The use of thoracoscopy for division of the splanchnic nerve has been reported for managing refractory abdominal pain from pancreatic cancer or from chronic pancreatitis [125]. The celiac plexus is innervated by the greater splanchnic nerve T5–T10, lesser splanchnic nerves T10–T11, and the least splanchnic nerve T12. By dividing these nerves, good results in pain management have been reported in 70 % of cases [91].

Vagotomy

Truncular vagotomy is easily performed by the thoracoscopic approach. For patients with recurrent ulcer disease and incomplete vagotomies, a transthoracic vagotomy can be performed by the left VATS approach [2, 14]. Laws and McKernan have reported on six patients with thoracoscopic vagotomies [68]. Champault reported on another 21 patients managed by this technique [13].

Spine

There has recently been interest in several centers using VATS to approach the thoracic spine [74, 75]. Thoracic disc herniation is the most common indication for thoracoscopic spine surgery, although most other surgical procedures can be performed by VATS. These include intervertebral disc

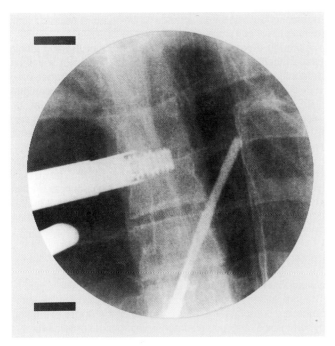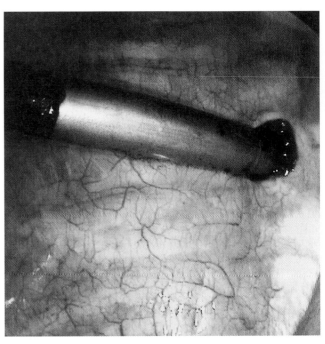

Figs. 6 A, B. Fluoroscope and intraoperative view of thoracoscopic placement of a BAK spinal fusion cage

space abscesses, biopsies of spinal masses or lytic lesions of the vertebral bodies, and corpectomies for cancer. Under development presently are fusion cages that will be capable of being placed by endoscopic techniques (Figs. 6A and B).

Contraindications

There are no true contraindications to VATS procedures, only relative ones. Patients who have had a previous thoracotomy or thoracoscopy may have pleural adhesions present. Only complete pleural symphysis is a contraindication. When pleural adhesions are present either due to pleurisy or previous surgery, the chest cavity can still frequently be entered in a limited space, and by sharp dissection, pleural adhesions lysed.

Preoperative Work-up

Preoperative assessment of the candidate for VATS procedures includes the standard history and physical examination. Although minimally invasive surgery, VATS should be considered a major operative procedure, because the thoracic cavity is entered. Because occasional conversion to an open thoracotomy may be necessary for a variety of reasons, particular attention to the cardiorespiratory system is relevant.

Patients are generally better able to undergo a VATS procedure than the same procedure performed by open techniques. In addition, there are several patients, especially with severe chronic obstructive pulmonary disease, who are not candidates for open thoracotomy, but are now operative candidates with the VATS procedures. Because of this, often patients undergoing the VATS procedures are poorer operative candidates than those previously considered for open tech-

niques. Because of extensive shunting due to underlying lung disease, we have found that even the patients with severe emphysema are able to tolerate the lung collapse necessary for VATS with minimal difficulty.

Anesthesia

Most VATS procedures are done under general anesthesia. Because collapse of the ipsilateral lung is necessary, single-lung ventilation must be maintained. For this a double lumen endotracheal tube is placed. A left-sided tube is preferable because of the short distance between the carina and the right upper lobe bronchus. Either lung can be collapsed with a left-sided tube placed. For pediatric or smaller adult patients in which a double lumen endotracheal tube cannot be placed, an endotracheal tube with a bronchial blocker (Univent) tube can be used. However, a double-lumen tube is preferable whenever possible because of the more rapid egress of air as well as the better ability to suction retained secretions compared with a bronchial blocker.

In the pediatric age group anesthetic management is best performed by single-lumen endotracheal tube with small tidal volumes. Manual retraction in the chest is usually sufficient to allow exposure. If this is not effective, the endotracheal tube can be selectively placed in one main-stem bronchus intermittently to allow thoracoscopy [44].

Some simple procedures can be performed under local anesthesia. Infiltration with 1 % Xylocaine or 0.5 % Marcaine in the intercostal space along with an intercostal nerve block is sufficient to perform a simple procedure such as a directed biopsy of a pleural-based mass or drainage of loculated pleural effusions. Several series reporting on sympathectomies performed under local anesthesia have been published [15, 60].

Operative Technique

Positioning

The majority of VATS operations are performed with the patient placed in the lateral decubitus position as is standard for a posterolateral thoracotomy. Depending on the procedure it may be helpful to tilt the patient either anteriorly or posteriorly to allow better placement of trocars. Similarly, Trendelenburg or reverse Trendelenburg positions may be helpful to allow gravity to help retract the lung out of the way so that better intraoperative exposure can be obtained.

It is also helpful to flex the operating table at the hip so that camera scope or operative instrumentation can easily be manipulated (Fig. 7). This positioning also allows the intercostal spaces to open wider allowing easier placement of trocars in the interspaces and presumably less pressure on the intercostal nerve while the trocar is in place [63].

Equipment

The standard video equipment used for laparoscopy, including telescopes and imaging systems, are the same for thoracoscopy, with a few exceptions. The standard telescope used is a 0°, 10-mm scope. There are some modifications that are helpful for VATS procedures. The standard telescope used for laparoscopy is longer than is necessary for thoracoscopic procedures. Some manufacturers have accommodated this by developing specific "thoracoscopes" that are approximately two-thirds the length of the standard telescopes used for laparoscopy. There are certain procedures, especially on the thoracic spine, in which the angle of 30° is optimal. Although most procedures are done with an end-viewing 0° scope, this angled viewing allows the surgeon to see around corners and specifically down into intervertebral disc spaces without interfering with operative instrumentation.

Carbon dioxide insufflation, which is standard in the abdomen, is seldom necessary in the chest [63]. When it is used because of inadequate collapse of the lung or to enhance the initial resorptive atelectasis, the pressure should be kept under 10–15 mmHg to avoid significant mediastinal shift [124].

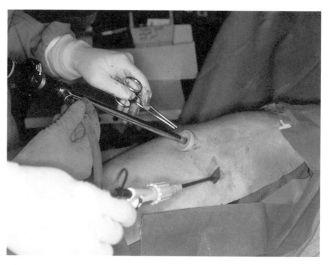

Fig. 8. Thoracoscopy being performed without trocars, with instruments placed directly through the chest wall in a thin patient

Instrumentation

Trocars are devices that are used as portals of entry to the thoracic cavity. Whereas sealed trocars are necessary because of carbon dioxide insufflation in the abdomen, an open system is sufficient in the chest. Standard open trocars are plastic tubes that are available in a variety of diameters from 3 to 15 mm. These devices allow placement of the telescope and operative instrumentation as well as stapling devices. Flexible trocars allow adaptation to the intercostal space, theoretically causing less pressure on the intercostal nerve. They also allow for placement of standard open thoracic instrumentation into the chest cavity.

In thin people a "trocarless" system can be used in which the instruments are placed directly through the chest wall (Fig. 8). When trocars are necessary, several reusable trocars are available. When possible, standard thoracic instrumentation is used. A useful modification is a set of long, curved ring forceps (Kaiser Pilling, Philadelphia, PA), which come in a variety of lengths and curvatures. This allows wide access to the chest cavity at a variety of different angles. These instruments have also proved very helpful in open thoracic procedures.

About half of the VATS procedures performed are lung resections. Standard lung resection is most easily performed by an endoscopic stapling device. The first device utilized for thoracoscopy was the Endo-GIA (see Chap. 4). The endoscopic stapler is also available in a 6-cm length and power-fired by a carbon dioxide cartridge. The length makes maneuvering in the chest cumbersome. The diameter of 15 mm compared with 12 mm for the Endo-GIA 30 can make placement in the intercostal spaces difficult.

Intercostal Approach Strategies

The standard approach to the thoracic cavity from a lateral position involves accurate placement of trocar sites. Most VATS procedures require three portals of entry, one for the telescope and two for hand instruments. If an operating scope, which includes a working port as well as a viewing port, is used, some procedures can be done through two, and

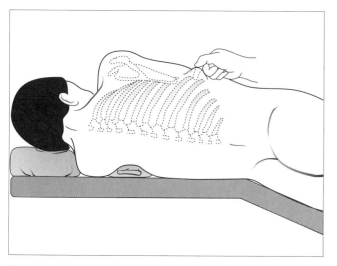

Fig. 7. The operating table is flexed at the hip to allow wide excursion of the thoracoscope and instruments. It also widens the intercostal spaces to allow easier access

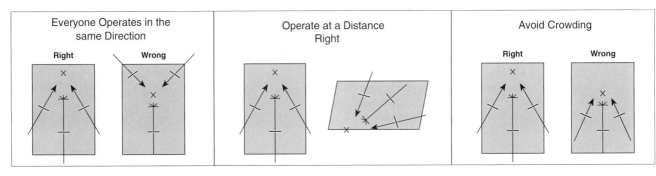

Fig. 9.   Rules for trocar position in thoracoscopy

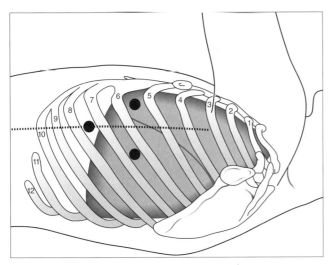

Fig. 10.   Standard arrangement of trocars for most thoracoscopic procedures

pleural procedures through only one, port. However, if anything more than a pleural procedure is planned, and a viewing-only scope is used, three ports are necessary. For some of the more complex procedures, including esophagomyotomy, which requires retraction of the lung and diaphragm, four or even five incisions may be necessary.

There are three principles that should be kept in mind when planning correct placement of trocars (Fig. 9). Firstly, the viewing telescope and instrumentation should all be placed so that they are facing in the same direction. If placement is such that the direction of the instrumentation comes back toward the viewing scope, mirror imaging occurs making correct movement of instruments within the chest virtually impossible. Secondly, the tendency to place the ports close to or immediately adjacent to the target area should be avoided. If the viewing scope and instruments are placed right on top of the target area, the panoramic view cannot be obtained and there is not enough room to maneuver the instrumentation. The trocar sites should be placed at a significant distance from the target area. Thirdly, there should be a significant distance between the viewing ports and the working ports. If the working ports are placed too close to the viewing port, the operative field will be obscured by the instrumentation. Also, the angle of retraction is not significant enough. Wide placement of the trocars allows instruments to be placed at the widest angles of retraction and placement possible.

With these principles in mind, the three trocars are placed. The typical arrangement is in an inverted triangle with the apex of the triangle being the lowest trocar site and the viewing scope being placed through this (Fig. 10). Working ports are then placed at the ends of the base of the inverted triangle.

For placement of the first trocar site, the seventh intercostal space is chosen. This is low enough in the chest so that a

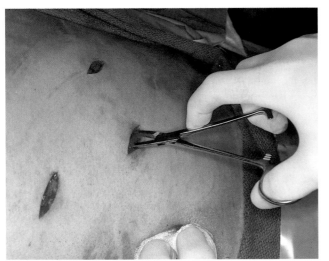
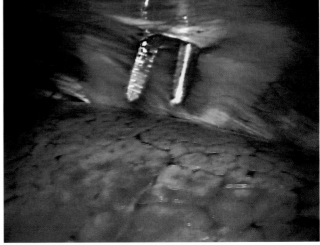

Figs. 11A, B.   Initiation of thoracoscopy by entry through the chest wall

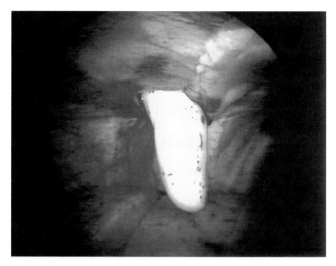

Fig. 12. Exploring digit to ensure that a free pleural space exists

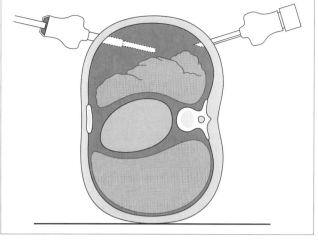

Fig. 13. Second trocar placed under direct vision

panoramic view of the thoracic cavity can be obtained, but high enough so that it is still above the diaphragm when the patient is in the lateral position. A 1-cm incision is made, and careful dissection through the intercostal muscles is performed with a hemostat (Figs. 11A and B). Once the pleural cavity is entered an exploring digit is placed through the incision to be sure that pleural symphysis is not present, and that the lung has dropped away from the chest wall (Fig. 12). Only when it is ascertained that a free pleural space is present should a trocar be introduced through the incision. Careful hemostasis is important, otherwise blood will drip down the trocar and onto the telescope continuously obscuring the lens. Once the initial trocar has been placed, a telescope is introduced through it. All further trocars are placed under direct vision in the thoracic cavity to avoid inadvertent injury to thoracic structures (Fig. 13). If there is difficulty ascertaining where correct placement of a trocar should be, an 18-gauge needle can be placed through the chest wall and its position located with the endoscope in the chest.

The standard position for the first trocar is usually in the seventh intercostal space in the midaxillary line. The second trocar is usually placed in the sixth intercostal space in the posterior axillary line, and the third in the fifth intercostal space in the anterior axillary line. The standard placement is modified based on the procedure being performed, e. g., all three trocar sites are moved one or two interspaces cephalad for performance of an apical blebectomy or a dorsal sympathectomy. All trocar sites are moved slightly more anterior for approaching posterior structures in the chest. For approaching anterior structures, such as the pericardium, trocars are placed more posteriorly so that there is more room for maneuverability. For procedures in the lower part of the chest, e. g., an esophagomyotomy on the distal esophagus or procedures around the diaphragmatic hiatus, placement of a monitor at the feet of the patient with the surgeon and assistant facing in that direction is preferred.

For most procedures we find it helpful to have the surgeon on one side of the table with his vision directed toward a video monitor on the opposite side of the table in line with the operative direction. The surgical assistant is usually on the opposite side of the table, again with the monitor directly facing him on the other side of the patient. For an increasing number of

procedures, however, we are finding it helpful to have the surgeon and assistant on the same side of the table. For instance, for thoracic spinal procedures as well as VATS lobectomy, it is helpful for both the surgeon and assistant to be on the same side of the table so that all work can be performed in the same direction (Fig. 14) [74].

At the initiation of the procedure, carbon dioxide insufflation is seldom necessary. However, if inadequate collapse of the lung exists, due to improper placement of the double-lumen tube or due to extensive mucous secretions obstructing resorptive atelectasis of the lung, a short period of carbon dioxide insufflation up to 10–15 mmHg may be helpful to enhance collapse. If visualization is still not adequate, a fan-type retractor can be used to retract the lung out of the way. Sometimes this is necessary only at the initiation of the procedure, and then subsequently the port through which the retractor was placed can be used for other purposes.

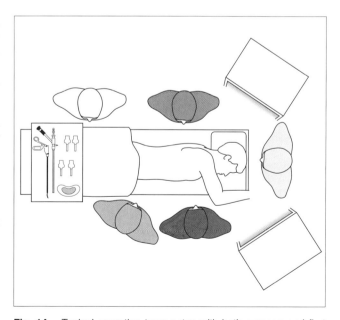

Fig. 14. Typical operative team setup with both surgeon and first assistant on the anterior side of the patient

Upon completion of the planned procedure, a chest tube is usually placed through one of the trocar sites. Since the thoracotomy incision with associated rib spreading has been eliminated, the role of the chest tube in causing postoperative pain has become more obvious. We have therefore significantly downsized the size of the chest tubes. We routinely employ size 20–24 Fr Argyle chest tubes if fluid accumulation or air leak is anticipated. For some procedures in which air or fluid is not anticipated, we do not use a chest tube; we simply watch to be sure that the lung is fully inflated at the end of the procedure and then ascertain complete expansion on a chest X-ray in the recovery room. Our routine practice for lung resections in which there is no air leak is placement of a chest tube at the end of the procedure. If there is no air leak after the patient has been coughing in the recovery room and the chest X-ray shows the lung to be fully expanded, the chest tube is immediately removed.

Postoperative Care

Surveillance in an intensive care unit is seldom necessary. Most patients are transferred from the recovery room to a general surgical floor, unless the patient has significant underlying medical problems or a general debilitated medical condition. We have found the intensive care unit to be necessary in less than 5 % of VATS procedures.

Postoperative pain management is through patient-controlled analgesia (PCA) pump. Morphine or meperidine is administered as long as a chest tube is in place. Once the chest tube is removed, parenteral narcotics are seldom necessary. Sometimes it is helpful to use an intercostal nerve block at the end of the procedure with 0.5 % Marcaine, which helps significantly in the first 24 h. Routine use is also made of nonsteroidal anti-inflammatory agents for postoperative pain management. Once the chest tube has been removed, oral pain medication is usually sufficient. Routine hospitalization after a VATS procedure varies with the procedure being performed, but is generally approximately 2 days. Outpatient treatment is possible for simple procedures performed early in the day such as lung biopsy or sympathectomy. Longer hospitalization is necessary for some of the more complex operations,

including VATS lobectomy, in which the duration of hospital stay is determined by chest tube duration. The average hospital stay after VATS lobectomy is 3–4 days.

Technique for Specific Procedures

Pleura

The standard VATS approach for pleural procedures involves usually only two trocars. If an operating scope is used that incorporates a working channel along with a viewing channel, only one port is necessary. If the procedure is being performed for a pleural effusion and loculations may be present, it is often helpful to ascertain the location of the effusion by needle aspiration so that the initial trocar can be placed in the proper position.

If the indication is given by an empyema, it is often helpful to enlarge one of the trocar sites to approximately 2 cm. This enlarged incision allows more efficacious débridement of the pleural peel and easy removal from the thoracic cavity. It also allows standard suction devices as well as copious amount of irrigation to be used.

When the VATS procedure is being performed for the diagnosis of indeterminate pleural effusion, the effusion is usually due to malignant involvement of the pleura [62]. Characteristic location of pleural involvement is somewhat dependent on the location of the primary tumor. Intra-abdominal malignancies, especially colon carcinoma, tend to spread through the diaphragmatic lymphatic and involve the diaphragm and lower portion of the lung. Breast cancer usually involves the chest wall lymphatics, and the anterior chest wall is most commonly involved. There is frequently no posterior chest wall involvement explaining the indeterminate nature of the effusion after blind percutaneous pleural biopsies.

When a pleurodesis is being performed for malignant effusions, talc is our sclerosing agent of choice. Although a number of other sclerosing agents have been used, including bleomycin, quinacrine, and tetracycline and derivatives, sterile talc is inexpensive, easy to administer, and has superior results than any of the other agents being effective

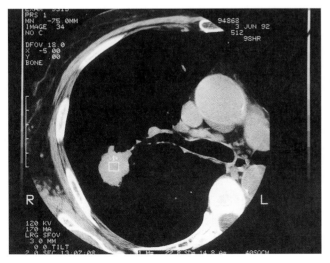
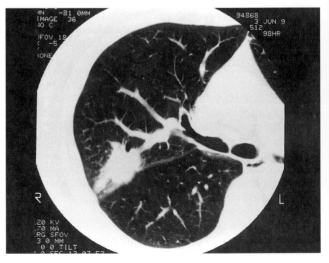

Figs. 15. A, B. **A.** A CT scan showing lung mass apparently deep within the lung and not accessible by VATS. **B.** Lung windows showing mass is adjacent to a fissure and therefore resectable by VATS

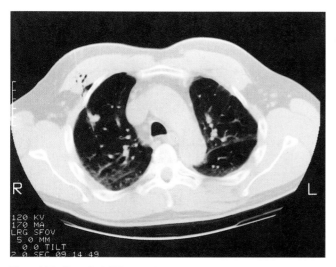

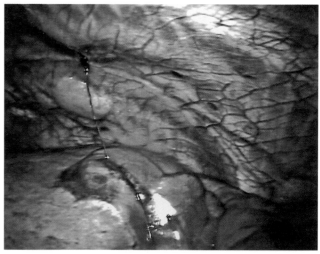

Figs. 16A, B. **A.** A CT scan showing preoperative placement of a localizing wire; **B.** Intraoperative view of localizing wire entering lung

in over 90 % of cases [8]. Usually, 4–6 g sterile talc is insufflated with a syringe through a dry suction device and aerosolized in the chest cavity ensuring complete coverage of both the parietal and visceral pleura (Fig. 2). As has been mentioned previously, for successful prevention of recurrence it is mandatory that pleural symphysis be obtained. If the lung is trapped secondary to tumor, the sclerosis will be ineffective.

Lung Resection

Wedge Resection
Wedge resection of the lung, whether being performed for resection of nodules or as a biopsy for diffuse disease, is most easily performed using endoscopic stapling devices. These allow a large sampling of lung tissue to be obtained in a minimal amount of time. The negative aspect, however, is the expense associated with endoscopic staplers.

Nodules that are candidates for resection are those that are located in the outer third of the lung and 1 cm in diameter or larger (Fig. 4). Some nodules that appear deep within the parenchyma of the lung upon initial inspection are in fact adjacent to the visceral pleura in one of the fissures upon closer examination of the CT scan (Figs. 15A and B). Lesions that are less than 1 cm in diameter and located more than 1 cm from the pleural surface should undergo some type of preoperative needle localization study (Figs. 16A and B). Techniques have been well described using needle localization similar to the system used for localizing nonpalpable breast cancer as well as injection of methylene blue in the visceral pleura adjacent to the lesion. Placement of the wire or injection of methylene blue allows prompt visual identification of the occult nodule at the time of thoracoscopy. With experience preoperative localization techniques are necessary in less than 5 % of nodules.

Nodules that are difficult to resect by VATS techniques include those that are in the suprahilar area along the medial aspect of the upper lobes as well as nodules in some of the basilar segments of the lower lobes that are not near an acute margin (Fig. 17). Because of this, it is sometimes difficult to apply the endoscopic stapler. Laser resective techniques are more appropriate for these nodules.

When the endoscopic stapler is used, a triangular-shaped portion of the lung is removed with at least a 1-cm margin around the tumor. The 3.5-mm staple length is typically used. The technique is easiest performed by alternating the stapler between the two working ports, one on each side of the nodule (Figs. 18A and B).

By a back-and-forth repetitive interchange between the two working ports, almost all lung nodules can be resected with this technique. If the correct angle of application of the stapler cannot be obtained through these two ports, sometimes interchanging the scope port with one of the stapler ports will allow easier resection.

It should also be mentioned that a finger can be introduced through one of the trocar sites to digitally palpate the lung (Fig. 19). If difficulty is anticipated in locating one of the nodules at the time of surgery, one of the trocar sites should be placed in the chest adjacent to the lung in which the nodule is anticipated to be located. The lung can then be brought into apposition with a probing index finger and most occult nodules can be palpated by this technique.

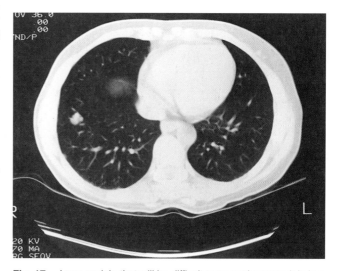

Fig. 17. Lung nodule that will be difficult to resect because it is in a basilar segment near a flat surface of the lung

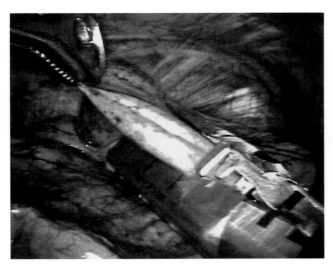 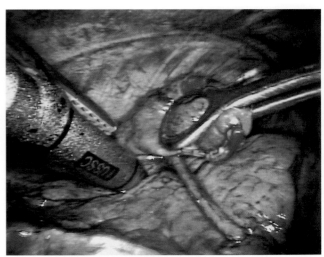

Figs. 18A, B. **A.** Technique for VATS stapled lung resection with grasper placed from the left and stapler from the right; **B.** Stapler and grasper are then alternated through opposite ports

When the endoscopic stapler cannot be easily applied to the lung, the nd:YAG laser can be used. The laser is used in the noncontact mode at approximately 30–35 mW of energy. In our experience, the laser is more effective than either the argon beam coagulator or precision electrocautery for resecting the nodule and preventing air leaks after resection. If a raw surface of the lung remains after laser resection, application of fibrin glue may help prevent postoperative air leaks.

VATS Lobectomy

The placement of incisions for a VATS lobectomy includes two trocars in the seventh and eighth intercostal spaces in the mid- and posterior axillary lines as well as an "accessory" or "utility" incision in the fifth intercostal space in the anterior axillary line approximately overlying the major fissure (Fig. 20). For upper lobectomies the placement of an additional port in the third intercostal space on the anterior axillary line is helpful for visualization of the superior aspect of the hilum, specif-

ically the anterior and apical posterior segmental pulmonary arteries.

The technique for lower lobectomies begins with division of the inferior pulmonary ligament and division of the inferior pulmonary vein with a vascular endostapler. Dissection is continued up on the posterior aspect until the bronchus is identified and divided with a 3.5-mm endoscopic stapler (Fig. 21). We have found that this inferior approach, rather than through the fissure, significantly expedites dissection and diminishes postoperative air leaks. Only after the vein and bronchus have been divided is the pulmonary artery managed. The superior segmental pulmonary artery is usually taken separately, and then the remaining pulmonary artery is also divided with a vascular endoscopic stapler. Any lung tissue at the fissure is also divided with the stapler to prevent postoperative air leaks.

If a lot of tissue remains, a 60-mm endoscopic stapler may occasionally be used; however, this is not our routine practice.

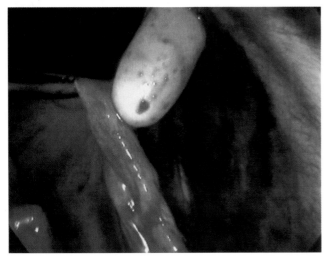 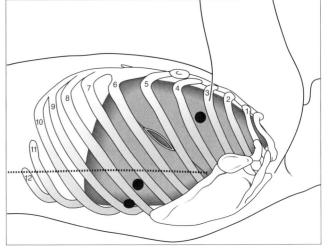

Fig. 19. Digital palpation of the lung with finger placed through a trocar site

Fig. 20. Incisions for VATS lobectomy

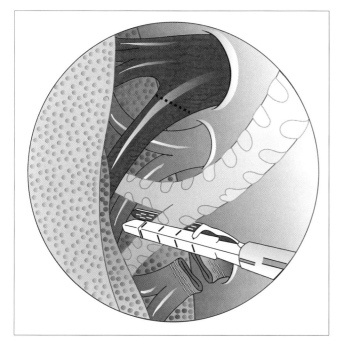

Fig. 21. Technique of VATS left lower lobectomy approached from the inferior aspect

For a right middle lobectomy the pulmonary vein is first divided, followed by the bronchus, and lastly, the artery. Again, none of the dissection is done through the fissure so that postoperative air leak is minimized.

The technique for upper lobectomy is similar involving division of the upper lobe vein first from the anterior aspect, then the upper lobe bronchus is divided from the posterior aspect, and lastly, the arteries.

If the fissure is incomplete, dissection can be very difficult and assessment is made early in the procedure of whether conversion to an open thoracotomy is necessary. In addition, the presence of extensive hilar lymphadenopathy makes dissection of the pulmonary artery difficult and sometimes hazardous. If the surgeon feels uncomfortable with the dissection because of lymphadenopathy, again, conversion to an open procedure should be considered.

At the completion of resection, the specimen is removed through the "accessory" incision (Fig. 22). No rib spreading is used if possible neither at the time of specimen removal nor at any time during the procedure. Postoperative pain is related to rib spreading, and any traction on the intercostal spaces negates the advantages of the VATS technique.

Several pneumonectomies have also been performed and reported by the VATS technique [110]. As with the open procedure, the technique is simpler and more straightforward than a lobectomy. The following maneuvers are helpful for a VATS pneumonectomy: Firstly, for safety reasons, when the right or left main pulmonary artery is divided with an endoscopic stapler, a vascular clamp should first be placed proximal to the stapler in case of inadvert misfiring or malfunction. Secondly, although a 3.5-mm endoscopic stapler is of sufficient staple length for a lobar bronchus, it is too short for the mainstem bronchus.

Secure closure of the mainstem bronchus requires placement of a TA 30 4.8-mm stapler across the bronchus. This stapler is difficult to place with the specimen in place; therefore, Roviaro and associates have advised removing the specimen by dividing the bronchus more distally with the endoscopic stapler, and once the specimen has been removed, the 4.8-mm TA stapler can be easily placed across the mainstem bronchus and the bronchus is completely resected leaving no significant bronchial stump.

Although we have come to believe that there are significant advantages to the VATS technique for lobectomy in terms of lessened postoperative pain and morbidity, it is a technically difficult procedure to master, and significant endoscopic experience is necessary.

Mediastinal Procedures

Thymectomy
A total thymectomy can be performed through either side of the chest, but it has been our preference to perform it from the left. Three trocars are necessary and are placed as shown in

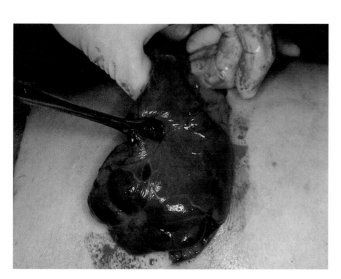

Fig. 22. Extraction of the resected lobe through the accessory incision without rib spreading

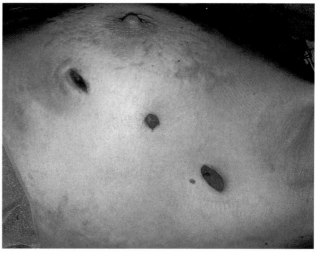

Fig. 23. Incisions for VATS thymectomy

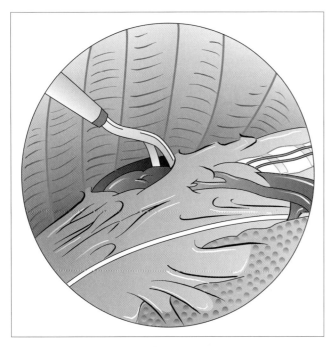

Fig. 24. Thymectomy by VATS from the left chest. Thymus gland is dissected from the retrosternal area

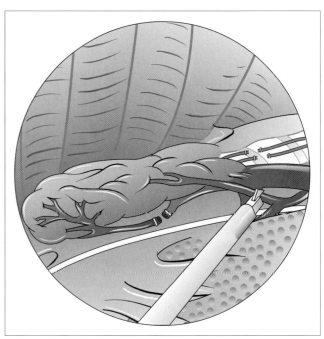

Fig. 26. The arterial supply to the thymus gland from the internal mammary artery is then doubly clipped

Figure 23 [51]. Dissection is begun at the inferior aspect on the left side and is carried just anterior to the left phrenic nerve. By a combination of sharp and blunt dissection, the thymus gland is dissected off the pericardium across to the right pleura.

At this point it is most helpful to dissect the thymus off the retrosternal area (Fig. 24). Next, from the inferior aspect the thymic vein branches from the innominate vein are identified and closed with endoscopic clips (Fig. 25). The arterial blood supply from the left and right internal mammary arteries are identified and doubly clipped (Fig. 26). The remainder of the thymectomy involves dissection of the superior poles in the cervical area above the innominate vein (Fig. 27). Complete extracapsular dissection of the thymus gland with total exenteration of all anterior mediastinal tissue should be performed (Figs. 28A and B).

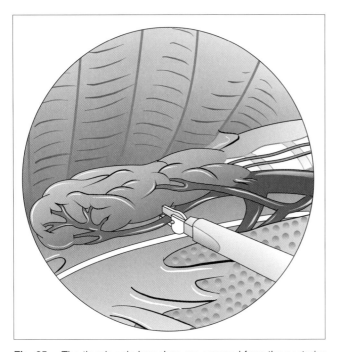

Fig. 25. The thymic vein branches are exposed from the posterior aspect and clipped

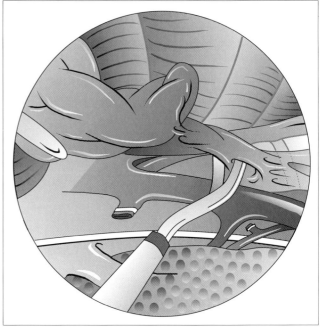

Fig. 27. Superior poles of the thymus gland in the cervical area above the innominate vein are dissected last

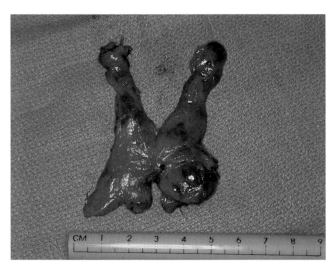
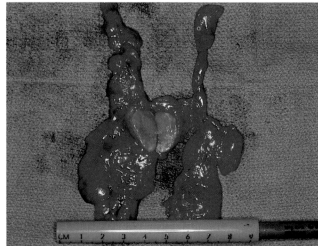

Figs. 28A, B. Resected thymus specimens

The specimen is then removed through one of the anterior trocar sites, and the bed of the thymus gland is examined to be sure that complete hemostasis has been obtained. A chest tube is usually not necessary.

Mediastinal Masses
Access to the anterior mediastinum is gained through trocars placed posterior to the midaxillary line (Fig. 29). In a similar manner, for operations in the posterior mediastinum, trocars are placed anterior to the midaxillary line as shown in Figure 30 [48]. Whether the procedure is being performed for biopsy of a mediastinal mass, excision of mediastinal cysts, or excision of a posterior mediastinal mass, the dissection is relatively straightforward once the trocars are well placed. As mentioned previously, left thoracoscopy has replaced anterior mediastinotomy (Chamberlain procedure) for performing staging of left-sided lung cancer [79]. Better visualization and access to the aortopulmonary window, anterior mediastinum, and subcarinal and inferior pulmonary ligament areas offers a superior method of staging.

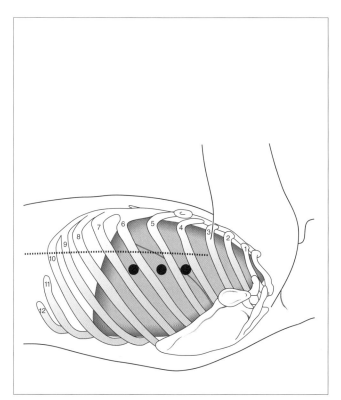

Fig. 29. Trocar placement posterior to the midaxillary line used for approaching the anterior mediastinum

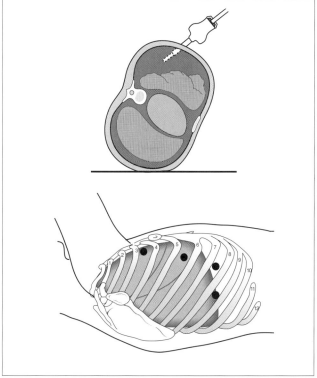

Fig. 30. Trocars are placed anterior to the midaxillary line for approaching the posterior mediastinum

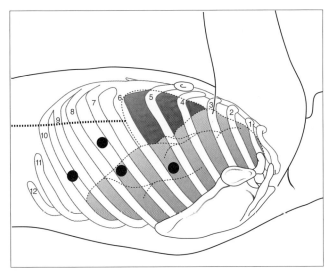

Fig. 31.   Trocar placement for VATS pericardiectomy

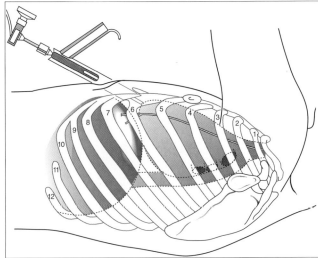

Fig. 33.   Approach for "video" subxiphoid pericardiectomy

Pericardiectomy

VATS pericardiectomy can be performed from either side of the chest. Trocars are placed posterior to the midaxillary line especially on the left side to avoid the distended pericardium (Fig. 31).

Some surgeons prefer to perform a pericardiectomy through the right chest because of the larger space for handling of instruments and visualization. Extensive pericardiectomy can be performed from both sides. If there is associated pleural effusion or parenchymal lung pathology, we usually select that side as the preferred method for approach. Upon entry into the chest the phrenic nerve is identified, and large swatches of pericardium are removed both anterior and posterior to the phrenic nerve leaving a bridge of pericardium beneath (Fig. 32). Electrocautery may be used cautiously for hemostasis from a bleeding pericardial edge being careful to retract the pericardium away from the heart.

For malignant pericardial effusions the subxiphoid approach is preferred obviating the need for general endotra-

cheal anesthesia with a double-lumen tube, arterial line, monitoring, etc. We recently have tried a video mediastinoscope for the subxiphoid approach in which a more extensive portion of pericardium can be removed than by traditional subxiphoid approaches (Fig. 33).

Trauma

As mentioned previously, the role of VATS in trauma includes nonexsanguinating hemothorax, retained or clotted hemothorax , and possible examination for injury to major vessels. The technique for management of hemothorax is similar to that of empyema.

A standard suction device is used to evacuate clotted blood. The curved-ring Kaiser-Pilling forceps are very helpful for extraction of clots out of the posterior gutter. If ongoing bleeding is a problem, an intercostal vessel can usually be controlled and ligated. Occasionally, a continuing hemorrhage from a lung injury can be either sealed with an endoscopic stapler for oversewn using endoscopic suturing techniques if the lesion is peripheral.

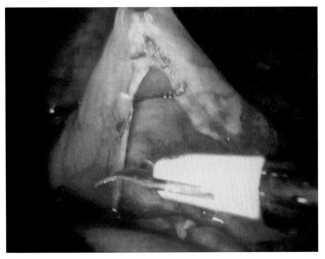

Fig. 32.   Wide swatch of posterior pericardium being resected

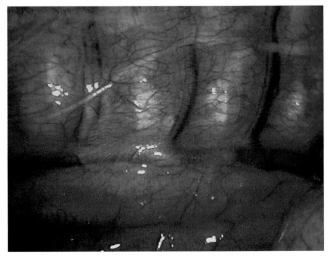

Fig. 34.   VATS view of the thoracic spine

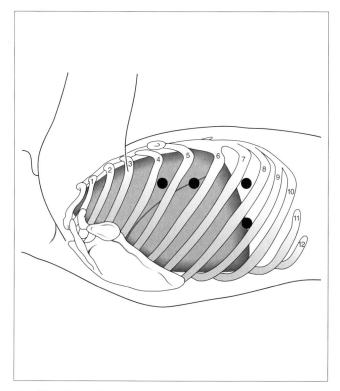

Fig. 35. Trocar placement in a reverse "L" arrangement for spine procedures

Spine
The technique for thoracoscopic spine surgery varies somewhat from the standard VATS techniques. The position of trocars is rotated 90 ° so that the view of the spine is horizontal across the operative field (Fig. 34). Trocar placement as shown in Figure 35 involves three trocars in the anterior axillary line usually in the third, fifth, and seventh intercostal spaces as well as a port in the seventh intercostal space in the midaxillary line for the camera. We find that these procedures are best carried out with both the surgeon and the assistant on the same side of the table (Fig. 14). The majority of thoracic spine procedures, including discectomy, corpectomy, drainage of intervertebral disc space abscesses as well as placement of fusion cages can now be done by endoscopic techniques. Modifications of standard orthopedic instrumentation is necessary, however, to facilitate the endoscopic approach. Pituitary rongeurs, Kerrisons, and Cobb elevators have all been elongated and modified for endoscopic use. The same operative technique as is standard for open operations is performed through this minimally invasive method of access. We have found that the 30 ° angled telescope is most helpful for spine procedures allowing direct viewing into the intervertebral disc space without interfering with operative instrumentation [103].

Complications

The same complications that have been observed after standard open thoracic surgery may occur with VATS [52]. However, because VATS is a less invasive approach and postoperative pain has been demonstrated to be less, hopefully the

Table 6. Complications of VATS common to any thoracic procedure

Death
Wound infection
Respiratory insufficiency
Prolonged air leak
Arrhythmia
Postoperative bleeding

postoperative morbidity will also be diminished. Table 6 lists the standard complications common to any thoracic procedure. All of these complications, including pain and respiratory insufficiency, are indeed less common with VATS than after open procedures. The exception, however, is prolonged air leak. Prolonged air leak seems to be more of a problem with VATS than with open procedures for several reasons: Firstly, endoscopic management of air leaks can be very difficult. Thoracoscopic surgeons, for the most part, are not always as familiar with endoscopic suturing techniques for oversewing lesions to the lung as they are in the open situation. Secondly, because VATS is less invasive, patients with severe bullous emphysema that were not candidates for traditional open surgery have now become accessible to therapy. Therefore, the underlying lung substrate being operated upon tends to leak more in the VATS patient than in the open situation.

Numerous techniques have been described for management of air leaks in the VATS situation. Among these are the use of the nd:YAG laser for obliteration of the raw surface of lung or bullous that is leaking. The laser seems to be more effective than either precision electrocautery or the argon beam coagulator for obtaining pneumostasis. Once the area of lung has been treated with the laser, application of fibrin tissue glue adds to the safety in preventing postoperative air leaks.

The use of bovine pericardium to reinforce staple lines as well as for the use as suture pledgets to bolster the suture used to oversew the leak has been very useful for managing air leaks in bullous emphysema. If the air leak persists, an apical pleural tent that can be taken down by VATS has been found very helpful in managing the leak.

The second type of complications associated with VATS are those that are specifically related to the procedure. They are listed in Table 7. The risk of uncontrolled hemorrhage is a real one, especially during VATS lobectomies in which operative maneuvers are performed on major vascular structures without the ability to immediately control them. Fortunately, in the initial series of VATS lobectomies from four major centers encompassing over 300 VATS lobectomies, there have been only two conversions to open procedures because of bleeding with no mortality.

Table 7. Complications specific to VATS

Uncontrolled bleeding
Hemodynamic compromise
Tumor seeding in the chest wall
Intercostal neuralgia
Inability to locate nodule
Incomplete staging
Compromise of procedure

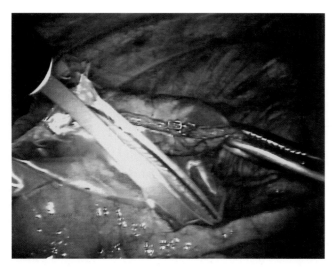

Fig. 36. Specimen containing a possibly malignant tumor being placed in a specimen bag to prevent potential tumor seeding during extraction

Other complications specific to VATS include intercostal neuralgia from trocar placement, which is due to pressure on the nerve at the time of the procedure. This can be minimized by using as small a trocar as possible and applying as little levering as possible. Levering can be minimized by curved instrumentation and angled scopes.

Another complication distressingly frequently being seen with VATS is the tumor seeding in the chest wall. With the removal of unprotected lung specimens containing tumor through the chest wall, tumor implantation along the track has been reported. It is mandatory when a lung is resected for malignancy, and a tumor will potentially be in contact with the chest wall during extraction from the thoracic cavity that the specimen be placed in a protective bag (Fig. 36). Numerous endoscopic specimen bags are available for protected removal of a specimen through a trocar site, and thus hopefully avoiding the complication of tumor seeding.

Table 8 lists hazards to be avoided, rather than true complications of the procedure. In the initial stages of the learning curve of VATS procedures, there is the tendency for operative times to be longer than the equivalent procedure being performed by open techniques. As the surgeon becomes more familiar with the VATS procedures, typically these operative times are shorter than the same procedure performed by open techniques.

If, however, it is apparent that the operative time is significantly prolonged by the VATS procedures, consideration should be given to conversion to an open technique so that the procedure can be completed within a reasonable period of time.

Table 8. Hazards to be avoided during VATS

Avoid prolonged operative time
Be aware of your place on the "learning curve"
Do not compromise procedure
Conversion to open procedure does not mean failure
"Can" does not mean "should"

In a similar manner the surgeon should be aware of his place in the learning curve. The complex or advanced VATS procedures should not be attempted early in the surgeon's experience. The surgeon should not feel pressured to accomplish a procedure solely by VATS techniques. If surgical principles have to be compromised in order to accomplish a procedure via a minimally invasive access, the VATS approach should be abandoned and conversion to an open procedure preferred. Conversion to an open operation should not be viewed as a failure on the part of the surgeon, but rather the exercise of mature surgical judgment.

Training

Numerous opportunities exist for the training of the inexperienced thoracic surgeon to VATS techniques. The surgeon who has no experience with endoscopic surgical techniques should begin his training in the inanimate trainer model. A thoracic trainer helps the surgeon to convert from the traditional surgical techniques with which the procedure has been performed with the surgeon looking directly at his instrumentation to a situation in which the only visualization is on a two-dimensional video monitor. The hand/eye coordination required for this surgical technique is different from that for open techniques. The inexperienced surgeon should become an expert in endoscopic techniques before proceeding on to a live situation.

The animal laboratory offers a unique experience for the surgeon to gain knowledge of endoscopic techniques. A live animal model is an opportunity for the inexperienced surgeon to develop the new hand/eye coordination necessary to perform endoscopic procedures as well as to become familiar with all the necessary equipment in a live nonhuman situation.

In the further course surgeons who have practice in simple procedures may become more experienced in the advanced procedures before attempting them in the human situation. For example, most experienced laparoscopic surgeons have become trained in the laparoscopic Nissen procedure by extensive animal laboratory experience first. For thoracic procedures the surgeon who is already experienced in VATS techniques and is considering performing a VATS lobectomy or a Heller myotomy for achalasia should first feel comfortable performing these operations in the animal model.

When the training and preceptor requirements have been satisfied, the surgeon should first attempt simple cases such as drainage of pleural effusions with pleurodesis, biopsy of pleural masses, or simple lung biopsies. After he or she becomes more experienced with the simple procedures, gradual advancement of the degree of complexity is appropriate. For example, in our own institution we had experience with 150 VATS procedures before we attempted our first VATS lobectomy.

We have also found it helpful in training to perform video-assisted open procedures. It is very helpful for a surgeon training himself to do a procedure by the open technique and place a video camera and scope through the open incision. He can then gain experience with the video-assisted techniques in the open situation in which he is more comfortable operating. By doing a "video-assisted" open procedure, the surgeon will gradually become more comfortable performing the procedure while using the video monitor, rather than direct visualization through the incision. Similarly, when the experienced thoracoscopic surgeon is attempting advanced procedures, the same type of "video-assisted" open procedure may again be appropriate. For instance, when attempting a VATS lobectomy, an open incision should be used first with the video camera placed in the chest and the procedure performed by a combination of open and video-assisted techniques. By this combination of both open and video-assisted techniques, gradually the thoracic surgeon will be able to progress to totally VATS techniques.

Credentialing

Only surgeons who are entitled to perform thoracic procedures by the open technique should proceed to perform thoracic procedures by the endoscopic techniques. Although the operation is less invasive than the open technique, major intrathoracic procedures with all the attendant complications are still present. The ability to convert a VATS procedure to an open procedure to manage a complication should be in the armamentarium of a surgeon. In order to be credentialed in VATS surgery, the surgeon should either be a thoracic surgeon or a general surgeon who already has thoracic privileges and has been experienced in thoracic techniques [85].

Proper credentialing should also include a laboratory course with an inanimate trainer portion as well as an animal laboratory portion. It is also appropriate depending on the local situation for a period of preceptorship involving somewhere between 5 and 10 proctored cases before full credentialing is obtained.

Conclusions and Future Directions

Video-assisted thoracic surgery has been a valuable addition to the specialty of thoracic surgery. However, like any new development in medicine or medical technology, it takes a period of time to ascertain the proper role for a procedure. The stages of development of new advancements in medical tech-

Table 9. Stages of development of medical technology

Discovery of new technology
Isolated successful application
Discovery of limitations
Definition of clinical usefulness

nology are listed in Table 9. As a procedure is introduced it is found to have an appropriate clinical application. Once it is found to have an isolated application, it is attempted in multiple other situations. In this manner the limitations of the procedure are developed and a definition of clinical usefulness is obtained. However, this definition of appropriateness is not a static position. As a surgeon becomes more experienced and advances along the learning curve, and as medical technology improves and makes the procedures more surgeon-friendly, the definition is a continuum that changes. What is not appropriate presently may in fact be appropriate in a few years from now as technological advancements and surgeon experience make the operation easier. As an example certain diseases, such as recurrent spontaneous pneumothorax and malignant pleural effusions, are optimally managed by VATS techniques. Other procedures, such as VATS lobectomy, although it has been demonstrated in fairly large experiences

that it can be performed safely, have not been demonstrated to have significant benefits that outweigh the risk, and in our opinion should remain investigational presently [57]. However, as more surgeons become more experienced, as the technique of VATS lobectomy is further refined and technical advancement continues, such as articulating staplers, then 2 years from now VATS lobectomy *may* become the optimal method of performing formal lung resections.

There will be a gradual evolutionary process in the years to come during which a larger percentage of thoracic procedures will be performed by the video-assisted approach. It will not be an explosive process, but it will be gradual assimilation of video-assisted techniques into the mainstream of thoracic surgery. Laparoscopic cholecystectomy was a revolution in general surgery, an introduction that is not likely to be repeated in the foreseeable future. Whereas laparoscopic cholecystectomy was a *revolution,* everything else is an *evolution.*

Several technological advances would appear to make all endoscopic surgery somewhat more surgeon-friendly in the future. Three-dimensional imaging technology is rapidly improving, which will remove the negative aspects of current two-dimensional imaging. Endoscopic suturing techniques will become technically easier with three-dimensional imaging.

Real-time magnetic resonance imaging (MRI) promises to make some procedures, including thoracoscopic spine surgery, able to be performed while the surgeon is watching an MR image, rather than a visual image, in real time. Ultimately, this technology may be used for locating occult lung nodules, also by giving the surgeon truly "X-ray vision."

Articulating staplers promise to make lung resection easier.

Virtual reality offers promise for educational purposes similar to airplane pilot training in jet trainers, and the endoscopic surgeon of the future will be able to develop and practice endoscopic procedures in a virtual reality trainer before attempting them in a live patient.

Several laboratories worldwide are examining cardiac applications of video-assisted techniques including coronary artery bypass, valve replacement, and intracardiac defect repairs. Although some of these techniques hold promise, they are all in the very early stages of development and await significant improvement in both the technology arena as well as surgeon expertise.

The past 4 years have been an exciting time in thoracic surgery due to the introduction of a new method of approach to thoracic procedures. By offering a less invasive approach to our standard operations, which hopefully results in less morbidity, especially in postoperative pain, thoracic surgical procedures will become more widely used. The same surgical principles that we have all learned and adhered to should be held intact. If we are able to perform our time-honored procedures by more patient-friendly techniques, our patients will be the true beneficiaries of the development of video-assisted thoracic surgery.

References

1. Aelony Y, King R, Boutin C: Thoracoscopic talc poudrage pleurodesis for chronic recurrent pleural effusions. Ann Intern Med 115 (1991) 778–782.
2. Axford T C, Clair D G, Bertagnolli M M, Mentzer S J, Sugarbaker D J: Staged antrectomy and thoracoscopic truncal vagotomy for perforated peptic ulcer disease. Ann Thorac Surg 55 (1993) 1571–1573.

3. BENSARD D D, MCINTYRE R C, WARING B J, SIMON J S: Comparison of video-assisted lung biopsy to open lung biopsy in the evaluation of interstitial lung disease. Chest 103 (1993) 765.

4. BERGQUIST S, NORDENSTAM H: Thoracoscopy and pleural biopsy in the diagnosis of pleurisy. Scand J Respir Dis 47 (1966) 64.

5. BRANDT H J: Diagnostic methods in pleural disease including thoracoscopy and biopsy. Thorax Chirg 22 (1947) 371.

6. BRANDT H, LODDENKENPER R, J. MAI: Atlas of diagnostic thoracoscopy: indications-techniques. Thieme Medical Publishers, New York (1985) 1–46.

7. BRANTIGAN O C, MUELLER E: Surgical treatment of pulmonary emphysema. Am Surg 23 (1957) 789–804.

8. BRESTICKER M A, OBA J, LOCICERO J, GREENE R: Optimal pleurodesis: a comparison study. Ann Thorac Surg 55 (2) (1993) 264–266.

9. CALHOUN P, FELDMAN P S, ARMSTRONG P ET AL.: The clinical outcome of needle aspirations of the lung when cancer is not diagnosed. Ann Thorac Surg 41 (1986) 592.

10. CANNON W B, VIERRA M A, CANNON A: Thoracoscopy for spontaneous pneumothorax. Ann Thorac Surg 56 (1993) 686–687.

11. CERFOLIO R J, ALLEN M S, TRASTEK V F ET AL.: Pulmonary resection of metastatic hypernephroma. Ann Thorac Surg (in press).

12. CHAMBERS A F, TUCK A B: ras-Responsive genes and tumor metastasis. Crit Rev Oncog 4 (2) (1993) 95–114.

13. CHAMPAULT G, BELHASSEN A, RIZK N, BOUTRLIER P: Duodenal ulcer: value of truncal vagotomy through thoracoscopy. Ann Chir 54 (1993) 240–243.

14. CHISHOLM M., CHUNG S C, SUNDERLAND T, LEONG H T, LI A K: Thoracoscopic vagotomy: a new role for the laparoscope. Br J Surg 79 (1992) 254.

15. CLAES G, DROTT C, GOTHBERG G: Thoracoscopy for autonomic disorders. Ann Thorac Surg 56 (1993) 715–716.

16. COLLARD J M, LENGELE B, OTTE J B, KESTENS P J: En bloc and standard esophagectomies by thoracoscopy. Ann Thorac Surg 56 (1993) 675–679.

17. COOPER J D, TRULOCK E P, TRIANTAFILLOU A N ET AL.: Bilateral pneumectomy (volume reduction) for chronic obstructive pulmonary disease. J Thorac Cardiovasc Surg 1995 (in press).

18. CROW J, SLAVIN G, KREEL L: Pulmonary metastases: a patho-logic and radiologic study. Cancer 47 (1981) 2595.

19. DANIEL T M, TRIBBLE C G, RODGERS B M: Thoracoscopy and talc poudrage for pneumothoraces and effusions. Ann Thorac Surg 50 (1990) 186–189.

20. DESLAURIERS J, MEHRAN R J: Role of thoracoscopy in the diagnosis and management of pleural diseases. Semin Thorac Cardiovasc Surg 5 (4) (1993) 284–293.

21. DOWLING R D, FERSON P F, LANDRENEAU R J: Thoracoscopic resection of pulmonary metastases. Chest 102 (1992) 1450.

22. DOWLING R D, KEENAN R J, FERSON P F, LANDRENEAU R J: Video-assisted thoracoscopic surgery for pulmonary metastases. Ann Thorac Surg 56 (1993) 772.

23. FEINS R H: The role of thoracoscopy in the AIDS/immunocompromised patient. Ann Thorac Surg 56 (1993) 649–650.

24. FERGUSON M K, LITTLE A G, SKINNER D B: Current concepts in the management of postoperative chylothorax. Ann Thorac Surg 40 (1985) 542–545.

25. FERGUSON M: Thoracoscopy for empyema, bronchopleural fistula, and chylothorax. Ann Thorac Surg 54 (1993) 644–645.

26. FERSON P F, LANDRENEAU R J, DOWLING R D ET AL.: Thoracoscopic vs. open lung biopsy for the diagnosis of diffuse infiltrative lung disease. J Thorac Cardiovasc Surg 105 (1993) 194.

27. FLEISHER A G, MCELVANEY G, LAWSON L ET AL.: Surgical management of spontaneous pneumothorax in patients with acquired immunodeficiency syndrome. Ann Thorac Surg 45 (1988) 21–23.

28. FORESTIER M, DURET M: Nécessité de la biopsie pleurale pour le diagnostic de l'endotheliome de la plèvre. Presse Med 32 (1943) 467.

29. GAENSLER E A, CUGELL D W, KNUDSON R J, FITZGERALD M X: Surgical management of emphysema. Clin Chest Med 4 (1983) 443–463.

30. GINSBERG R J, RUBINSTEIN LV: Patients with T1NO non-small-cell lung cancer (abstract 304). Lung Cancer 7 (Suppl) (1991) 83.

31. GORENSTEIN L A, PUTNAM J B, NATARAJAN M A ET AL.: Improved survival after resection of pulmonary metastases from malignant melanoma. Ann Thorac Surg 52 (1991) 204.

32. GOSSOT D, FOURQUIER P, CÉLÉRIER M.: Thoracoscopic esophagectomy: technique and initial results. Ann Thorac Surg 56 (1993) 667–670.

33. GRAEBER G M, JONES D R: The role of thoracoscopy in thoracic trauma. Ann Thorac Surg 56 (1993) 646–648.

34. GRANKE K, FISCHER C R, GAGO O ET AL.: The efficacy and timing of operative intervention for spontaneous pneumothorax. Ann Thorac Surg 42 (1986) 540–542.

35. GUIDICELLI R, THOMAS P, LONGON T ET AL.: Comparative study of lobectomy through conventional thoracotomy and video-assisted thoracoscopy. Ann Thorac Surg 1995 (in press).

36. HARPOLE D H, JOHNSON C M, WOLFE W G ET AL.: An analysis of 945 cases of pulmonary metastatic melanoma. J Thorac Cardiovasc Surg 103 (1992) 743.

37. HARTMAN D L, GAITHER J M, KESSLER K A, MYLET D M, BROWN J W, MATHUR P N: Comparison of insufflated talc under thoracoscopic guidance with standard tetracycline and bleomycin pleurodesis for control of malignant pleural effusions. J Thorac Cardiovasc Surg 105 (4) (1993) 743–747.

38. HAZELRIGG S R, MACK M J, LANDRENEAU R J, ACUFF T E, SEIFERT P, AUER J E: Thoracoscopic pericardiectomy for effusive pericardial disease. Ann Thorac Surg 56 (1993) 792–795.

39. HAZELRIGG S R, MACK M J, LANDRENEAU R J: Video-assisted thoracic surgery for mediastinal disease. Chest Surg Clin North Am 3 (2) (1993) 283–297.

40. HAZELRIGG S R, MACK M J: Thoracoscopic surgery. Surger for Autonomic Disorders 15 (1992) 189–202.

41. HAZELRIGG S R, LANDRENEAU R J, MACK M J, ACUFF T, SEIFERT P E, AUER J E, MAGEE M: Thoracoscopic stapled resection for spontaneous pneumothorax. J Thorac Cardiovasc Surg 105 (1993) 389–393.

42. HAZELRIGG S R, LANDRENEAU R J, MACK M J, ACUFF T E: Thoracoscopic resection of mediastinal cysts. Ann Thorac Surg 56 (1993) 659–660.

43. HAZELRIGG S R: Thoracoscopic management of pulmonary blebs and bullae. Semin Thorac Cardiovasc Surg 5 (4) (1993) 327–331.

44. HORSWELL J L: Anesthetic techniques for thoracoscopy. Ann Thorac Surg 56 (1993) 624–629.

45. HUCKER I, BHATNAGAR N K, AL-JILAIHAWI A N, FORRESTER-WOOD C P: Thoracoscopy in the diagnosis and management of recurrent pleural effusions. Ann Thorac Surg 52 (1991) 1145– 1147.

46. INDERBITZI R G, FURRER M, STRIFFELER H, ALTHAUS U: Thoracoscopic pleurectomy for treatment of complicated spontaneous pneumothorax. J Cardiovasc Surg 105 (1993) 84–88.

47. INDERBITZI R G, KREBS T, STIRNEMANN P, ALTHAUS U: Treatment of postoperative chylothorax by fibrin glue application under thoracoscopic view with use of local anesthesia. J Thorac Cardiovasc Surg 104 (1992) 209–210.

48. JACOBAEUS H C: Endopleural operations by means of a thoracoscope. Beitr Klin Tuberk 35 (1915) 1.

49. JACOBAEUS H C: Possibility of the use of the cystoscope for investigation of serous cavities. Münch Med Wochenschr 57 (1910) 2090.

50. JACOBAEUS H C: The cauterization of adhesions in pneumothorax treatment of tuberculosis. Surg Gynecol Obstet 32 (1921) 493.

51. JACOBAEUS H C: The practical importance of thoracoscopy in surgery of the chest. 34 (1922) 209.

52. KAISER L R, BAVARIA J E: Complications of thoracoscopy. Ann Thorac Surg 56 (3) (1993) 796–798.

53. KAISER L R: Diagnostic and therapeutic uses of pleuroscopy (thoracoscopy) in lung cancer. Surg Clin North Am 67 (1987) 1081.

54. KEENAN R J, LANDRENEAU R J, MACK M J ET AL.: Video-assisted thoracoscopy for the diagnosis and management of pleural diseases. Ann Rev Respir Dis 147 (1993) 1737.

55. KERN K A, PASS H I, ROTH J A: Treatment of metastatic cancer to lung. In: DeVita V T, Hellman S, Rosenbert S A (eds.): Cancer principles and practice of oncology. J. B. Lippincott, Philadelphia (1989) 69–100.

56. KIRBY T J, MACK M J, LANDRENEAU R J, RICE T R: Lobectomy: VATS vs. thoracotomy. A randomized study. J Thorac Cardiovasc Surg 1995 (in press).

57. KIRBY T J, MACK M J, LANDRENEAU R J, RICE T W: Randomized comparison of VATS lobectomy versus lobectomy performed through muscle-sparing thoracotomies. J Thorac Cardiovasc Surg 1995 (in press).

58. KIRBY T J, RICE T W: Thoracoscopic lobectomy. Ann Thorac Surg 56 (1993) 784–786.

59. KRASNA M J, MCLAUGHLIN J S: Thoracoscopic lymph node staging for esophageal cancer. Ann Thorac Surg 56 (1993) 671–674.

60. KUX M: Thoracoscopic endoscopic sympathectomy in palmar and axillary hyperhidrosis. Arch Surg 113 (1978) 264.

61. LANDRENEAU R J, MACK M J, HAZELRIGG S R ET AL.: Video-assisted thoracic surgical resection of benign pulmonary lesions. Chest Surg Clin North Am 3 (1993) 283.

62. LANDRENEAU R J, MACK M J, HAZELRIGG S R, NAUNHEIM K S, KEENAN R J, FERSON P F: Video-assisted thoracic surgery: a minimally invasive approach to thoracic oncology. In: Rosenberg, S. A. (ed.): Cancer principles and practice of oncology. J. B. Lippincott, Philadelphia (1989) 2–14.

63. LANDRENEAU R J, MACK M J, HAZELRIGG S R, DOWLING R D, ACUFF T E, MAGEE M J, FERSON P F: Video-assisted thoracic surgery: basic technical concepts and intercostal approach strategies. Ann Thorac Surg 54 (4) (1992) 800–807.

64. LANDRENEAU R J, DOWLING R D, CASTILLO W, FERSON P F: Thoracoscopic resection of an anterior mediastinal mass. Ann Thorac Surg 54 (1992) 142.

65. LANDRENEAU R J, HAZELRIGG S R, MACK M J, FITZGIBBON L D, DOWLING R D, ACUFF T E, KEENAN R J, FERSON P F: Thoracoscopic mediastinal lymph node sampling: a useful approach to mediastinal lymph node stations inaccessible to cervical mediastinoscopy. J Thorac Cardiovasc Surg 105 (1993) 554–558.

66. LANDRENEAU R J, HAZELRIGG S R, MACK M J: The role of thoracoscopy in the management of intrathoracic neoplastic processes. Semin Thorac Cardiovasc Surg 5 (1993) 219.

67. LANZA L A, NATARJAN G, ROTH J A, PUTNAM J B: Long-term survival after resection of pulmonary metastases from carcinoma of the breast. Ann Thorac Surg 54 (1992) 244.

68. LAWS H L, MCKERNAN J B: Endoscopic management of peptic ulcer disease. Ann Surg 217 (1993) 548–556.

69. LEWIS R J, CACCAVALE R J, SISLER G E: VATS-argon beam coagulator treatment of diffuse end-stage bilateral bullous disease of the lung. Ann Thorac Surg 55 (1993) 1394–1399.

70. LILLINGTON G A: Management of solitary pulmonary nodules. Dis Mon 37 (1992) 271.

71. LILLINGTON G A: Pulmonary nodules: solitary and multiple. Clin Chest Med 3 (1982) 361.

72. LOCICERO J: Thoracoscopic management of malignant pleural effusion. Ann Thorac Surg 56 (1993) 641–643.

73. MACK M J, SHENNIB H, LANDRENEAU R J, HAZELRIGG S R: Techniques for localization of pulmonary nodules for thoracoscopic resection. J Thorac Cardiovasc Surg 106 (1993) 550.

74. MACK M J, REGAN J J, MCAFEE P ET AL.: Video-assisted thoracic surgery (VATS) for the anterior approach to the thoracic spine. Ann Thorac Surg 1995 (in press).

75. MACK M J, REGAN J J, BOBECHKO W P, ACUFF T E: Application of thoroscopy for diseases of the spine. Ann Thorac Surg 56 (1993) 736–738.

76. MACK M J, ARONOFF R J, ACUFF T E, DOUTHIT M B, BOWMAN R T, RYAN W H: Present role of thoracoscopy in the diagnosis and treatment of diseases of the chest. Ann Thorac Surg 54 (1992) 403–409.

77. MACK M J, LANDRENEAU R J, HAZELRIGG S R, ACUFF T E: Malignant pericardial effusions. Basic management concepts of the role of thoracoscopic pericardiectomy. Chest 103 (Suppl) (1993) 390.

78. MACK M J, HAZELRIGG S R, LANDRENEAU R J, ACUFF T E: Thoracoscopy for the diagnosis of the indeterminate solitary pulmonary nodule. Ann Thorac Surg 56 (1993) 825.

79. MACK M J: Thoracoscopy and its role in mediastinal disease and sympathectomy. Semin Thorac Cardiovasc Surg 5 (4) (1993) 332–336.

80. MANCINI M L, SMITH M, NEIN A, BUECHTER K J: Early evacuation of clotted blood in hemothorax using thoracoscopy: case reports. J Trauma 34 (1) 144–147.

81. MAO L, BRUBAN R H, BOYLE J O ET AL.: Detection of oncogene mutations in sputum precedes diagnosis of lung cancer. Cancer Res 54 (7) (1994) 1634–1637.

82. MARTS B C, NAUNHEIM K S, FIORE A C, PENNINGTON D G: Conservative versus surgical management of chylothorax. Am J Surg 164 (1992) 532–535.

83. MCAFEE M K, ALLEN M S, TRASTEK V F ET AL.: Colorectal lung metastases: results of surgical excision. Ann Thorac Surg 53 (1992) 780.

84. MCKENNA R J JR: Lobectomy by video-assisted thoracic surgery with mediastinal node sampling for lung cancer. J Thorac Cardiovasc Surg 107 (1994) 879–882.

85. MCKNEALLY M F: Statement of the AATS/STS joint committee on thoracoscopy and video-assisted thoracic surgery. J Thorac Cardiovasc Surg 104 (1) (1992) 1.

86. MCKNEALLY M F: Video-assisted thoracic surgery: standards and guidelines. Chest Surg Clin North Am 3 (1993) 345.

87. MENZIES R, CHARBONNEAU M: Thoracoscopy for the diagnosis of pleural disease. Ann Intern Med 114 (1991) 271.

88. MIDTHUN D E, SWENSON S J, JETT J R: Clinical strategies for solitary pulmonary nodules. Ann Rev Med 41 (1992) 195.

89. MILLER J I, HATCHER C R: Thoracoscopy: a useful tool in the diagnosis of thoracic disease. Ann Thorac Surg 46 (1978) 68.

90. MIYAMOTO H, HARADA M, ISOBE H ET AL.: Prognostic value of nuclear DNA content and expression of the ras oncogene product in lung cancer. Cancer Res 51 (1991) 6346–6350.

91. MOCKUS M B ET AL.: Sympathectomy for causalgia. Arch Surg 122 (1987) 668.

92. MOUNTAIN C F, MCMURTEY M J, HERMES K E: Surgery for pulmonary metastases: a 20-year experience. Ann Thorac Surg 38 (1984) 323.

93. NATHANSON L K, SHIMI S M, WOOD R A, CUSCHIERI A: Videothoracoscopic ligation of bulla and pleurectomy for spontaneous pneumothorax. Ann Thorac Surg 52 (1991) 316–319.

94. NAUNHEIM K S, KESLER K A, FIORE A C, TURRENTINE M, HAMMEL L M, BROWN J W, MOHAMMED Y, PENNINGTON D G: Pericardial drainage subxiphoid vs. transthoracic approach. Eur J Cardiothorac Surg 5 (1991) 99–104.

95. NAUNHEIM K, HAZELRIGG S R, LANDRENEAU R J, MACK M J ET AL.: Safety and efficacy of video-assisted thoracic surgical techniques for the treatment of spontaneous pneumothorax. J Thorac Cardiovasc Surg (in press).

96. OLCOTT C IV ET AL.: Reflex sympathetic dystrophy – the surgeon's role in management. J Fasc Surg 14 (1991) 488.

97. PAGE R D, JEFFREY R R, DONNELY R J: Thoracoscopy: a review of 121 consecutive surgical procedures. Ann Thorac Surg 48 (1989) 66.

98. PELLEGRINI C A, LEICHTER R, PATTI M, SOMBERT K, OSTROFF J W, WAY L: Thoracoscopic esophageal myotomy in the treatment of achalasia. Ann Thorac Surg 56 (1993) 680–682.

99. PLUNKETT M B, PETERSON M S, LANDRENEAU R J ET AL.: CT-guided preoperative percutaneous needle localization of peripheral pulmonary nodules. Radiology 185 (1992) 274.

100. PUTNAM J B, ROTH J A, WESLEY M N ET AL.: Analysis of prognostic factors in patients undergoing resection of pulmonary metastases from soft tissue sarcoma. J Thorac Cardiovasc Surg 87 (1984) 260.

101. PUTNAM J B, ROTH J A, WESLEY M N: Survival following aggressive resection of pulmonary metastases from osteogenic sarcoma: analysis of prognostic factors. Ann Thorac Surg 36 (1983) 516.

102. REDDICK E L, OLSEN D O: Laparoscopic laser cholecystectomy: a comparison with mini-lap cholecystectomy. Surg Endosc 3 (1989) 131–133.

103. REGAN J J, MACK M J, MCAFEE P (EDS.): Atlas of endoscopic spine surgery. Quality Medical Publishing, St. Louis 1995 (in press).

104. RIDLEY P D, BRAIMBRIDGE M V: Thoracoscopic débridement and pleural irrigation in the management of empyema thoracis. Ann Thorac Surg 51 (1991) 461–464.

105. ROBINSON L A, MOULTON A L, FLEMING W H, ALONSO A, GOLBRAITH T A: Intrapleural fibrinolytic treatment of multiloculated thoracic empyemas. Ann Thorac Surg 47 (1994) 803–814.

106. RODGERS B M, MOAZAM F, TALBERT J L: Thoracoscopy: early diagnosis of interstitial pneumonitis in the immunologically suppressed child. Chest 75 (1979) 126.

107. RODGERS B M, TALBERT J L: Thoracoscopy for diagnosis of intrathoracic lesions of children. J Pediatr Surg 11 (1976) 703.

108. ROTH J A, PASS H I, WESLEY M N ET AL.: Comparison of median sternotomy and thoracotomy for resection of pulmonary metastases in patients with soft tissue sarcoma. Ann Thorac Surg 42 (1986) 143.

109. ROTH J A: Treatment of metastatic cancer to lung. In: DeVita, V. T., S. Hellman, S. A. Rosenbert (eds.): Cancer principles and practice of oncology. J. B. Lippincott, Philadelphia (1989) 2261–2275.

110. ROVIARO G, VAROLI F, REBUFFAT C, VERGANI C, D'HOORE A, SCALAMBRA S M, MACIOCCO M, GRIGNANI F: Major pulmonary resections: pneumonectomies and lobectomies. Ann Thorac Surg 56 (1993) 779–783.

111. SALAZAR A M, WESTCOTT J L: The role of transthoracic needle biopsy for the diagnosis and staging of lung cancer. Clin Chest Med 14 (1993) 99.

112. SANCHEZ-AMRENGOL A, RODRIGUES-PANADERO F: Survival and talc pleurodesis in metastatic pleural carcinoma, revisited. Chest 104 (1993) 1482–1485.

113. SHENNIB H, LANDRENEAU R J, MACK M J: Video-assisted thoracoscopic wedge resection of T1 lung cancer in high-risk patient. Ann Surg 218 (1993) 555.

114. SLEBOS R J C, KIBBELAAR R E, DASESIO O ET AL.: Kras oncogene activation as a prognostic marker in adenocarcinoma of the lung. N Engl J Med 323 (9) (1990) 561–565.

115. SMITH R S, FRY W R, TSOI E K, MORABITO D J, KOEHLER R H, REINGANUM S J, ORGAN C H: Preliminary report on videothoracoscopy in the evaluation and treatment of thoracic injury. Am J Surg 166 (1993) 690–693.

116. SUGARBAKER D J: Thoracoscopy in the management of anterior mediastinal masses. Ann Thorac Surg 56 (1993) 653–656.

117. SWIERENGA J, WAGENAAR J P, BERGSTEIN P G: The value of thoracoscopy in the diagnosis and treatment of diseases affecting the pleura and the lung. Pneumologie 151 (1974) 11.

118. VAN DONGEN J A, VAN SLOOTEN E A: The surgical treatment of pulmonary metastases. Cancer Treat Rev 4 (1978) 29.

119. WAKABAYASHI A, BRENNER M, WILSON A F, TADIR Y, BERNS M: Thoracoscopic treatment of spontaneous pneumothorax using carbon dioxide laser. Ann Thorac Surg 50 (1990) 786–790.

120. WAKABAYASHI A, BRENNER M, KAYALEH R A, BERNS M W, BARKER S J, RICE S J, TADIR Y, BELLA L D, WILSON A F. Thoracoscopic carbon dioxide laser treatment of bullous emphysema. Lancet 337 (1991) 881–883.

121. WAKABAYASHI A: Thoracoscopic ablation of blebs in the treatment of recurrent or persistent spontaneous pneumothorax. Ann Thorac Surg 48 (1989) 651–653.

122. WAKABAYASHI A: Video-assisted laser resection is the best treatment for bullous emphysema. American College of Surgeons, 79th Annual Clinical Congress, 10–15 October 1993, San Francisco, pp 46–47.

123. WESTCOTT J L: Percutaneous transthoracic needle biopsy. Radiology 160 (1986) 319–327.

124. WOLFER R S, KRASNA M J, HASNAIN J U, MCLAUGHLIN J S: Hemodynamic effects of carbon dioxide insufflation during thoracoscopy. Ann Thorac Surg 58 (2) (1994) 404–407.

125. WORSEY J, FERSON P F, KEENAN R J, LANDRENEAU R J: Thoracoscopic pancreatic denervation for pain in unresectable pancreatic cancer. Br J Surg 80 (1993) 1051.

126. YAMAGUCHI A, SHINONAGA M, TATEBE S, SOUMA T, TSUCHIDA M, SAITO A: Thoracoscopic stapled bullectomy supported by suturing. Ann Thorac Surg 56 (1993) 691–693.

127. YIM A, HO J K, LEE T W, CHUNG S S: Thoracoscopic management of pleural effusions revisited. Surg Endosc 1995 (in press).

Laparoscopic Surgery in Urology

Critical Comments

A. D. Smith

Unfortunately, the development of urologic laparoscopy in the United States has become entangled in the issues of outcome analysis and cost containment efforts. Outcome analysis is concerned primarily with hospital stay and expense as it relates to the procedure and its complications: it pays little heed to the rapidity with which the patient returns to his or her usual occupation. The explanation lies in the fact that health care and disability policies are invariably written by different insurance companies. In considering cost containment, it must be remembered that every 1 hour in the operating room costs about $1000 to $1500 – about the same as a day of hospitalization. Therefore, in order for a new laparoscopic procedure to be cost effective, if it entails an additional 3 hours in the operating room (which is not an unreasonable assumption), it must diminish the hospital stay by at least 3 days. Moreover, its usual competition, the open operation, is becoming less costly. In the past, the average length of stay for open surgery was 10 to 12 days. Now, it ranges from 3.5 to 7 days.

The new financial realities are complicating the adoption of laparoscopy in another way. The remuneration of surgeons working in managed care arrangements is progressively decreasing, and urologists find that they are working far harder and generating a lower income. Because they are paid the same whether they perform the procedure laparoscopically or in the usual open technique; the financial incentive for the urologist in private practice is to perform as many procedures as possible as quickly and safely as possible. This pressure greatly reduces the appeal of laparoscopic alternatives. Consequently, most laparoscopic procedures are being conducted in academic medical centers by full-time staff.

All of this could change dramatically if there is a significant technical advance that enables one to expedite major laparoscopic ablative and reconstructive procedures. Where do we stand now with procedures on various organs?

Adrenal Gland

Initially restricted to pathologic conditions other than pheochromocytoma, this hurdle for laparoscopic adrenalectomy has now been overcome. The techniques are well established, and the operative times of experienced surgeons, which are 1 to 2 hours longer than those of open surgery, are offset by a reduction in the hospital stay of nearly a week. The turf battle between the urologist and the general surgeon over the adrenal gland therefore will intensify, and the outcome will depend on who can do the procedure most effectively laparoscopically.

Kidney

Removal of the kidney laparoscopically is now a well-established technique, but the indications are limited because the potential benefits are not particularly impressive. Small kidneys are most effectively removed retroperitoneally, as this technique obviates mobilization of the colon and avoids peritoneal contamination. Retroperitoneal laparoscopic nephrectomy is not suitable for larger kidneys or in obese patients, as

one needs the requisite space in the peritoneal cavity to unroll the specimen bag and position the pathologic kidney in it.

The experienced laparoscopist takes about 2 to 3 hours for a relatively easy case. Some of these patients could merely undergo angioinfarction and not have the kidney removed. More complicated cases may take considerably longer than the 1 to 2 hours generally needed for open surgery. This would not matter if the outcome were significantly better, yet the hospital stay is 3 to 9 days (vs. 7 to 14 days after open surgery), and the complication rate is similar to that of open surgery. In addition, the learning curve is long; indeed, it seems to get longer every time I speak to the experts!

At present, it is fair to say that although purists might not want to accept laparoscopically assisted nephrectomy, there may be a place for it provided that studies show a significant benefit of a small incision over the standard one. There is preliminary evidence, for example, of better postoperative lung function in patients having the minimally invasive procedure.

The standard management for a benign renal cyst is periodic evaluation alone. If the cyst becomes symptomatic, the least invasive procedure is aspiration and sclerotherapy. If this technique fails, as it often does, one can consider laparoscopic unroofing of the cyst. Care must be taken not to unroof a malignant lesion, as has been reported in the literature.

Ureteropelvic Junction

Relief of ureteropelvic junction obstruction with the laparoscope is a technically demanding procedure that is very time consuming, although a great deal of headway has been made by using the new suturing devices. Still, endopyelotomy, the original percutaneous operation, is quick and simple and has a success rate of 85 %. If laparoscopic pyeloplasty can yield the same success rate as open surgery, which is approximately 95 %, the newer procedure may be justified, but at present, its role appears questionable.

We can hope that over the course of time, we will be able to identify suitable candidates for both procedures with greater accuracy than is now possible. We may then be able to produce higher success rates.

Ureter

Laparoscopic cutaneous ureterostomy is a simple and safe procedure. Although it has limited applications, it certainly should be considered in appropriate patients. Ureterolithotomy is easily accomplished laparoscopically, but it too is indicated in only a few patients. An example would be a patient with a large calcium oxalate stone in the middle of the ureter; in such a case, other available methods have a high failure rate. Laparoscopic ureteroneocystostomies are technically demanding but should be considered for the repair of iatrogenic ureteral injuries or for the correction of vesicoureteral reflux in children.

Testis

Laparoscopic diagnostic studies of the undescended testis were the first widely accepted use of the laparoscope in urology. Today, they are undoubtedly the accepted state of the art.

The role of laparoscopic varicocelectomy is far more controversial, as this approach is difficult to justify. Both open and laparoscopic varicocelectomy are performed as outpatient procedures, and both are associated with a rapid return to work. A laparoscopic procedure may be slightly less painful, but it is more expensive and can be associated with a greater risk of complications.

Laparoscopic sampling of the para-aortic lymph nodes for diagnostic purposes may be as effective as open surgery in testicular tumors. However, it is not recommended after several courses of chemotherapy, which makes it inappropriate for many patients.

Prostate

Laparoscopic pelvic lymphadenectomy is worthwhile in selected cases. For example, in men with moderately or poorly differentiated primary tumors and those with elevated serum concentrations of prostate specific antigen, the likelihood of metastases justifies the procedure. If the biopsy is negative, then perineal prostatectomy or radioactive seed implantation should be carried out during the same anesthesia, whereas if the nodes are positive for tumor, then bilateral orchidectomy should be contemplated. (Laparoscopic pelvic lymphadenectomy should not be done as a separate operation in the United States, as the interval between the diagnostic and therapeutic procedures is wasted time that will only add to the patient's length of stay.) Teichman et al. [1] have recently shown that the combination of laparoscopic pelvic lymphade-nectomy and laparoscopically assisted total perineal prostatectomy compares favorably with radical retropubic prostatectomy in outcome analysis. However, if one routinely performs retropubic radical prostatectomy, laparoscopic pelvic lymphadenectomy becomes less useful.

Penis

The benefit of laparoscopic lymph node sampling for staging in carcinoma of the penis is unquestionable.

Conclusion

From this review, it is apparent that although urologic laparoscopy is valuable for many procedures, its practical use is limited. We need significant technologic breakthroughs for laparoscopy to become accepted among the practicing urologists. If the indications are so few, it becomes difficult to find enough cases to train resident fellows adequately, and that limitation of experience will make them more reluctant to contemplate laparoscopic surgery when they begin independent practice. We must therefore conclude that the prognosis for urologic laparoscopy is somewhat guarded.

References

1. TEICHMAN JMH, REDDY PK, HULBERT JC: Laparoscopic pelvic lymph node dissection, laparoscopically assisted seminal vesicle mobilization, and total perineal prostatectomy versus radical retropubic prostatectomy for prostate cancer. Urology 45 (1995) 823–830.

30. | Laparoscopic Pelvic Lymph Node Dissection

J. J. RASSWEILER, M. J. COPTCOAT, AND R. TSCHADA

Introduction

The laparoscopic pelvic lymphadenectomy (LPL) has become an established procedure in some urological and gynecological departments for the staging of early carcinoma of the prostate, bladder, uterus, and cervix [3, 6, 16, 36, 42]. There is no doubt that LPL is both a reasonable and feasible procedure, but this does not justify its use unless the finding of micrometastases in regional lymph nodes alters the management of a particular case. In the case of prostate cancer, the probability of finding positive lymph nodes significantly rises when the tumor marker PSA (prostate specific antigen) is above 25 μg/ml (Fig. 1). However, before discussing the indications and technique of LPL we demonstrate the anatomical basis for this procedure.

Basic Anatomy of Pelvic Lymphatics

The common iliac nodes are grouped around the artery one or two centimeters inferior to the aortic bifurcation and anterior to the fifth lumbar vertebra and sacral promontory. They drain the external and internal iliac nodes and send efferents to the lateral aortic nodes. They usually form a medial, lateral, and intermediate (anterior) chain, the lateral being the main route.

The external iliac nodes are usually divided into three subgroups lateral, medial, and anterior to the external iliac vessels, the anterior one being constant. The medial nodes are considered the main channel of drainage collecting from the inguinal nodes, deeper layers of the infraumbilical abdominal wall, adductor region of the thigh, glans penis, or clitoris, membranous urethra, prostate, vesical fundus, cervix, uterus,

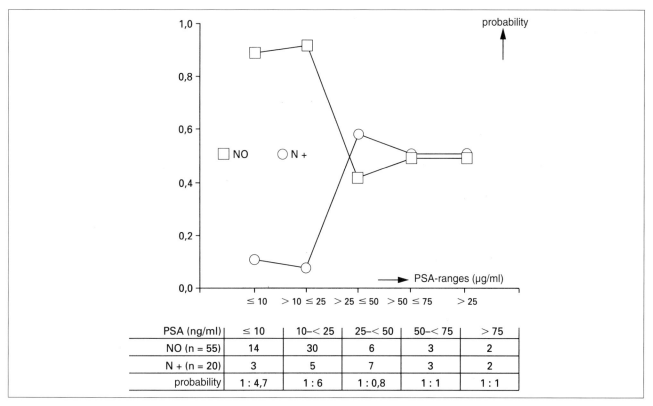

PSA (ng/ml)	≤ 10	10–< 25	25–< 50	50–< 75	> 75
NO (n = 55)	14	30	6	3	2
N + (n = 20)	3	5	7	3	2
probability	1 : 4,7	1 : 6	1 : 0,8	1 : 1	1 : 1

Fig. 1. Probability of positive lymph nodes of a prostate cancer depending on the preoperative prostatic specific antigen (PSA) level. Significant rise in positive lymph nodes if PSA is more than 25 μg/ml

and upper vagina. Their efferents pass to the common iliac nodes. Inferior epigastric and circumflex iliac nodes are associated with their vessels and drain the corresponding areas being outlying members of the external iliac group and inconstant in number. The internal iliac nodes surround the vessels receiving afferents from all the pelvic viscera, deep parts of the perineum, gluteal, and posterior femoral muscles. Efferents pass to the common iliac nodes. Sacral nodes along the median and lateral sacral vessels, and an obturator node sometimes occurring in the obturator canal, are outlying members of the internal iliac group.

Lymphatic Drainage of the Pelvis

There is considerable bypassing in the iliac groups of lymph nodes. Lymphangiographic studies have demonstrated the connections between the right and left groups.

Lymphatic Drainage of the Bladder
Bladder lymphatics begin in the mucosal, intramuscular and extramuscular plexuses. Collecting vessels nearly all ending in the external iliac nodes are in three sets; vessels from the trigone emerge on the vesical exterior to run superolaterally; those from the superior surface converge to the posterolateral angle and pass superolaterally across the lateral umbilical ligament to the external iliac nodes (one may go to the internal or common iliac group); the nodes from the inferolateral surface join those from the superior surface.

Lymphatic Drainage of the Prostate
Collecting vessels from the ductus deferens end in the external iliac nodes while those from the seminal vesicles go to the internal and external iliac nodes. Prostatic vessels end mainly in internal iliac and sacral nodes. A vessel from the posterior surface accompanies the vesicle vessels to the external iliac nodes, and one from the anterior surface gains the external iliac group by joining vessels of the membranous urethra.

Lymphatic Drainage of the Uterus and Cervix
Uterine lymphatics are superficial and deep in the uterine wall. Collecting vessels from the cervix pass laterally in the perimetrium to the external iliac nodes, posterolaterally to the internal iliac nodes and posteriorly to the sacrogenital fold to the rectal and sacral nodes. Some cervical efferents may reach the obturator gluteal nodes. Vessels from the lower part of the uterine body pass mostly to the external iliac nodes with those from the cervix. From the upper part of the body, fundus, and uterine tubes, vessels accompany those of the ovaries to the lateral aortic and pre-aortic nodes, a few passing to the external iliac nodes. The region surrounding the isthmic part of the uterine tube is drained along the round ligament to the superficial inguinal nodes.

Extent of Laparoscopic Pelvic Lymph Node Dissection

Although various sentinel nodes have been described for particular pelvic cancers, it can be seen from the above description that reasonable samples of nodal tissue must be taken from the obturator internal iliac and external iliac node groups, and on both sides, to provide a sensitive regional nodestaging of prostatic, bladder, urethral, penile, uterine, and cervical cancer (Table 1).

Table 1. Dissection area of (laparoscopic) pelvic lymphadenectomy depending on site of the tumor

Tumor	Obturator chain	External iliac chain	Common iliac chain
Prostate	Obligatory	Optional	Not included
Urethra	Obligatory	Obligatory	Optional
Bladder	Obligatory	Obligatory	Obligatory
Penis	Not included	Obligatory	Obligatory
Cervix	Obligatory	Obligatory	Not included
Corpus	Obligatory	Obligatory	Obligatory

The extent of the dissection recommended in LPL is based on the expected lymphatic drainage of a pelvic cancer, but is also influenced by the historical development of the open pelvic lymphadenectomy. The earlier approach of such an open lymphadenectomy was an extensive dissection lateral to the genitofemoral nerve, removing all fibrolymphatic tissue of the external iliac vessels, extending proximally to the common iliac vessels and medially to skeletonize the obturator vessels and nerve as well as the internal iliac artery and branches. Finally, the dissection included the presacral and lateral sacral lymph nodes.

The distal extent of the dissection included Cloquet's inguinal node and extended inferiorly to the pelvic bone where the circumflex vein crosses over the external iliac artery. Over the past 10 years many urological surgeons at least have become less radical and have recommended a modified open pelvic lymphadenectomy that includes primarily the nodal and fibrofatty tissue within the obturator fossa surrounding the obturator vessels and nerve. The lateral and medial borders of this dissection include the external iliac vein and hypogastric artery, respectively. The cranial and caudal limits are the bifurcation of the iliac vessels and Cloquet's node or Cooper's ligament, respectively.

A major reason in urology for this modification was that 86–94 % of the positive nodes from prostate cancer were within the obturator/internal iliac artery region with only 6–14 % of cases showing skip lesions involving only the presacral or common iliac regions [12]. A second reason is that postoperative complications are more significant especially when followed by radiotherapy [28]. Such developments in open surgery have influenced our technique for LPL.

Indications

The indications for laparoscopic pelvic lymphadenectomy are described in Table 2. Contraindications are given when the patient's general condition does not allow anesthesia or when important previous abdominal operations (i. e., adhesiolysis) lead the surgeon to expect extensive adhesions.

Instrumentation

The main equipment required for the procedure is listed on Table 3. Under a general anesthesia with muscle paralysis and assisted ventilation, the patient is placed in a supine posi-

Table 2.   Indications for laparoscopic pelvic lymphadenectomy (LPL)

Prostatic carcinoma

Stage T_{2-3} N_x M_{CT0} (= A_2, B, C)

Prior to radical retropubic prostatectomy in case of pathological PSA* value (> 25 μg/ml)

Prior to radical perineal prostatectomy or irradiation (brachytherapy, high voltage small volume) independent from PSA* value

Bladder cancer

Stage T_{2-3} N_x M_{CT0}

After neoadjuvant chemotherapy prior to curative cystectomy, if in case of positive nodes no palliative cystectomy is indicated (i.e., due to limited local disease, no urgency, no severe hematuria)

After neoadjuvant chemotherapy in case of an organ-preserving approach (TUR, segmental resection of the bladder) and clinical complete remission(CRc)

Prior to definitive radiotherapy

*PSA prostatic specific antigen

tion with a 20–25 ° head-down tilt. A bladder catheter is routinely placed during the procedure. Hip flexion is not required. Heparinization is recommended and thromboembolic deterrent stockings should be worn for deep venous thrombosis (DVT) prophylaxis.

Table 3.   Instruments for LPL

Armamentarium

Electronic high-flow laparoflator (Storz)

Xenon cold-light source (Storz)

HF generator with foot pedal (Erbotom Acc 450)

One (three)-chip CD camera auto exposure (Storz)

Irrigation and suction unit (Storz Pelvi-Cleaner)

Video unit (Sony U-matic VO-7360/ super VHS/ Betacam) including two monitors and videocart

Instruments

Veress needle with safety device

First trocar (10 mm) with safety shield (transperitoneal approach) or only reusable metal trocars with clap valve (Storz)

For normal-sized patients: 2- x 10-mm, 2- x 5-mm ports (rhomboid arrangement)

For obese patients: 2- x 10-mm, 3- x 5-mm (U-shape arrangement)

One endoshears (Metzenbaum) with rotatable blades connected to monopolar coagulation

One endodissector with rotatable blades

One endobowel clamp (Storz)

One endoretract (USSC)

One irrigation–suction probe (Storz)

Endoclips (medium and large), i. e., reusable applicator ligaclip

Small lapsac (Cook, Europe)

30 ° telescope (10 mm; Storz)

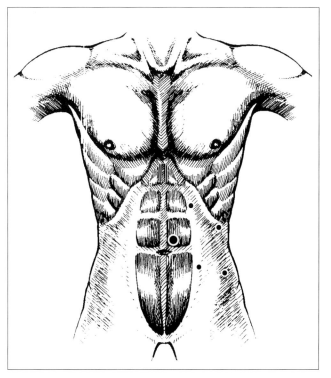

Fig. 2.   Trocar arrangement for laparoscopic pelvic lymphadenectomy (LPL)

Operative Technique

Creation of the Pneumoperitoneum

The Veress needle is inserted at a 45 ° angle. The position should be checked by aspiration and injection of 5 ml saline, and the intra-abdominal pressure should be carefully observed to remain below 12 mmHg during insufflation. The disposable Veress needle with a safety shield is safer in the hands of inexperienced laparoscopists. Previous major abdominal surgery is a relative contraindication to blind needle insertion and an open access (Hasson technique) should be used for the first port, which should be inserted well away from the scar so that adhesions can be seen and taken down.

Placement of Trocars

Two 10-mm and two to three 5-mm ports are placed according to Figure 2. The subumbilical port is used for the telescope (preferably 30 ° angle view). The two lateral ports along the edge of the rectus sheath are used for dissecting instruments. The central port 3–4 cm above the symphysis pubis can be used for the endoclip applicator or for retracting devices (bowel forceps, fan retractor) pushing the bladder medially and thus opening the operative field in the obturator fossa. The ports can be fixed with a combination of sutures and sterile adhesive strips or surgigrips (see Chap. 4). The universal use of 10-mm ports allows greater options for the telescope (necessary if a 0 ° telescope is used), endoclip, and 10-mm instrument (i.e., fan retractor) introduction. The surgeon stands on the contralateral side of the patient while the camera holder is placed on the ipsilateral side. The monitors should be at the bottom corners of the operating table.

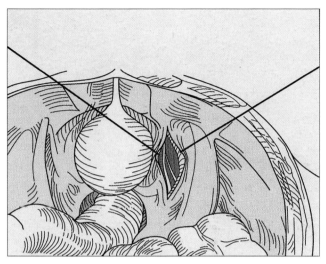

Fig. 3. Transperitoneal laparoscopic pelvic lymph node dissection. Peritoneal incision lateral to the lateral umbilical ligament

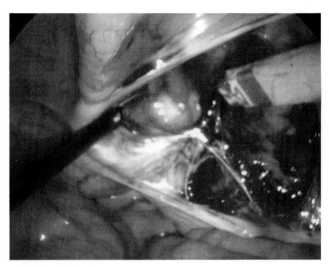

Fig. 4. Transperitoneal laparoscopic pelvic lymph node dissection. Clipping and transection of the vas deferens

Lymph Node Dissection

The landmarks of dissection are the umbilical ligament medially, the pubic bone anteriorly, and the external iliac vessels laterally (Table 4). The vas deferens or round ligament courses across this triangle and sometimes requires division for easier access to the obturator fossa.

Table 4. LPL landmarks of dissection

Lateral: External iliac artery
Caudal: Pubic bone
Medial: Bladder
Dorsal: Obturator nerve
Cranial: Hypogastric vein

The dissection is begun by incising the peritoneum lateral to the lateral umbilical ligament (Fig. 3) thereby gaining access to the extraperitoneal space. After clipping and transection of the vas deferens (Fig. 4), the lateral umbilical ligament is pushed medially and the dissection starts along the medial border of the external iliac vein (Fig. 5), and fibro-fatty tissue is removed from around this vessel until it can be clearly exposed between the inguinal ligament and a region 2–3 cm proximal to its bifurcation. Moreover, the pubic bone is identified and the lymphatic chain above it clipped distally and transected for the caudal landmark of lymphadenectomy (Fig. 6). The dissection then begins in the obturator fossa and all fibro-fatty tissue is removed until the obturator nerve is exposed (Figs. 7–9). The obturator artery and vein can usually be left intact. The circumflex vein and an aberrant obturator artery sometimes run across this space, and these usually have to be clipped and cut. Minimizing the use of diathermy in the obturator fossa helps to prevent obturator nerve injury.

The dissection always stays lateral to the medial umbilical ligament, and care must be taken closer to the iliac bifurcation

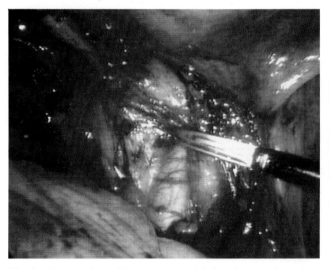

Fig. 5. Transperitoneal laparoscopic pelvic lymph node dissection. Medial retraction of the lateral umbilical ligament and identification of the external iliac vessels with the external iliac artery (lateral border of dissection)

where the ureter is crossed by the ligament. Many of the lymphatics are small and can be sealed with diathermy, but larger vessels require endoclips (Fig. 9). Ideally, the fibro-fatty tissue will have been removed en bloc, but sometimes it comes away in several pieces. The number of pieces should be noted by a nurse, and they can be easily left on one side in the paracolic gutter until they are all placed in a retrieval bag (Figs. 10 and 11).

Retrieval of Lymph Nodes

The fibro-fatty tissue dissected should be placed in a retrieval bag inserted through a port from the opposite iliac fossa (Figs. 10 and 11). The neck can be held open with two sets of forceps while a third places the tissue inside the bag. It is advisable to mark the retrieval bags as left and right for future audit of the dissection. In case of smaller lymph node packag-

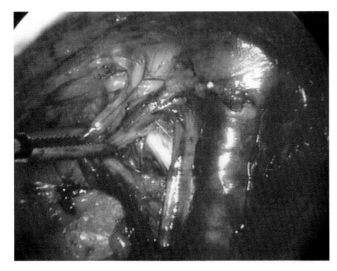

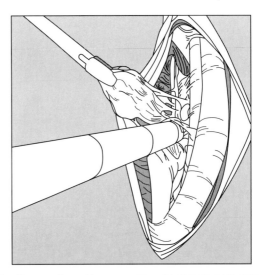

Fig. 6. Transperitoneal laparoscopic pelvic lymph node dissection. Distal clipping of the lymphatic chain above the pubic bone representing the distal border of lymphadenectomy. On the right the external iliac artery and collapsed external iliac vein can be seen.

Fig. 7. Transperitoneal laparoscopic pelvic lymph node dissection. Blunt and sharp dissection of the lymphatic chain from the lateral pelvic wall thereby isolating the obturator nerve

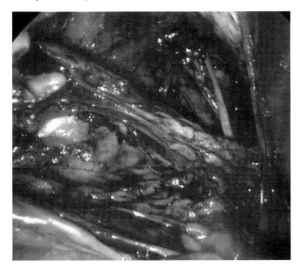

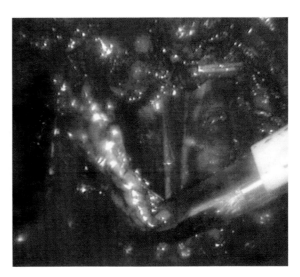

Figs. 8 and 9. Transperitoneal laparoscopic pelvic lymph node dissection. Proximal clipping and transection of the lymphatic chain at the branching of the internal iliac vein representing the proximal border of lymphadenectomy

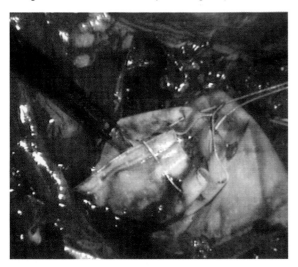

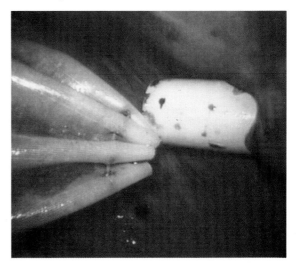

Figs. 10 and 11. Transperitoneal laparoscopic pelvic lymph node dissection. Entrapment of the lymphatic tissue in a small lapsac

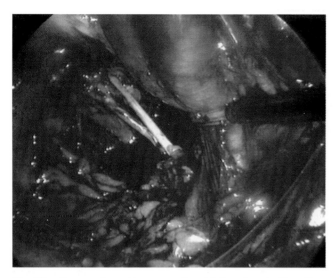

Fig. 12. Transperitoneal laparoscopic pelvic lymph node dissection. Endoscopic view into the obturator fossa with the obturator nerve after complete removal of lymphatic tissue

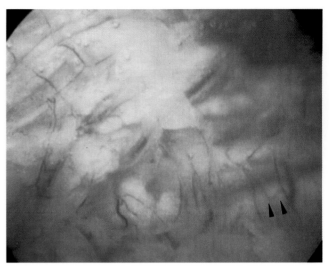

Fig. 14. Extraperitoneal pelvic lymph node dissection. Endoscopic view through the dissecting balloon filled with 900 cc normal saline on the pubic bone (arrows)

es they may be retrieved directly through the trocar via an inserted 10-mm retrieval sheath. Both sides are irrigated. If there is any oozing, a swab can be pressed over the area. After completing the dissection on the opposite side (Fig. 12), in the same way the instruments can be removed and the ports taken out under direct vision. All carbon dioxide is evacuated. A drain may be helpful indicating delayed bleeding, but is usually not required.

Wound Closure

All 10-mm trocar wounds require a deep fascial suture to prevent wound herniation. The skin can be either sutured with a subcuticular absorbable suture or adapted with a wound dressing. The patients require 2–3 h to recover, and can usually then be discharged if they can demonstrate effective micturition and do not feel discomfort or nausea.

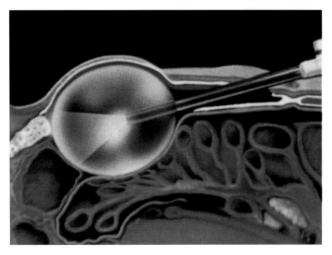

Fig. 13. Extraperitoneal pelvic lymph node dissection. Video-optic controlled balloondissection using a disposable balloon trocar

Extraperitoneal Approach

Recently, we have successfully applied an extraperitoneal approach for pelvic lymphadenectomy using a modification of the technique described by Gaur et al. [15] for retroperitoneal nephrectomy using a balloon-trocar system (Fig. 13). After a 15-mm subumbilical skin incision, the transverse fascia is explored through a blunt midline dissection. We use the index finger for preliminary dissection of the extraperitoneal space. Then a balloon-trocar system is introduced. The balloon is filled continuously with 1000–1200 cc saline according to patient size. The balloon dissection can be monitored endoscopically with the laparoscope inserted in the balloon-trocar sheath (Fig. 14).

Moreover, we monitor the insufflation pressure manometrically which should not exceed 110 cm H_2O to avoid rupture of the latex balloon. The balloon is kept inflated for 5 min to provide adequate hemostasis. After desufflation and retrieval of the balloon catheter, an 11-mm metal trocar is inserted coaxially via the laparoscope, fixed with an air-tight matress suture, and connected to the high-flow laparoflator (maximum pressure 15 mmHg). It is then possible to insert the subsequent trocars similar to the transperitoneal approach.

Lymph node dissection can be performed more equivalent to the open technique; the principle anatomical landmarks, however, are the same as for the transperitoneal laparoscopic procedure (external iliac vein, pubic bone, obturator nerve, and vessels). It is impressive to note how easily the pubic bone can be identified (Fig. 15). The lymph node dissection therefore starts at the pubic bone and continues proximally (Figs. 16 and 17) to the branching of the hypogastric vein (Fig. 17).

One major advantage of this approach is the fact that no disposable instruments are needed. Moreover, the access is exactly the same as in open surgery, thus excluding the risk of intraperitoneal spread of tumor cells (Figs. 18 and 19). However, the final value of this technique has to be evaluated in controlled clinical trials.

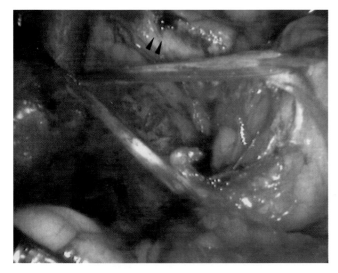

Fig. 15. Extraperitoneal pelvic lymph node dissection. Endoscopic view of pubic bone (arrow) after establishment of a pneumoretroperitoneum during extraperitoneoscopy ("retzioscopy"), clipping of vas deferens

Results

In both centers more than 100 procedures have been performed, and worldwide more than 1000 pelvic lymphadenectomies have been reported. The indications were mainly given by staging of prostate cancer. The mean operative time in our experience was 124 min (range 75–185 min). The diagnostic sensitivity of the procedure was as high as 97–98 % (2–3 % undetected positive nodes when radical prostatectomy was performed) which corresponds to the experience of other authors (Tables 5 and 6).

The LPL can usually be carried out as a day case procedure. Only 6 % of the patients in King's College Hospital have required overnight stay. This was mostly due to persistent nausea. Some of our early patients received preoperative opiate analgesia, and this was identified as a cause of their nausea. Further eradication of this problem has come with the introduction of Ondansetron. This is not given routinely, but only to those patients who still feel nauseous 2–3 h after their procedure. Complications can otherwise be general to laparoscopy and specific to this procedure.

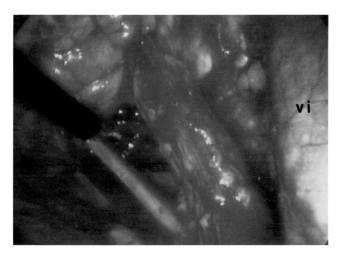
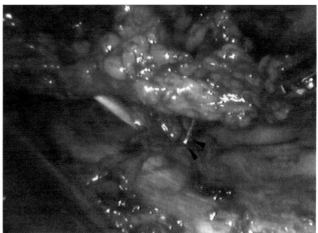

Figs. 16 and 17. Extraperitoneal pelvic lymph node dissection. Identification of external iliac vein (vi) lateral to the pubic bone and lymphatic chain. Blunt and sharp dissection of the lymphatic chain in the obturator fossa with isolation of obturator nerve and proximal clipping of lymphatic chain at branching of hypogastric vein

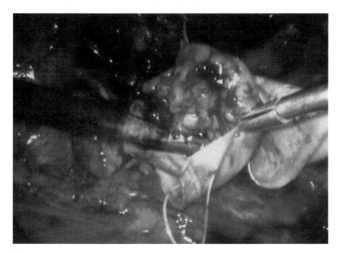
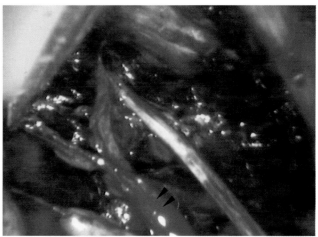

Fig. 18. Extraperitoneal pelvic lymph node dissection. Entrapment and retrieval of lymph nodes (positive histology) with a small lapsac

Fig. 19. Extraperitoneal pelvic lymph node dissection. Final view into the empty obturator fossa after complete removal of all lymph nodes

In Mannheim/Heilbronn therapeutic strategy is a little different, because in case of negative frozen section a retropubic prostatectomy is performed under the same anesthesia. However, for those patients with positive nodes receiving simultaneous orchidectomy and delayed brachytherapy with iodine seed implantation (Table 5), the postoperative stay was 3 days on average.

Table 5. LPL Mannheim experience (February 1992 – September 1994; n = 47)

Transperitoneal access	29
Operating time (80–190) min	117
Extraperitoneal access	18
Operating time (115–180) min	138
Mean number of lymph nodes (4*–12)	9.7
Positive lymph nodes	13 (29%)
Orchidectomy, flutamide, and iodine^{125} seed implantation	11
Orchidectomy plus flutamide	2
Radical prostatectomy in one session	27 (57%)
Radical prostatectomy delayed	7 (15%)
Total complications	4 (8.7%)
Laceration of mesosigma	1
Injury of the bladder	1
Pelvic hematoma	1
Temporary neuropathy	1

* Only one side operated on because of positive frozen section

Complications

Ruckle et al. [35] reported a 14 % specific complication rate that included two patients with a DVT, an obturator nerve palsy, a retroperitoneal abscess, and an accidental cystotomy. The King's and Mannheim experience with this procedure has an 8 % complication rate. DVTs have not been experienced in our series, possibly due to the universal use of thromboembolic deterrent stockings. Three patients required immediate open exploration: one because of arterial bleeding during dissection. This was identified at the junction between the supposedly obliterated umbilical artery and the internal iliac artery. It was a reminder not to take the dissection too proximal-

Table 6. LPL worldwide experience

Transperitoneal laparoscopic vs open lymphadenectomy [42]

Criteria	LPL	Open
Patients	66	27
Number of nodes	9.6	11
Blood loss (ml)	100	215
Operative time (min)	150	124
Postoperative stay (days)	1.5	6.5

Complications (U. S. experience with LPL; n = 372) [20]

	n	%
Vascular injury	11	3
Visceral lesion	8	2
Subileus	7	2
Wound infection	5	1
Lymphocele	5	1
Open revision	13	3.5

ly in the future, because this is also the point at which the ureter may be cut accidentally where it crosses beneath the obliterated umbilical artery. Winfield et al. [42] reported a 6 % incidence of perioperative hemorrhage. Two of these four cases required urgent exploration. This slightly high incidence probably reflects the variety in radicality of the lymphadenectomy.

In another case bleeding occurred after trocar insertion due to blunt trauma of the sigmoidal mesocolon, and in the last case accidental cystotomy occurred. Overall, all these complications occurred within the first 20 cases. This corresponds to the experience of the major centers in the United States (Table 6) [20]. Once laparoscopic experience and expertise are acquired, the morbidity of LPL is much less than after an open procedure [24, 42].

One other patient went into urinary retention, which can always happen if routine catheterization is used in elderly men. One would have imagined that carbon dioxide absorption through the dissection sites would be high, but the continual measurement of end-tidal carbon dioxide levels and correction with assisted ventilation has not led to any such complications. Minor complications, such as the formation of a pneumoscrotum, do occur occasionally, but these all settle within a few hours of the procedure and do not seem to cause the patient any discomfort.

Discussion

Importance of Laparoscopic Pelvic Lymphadenectomy

Laparoscopic pelvic lymphadenectomy has been accepted increasingly; however, the procedure is still regarded by some urologists as "a nice procedure looking for an indication." The main reason for this is the fact that actually the indication for retropubic radical prostatectomy has been extended also to patients with positive, but resectable, lymph nodes with nodal-positive patients receiving additional antiandrogen therapy. Therefore, the question may be: Is laparoscopic staging necessary?

The answer to this question varies slightly with each type of pelvic cancer, but more importantly with each individual patient. It can generally be said that surgical staging of lymph nodes is an attractive alternative to clinically noninvasive staging in the planning of therapy for such pelvic cancers, because it is more accurate and provides precise histological documentation of disease extent, and it permits individualization of therapy on the basis of specific patterns of disease spread.

Various diagnostic modalities have been employed as alternatives to surgical exploration such as lymphangiography, computed tomography (CT), and magnetic resonance imaging (MRI); all are limited in their ability to delineate disease extent and cannot compare with the accuracy of surgical staging [4, 11, 22, 34]. This preliminary thesis should apply only if the combined morbidity and mortality of a laparoscopic exploration and definitive therapy do not outweigh the benefits gained by the precise definition of disease.

A wider acceptance of LPL may directly benefit many patients who were referred for radiotherapy. In the past surgeons and radiation oncologists have been hesitant to encourage an open pelvic lymphadenectomy strongly for patients who undergo external or interstitial radiotherapy [33].

The problem with this philosophy has been that many patients will have been understaged, and therefore inappropriately receiving therapy with its attendant side effects and not cured. Radiation oncologists will often argue that their 5-, 10-, and 15-year results are comparable to those of most surgical series for all pelvic cancers, despite the fact that radiotherapy patients were not pathologically staged or not technically or medically fit for surgery [1]. This is a contentious statement, and many surgeons would point to so-called definitive papers that show that surgery provides superior results [29].

Whatever the specific argument in each type of cancer, there is every reason to believe that the introduction of LPL for patients referred for radiotherapy would lead to better patient selection, and ultimately improve the stated results in radiotherapy reports.

LPL is an accurate staging procedure only, and is in no way therapeutic. It cannot be seen as a complete clearance of all relevant nodes in all patients, and therefore cannot fit into the management protocol of patients where radical surgery and a radical lymphadenectomy is pursued in the presence of positive lymph nodes as suggested by Zincke [41] for advanced prostatic cancer.

Patient Selection for Laparoscopic Pelvic Lymphadenectomy

Laparoscopic pelvic lymphadenectomy has had the greatest impact in cases of prostatic cancer. The incidence of lymph node metastases in patients who are thought to otherwise have confined, localized prostate cancer and are eligible for radical prostatectomy is approximately 20–30 % [19, 24]. The likelihood of positive node metastases correlates with both local tumor volume and the degree of differentiation [2]. Prostatic specific antigen (PSA) levels between 20 and 50 µg/ml usually have a 65 % risk of nodal metastases or seminal vesicle involvement [18]. This latter finding has led us to develop the following protocol for patients with localized prostate cancer: A patient with a PSA level over 20 µg/ml who would still have been considered for radical surgery will undergo a staging pelvic lymphadenectomy as a separate day case procedure [31]. The likelihood of positive nodes is high (Fig. 1), and the patient is unlikely to experience the psychological trauma of recovering to find that his definitive procedure has not gone ahead.

Patients with a PSA level lower than this will undergo LPL in the same session as their planned definitive surgery. Frozen sections will be examined, and the most likely outcome is that the sections will be negative and definitive surgery can go ahead. The only concern with this protocol is that frozen sections have a false-negative rate of up to 19 % and are not as reliable as paraffin sections for the diagnosis of micrometastases [5]. The obvious advantages of only one anesthesia outweigh this when positive nodes are unlikely to be found. It must be stressed that such a protocol is only used after CT or MRI scanning of the abdomen and pelvis did not reveal enlarged lymph nodes. There is absolutely no point in carrying out LPL when macroscopically enlarged nodes can be identified on noninvasive scans. Such nodes can be easily assessed with fine-needle aspiration [7]. Use of laparoscopic lymphadenectomy is reserved for those cases where either CT or MRI is negative for nodes.

Extraperitoneal Approach

An alternative option for minimally invasive staging of pelvic nodes is the extraperitoneal pelviscopy [17, 38, 39]. The Ve-

ress needle in this procedure is placed suprapubically but extraperitoneally. The extraperitoneal space can be easily insufflated, but its lateral restriction is at the point of the deep inguinal ring, and dissection in this area is more difficult than through a transperitoneal approach. Shafik [38, 39] describes a new approach whereby the telescope is actually introduced through a second incision over the superficial inguinal ring and passed through the inguinal canal to enter the pelvis through the deep inguinal ring. The number of lymph nodes removed with this alternative technique and the sensitivity and specificity are comparable to all reports of the transperitoneal LPL. Nevertheless, we feel that the hydraulic dissection of the extraperitoneal space using the Gaur balloon is much more effective and offers a great view of the operative field allowing to perform the lymphadenectomy similar to the transperitoneal approach.

One theoretical advantage of this extraperitoneal technique is that there is the ability to come back for a second look after neoadjuvant treatment is commenced. This second look would probably be impossible through the same portal of entry, but one could then revert easily to a transperitoneal approach. Unfortunately, once a transperitoneal LPL has been undertaken, significant adhesions to the sites of dissection may be expected, which precludes a further second-look dissection by either a transperitoneal or extraperitoneal route. Unfortunately, one of the greatest complications reported after an extraperitoneal approach is lymphocele formation. This occurs in approximately 10 % of patients and requires some form of percutaneous drainage postoperatively. This complication does not occur with the transperitoneal approach, because the lymph drains into the open peritoneal cavity and is immediately absorbed. However, in our own series we have not experienced any lymphocele formation after extraperitoneal LPL. This may be due to the consequent clipping of all major lymphatic vessels, instead of simple electrocauterization.

The representation, but not the completeness, of this extraperitoneal approach has been shown. Both Winfield [42] and Coptcoat [6] assessed the validity of their transperitoneal laparoscopic procedure in 62 of 66 and 31 of 34 cases, respectively. Some remaining nodal tissue was then removed at open dissection, especially at the iliac bifurcation, but the false-negative rate was 4 and 0 %, respectively. Of course, the final value of the extraperitoneal approach including an analysis of sensitivity, specificity, costs, and complications has to be evaluated in a future clinical trial.

Extent of Pelvic Lymph Node Dissection

Previous reports of an open staging lymphadenectomy in gynecological cancer have shown a substantial disparity between the clinical and surgical disease extent. This has been reported as a 42 % difference for carcinoma of the cervix [21] and 52 % with carcinoma of the endometrium [8]. The risk of "skip" metastases (primitive iliac or para-aortic nodes without pelvic node involvement) is less than 2 % [9] and seems to occur only in patients with large tumor volumes. The introduction of minimally invasive staging of pelvic lymphadenectomy in itself allows reduction of open curative surgery for early cervical cancer (stages 1, 2a, or 2b) with negative nodes. These can probably be cured by vaginal surgery alone or by brachytherapy without the need for external radiotherapy. On the other hand, radical hysterectomy does not seem justified when positive nodes are known to be present [30]. The consequent reduction of risks and cost justifies the additional general anesthesia and the short hospital stay of a diagnostic laparoscopy. Patients with positive nodes should not have inappropriate and unnecessary extensive surgery or radiotherapy anymore, because as with bladder cancer, for this unfortunate group of patients no reasonable treatment is available. We await the refinement of neoadjuvant and adjuvant chemotherapy regimes, which will give this group of node-positive patients a chance of cure. Some stage A_2 cervical carcinomas without pelvic node metastases can be treated by cervical conization alone. When hysterectomy is not necessary for the local control of such tumors, laparoscopic lymphadenectomy helps identify women of reproductive age with microinvasive carcinomas who may benefit from conservative therapy. The rare cases with no metastases, which justify a radical treatment protocol, can be differentiated from cases with negative nodes in which cervical conization with preservation of fertility is an acceptable treatment.

Laparoscopic Lymphadenectomy and Radical Perineal Prostatectomy

The appearance of LPL has also changed the type of curative surgery that can now be offered to the patient. Radical perineal prostatectomy was first described by Hugh Hampton-Young in 1905 [43], but has not gained wide acceptance, because the open staging pelvic lymphadenectomy required an additional abdominal incision.

Thus, the standard form of radical prostate surgery has become the radical retropubic prostatectomy as pioneered by Walsh [41]. Now that we can carry out our staging pelvic lymphadenectomy laparoscopically, there is no need to continue with the retropubic dissection. The perineal approach is less invasive (Fig. 20), is associated with less blood loss, is still nerve-preserving, and in many series, no blood transfusion is used at all [13]. Patients can be discharged 3–4 days earlier with this type of surgery, and this will probably become the standard method now that LPL is gaining acceptance for its accuracy and specificity of node sampling.

The finding of positive nodes during radical prostatectomy is actually much less common than the finding of either prostatic capsular involvement or seminal vesicle involvement. Understaging in these two regards has caused great concern, and it is now possible to carry the laparoscopic dissection down through the pouch of Douglas toward the seminal vesicles and lateral and posterior aspects of the prostatic capsule. Biopsies can be taken from these regions, which should allow us to more correctly stage the local prostate cancer. The operation is therefore developing into a synchronous-combined laparoscopic and radical perineal prostatectomy in the same way as the synchronous combined abdomino-perineal resection for low rectal cancers. We have carried out four such procedures, and although the operative time for the staging laparoscopy was extended by up to an average of 60 min, the information of negative vesicle and capsular biopsies made the subsequent radical prostatectomy much more certain of cure. This is probably the way that all staging lymphadenectomies for pelvic cancer will go in that either whole or parts of the definitive curative surgery will also be undertaken in the same minimally invasive way.

On the other hand, laparoscopic radical prostatectomy, even if experimentally [26] and clinically [37] feasible, does not seem to be advantageous over the previously mentioned

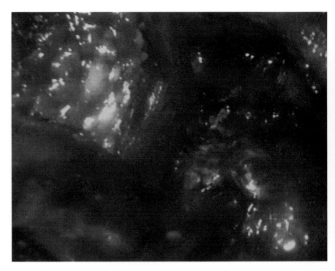

Fig. 20. Perineal radical prostatectomy with development of the prostate gland

combination of LPL and perineal radical prostatectomy. This is due mainly to the long operative time and the technical problems with the vesicourethral anastomosis.

Laparoscopic Pelvic Lymphadenectomy for Bladder Cancer

The role of LPL for bladder cancer is still unclear. Few authors have evaluated it because of the absence of any satisfactory treatment when positive nodes are found [10]. However, this argument is parallel to that in gynecological cancers, and surely the opportunity to prevent patients from going through inappropriate and unnecessary surgery or radiotherapy must make this staging procedure worthwhile [21, 23]. Skinner [40] has advocated that micrometastases in the pelvic nodes do not make any difference to overall survival following a radical cystectomy, but his series only contains 11 patients and it is difficult to understand why nodal metastatic bladder cancer would behave in such a benign way compared with other pelvic cancers.

Again, our hope would be that positive nodes would indicate neoadjuvant chemotherapy followed by a second-look sampling and radical surgery if the nodes become negative. This is still very speculative, but we should have some answers within the next few years.

Conclusion

In conclusion, one can say already that LPL is accurate and sensitive for the staging of lymph nodes affected by micrometastases from all pelvic cancers. Its present value lies in staging, rather than in therapy, but as laparoscopic techniques evolve, it may become part of a curative surgical procedure as in the case of the superior dissection of the prostate prior to a radical perineal prostatectomy and reanastomosis. Any staging lymphadenectomy will only be worthwhile if the finding of micrometastases alters the management of a particular patient. This is certainly true in early cervical cancer and prostate cancer, but we still await further development of neoadjuvant chemotherapy and/or radiotherapy for bladder cancer and more advanced endometrial cancer before the true impact in these cases can be felt. In these cases a second-look node sampling will be required, and a combination of preliminary laparoscopic extraperitoneal and secondary transperitoneal procedures may be considered. The LPL may be a simple, safe, day case procedure that surgically stages pelvic cancer.

References

1. BAGSHAW MA, RAY GR, COX RS: Selecting initial therapy for prostate cancer: Radiation therapy perspective. Cancer 60 (1987) 521.
2. BARZELL W, BEAN MA, HILARIS BS, WHITMORE WF JR: Prostatic adenocarcinoma: Relationship of grade and local extent to the pattern of metastases. J Urol 118 (1977) 278.
3. BEER M: Laparoskopische pelvine Lymphadenektomie. Uroimaging 1 (1991) 167–175.
4. BENSON KH, WATSON RA, SPRING DB, AGEE RE: The value of computerised tomography in evaluation of pelvic lymph nodes. J Urol 126 (1981) 63.
5. CATALONA WJ, STEIN AJ: Accuracy of frozen section detection of lymph node metastases in prostatic carcinoma. J Urol 127 (1982) 460.
6. COPTCOAT MJ, WICKHAM JEA: Laparoscopy in urology. Minimally Invasive Therapy 1 (1992) 337–342.
7. CORREA RS JR, KIDD CR, BURNETT L, BRANNEN GE, GIBBONS RP, CUMMINGS KB: Percutaneous pelvic lymph node aspiration in carcinoma of the prostate. J Urol 126 (1981) 190.
8. COWLES TA, MAGRINA JF, MASTERSON BJ, CAPEN CV: Comparison of clinical and surgical staging in patients with endometrial carcinoma. Obstet Gynecol 66 (1985) 413.
9. DARGET D, SALVAT J: L'envahissement ganglionnaire pelvien. Paris 1989; MEDSI.
10. DRETLER SP, RAGSDALE BD, LEADBETTER WF: The value of pelvic lymphadenectomy in the surgical treatment of bladder cancer. J Urol 109 (1973) 414.
11. FEIGEN M, CROCKER EF, READ J, CRANDON AJ: The value of lymphoscintigraphy, lymphangiography and computer tomography scanning in the pre-operative assessment of lymph nodes involved by pelvic malignant conditions. Surg Gynecol Obstet 165 (1987) 107–110.
12. FLOCKS RH, CULP D, PORTO R: Lymphatic spread from prostate cancer. J Urol 81 (1959) 194.
13. FRAZIER HA, ROBERTSON JE, PAULSON DE: Radical prostatectomy: the pros and cons of the perineal versus retropubic approach. J Urol 147 (1992) 888–890.
14. GAUR D: Laparoscopic operative retroperitoneoscopy. J Urol 148 (1992) 1137–1139.
15. GAUR DD, AGARWAL DK, PUROHIT KC: Retroperitoneal laparoscopic nephrectomy: initial case report. J Urol 149 (1993) 103–105.
16. GERSHMAN A, DAYKHOVSKY L, CHANDRA M, DANOFF D, GRUNDFEST W: Laparoscopic pelvic lymphadenectomy. J Laparoendosc Surg 1 (1) (1990) 63–68.
17. HALD T, RASMUSSEN F: Extraperitoneal pelviscopy: a new aid in staging of lower urinary tract tumours; a preliminary report. J Urol 124 (1980) 245.
18. HUDSON MA, BAHNSON RB, CATALONA WJ: Clinical use of prostate and specific antigen in patients with prostate cancer. J Urol 142 (1989) 1011.
19. JEWETT HJ, EGGLESTON JC, YAWN DH: Radical prostatectomy in the management of carcinoma of the prostate: probable causes of some therapeutic failures. J Urol 107 (1972) 1034.
20. KAVOUSSI LR, SOSA E, CHANDHOKE P, CHODAK G, CLAYMAN RL, HADLEY HR, LOUGHLIN KR, RUCKLE HC, RUKSTALIS D, SCHUESSLER W, SEGURA J, VANCAILLE T, WINFIELD H: Complications of laparoscopic pelvic lymph node dissection. J Urol 149 (1993) 322–325.
21. LAPOLLA JP, SCHLAERTH JB, GADDIS O, MORROW CP: The influence of surgical staging on the evaluation and treatment of patients with cervical carcinoma. Gynecol Oncol 24 (1986) 194.
22. LOENING SA, SCHMIDT JD, BROWN RC, HAWTRY CE, FALLON B, CULP DA: A comparison between lymphangiography and pelvic lymph node dissection in the staging of prostatic cancer. J Urol 117 (1977) 752.
23. MALKOWICZ SB, NICHOLS P, LIESKOVSKY G, BOYD SD, HUFFMAN J, SKINNER DG: The role of radical cystectomy in the management of high grade, superficial bladder cancer (PA, P1, PIS and P2). J Urol 144 (1991) 641–645.
24. MCCULLOUGH DL MCLAUGHLIN AP, GITTES RF: Morbidity of pelvic lymphadenectomy and radical prostatectomy for prostatic cancer. J Urol 145 (1977) 988–991.
25. MCCULLOUGH DL, PROUT GR, DALY JJ: Carcinoma of the prostate and lymphatic metastases. J Urol 111 (1974) 65.
26. MORAN ME, BOWYER DW, SZABO Z: Laparoscopic radical prostatectomy: a canine surgical model. J Endourol 6 (1992) S-166 (abstract no. V-60).
27. PARRA R, ADRUS C, BOULLIER: Staging laparoscopic pelvic lymph node dissection: comparison of results with open pelvic lymphadenectomy. J Urol 147 (1992) 875–878.
28. PAULSON DF: The prognostic role of lymphadenectomy in adenocarcinoma of the prostate. Urol Clin North Am 7 (1980) 615.
29. PAULSON DF, LIN GH, HINSHAW W, STEPHANI S: The Uro-Oncology Research Group: radical surgery versus radiotherapy for adenocarcinoma of the prostate. J Urol 128 (1982) 502.
30. POTTER ME, ALVAREZ RD, SHINGLETON HM, SOONG SJ, HATCH KD: Early invasive cervical cancer with pelvic lymph node involvement; to complete or not to complete radical hysterectomy? Gynecol Oncol 37 (1990) 78–81.
31. RASSWEILER JJ, HENKEL TO, POTEMPA DM, ALKEN P: Laparoskopische Eingriffe in der Urologie. Laparo-endosk Chir 1 (1992) 121–140.
32. RASSWEILER JJ, HENKEL TO, POTEMPA DM, COPTCOAT MJ, ALKEN P: The technique of transperitoneal laparoscopic nephrectomy, adre-nalectomy and nephroureterectomy. Eur Urol 23 (1993) 425–430.
33. RAY GR, PISTENMA DA, CASTELLINO RA, KEMPSON R, MEARES E, BAGSHAW MA: Operative staging of apparently localized adenocarcinoma of the prostate: results in fifty selected patients 1; experimental design and preliminary results. Cancer 38 (1976) 73.
34. RIFKIN MC, ZERHOUNI EA, GATSONIS CA ET AL.: Comparison of magnetic resonance imaging and ultrasonography in staging early prostate cancer. N Engl J Med 323 (1990) 621.
35. Ruckle H, Hadley R, Lui P, Stewart S: Laparoscopic pelvic lymph node dissection: assessment of intra-operative and early post-operative complications. J Endourol 6 (2) (1992) 117–119.
36. SCHUESSLER WW, VANCAILLIE TG, REICH H, GRIFFITH DP: Transperitoneal endosurgical lymphadenectomy in patients with localised prostate cancer. J Urol 145 (1991) 988.
37. SCHUESSLER WW, KAVOUSSI LR, CLAYMAN RV, VANCAILLIE TG: Laparoscopic radical prostatectomy: initial case report. J Urol 147 (1992) 246 A (abstract no. 130).
38. SHAFIK A: Inguinal pelviscopy: a new approach for examining the pelvic organs. Gynecol Obstet Invest 30 (1990) 159.
39. SHAFIK A: Extraperitoneal laparoscopic lymphadenectomy in prostatic cancer: preliminary report of a new approach. J Endourol 6 (2) (1992) 113–116.
40. SKINNER DG: Management of invasive bladder cancer: a meticulous pelvic node dissection can make a difference. J Urol 128 (1982) 34.
41. WALSH PC, LEPOS H, EGGLESTON JD: Radical prostatectomy with preservation of sexual function; anatomical and pathological considerations. Prostate 4 (1983) 473.
42. WINFIELD HN, DONOVAN JF, SEE WA, LOENING SA, WILLIAMS RD: Laparoscopic pelvic lymph node dissection for genitourinary malignancies: indications, techniques and results. J Endourol 6 (2) (1992) 103–112.
43. YOUNG HH: The early diagnosis and radical cure of carcinoma of the prostate; being a study of 40 cases and presentation of a radical operation which was carried out in four cases. Bull Johns Hopkins Hosp 16 (1905) 315.
44. ZINCKE H, FLEMING TR, FURLOW WL ET AL.: Radical retropubic prostatectomy and pelvic lymphadenectomy for high stage cancer of the prostate. Cancer 47 (1981) 1901.
45. ZINCKE H: Extended experience with surgical treatment of stage D1 adenocarcinoma of prostate. Urology 33 (1989) (Suppl) 27–35.

31. Laparoscopic Nephrectomy, Nephroureterectomy, and Adrenalectomy

J. Rassweiler, T. O. Henkel, O. Seemann, and P. Alken

Introduction

Laparoscopic surgery [15, 17, 19, 30, 45] has also found acceptance in urological surgery, e. g., cryptorchidism [14, 52], pelvic lymphadenectomy [43, 55], and varicocelectomy [16, 27]. Coptcoat, Wickham, and others began experimenting toward the end of the 1980s with percutaneous nephrectomy techniques [2, 5, 11, 13, 47, 51, 54]. However, the final breakthrough was achieved by Clayman who, in 1990, carried out the first transperitoneal laparoscopic nephrectomy [7]. After assisting Coptcoat with the first European transperitoneal laparoscopic tumor nephrectomy in London [12], we set up our own step-by-step training program in order to acquaint our clinic with this new surgical approach [28, 39]. Experimental standardization of all operative steps could definitely ease the clinical introduction of this minimally invasive technique, which has become a part of our clinical routine for many indications (Table 1).

Table 1. Laparoscopic procedures performed in the Department of Urology, Klinikum Mannheim (January 1992–October 1994)

Operation	n
Laparoscopic varicocelectomy	41
Laparoscopy for cryptorchidism	20
Laparoscopic pelvic lymphadenectomy	47
Laparoscopic nephrectomy	57
Laparoscopic tumor nephrectomy	10
Retroperitoneoscopic nephropexy	5
Laparoscopic nephroureterectomy	8
Laparoscopic adrenalectomy	12*
Laparoscopic retroperitoneal lymphadenectomy	18
Other procedures (i. e., ureterolithotomy, pyeloplasty, ureterostomy, etc.)	12
Total	230

* Including 9 adrenalectomies during radical tumor nephrectomy

One major criticism about laparoscopic nephrectomy for benign disease, however, is that it requires a transabdominal approach in contrast to open surgery. Therefore, both Clayman et al. [20] and Wickham et al. [50, 53] started experimental and clinical studies to realize retroperitoneal laparoscopic nephrectomy. However, their attempts have proved to be difficult, due to the inability to create an effective pneumoretroperitoneum [34, 47, 48] because of the dense areolar tissue binding the fat in the retroperitoneum, which could not be broken down merely by the technique of pneumoinsufflation (Table 2).

In 1992 Gaur [22] developed a pneumatic dissection technique of the retroperitoneum based on balloon insufflation (maximum 110 mmHg). He could successfully apply this approach for multiple procedures in the upper retroperitoneum including simple nephrectomy, renal biopsy, ureterolithotomy, and varicocelectomy [23–26]. In the meantime other authors [29, 32, 33] presented their experience with the Gaur-balloon for further indications, i. e., radical tumor nephrectomy, nephrectomy in children or lumbar sympathectomy using either pneumatic or hydraulic balloon dissection (Table 2).

Table 2. History of retroperitoneoscopy in urology

Author	Procedure
Sommerkamp (1974)	Renal biopsy (no pneumoretroperitoneum)
Wickham (1979)	Ureterolithotomy
Hald and Rasmussen (1980)	Pelvic lymph node biopsy (no pneumoretroperitoneum)
Bay-Nielsen and Schultz (1982)	Ureterolithotomy (no pneumoretroperitoneum)
Wickham (1983)	Diagnostic procedures for renal disease
Mazman (1985)	Pelvic lymphadenectomy (no pneumoretroperitoneum)
Shafik (1992)	Pelvic lymphadenectomy
Gaur (1992)	Ureterolithotomy, nephrectomy, renal biopsy, varicocelectomy (1992) (with dissecting balloon)
Rassweiler and Preminger (1993)	Radical tumor nephrectomy
Mandressi (1993)	Nephrectomy, adrenalectomy
Rassweiler (1993)	Nephrectomy, nephropexy, renal cyst resection, ureterocutaneostomy, pyeloplasty, heminephrectomy (video-optically controlled balloon dissection)

We have modified this procedure into a hydraulic endoscopically controlled balloon-dissection technique [40, 41] of the retroperitoneal space (Table 3), which has enabled us to perform successfully more than 100 procedures in the upper retroperitoneum including simple nephrectomy, heminephrectomy, nephropexy, renal cyst resection, ureterocutaneostomy, and dismembered pyeloplasty (Table 1).

Table 3. Technical development of retroperitoneoscopy

Lumboscopy without pneumoretroperitoneum utilizing
a mediastinoscope or laryngoscope

Retroperitoneoscopy after CO_2 insufflation to create
an operative space in the retroperitoneum

Retroperitoneoscopy after balloon dissection of the retroperitoneal
space followed by a pneumoretroperitoneum

Retroperitoneoscopy after hydraulic endoscopically controlled
dissection of the retroperitoneum utilizing a balloon-trocar system

Indications and Patient Selection

The list of indications for the 100 laparoscopic nephrectomies
is shown in Table 4. This includes mainly removal of nonfunctioning kidneys due to chronic hydronephrosis, chronic pyelonephritis, renovascular disease, end-stagestone disease, reflux nephropathy, and renal dysplasia. However, we have also
treated localized renal cell carcinoma and transitional cell carcinoma of the upper urinary tract laparoscopically. Of these
procedures, 46 have been performed transperitoneally,
whereas in 54 cases the retroperitoneal route was used.
Moreover, 26 further retroperitoneoscopical operations have
been performed.

Table 4. Indications for laparoscopic nephrectomy

Benign renal disease

Nonfunctioning infected kidneys due to:
  Chronic pyelonephritis
  End-stage stone disease
  Reflux nephropathy (with ureterectomy)

Renal hypertension due to:
  Renovascular disease (i. e., malignant nephrosclerosis)
  Renal dysplasia
  Renal artery embolism

Chronic hydronephrosis due to:
  Ureteral stenosis
  Urolithiasis

The indication for laparoscopic radical tumor nephrectomy
was restricted to smaller T_2 tumors. Routinely, this procedure
includes adrenalectomy. Additionally, we have performed another transperitoneal laparoscopic adrenalectomy for a cortical adenoma of the left adrenal.

Relative contraindications for the transperitoneal approach
are previous renal surgery or a history of multiple transabdominal incisions. Absolute contraindications are acute septi-
cemia, coagulations disorders, and chronic respiratory disease with poor pulmonary function (evaluated preoperatively).

Patient Preparation and Positioning

All patients receive similar preoperative preparation as performed prior to open surgery (including informed consent,
bowel preparation with 10 mg bisacodyl p.o., thromboembolic
prophylaxis with elastic stockings, and low-molecular heparin). Retrograde stenting of the respective ureter has been
done prior to the procedure in the first cases in order to facili-

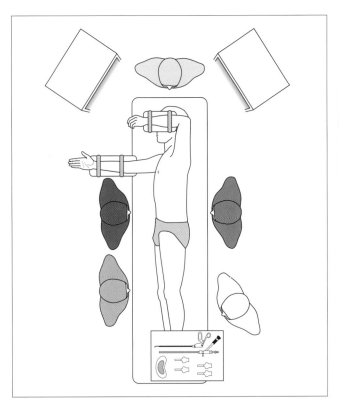

Fig. 1. Positioning of patient for transperitoneal laparoscopic nephrectomy. Arrangement of the two video carts at the head of the patient, surgeon and camera assistant on ventral side, second assistant
and nurse on dorsal side of patient

tate intraoperative identification of the ureter. However, with
increasing experience we stent the ureter only in selected
cases (i. e., history of periureteritis, previous surgery). The
urinary bladder is catheterized, but the catheter is removed at
the end of the operation in most of the cases.

Before creating a pneumoperitoneum, a nasogastric tube is
inserted with the patient placed in the typical flank position
with a 30 ° decline (Trendelenburg) under general anesthesia
with the two video monitors mounted on two video carts in an
oblique position lateral to the patient's head (Fig. 1).

Operative Technique

Transperitoneal Laparoscopic Nephrectomy (TLN)

Trocar Placement
After a pneumoperitoneum was obtained with the inserted
Veress needle placed lateral to the rectus abdominis muscle
on one line with the umbilicus, trocars were inserted through
the abdominal wall as depicted in Figure 2:
Port I: 10 mm periumbilical (edge of M. rectus abdominis)
Port II: 11/12 mm subcostal (mamillary line) for right kidney,
          5 mm for left side
Port III: 11/12 mm above Spina iliaca superior (mamillary
          line) for left kidney, 5 mm for right side

The laparoscope is passed through port I and used to intra-
abdominally inspect the trocar insertion of ports II and III. The
ports are secured with a sterile adhesive tape and sutured to

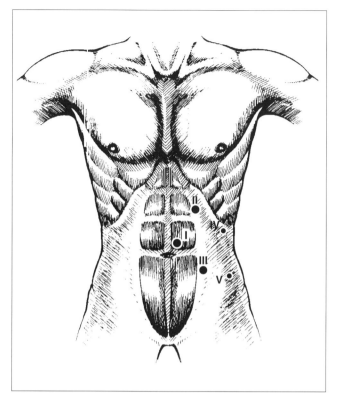

Fig. 2. Size and sites of trocars for laparoscopic procedures in upper retroperitoneum for left side

the skin. After complete inspection of the intra-abdominal situs, either the ascending (right kidney) or descending (left kidney) colon is mobilized through laterocolic incision of the peritoneum along the line of Toldt. We prefer a bimanual dissec-

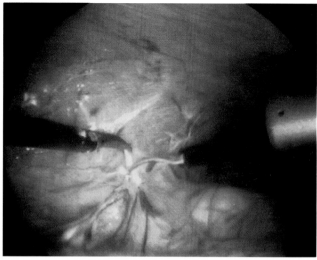

Fig. 4. Same as Figure 3

tion technique. Therefore, the left-hand port has only to be 5 mm, whereas the right-hand port needs to be 12 mm for insertion of a multifire clip applicator and the endoscopic stapler (Endo-GIA). Once the respective colon is free to fall off medially (Figs. 3 and 4), one or two further ports can be inserted through the newly exposed retroperitoneum:

Port IV: 5 mm along the lateral abdominal wall parallel to port II
Port V: 5 mm along the lateral abdominal wall parallel to port III

These two ports are mainly used to grasp the kidney during dissection and kidney retrieval. For small kidneys and slim patients only one port may be necessary.

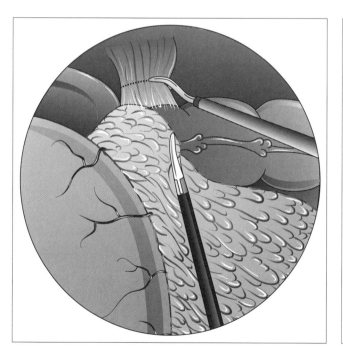

Fig. 3. Dissection of retroperitoneum. Laterocolic incision at the line of Toldt. Anatomy and endoscopic picture of technique for left side nephrectomy

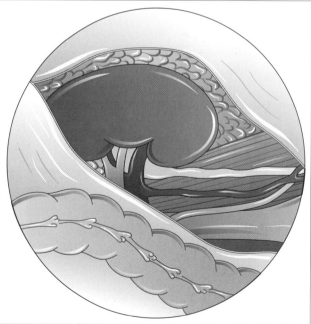

Fig. 5. Dissection of ovarian/spermatic vein. Retroperitoneal anatomy after deflection of descending colon

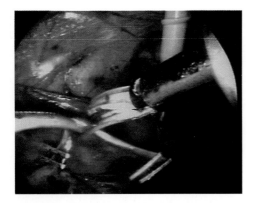

Fig. 6. Clipping and transection of the gonadal vein

Clipping the Ureter

The ovarian/spermatic vein is identified in proximity to the sacral promontory, clipped, and dissected (Figs. 5 and 6), as is the ureter thereafter (Figs. 7 and 8). In our first case, however, extensive periureteral inflammation (periureteritis) necessitated use of the Endo-GIA in contrast to the typical double clipping done in normal cases. Retraction of the ureter can be established either with a transcutaneous suture using a straight needle through the lateral abdominal wall (see Fig. 28), which allows further use of ports IV and V for retraction of the kidney and adjacent organs, or simply with an endobowel clamp inserted through ports IV or V. We use the transcutaneous suture of the ureter only in complicated cases or when performing nephroureterectomy when distal ureter tension is needed.

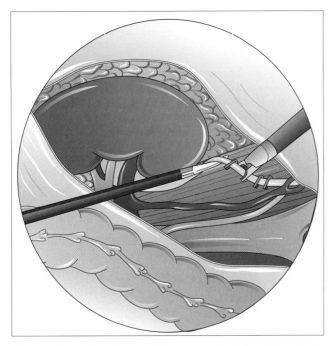

Fig. 7. Dissection of ureter. Dissection and clipping of previously stented ureter

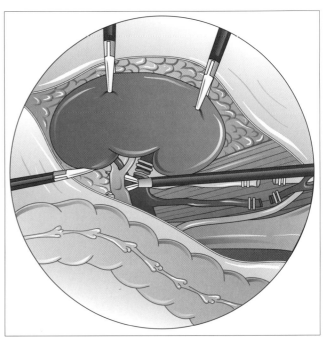

Fig. 9.

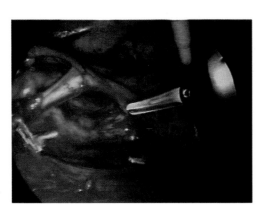

Fig. 8. Transsection of clipped ureter with scissors

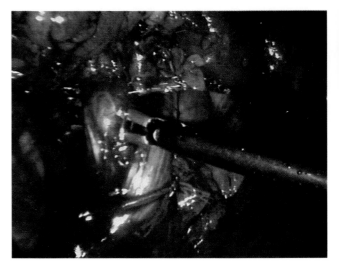

Figs. 9 and 10. Careful dissection of a second branch of renal artery

Renal Vessel Clipping

The main renal artery and vein are stapled with the Endo-GIA 30 (Figs. 9–15) while smaller vessels can be clipped. For cost reduction the main renal vessels can be dissected between large double clips (12 mm) on each side. It must be emphasized that arterial and venous vessels should not be stapled together, due to the possible complication of arteriovenous fistula [21]. Dissection of the renal vessels is carried out bimanually with endoshears and endodissector, very similar to open surgery (Fig. 9).

Organ Retrieval

The kidney, including the Gerota fascia, is dissected free of the respective adrenal gland and the surrounding peritoneum. Next, it is grasped in the hilar region and moved down into the

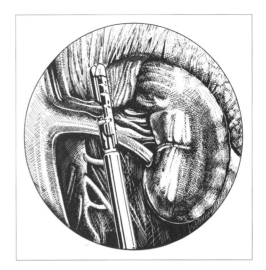

Fig. 13. Same as Fig. 12

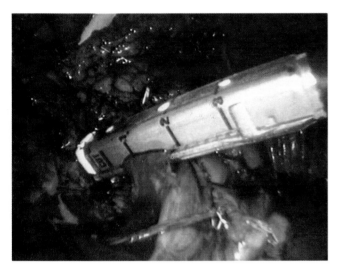

Fig. 11. Transection of the renal artery with an endoscopic stapler (Endo-GIA 30, white cartridge)

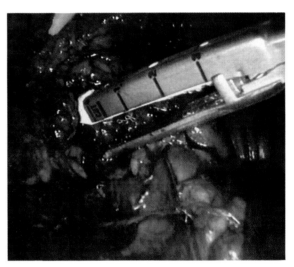

Fig. 14. The renal vein has been safely closed with a triple row of staples

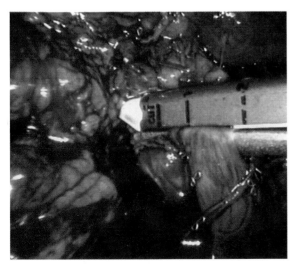

Fig. 12. Ligation of renal vein. Placement of Endo-GIA

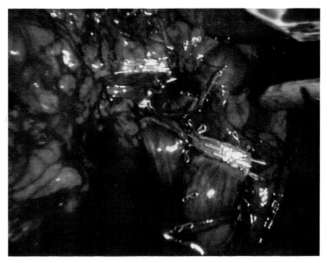

Fig. 15. Proximal stump of transected renal vein with three rows of titanium staples

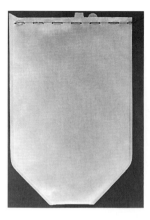

Fig. 16. Entrapment of kidney. The self-defolding organ bag (lapsac)

pelvic area preventing any interference with intra-abdominal introduction of the organ bag (Figs. 16–18). The lapsac is twirled around on a previously 4.5-mm converter-reduced endograsp and passed through port III. The organ bag unfolds intraabdominally and is held open by three endoforceps (via ports II , IV, and V) while the kidney is maneuvered into the lapsac (Figs. 19 and 20).

Recently, we have developed a new type of organ bag, the "lapbag", which opens intra-abdominallly because of a built-in nitenol ring, and therefore no further endoclamp is needed. This has significanty improved the procedure of organ entrapment.

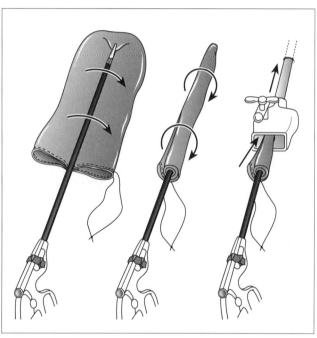

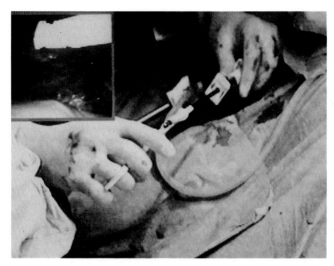

Figs. 17 and 18. Entrapment of kidney. Folding the bag over an endoforceps and insertion via the 12-mm port

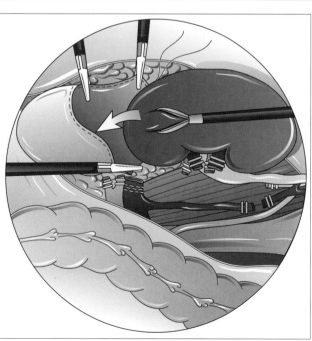

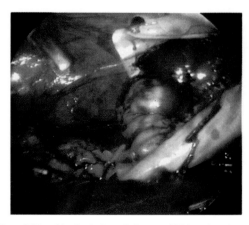

Figs. 19 and 20. Manipulation of dissected kidney into lapsac. Two or three clamps keep the organ bag open (triangle with base on the psoas muscle) while one or two pairs of forceps are necessary for entrapment of kidney

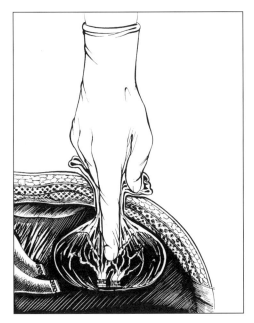

Fig. 21. Digital morcellation of kidney within the organ bag with index finger

Digital Fragmentation

After the endodissector pulls the drawstring thereby closing the bag, the trocar sleeve is removed and the neck of the bag is pulled out over the surface of the abdomen (subcostal port II for right kidney, suprailiacal port for the left side) under endoscopic control. The port wound is further incised (20 mm) making forceps removal of fatty tissue and digital fragmentation of the kidney into 3–5 pieces possible (Figs. 21 and 22). We never used a mechanical liquidizer, aspirator, or morcellating device during clinical or experimental cases.

Wound Closure

Before the trocars are removed under direct vision, the nephrectomy situs is inspected to rule out any active bleeding. Similar to open surgery, a drainage tube is placed routinely through ports IV or V. This permits drainage of blood and irrigation fluid and may reveal postoperative bleeding. The enlarged port incision is closed with fascia and skin suture. All other port incisions are sutured intracutaneously or covered with adhesive strips resulting in a favorable postoperative cosmetic appearance (Fig. 23).

Laparoscopic Nephroureterectomy

If additional ureterectomy is indicated (i. e., reflux nephropathy, organ-confined transitional cell carcinoma of the upper urinary tract), we first circumsize the orifice transurethrally with the electrohook following insertion of a ureteral stent (Figs. 24–27). Then, after transperitoneal laparoscopic nephrectomy, the distal ureter is dissected down to the bladder. By gently pulling on the ureter the previously circumsized intramural part can be antegradely extracted (Figs. 30–32) and removed from the abdominal cavity. Finally, the kidney specimen with the upper ureteral stump is retrieved by use of an organ bag and digital morcellation. After the procedure the bladder catheter is kept in place for 5–7 days providing healing of the urinary bladder.

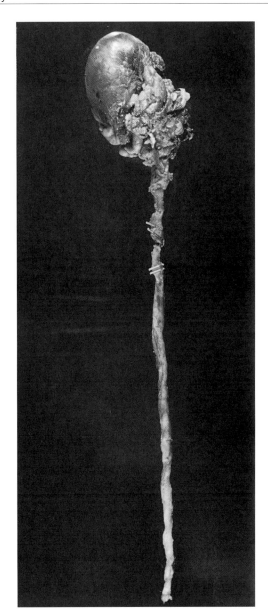

Fig. 22. Specimen of a laparoscopically removed reflux nephropathy

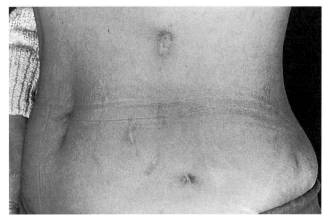

Fig. 23. Trocar wounds 4 weeks after transperitoneal laparoscopic nephrectomy (TLN)

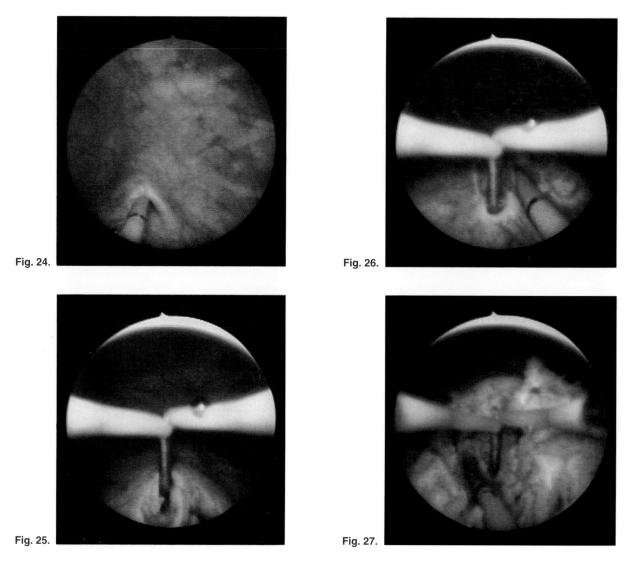

Fig. 24.

Fig. 26.

Fig. 25.

Fig. 27.

Figs. 24–27. Laparoscopic nephroureterectomy: transurethral circumcision of right orifice with the electrohook until intramural part of ureter is totally dissected

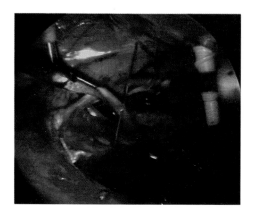

Fig. 28. Laparoscopic nephroureterectomy: fixation of the ureter by a transcutaneous suture

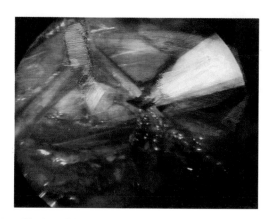

Fig. 29. Clipping of the ureter

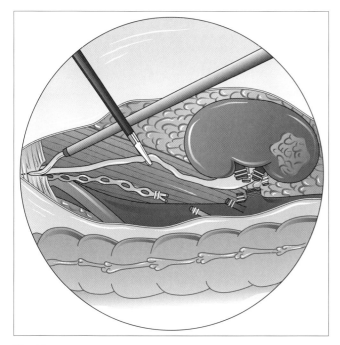

Fig. 30.

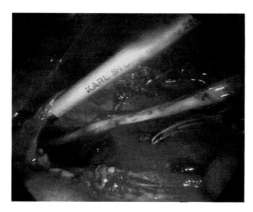

Fig. 31.

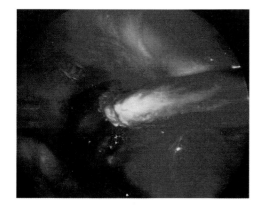

Fig. 32.

Figs. 30–32. Laparoscopic nephroureterectomy – antegrade dissection of the distal ureter under gentle traction until the previously circumcized orifice appears

Transperitoneal Laparoscopic Adrenalectomy

With the same access laparoscopic adrenalectomy can be performed (Figs. 33–36). Whereas on the left side complete mobilization of the descending colon is necessary to dissect the renal hilum for transection of the inferior suprarenal vein, for right-sided tumors subhepatic incision of the peritoneum over the inferior vena cava may be sufficient for adequate exposure of the gland. Retrieval of the organ can be performed with use of a small lapsac (Cook, Europe; Fig. 35).

Retroperitoneoscopy

Retroperitoneal Laparoscopic Nephrectomy (RLN)

Balloon-trocar System
The balloon-trocar system consists of a latex balloon ligated to an 11-mm metal trocar sheath (Fig. 37). A specially designed disposable balloon-trocar system is commercially available. However, in our experience the described cheap modification of this system proved to be sufficient when used according to the described manner. The balloon can be filled via the insufflation canal of the trocar sheath (Fig. 37).

For monitoring of the dissecting pressure during inflation we use a three-way system connected to the filling syringe (50 cc) and a manometer (i. e., hydraulic manometer as used for cystotonometry). As a cheaper solution the tube that is connected to the insufflation channel of the trocar sheath can be permanently marked with sterile bands every 10 cm. For measurements of the pressure existing in the balloon, the tube is then disconnected from the syringe and held vertically: The height of the water column in the tube in relation to the level of the kidney can thereby be estimated.

Once the latex balloon is filled with about 50 cc of normal saline the telescope is inserted into the trocar sheath. Because of its distension, the balloon becomes transparent and the process of dissection can be monitored under direct vision (see Fig. 41). The balloon is blocked with 400–1000 cc according to patient size (children 400–700; adults 700–1000 cc). In our studies the maximal capacity of the balloon (until rupture) amounted to 2000–2400 cc. But spontaneous rupture of the balloon may occur earlier, particularly if the intraluminal pressure increases due to significant adherences in the retroperitoneum (more than 130 cm H_2O). Therefore, the pressure in the balloon should not exceed 110 cm H_2O (Fig. 40).

Access to Retroperitoneum
Under general anesthesia, the patient is placed in the typical "kidney position" (see Fig. 43). No Trendelenburg position is necessary. A 15- to 18-mm incision (Fig. 38) is made in the "muscle-free" triangle between the 12th rib and the anterior iliac spine (between the lateral edges of the M. latissimus dor-

Fig. 33–36. Transperitoneal laparoscopic adrenalectomy

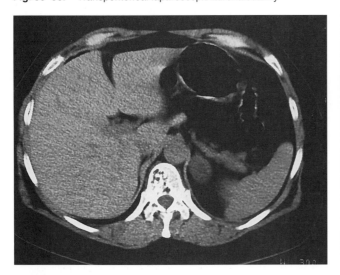

Fig. 33. Computertomography showing a 3 cm sized tumor in the left adrenal

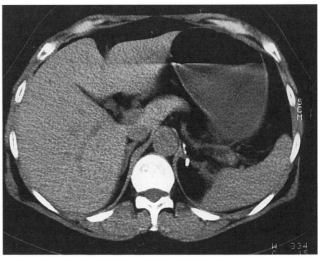

Fig. 36. CT-scan after laparoscopic removal of the tumor (cortical adenoma) demonstrating the Endoclips

Figs. 37–42. Balloon-trocar system for endoscopically controlled hydraulic dissection of the retroperitoneum

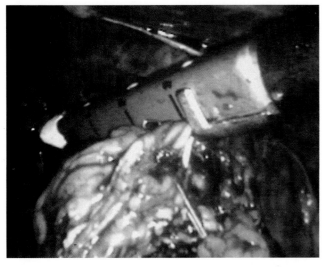

Fig. 34. Transsection of the adrenal using the Endo-GIA

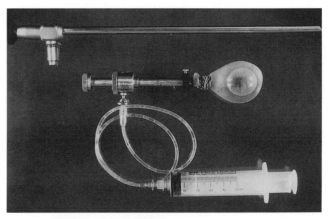

Fig. 37. A latex balloon is ligated to a fixation grip of a 11/12 mm metal trocar sheath. This balloon can be filled via the insufflation channel using a bladder syringe. During insufflation the telescope can be inserted to monitor the balloon dissection

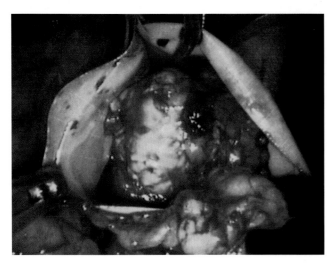

Fig. 35. Entrapment of the gland with small LapSac®

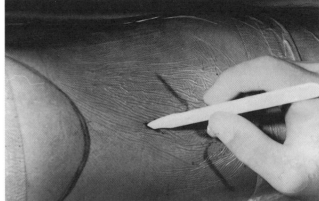

Fig. 38. 15 mm lumbodorsal incision at the "muscle-free" triangle between the edges of M. latissimus dorsi and M. obliquus externus. Subsequently a canal down to the retroperitoneal space is created by use of a dissecting forceps

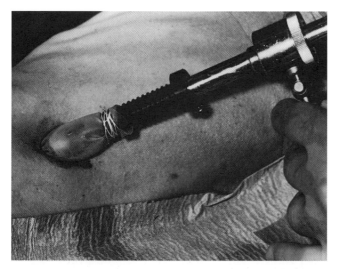

Fig. 39. Insertion of the balloon-trocar system after blunt dissection of the retroperitoneal space with the index finger pushing the peritoneum medially

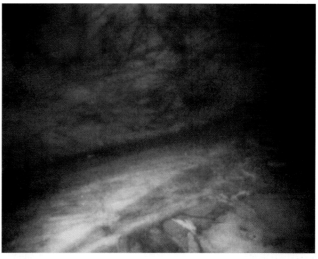

Fig. 41. Endoscopic view during balloon-dissection: The dense areolar tissue binding the fat in the retroperitoneum is pushed away by the balloon. Psoas muscle as well as Gerota's fascia can be identified through the balloon

si and M. obliquus externus). Then by blunt dissection with an Overhold forceps a canal is created down to the retroperitoneal space. The canal is dilated until the index finger can be introduced to push forward the peritoneum, thus creating a retroperitoneal cavity for correct placement of the balloon-trocar system (Fig. 39).

Hydraulic Balloon-Dissection
The balloon is filled with warmed normal saline (37 °C) using a 50 cc-syringe with Luer lock. Simultaneously, the dissection is endoscopically controlled with the telescope introduced via the trocar sheath into the balloon. It is of major importance

that the process of dissection be observed continously, i. e., separating Gerota's fascia from the psoas muscle (Fig. 41). If this is not the case, the pressure in the system has to be checked manometrically. It should not increase over 110 cm H_2O, otherwise the balloon has to be deflated to avoid its rupture. The total volume of the balloon depends mainly on the size of the patient. The filling is maintained for 5 min to achieve adequate haemostasis within the retroperitoneal space (Fig. 40).

After desufflation of the balloon, the balloon-trocar system is withdrawn. We then insert a sterile gauze into the retroperitoneal space to keep it dry. Additionally, the trocar sheath has to be cleaned and dried before placement. Then the trocar wound is closed around the sheath to avoid gas leakage (purse-string suture). The trocar is connected to the CO_2 insufflator to establish a pneumoretroperitoneum (15 mmHg, 3.5 l/min), and retroperitoneoscopy is performed (Fig. 42).

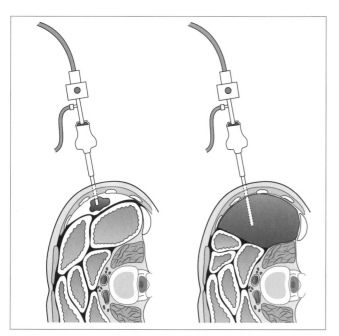

Fig. 40. Schematic drawing of video-optic controlled hydraulic balloon-dissection of the retroperitoneum (400–1000 cc normal saline). The intraluminal pressure can be measured manometrically and should not exceed 110 cm H_2O

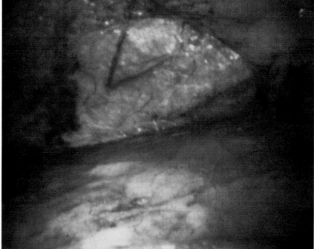

Fig. 42. Retroperitoneoscopy after removal of the balloon-trocar system and establishment of a pneumoretroperitoneum (12 mmHg) showing the ileo-psoas muscle

Fig. 43–45. Retroperitoneoscopic surgery – Patient's position, arrangement of armamentarium, site and size of trocars

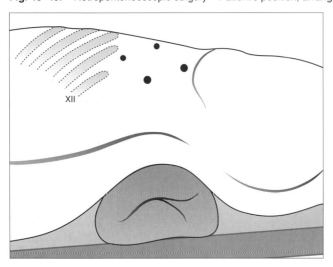

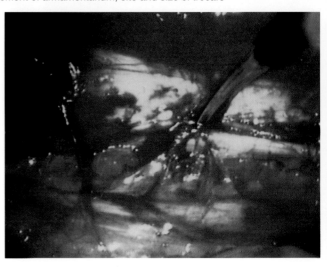

Fig. 43. Patient lies in typical flank position. Surgeon stands on the backside

Fig. 45. First operative step of retroperitoneoscopic surgery: incision of Gerota's fascia and dissection of the ureter

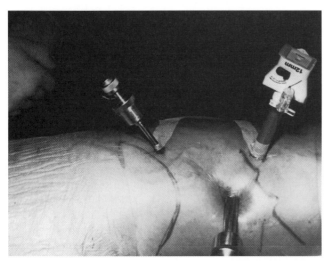

Fig. 44. Port I (12/13 mm for telescope), Port II (12 mm for Endo-GIA, alternatively 10/11 mm for right hand of surgeon), Port III (5 mm for left hand), Port IV (5 mm for assistant)

Placement of Secondary Trocars

In most cases four ports are used: port II (10/11 mm) for the right hand of the surgeon (use of endoshears and endoclip applicator) and port III (5 mm) for the left hand of the surgeon (use of endodissector). Finally, medially to the rim of the peritoneum, another 5-mm trocar is inserted (Port IV) serving for retraction of the kidney during the dissection. After placement of all trocars, the maximal insufflation pressure is decreased to 12 mmHg. As in the open procedure, the surgeon and the camera assistant stand on the dorsal side of the patient (Figs. 43 and 44).

First step of almost all procedures in the upper retroperitoneum represents the incision of Gerota's fascia (Fig. 45). The further technical steps of retroperitoneal laparoscopic nephrectomy (RLN) are the same as for the transperitoneal approach (Figs. 46-48).

Retroperitoneoscopic Heminephrectomy

Dissection of Ureter and Corresponding Vessels

Prior to retroperitoneoscopy we performed a retrograde pyelogram showing a stenosis of the ureteropelvic junction (UPJ) of the lower part of a duplicated right kidney (Fig. 49). Subsequently, the respective ureter was stented. Because the patient was very slim, the stented ureter was already visible via the balloon during dilatation of the retroperitoneum. The ureter was isolated and followed to the hilum where a crossing lower pole artery could be dissected and clipped (Figs. 50 and 51). In the following, all arterial and venous branches feeding the lower pole were isolated and transected between endoclips. This resulted in a purple color of the lower part of the kidney (Fig. 52) defining the line of resection.

Partial Resection of Kidney

We then started to transect the lower pole of the kidney with endoshears, whereas most of the heminephrectomy was performed with an endoscopic stapler in order to achieve adequate haemostasis (Fig. 53). The residual part of the resection plane was then sealed with a new haemostyptic collagen patch covered on one side with fibrin glue (TachoComb®, Nycomed Germany). For adequate haemostasis the patch has to be pressed on the resection plane for 5 min, thus controlling all minor bleeders. Of course, the same can be achieved utilizing an argon beam coagulator. The postoperative intravenous pyelogram showed an optimal function of the remnant upper pole (Fig. 54).

Retroperitoneoscopic Renal Biopsy and Cyst Marsupialization

Both procedures are technically not difficult. They mostly require only three ports. For retroperitoneoscopic renal biopsy, after incision of Gerota's fascia, the lower pole of the kidney is isolated and a spring-loaded biopsy needle is inserted transcutaneously parallel to port II. Thus, the biopsy can be performed under vision and the surface of the kidney fulgurated after withdrawal of the biopsy needle (Figs. 55 and 56).

Figs. 46–48. Dissection, clipping and division of the lumbar ureter

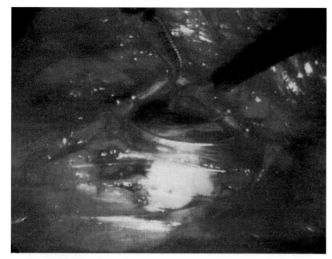

Fig. 46. Dissection, clipping and division of the lumbar ureter

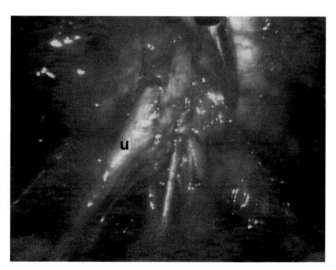

Fig. 47. Dissection of the renal hilum with ureter (u), and renal vessels

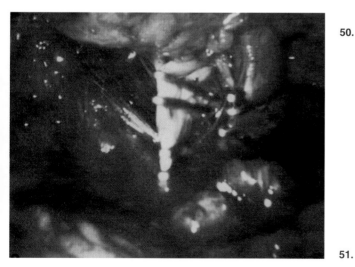

Fig. 48. Transsection of renal vein and artery between clips

Figs. 49–54. Retroperitoneoscopic heminephrectomy

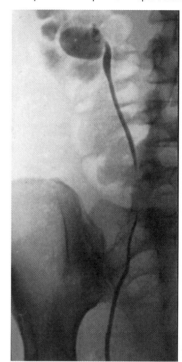

Fig. 49. Retrograde pyelogramm revealing stenosis of ureteropelvic junction of the lower collecting system of a duplicated right kidney

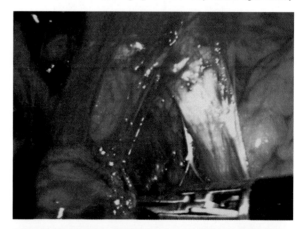

50.

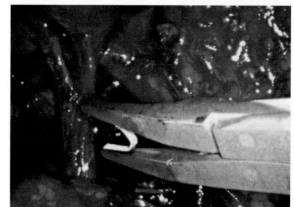

51.

Figs. 50 and 51. Dissection and clipping of a crossing lower pole artery causing the UPJ-stenosis

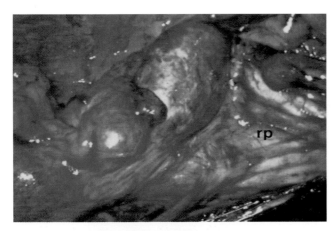

Fig. 52. Purple colour of the completely devascularized lower part of the kidney with its redundant renal pelvis (rp)

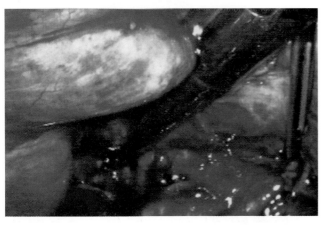

Fig. 53. The major part of heminephrectomy has been performed with an endoscopic stapler

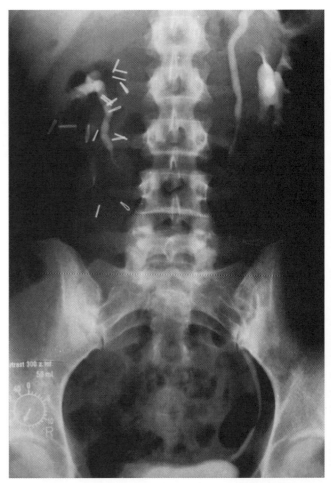

Fig. 54. Intravenous pyelogram on fourth postoperative day with optimal function of the residual upper part of the right kidney

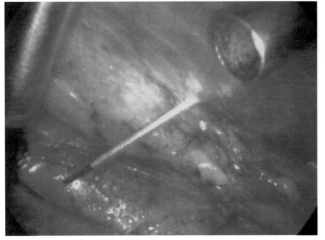

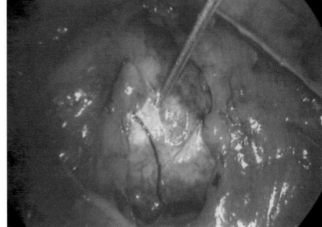

Figs. 55 and 56. Retroperitoneoscopic renal biopsy: Transcutaneous endoscopically guided puncture of the renal parenchyma with a spring-loaded needle.

Fig. 57–59. Retroperitoneoscopic marsupialisation of a right renal cyst with suspicious computertomographic finding.

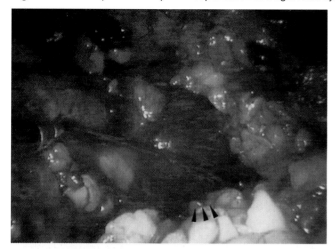

Fig. 57. Dissection of the cyst

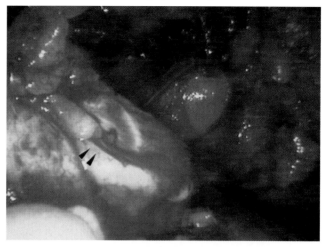

Fig. 59. Inspection and fulguration of the basis of the cyst

For renal cyst marsupialization the relevant part of the kidney has to be isolated from the overlying fatty capsule. After its identification (Fig. 57), the cyst is punctured or incised, and the containing fluid is aspirated and sampled for biochemical and cytological analysis. Thereafter, the cyst is resected "en niveau" with coagulation of the remnant cystic wall and floor (Figs. 58 and 59).

Retroperitoneoscopic Nephropexy

After placement of the trocars, the kidney is completely dissected within Gerota's fascia. Finally, the lower pole is fixed with two sutures (3/0 vicryl) to the psoas muscle. The suture has to include the fibrous renal capsule (Fig. 60). The knots are tied endoscopically using a technique similar to microsurgery (Fig. 61). For this purpose the length of the suture should not exceed 20 cm. We prefer a standard curved needle that is introduced via a 5/10-mm reducer sheath. After the procedure, the patient has absolute bedrest for 5 days.

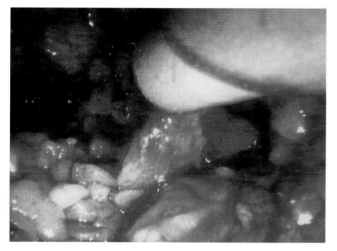

Fig. 58. Removal of the cystic wall via a reducer sheath

Figs. 60 and 61. Retroperitoneoscopic nephropexy

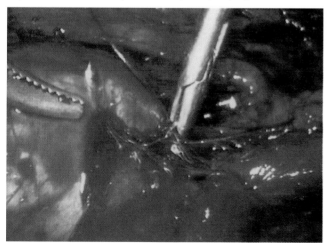

Fig. 60. Endoscopic suture taking the fibrous capsule and the psoas muscle

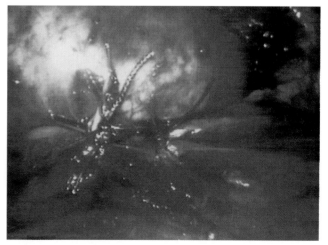

Fig. 61. Retroperitoneoscopic view after nephropexy using two endoscopic knots (vicryl 3/0)

Retroperitoneoscopic Dismembered Pyeloplasty

Dissection of Ureter and Aberrant Lower Pole Artery

Prior to retroperitoneoscopy a retrograde pyelogram was performed showing a crossing vessel causing the stenosis at the UPJ in both cases. We then placed an indwelling ureteral catheter (double-J stent). After having established the pneumoretroperitoneum, the upper ureter and the lower-pole artery crossing the ureter at the level of the UPJ are isolated (Fig. 62). In one case the artery was transected between two endoclips because the renal circulation seemed to be unaffected during temporary clamping of the vessel. In the other case the artery was left in place while reanastomosis of the renal pelvis was performed anteriorly.

Dismembered Pyeloplasty

After placement of a transcutaneous stay suture using a straight needle, the ureter is divided and spatulated. If necessary, the renal pelvis is trimmed and sutured (continuous suture). For reanastomosis of the ureteropelvic junction two interrupted sutures (Fig. 63) are placed endoscopically at the top and bottom of the anastomosis which is then accomplished with two continuous suture lines (Fig. 64). Finally, a drain is placed for 5 days. The bladder catheter is removed on the fifth day and the double-J stent on the 21st day.

Retroperitoneoscopic Ureterolithotomy

In case of the retroperitoneoscopic ureterolithotomy after failure of extracorporeal shockwave lithotripsy and ureteroscopy, the lumbar ureter was isolated and lifted with a vessel loop. Both ends of the loop were brought out alongside the trocar sheath of port II. After reinsertion of the trocar sheath, the ureter was longitudinally incised over the stone (Fig. 65), which was then extracted via an 11- to 5-mm reducer sheath. Finally, the ureter was closed by three interrupted endoscopic sutures of the adventitia (Figs. 66 and 67) and a drain placed for 3 days. The preoperatively placed ureteral stent was removed on the seventh day.

Retroperitoneoscopic Ureterocutaneostomy

For retroperitoneoscopic ureterocutaneostomy the lumbar ureter is isolated, clipped, and transected below its crossing with the iliac vessels. The distal tip of the ureter is then carefully pulled out to the surface of the trocar wound of port IV, which is used as the site of the ureterostomy. For this purpose the pneumoperitoneum has to be deflated. The ureter is then spatulated, stented (6F ureteral catheter), and sutured to the skin creating a ureteral nipple. The ureteral stent is removed on the tenth postoperative day.

Foreign-Body Extraction of Retroperitoneum

With the same technique it was possible to extract the tip of a ureteral catheter, which had perforated the ureter during ureteroscopy and accidentally was cut off by the sharp edge of the ureteroscope. It was then impossible to extract the catheter tip endoscopically without major risk of further ureteral damage. Retroperitoneoscopy using three ports followed by a gentle dissection of the periureteral tissue easily showed the tip of the stent so that the lost part of the catheter could be removed.

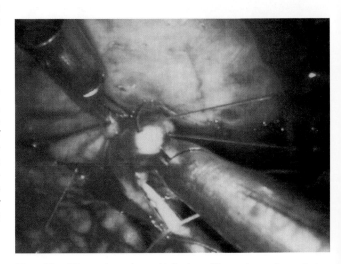

Fig. 63. Dismembered pyeloplasty with endoscopic suturing technique

Figs. 62–64. Retroperitoneoscopic pyeloplasty

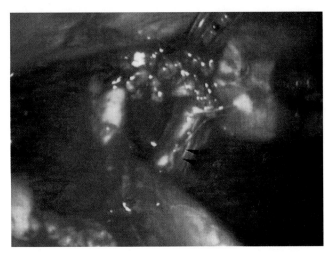

Fig. 62. Crossing lower pole vessel (arrows) causing UPJ-stenosis

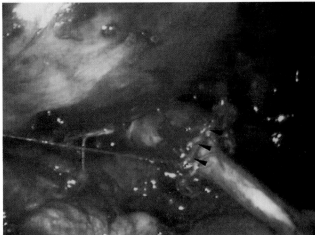

Fig. 64. Postoperative result showing the suture line (arrows)

Results

We performed the first successful laparoscopic nephrectomy on February 5, 1992. In the meantime we have performed a total of 58 nephrectomies, 10 radical tumor nephrectomies, 3 adrenalectomies, 7 nephroureterectomies, and 18 modified retroperitoneal lymphadenectomies for stage I testicular cancer (Figs. 68–72).

The operation time varied from 50 to 90 min (renal biopsy, renal cyst marsupialization, foreign-body extraction), 120–190 min (simple nephrectomy, nephropexy, heminephrectomy), to 360–400 minutes (tumor nephrectomy, pyeloplasty, retroperitoneal lymphadenectomy). The mean blood loss amounted to 125 (0–1200) cc. This included four cases that required open intra- or postoperative revision due to severe bleeding (Table 5). Three other cases with subcutaneous or retroperitoneal hematoma were treated conservatively. In four further instances open revision was necessary due to massive inflammatory adhesions of the kidney with the right lobe of the liver and in the other case due to bowel injury during adhesiolysis.

All these cases had an uneventful postoperative course. The mean postoperative stay was 6 days ranging from 3 to 18 days.

Using the retroperitoneal access (RLN), we were able to further reduce the postoperative morbidity (i. e., amount of analgetics) of the procedure compared with the transperitoneal laparoscopic and open nephrectomy (Table 5). In two instances we encountered a rupture of the balloon after instillation of 900 cc. In both cases all of the fluid was aspirated and the dissecting maneuver repeated up to 1000 and 1100 cc, respectively. After monitoring of the dissecting pressure (maximum 110 cm H_2O) this could be avoided.

On average, drainage tubes could be removed on the third day after minimal fluid secretion (150–300 ml). Morphinoid analgetics required for relief of postoperative pain on the ward

Table 5. Transperitoneal (TLN) vs retroperitoneal laparoscopic nephrectomy (RLN) for benign renal disease. Comparison with open nephrectomy (Nx)

	TLN ($n = 22$)	RLN ($n = 23$)	Nx ($n = 19$)
Indication			
Hydronephrosis	9	11	11
Chronic pyelonephritis	4	5	
Renovascular disease	2	4	1
Renal dysplasia	1	2	–
Reflux nephropathy	2	3	1
End-stage nephrolithiasis	3	1	
Previous surgery			
Abdominal	1	3	3
Retroperitoneal	–	1	1
Results			
Mean duration (min)	202	168	117
Complications (III/IV)	5	1	2
Need of analgetics			
Amount (vial/pat)	1.8	0.7	3.3
Duration (postop. days)	2.5	1.0	4.0
Postoperative stay (days)	6.9	4.7	10.3

Figs. 65–67. Retroperitoneoscopic ureterolithotomy for an impacted calculus in the upper ureter

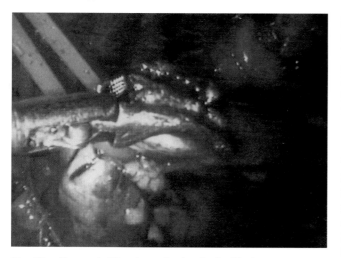

Fig. 65. Removal of the stone after longitudinal incison

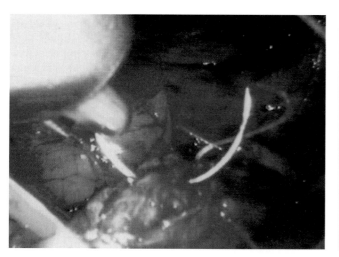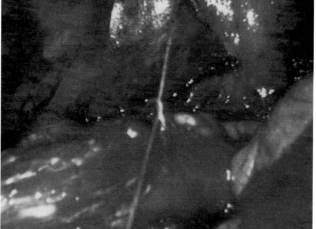

Figs. 66 and 67. Closure of the ureteral wall by three endoscopic sutures (Vicryl, 4/0)

Figs. 68–72. Laparoscopic retroperitoneal lymphadenectomy for stage I non-seminomatous testicular cancer

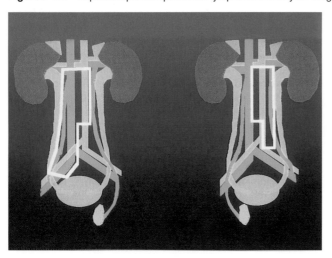

Fig. 68. Template of modified lymph node dissection for left and right testicular tumor (according to Weißbach 1987)

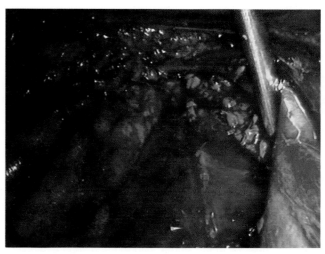

Fig. 71. Complete removal of paracaval lymphatic tissue

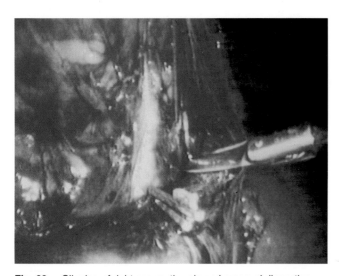

Fig. 69. Clipping of right spermatic vein and precaval dissection.

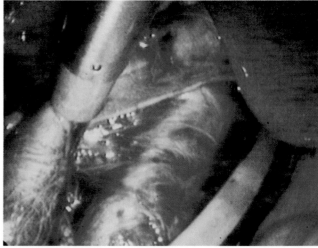

Fig. 72. Complete removal of interaortocaval lymph nodes, placement of drainage tube

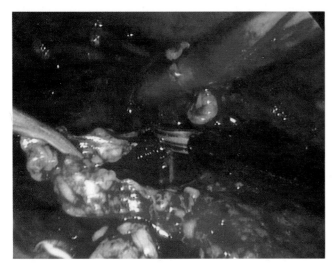

Fig. 70. Paracaval lymph node dissection

averaged 1.15 vials per patient within 2.1 days. Thus, patients could be quickly mobilized and were discharged after uneventful recovery on the sixth (4-10) postoperative day. Figure 23 demonstrates the minor scarring that was seen 4 weeks after laparoscopic nephrectomy.

Laparoscopic Versus Open Nephrectomy

We have compared 22 transperitoneal laparoscopic case results with 23 retroperitoneoscopic and 19 matched open nephrectomies performed in our department. The main results, summarized in Table 5, indicate the longer operating time of laparoscopic nephrectomy, but also reveal the significant advantages of this approach with regard to postoperative pain and hospitalization. Furthermore, it demonstrates the further reduction of access trauma when using the retroperitoneoscopic approach.

Transperitoneal Laparoscopic Nephrectomy: Modification of Clayman's Technique

Laparoscopic nephrectomy was first successfully carried out in 1990 by Clayman [7]. After extensive preclinical work [6], Clayman solved two major problems: kidney retrieval with an organ bag and tissue morcellation to ease intra-abdominal bag removal. Like others [3, 57] we support most of his approach; however, certain steps, in our opinion, warrant modification:

Creation of Pneumoperitoneum and Trocar Placement in Flank Position

Clayman reported creation of the pneumoperitoneum in supine Trendelenburg position of the patient. Thereafter, all trocars are inserted and the patient is put in a flank position [7, 8]. In our experience, creation of the pneumoperitoneum and trocar placement can easily be performed with the patient in the standard flank position (Fig. 1) [46]. Moreover, port I is situated lateral to the umbilicus, not supraumbilically [7–9], thereby avoiding visual interference with displaced colon. Insertion of the lateral trocars in the retroperitoneum (ports IV and V) can be carried out safely after colon mobilization. The entire organ dissection is performed through ports II and III, and ports IV and V are mainly used for traction holding and organ retrieval.

Safe Individual Stapling of Renal Vessels with Endo-GIA Instead of Clipping Methods

We prefer to transect the main renal vessels with individual stapling using the Endo-GIA. Of course, this is a cost-intensive approach. However, the renal vein should be ligated with this device, because the diameter of the renal vein may exceed the length of the endoclips. On the other hand, smaller renal arteries may also be secured by use of the large endoclips presently available. It has to be emphasized that both vessels should be divided separately, because stapling of both of the renal vessels together with the Endo-GIA may lead to arteriovenous fistula as observed by Clayman and coworkers after Endo-GIA stapling in their animal studies [21].

Digital Fragmentation of the Kidney

Our experience with organ retrieval has convinced us that complete liquidization of the kidney is not necessary. Digital fragmentation as seen in transvesical prostate adenomectomy, avoids mechanical injury to the organ bag described by Figenshau [21] and on the other hand permits exact macroscopic and histological evaluation by the pathologist [37, 38]. In special cases however, e. g., uterus myomatosus, mechanical fragmentation may be inevitable. Newly developed instruments with rotating blades [6], tissue liquidizers, or ultrasonic aspirators (CUSA) may prove suitable in such cases [11]. Intra-abdominal kidney removal by means of an organ bag is, even in cases of malignant disease, a safe method of organ retrieval assuming that the bag is impermeable to tumor cells and bacteria. In this situation we increasingly prefer to retrieve the organ intact via a small lower abdominal or suprapubic incision [4].

Transabdominal Versus Retroperitoneal Approach

In most of our cases we have used the transabdominal approach. In our opinion, the major advantage of this technique in comparison with the retroperitoneal approach is that it per-

mits excellent intracavitary viewing of all adjacent organs. Experimental and clinical reports on complications after retroperitoneal laparoscopic nephrectomy [20, 50], report insufficient endoscopic viewing. However, all these authors created the retroperitoneal space only pneumatically by CO_2 insufflation via Veress needle.

Retroperitoneoscopy: Modification of Gaur's Technique

Recently, Gaur [22] described a very interesting modification to create the retroperitoneal space by use of a balloon catheter placed either outside or inside of Gerota's fascia. For adequate haemostasis the balloon was filled with 1–1.5 liters of air and kept in place for 15–20 min. We have had excellent results with this method, but in the meantime we have modified the Gaur technique in several ways [40, 41]:

1. We use the first trocar incision for digital dissection of the retroperitoneal space prior to balloon insufflation.

   In the beginning, when using the red rubber balloon catheter, we tried to minimize the size of the tract to the retroperitoneum. However, we have changed this approach completely: The first trocar incision is made to about 15 mm, which allows to introduce the index finger into the retroperitoneum and to push away the peritoneum as in open surgery. Thereby a considerable space can be created prior to insertion of the balloon-trocar system. Moreover, the kidney can also be localized already by palpation.

   The major advantage of this technique is that the dissection pressure inside the balloon is significantly reduced, and rupture of the balloon does not occur. On the other hand, the larger trocar incision can be later used for retrieval and morcellation of the kidney. In our approach now, the extension of the trocar incision is made at the beginning, not – as previously reported with transperitoneal laparoscopic nephrectomy [38, 39] – at the end of the procedure.

   Additionally, this technique of entering the retroperitoneal space proved to be very safe, easy, and reproduceable. We feel that it may obviate other approaches to retroperitoneoscopy, i. e., utilizing fluoroscopic-guided placement of the Veress needle [33].

2. We perform a preliminary blunt dissection only down to the psoas muscle and not inside Gerota's fascia.

   Gaur pointed out that it would speed up the operating time if Gerota's fascia was incised for subfascial placement of the balloon, because the total ureter would be already isolated by balloon dissection. We consider our approach safer and prefer the endoscopic dissection of the ureter with endoshears and endodissectors. In our experience, the incision of Gerota's fascia and isolation of the ureter after creation of the pneumoretroperitoneum represents a very straightforward procedure.

3. We control the balloon dissection endoscopically

   In the beginning with the balloon catheter [40], we used a coaxial introduction technique of the trocar sheath via the telescope. The balloon catheter was then inserted via the sheath. With the recently applied balloon-trocar-sheath technique this is no longer necessary. The balloon-trocar allows the endoscopic observation of the balloon dissection by simply introducing the telescope in the balloon-trocar sheath. A disposable balloon-dissecting trocar system has been developed mainly for extraperitoneal pelvic lymphadenectomy (s. Chap. 4), which proved to be very effective in our hands. However, a similar and much cheaper system can be self-made using a latex balloon tied to a metal trocar.

4. We use a hydraulic dissecting technique

Gaur [22] described a pneumatic balloon-dissecting technique utilizing air insufflation at a pressure up to 110 mmHg. We feel that filling the balloon with normal saline provides better dissecting properties because water is incompressible. However, the position of the balloon must be controlled exactly. In problematic cases (i. e., in case of previous surgery or in children) when using the balloon catheter, we interrupted the balloon insufflation, and after establishing a pneumoretroperitoneum, checked the amount of dissection in the retroperitoneal space or used an ultrasound scanner during balloon insufflation. However, with digital predissection using the index finger the amount of dense adhesions can now be estimated prior to insertion of the balloon-trocar system. In our experience, severe adhesions (i. e., after previous renal surgery) cannot be taken down sufficiently by hydraulic balloon dissection and need endoscopic dissection.

5. We monitor the pressure in the balloon-trocar system

To avoid rupture of the latex balloon and possible injury to the peritoneum, it is of major importance to monitor the dissecting pressure in the system. Because we use a hydraulic dissecting technique, manometry is very simple and provides exact data, rather than using a pneumatic balloon technique as proposed by Gaur [22]. The maximum intraluminal pressure should not exceed 110 cm H_2O. Adhesions that cannot be broken down at this level should be dissected under retroperitoneoscopic view.

There is no doubt that endoscopically controlled balloon dissection represents one of the major improvements for retroperitoneoscopic surgery. In our experience, it allows safe access to the retroperitoneal organs. Together with gas insufflation optimal anatomical exposure of the kidney and ureter can be accomplished, rather than using a gasless approach (i. e., with the Buess endoscope).

Advantages of Retroperitoneoscopy
One of the major advantages of this new technique represents the fact that it is exactly the same approach to the kidney as in open surgery. Thus, in contrast to the transperitoneal laparoscopic access, more or less the same surgical dissecting principles can be applied (i. e., primary isolation of the ureter and dissection of the kidney within Gerota's fascia in case of a simple nephrectomy). As a result, the learning curve of laparoscopic urological surgery is significantly reduced compared with the transperitoneal approach: It was interesting to note how easily the retroperitoneoscopic dissection could be performed by experienced urosurgeons with only minor laparoscopic experience.

In accordance with Kerbl and Clayman [32], our first experience with retroperitoneal laparoscopic nephrectomy (RLN) in-

dicated that this access enables further reduction of postoperative morbidity compared with transperitoneal laparoscopic nephrectomy (TLN) and open surgery (Table 5). We therefore currently use the previously described transperitoneal laparoscopic approach [38, 39] only for a tumor nephrectomy, adrenalectomy, and retroperitoneal lymphadenectomy. All other procedures in the upper retroperitoneum are performed retroperitoneoscopically.

Finally, the retroperitoneoscopic access is safer and cheaper than the transperitoneal approach: There is no need for a blind puncture with the Veress needle or the first trocar [7, 8, 38, 39]. Therefore, only reusable trocars and instruments are used. With the introduction of endoclip applicators making the use of the same clips as in open surgery possible, the need for disposable multiclip applicators has become questionable. As a result, in the future only endoscopic staplers may be necessary in some cases of larger renal veins as single disposable instruments.

Disadvantage of Retroperitoneoscopy
A little disadvantage of the retroperitoneoscopic approach represents the smaller operative field compared with the transperitoneal laparoscopic access. However, with the use of a 30° telescope we could successfully compensate this even in the case of children. Theoretically, in problematic situations the cranial working port could be placed transcostally (i. e., between 11th and 12th rip) as for thoracoscopic procedures. However, it must be emphasized that in case of major obesity with a large perirenal fatty capsule, the transperitoneal route should be preferred.

Perspectives of Retroperitoneoscopy
There is no doubt that most of the ablative procedures for benign disease of kidney, ureter, and adrenals can be performed using this access (Table 2). In this group RLN plays the most important role and has already become an established procedure in a few centers in the world (11th World Congress on Endourology and ESWL, Florence, October 20–23, 1993), whereas heminephrectomy and renal cyst marsupialization will be performed infrequently. In the case of adrenalectomy, the transperitoneal route [35, 38] may be preferable for larger cortical adenomas or pheochromocytomas. Another interesting, but also rare indication is the retroperitoneoscopic lumbar sympathectomy [29, 56].

Regarding reconstructive retroperitoneoscopic procedures, we and others (Table 2) have limited clinical experience with endoscopic suturing. However, most of the present open reconstructive operations on kidney and ureter have been performed laparoscopically including nephropexy, pyelo-lithotomy, dismembered pyeloplasty, ureterolithotomy, and ureterocutaneostomy [18, 24-26, 40, 41]. We feel that the retroperitoneoscopic access should be preferred for all these indications. However, presently there are considerable limitations either with regard to the indication for these procedures (i. e., laparoscopic pyelo- or ureterolithotomy in the area of extracorporeal shockwave lithotripsy and endourology) or regarding the laparoscopic expertise to perform complicated endoscopic suturing techniques (i. e., for dismembered pyeloplasty) resulting in long operating times.

Therefore, future studies are necessary to determine the definitive value of retroperitoneoscopy for all reconstructive procedures.

Laparoscopic Adrenalectomy

In the meantime several authors have shown that the same technique can be applied for removal of other organs in the retroperitoneum such as the adrenal glands [35, 38, 44, 49]. We have carried out nine adrenalectomies together with laparoscopic tumor nephrectomy and an additional three for a cortical adenoma (Figs. 33–36). Adrenalectomy may be difficult due to fragility of the organ, thus inducing diffuse bleeding. Therefore, new instruments or dissection techniques (i. e., with pulsed Neodym-YAG laser fiber) need to be developed.

Okada et al. [35] recently reported six adrenalectomies using the Buess endoscope in a retroperitoneal approach after making a 4-cm incision. In accordance with other authors, we feel that in contrast to this technique, the transperitoneal laparoscopic approach offers the advantage of a complete overview. This might be important at least in cases of larger adrenalomas or a pheochromocytoma, which was excluded by Okada and coworkers.

Laparoscopy for Renal and Upper Urinary Tract Tumors

Whereas laparoscopic adrenalectomy including only a small number of patients may be very accepted as indication, laparoscopic removal of renal malignancies is still strongly debated. The main concerns are directed toward the removal of the tumor specimen with the risk of intra-abdominal spillage of tumor cells. According to this we could demonstrate as others (Table 6) that all guidelines of radical tumor surgery, i. e., primary dissection of the artery, en bloc removal of kidney, Gerota's fascia, and the adrenal, can be fulfilled laparoscopically. Additionally, we could demonstrate that digital fragmentation of the specimen within the lapsac enables exact diagnosis by the pathologist even in case of a renal cell carcinoma, without the risk of damaging the bag during mechanical morcellation as reported by Figenshau [21]. Moreover, the risk of spillage of tumor cells or bacteria in case of a pyonephrosis can be avoided by shielding the neck of the lapsac with an adhesive foil.

Nevertheless, digital fragmentation does not represent a very elegant technique; therefore, further research activities are neccessary. In case of larger tumors, retrieval of the intact specimen within the lapsac via a 3- to 4-cm suprapubic incision may be an alternative [4]. This access can also be used during the procedure as a "manually assisted laparoscopic tumor nephrectomy," which, according to our experience, leads to further reduction of the operative time without a significant increase of postoperative morbidity. However, the coordination of the intra-abdominal hand with the laparoscope requires extended video-endoscopic experience.

Laparoscopic nephroureterectomy can be performed in combination with transurethral circumcision of the orifice (Figs. 24–27). We perform just an antegrade dissection and extraction of the previously intramurally transected ureter. In contrast to Clayman [31] and Chiu [4], we do not believe that the dissection of a bladder cuff with the Endo-GIA is needed.

We have applied our technique of antegrade ureterectomy in combination with open nephroureterectomy to avoid a second incision in more than 40 cases (unpublished data). In a 4-year follow-up, no local tumor recurrence was observed, and no complication occurred when the bladder catheter was removed on the seventh postoperative day. The major advantage of performing this technique laparoscopically is that the ureter can be dissected under excellent vision down to the bladder, thereby achieving complete haemostasis. We significantly cut down the operating time from 9–10 h, as reported by Clayman and Kerbl [31] to 4–5 h.

However, presently there is no doubt that laparoscopic surgery for tumor in the upper urinary tract is still experimental. Therefore, exact selection of patients and evaluation of postoperative data is required to determine the final value of laparoscopy for this indication.

Future of Laparoscopic Nephrectomy: Laparoscopic Training

The continuous spread of TLN with now more than 500 procedures carried out world-wide (Table 6) indicates that this technique is about to become a standard urological procedure. However, it has to be emphasized that TLN is difficult; therefore, adequate laparoscopic training is required [28]. We followed a step-by-step training program that enabled us to successfully perform our first case after a training period of 6 months (Table 7). Nevertheless, we very much appreciated the experienced assistance of Malcolm Coptcoat in our first case.

Table 7. Step-by-step training program for laparoscopic surgery

Lap simulator
Animal studies
Laptent-assisted surgery
Easy laparoscopic procedures
Transperitoneal laparoscopic nephrectomy

With increasing application of laparoscopy in urology, not only for ablative but also for reconstructive surgery, a standardized training program being organized by the different "Lap-centers" that exist in every country seems reasonable. This should include courses on the lap simulator and animal model. However, in addition "Lap-tent"-simulated surgery (Table 7) proved to be very useful to bridge the gap from "pig to person" [1, 28]. Finally, hands-on assistance during clinical

Table 6. Laparoscopic nephrectomy: worldwide experience

Author	n	Indications
Clayman and Kavoussi	80	Benign and malignant renal disease
Coptcoat and Joyce	93	Benign and malignant renal disease
El-Kappany	110	Benign renal disease
Rassweiler	100	Benign and malignant renal disease
Others*	100	Benign and malignant renal disease

* Beer, Bowsher, Chirpas, Chiu, Fahlenkamp, Hulbert, Janetschek, Künkel, Recker, Schuessler, Smith, Weber, Webb, Wickham, Winfield, Yamada

cases may be mandatory. Thereafter, the first steps should be supervised by a laparoscopically experienced urologist.

There is no doubt that even the most experienced laparoscopists in urology have not reached the end of their learning curve. However, the presently accumulated expertise should allow laparoscopists to avoid severe complications. In the end, laparoscopy may one day become a normal part of the urological teaching program as in the case of endourology presently. However, we are still far away from this point.

References

1. ALTMAN L: Surgical injuries lead to new rule. The New York Times, Sunday, June 14, 1992, 47.
2. BAY-NIELSEN H, SCHULTZ A: Endoscopic retroperitoneal removal of stones from the upper half of the ureter. Scand J Urol Nephrol 16 (1982) 227–228.
3. BOWSHER WG, CLARKE A, COSTELLO AJ: Laparoscopic nephrectomy. J Endourol 6 (1992) S152 (abstract no. V-1).
4. CHIU AW, CHEN MT, HUANG WJS, JUANG GD, LU SH, CHANG LS: Laparoscopic nephroureterectomy and endocopic incision of bladder cuff. Min Invas Therapy 1 (1992) 299–303.
5. CLAYMAN RV, PREMINGER GM, FRANKLIN JR, CURRY T, PETERS PC: Percutaneous ureterolithotomy. J Urol 133 (1985) 671–673.
6. CLAYMAN RV, KAVOUSSY LR, LONG SR, DIERKS SM, MERETYK S, SOPER NJ: Laparoscopic nephrectomy: initial report of pelviscopic organ ablation in the pig. J Endourol 4 (1990) 247–251.
7. CLAYMAN R, KAVOUSSI LR, SOPER NJ, DIERKS SM, MERETYK S, DARCY MD, ROEMER FD, PINGLETON ED, THOMSON PG, LONG SR: Laparoscopic nephrectomy: initial case report. J Urol 146 2 (1991) 278–282.
8. CLAYMAN RV, KAVOUSSI LR, SOPER NJ, ALBALA DM, FIGENSHAU RS, CHANDHOKE PS: Laparoscopic nephrectomy: review of the initial 10 cases. J Endourol 2 (1992) 127–132.
9. CLAYMAN RV, MCDOUGALL EM, KAVOUSSI LR, SOPER NJ, ALBALA D, FIGENSHAU RS, CHANDHOKE PS: Laparoscopic nephrectomy. J Endourol 6 (1992) 58 (abstract no. B-11).
10. CHIRPAZ A, PETIBON E: Nephro-uretérectomie gauche sous contrôle coelioscopique. J Coelio-chir 2 (1992) 32–34.
11. COPTCOAT MJ, ISON KT, WICKHAM JEA: Endoscopic tissue liquidization and surgical aspiration. J Endourol 2 (1988) 321–329.
12. COPTCOAT MJ, JOYCE A, RASSWEILER J, POPERT R: Laparoscopic nephrectomy: the Kings and Mannheim clinical experience. J Urol 147 (1992) 433 A (abstract no. 881).
13. COPTCOAT MJ: Endoscopic tissue liquidization of the prostate, bladder and kidney. ChM thesis, 1990, Liverpool University.
14. CORTESI N, FERRARI P, ZAMBARDA E, MANETTI A, BALDINI A, MORANO FP: Diagnosis of bilateral abdominal cryptorchidism by laparoscopy. Endoscopy 8 (1976) 33–37.
15. CUSCHIERI A, DUBOIS F, MOUIEL J, MOURET P, BECKER H, BUESS G, TREDE M, TROIDL H: the European Experience with laparoscopic cholecystectomy. Am J Surg 161 (1991) 385.
16. DONOVAN JF, WINFIELD HN: Laparoscopic varix ligation. J Urol 147 (1992) 77–81.
17. DUBOIS F, ICARD P, BERTHELOT G, LEVARD H: Coelioscopic cholecystectomy: preliminary report of 36 cases. Ann Surg 211 (1990) 60–62.
18. ESCOVAR P, REY M, LOPEZ JR, RODRÍGUEZ M, LARIVA F, GONZALES R: Ureterolitotomia laparoscopica. Urologia Panam 4 (1992) 29– 34.
19. ESPINER HJ, ELTRINGHAM WK: Organ retrieval system for laparoscopic surgery, Endo 1991, 25th Congress of S.M.I.E.R., Mannheim 27–30 November 1991.
20. FIGENSHAU RS, CLAYMAN RV, KAVOUSSI LR, CHANDHOKE P, ALBALA DM, STONE AM: Retroperitoneal laparoscopic nephrectomy: laboratory and initial clinical experience. J Endourol 5 (1991) S 130 (abstract no. P XIII-15).
21. FIGENSHAU RS, ALBALA DM, CLAYMAN RV, KAVOUSSI LR, CHANDHOKE P, STONE AM: Laparoscopic nephrourectomy: initial laboratory experience. Min Invas Therapy 1 (1991) 93–97.

22. GAUR DD: Laparoscopic operative retroperitoneoscopy. J Urol 148 (1992) 1137–1139.
23. GAUR D, AGARWAL DK, PUROHIT KC: Retroperitoneal laparoscopic nephrectomy: initial case report. J Urol 149 (1993) 103–105.
24. GAUR DD: Retroperitoneal laparoscopic ureterolithotomy. World J Urol 11 (1993) 175–177.
25. GAUR DD, PUROHIT KC, AGARWAL DK, DARSHANE AS: Laparoscopic ureterolithotomy for impacted lower ureteral calculi: initial case report. Min Invas Therapy 2 (1993) 267–269.
26. GAUR DD, AGARWAL DK, PUROHIT KC, DARSHANE AS: Retroperitoneal laparoscopic pyelolithotomy. J Urol 151 (1994) 927–929.
27. HAGOOD PG, MEHAN DJ, WORISCHEK JH, ANDRUS CH, PARRA RO: Laparoscopic varicocelectomy: preliminary report of a new technique. J Urol 147 (1992) 73–76.
28. HENKEL TO, POTEMPA DM, RASSWEILER J, MANEGOLD BC, ALKEN P: Lap simulator, animal studies and the Laptent: bridging the gap between open and laparoscopic surgery. Surg Endosc 7 (1993) 539–543.
29. JANETSCHEK G, FLORA G, BIEDERMANN H, BARTSCH G: Lumbar sympathectomy by means of retroperitoneoscopy. Min Invas Therapy 2 (1993) 271–273.
30. KELLING G: Über Ösophagoskopie, Gastroskopie und Coelioskopie. Münch Med Wschr 49 (1901) 21–24.
31. KERBL K, CLAYMAN RV, MCDOUGALL EM, URBAN DA, GILL I, KAVOUSSI LR: Laparoscopic nephroureterectomy: evaluation of first clinical series. Eur Urol 23 (1993) 431–436.
32. KERBL K, CLAYMAN RV: Advances in laparoscopic renal and ureteral surgery. Eur Urol 25 (1994) 1–6.
33. MANDRESSI A, BUIZZA C, ANTONELLI D, BELLONI M, CHISENA S, ZAROLI A, BERNASCONI S: Retro-extraperitoneal laparoscopic approach to excise retroperitoneal organs: kidney and adrenal gland. Min Invas Therapy 2 (1993) 213–220.
34. MAZEMAN E, LEMAITRE L, WURTZ A, GILIOT P: Lymph node staging in prostatic and bladder cancers. Progr Urol 1 (1991) 224–234.
35. OKADA K, YOSHIKAWA T, HIRAKATA H, HAMADA T: Endoscopic adrenalectomy. J Endourol 6 (1992) S56 (abstract no. B-2).
36. RASSWEILER J, RICHTER GM, KAUFFMANN GW, ALKEN P (1991): Capillary chemoembolization with Ethibloc: pharmacokinetical basis and results in a new model of renal rat tumors. Proceedings of Third International Congress of Minimally Invasive Therapy, Boston, 10–12 November, p. 68 (abstract no. G-134).
37. RASSWEILER JJ, HENKEL TO, POTEMPA DM, BECKER P, GNNTHER M, COPTCOAT M, ALKEN P: Die Technik der transperitonealen laparoskopischen Nephrektomie (TLN) – experimentelle Grundlagen und erste klinische Erfahrungen. Akt Urol 23 (1992) 220–228.
38. RASSWEILER JJ, HENKEL TO, POTEMPA DM, COPTCOAT M, ALKEN P: The technique of transperitoneal laparoscopic nephrectomy, adrenalectomy and nephroureterectomy. Eur Urol 22 (1993) 425– 430.
39. RASSWEILER J, HENKEL TO, POTEMPA DM, COPTCOAT MJ, MILLER K, PREMINGER GM, ALKEN P: Transperitoneal laparoscopic nephrectomy: training, technique and results. J Endourol 7 (1993) 505–516.
40. RASSWEILER JJ, HENKEL TO, STOCK CH, GRESCHNER M, BECKER P, PREMINGER GM, SCHULMAN CC, FREDE T, ALKEN P: Retroperitoneal laparoscopic nephrectomy and other procedures in the upper retroperitoneum using a balloon dissection technique. Eur Urol 25 (1994) 229–236.
41. RASSWEILER JJ, HENKEL TO, STOCK C, FREDE T, ALKEN P : Retroperitoneoscopic surgery – technique, indications and first experience. Min Invas Therapy 3 (1994) 179–195.
42. REDDICK EJ, OLSON DO: Laparoscopic laser cholecystectomy: a comparison with mini-lap cholecystectomy. Surg Endosc 3 (1989) 34–39.
43. SCHÜSSLER WW, VANCAILLIE TG, REICH H, GRIFFITH DP: Transperitoneal endosurgical lymphadenectomy in patients with localized prostrate cancer. J Urol 145 (1991) 988–991.
44. SCHÜSSLER WW, PHARAND D: Laparoscopic adrenalectomy: case report. J Endourol 6 (1992) 158 (abstract no. V-27).
45. SEMM K: Endoscopic appendectomy. Endoscopy 15 (1983) 59–64.
46. SMITH AD, WEISS G: The lateral oblique position for laparoscopic nephrectomy. J Endourol 6 (1992) 59 (abstract no. B-16).
47. SOMMERKAMP H.: Lumboskopie: ein neues diagnostisch-therapeutisches Prinzip der Urologie. Akt Urol 5 (1974) 183–185.

48. Sommerkamp H, Hederer R, Wagner S: Nierenbiopsie: Vergleichende Studie zwischen offener und halboffener (lumboskopischer) Technik. Urologe A 15 (1976) 288–292.
49. Suzuki K, Ihara H, Kurita Y, Kageyama S, Ueda D, Ushiyama T, Ohtawara Y, Kawabe K: Laparoscopic surgery for adrenal tumors. J Endourol 6 (1992) 57 (abstract no. B-5).
50. Watson GM, Ralph DJ, Timoney AG, Wickham JEA: Laparoscopic nephrectomy: initial experience. Eur Urol 20 (Suppl) (1992) 314 (abstract no. 225).
51. Weinberg JJ, Smith AD: Percutaneous resection of the kidney: preliminary report. J Endourol 2 (1988) 355–357.
52. Weiss RM, Seashore JH: Laparoscopy in the management of non-palpable testis. J Urol 138 (1987) 382–384.
53. Wickham JEA: The surgical treatment of renal lithiasis. In: Wickham JEA (ed.): Urinary calculus disease. Churchill Livingstone, New York (1979) 145–198.
54. Wickham JEA, Miller RA: Percutaneous renal access. In: Percutaneous renal surgery. Churchill Livingstone, New York (1983) 33–39.
55. Winfield HN, See WA, Donovan JF et al.: Laparoscopic pelvic lymph node dissection – a new staging technique for cancer of the prostate. J Endourol 5 (Suppl) (1991) 131.
56. Wittmoser R: Die Retroperitoneoskopie als neue Methode der lumbalen Sympathikotomie. Fortschr Endoskopie 4 (1973) 219– 223.
57. Yamada S, Ono Y, Sahashi M, Suenaga H, Ohshima S: Laparoscopic nephrectomy. J Endourol 6 (1992) 58 (abstract no. B-10).

32. | Laparoscopic Varix Ligation

J. F. DONOVAN JR. AND H. N. WINFIELD

Introduction

A varicocele is a cystic dilation of the pampiniform plexus. The venous dilation presumably occurs due to absent or incompetent venous valves. The greater frequency of left varicoceles is possibly due to increased pressures in the left spermatic vein secondary to anastomosis at a right angle with the left renal vein and/or hydrostatic pressure in the renal vein above that found in the inferior vena cava, the site of right spermatic vein drainage [37]. Varicoceles typically develop during adolescence and are present in 15 % of the male population [2, 36, 37].

Varicoceles are diagnosed primarily by physical exam. With the patient standing for 10–15 minutes in a warm room, one may observe or palpate the varicocele just above the testes. Varicoceles are graded by ease of detection: Large varicoceles are visible on inspection, medium varicoceles are palpable without Valsalva, and small varicoceles are identified by a palpable distention of the pampiniform during Valsalva [28]. One must take care to distinguish venous dilation from cord expansion due to shortening of the cremasteric muscle during contraction of the internal oblique muscle. The effect of the cremasteric contraction can be minimized by supporting the testes prior to Valsalva.

Small varicoceles may be difficult to detect on physical exam but may be no less responsible for decrease in male reproductive function when compared to medium or large varico-celes [9]. Other techniques may be used to assist in or confirm the diagnosis of varicocele [18, 28, 30, 40]. These include contact thermography, Doppler sonography, radionuclide angiography, color Doppler sonography, and venography. Each test may provide false negative results. As suggested by Nagler, sophisticated diagnostic techniques should not be used to carry out a "witch hunt" in search of subclinical varices [28] Treatment of the subclinical varicocele remains controversial. McClure has reported greater improvement in sperm motility in treating patients with subclinical varices when compared to treating patients with clinical varices [26]. We rely upon physical exam to identify clinically palpable varix and use color Doppler sonography to confirm the diagnosis or examine for evidence of a contralateral varix and in follow-up for patients who have undergone varix ablation as suggested by Petros [30].

Indications for Varix Ligation

Varix ligation is indicated in patients who demonstrate a palpable varix and at least one of the following: 1. male subfertility as demonstrated by abnormal seminal fluid analysis (SFA) and failure to impregnate a partner who is free of demonstrable female infertility; 2. adolescent testicular growth retardation which is persistent during a 6-month observation period; and 3. pain which is not attributable to other intrascrotal abnormalities. Special care in evaluation of the patient with orchalgia should include a careful history including a subjective description of the character of the pain and elucidation of precipitating and ameliorating factors (pain typically described as "dull" or "dragging" which increases with extended periods of standing or exertion and alleviated by recumbency – never present upon awakening). Neither ligation of subclinical varices nor prophylactic varicocelectomy in the adolescent have been used as sufficient indication for varix ligation in our series [2, 26].

Current Techniques

Techniques for ablation of varicocele may be categorized as operative and non-operative. The most popular operative techniques include the inguinal approach of Ivanissevitch and the retroperitoneal approach of Palomo [19, 29]. The inguinal approach identifies the spermatic vessels as they course through the inguinal canal, and careful dissection at this site permits the ligation of the spermatic veins and the cremasteric vein which some authors feel may contribute to the pathophysiology of the varicocele. Through the retroperitoneal approach, the cremasteric vein is not accessible. However, the Palomo procedure permits dissection of the spermatic vascular bundle without risk to the collateral arterial supply provided by the cremasteric and deferential arteries. The subinguinal and high scrotal approach to varix ligation offer the advantage of testicular cord dissection at a more superficial site but require ligation of more venous tributaries while maintaining diligence in preservation of testicular arterial vessels [15, 24].

Non-operative Methods

Non-operative varix ablation methods include transvenous embolization or sclerosis. Embolization may be accomplished with either balloons or coils while sclerosis utilizes boiling-hot contrast [33, 38, 39]. These procedures require the service of a skilled interventional radiologist. Performed under local anesthesia with intravenous sedation, the procedure is admittedly minimally invasive, but success rates are, in general, less than those achieved with operative varix ligation [12].

Patient Selection

The indications for laparoscopic varix ligation are identical to those listed above. Patient selection must address contraindications. An absolute contraindications is a previous failed varix ligation performed using the retroperitoneal approach. Patients who have failed a Palomo approach are best served by transvenous ablation or surgical correction using an inguinal or subinguinal dissection.

Previous abdominal surgery is a relative contraindication. Patients who have undergone abdominal surgery are at risk for intraperitoneal adhesions which make Veress needle insertion and insufflation more hazardous. With experience, the laparoscopic surgeon may chose to insert the Veress needle at a site away from the previous surgical incision. Alternatively, one may use the Hasson cannula in the open laparoscopy approach.

All reasonable measures should be utilized to reduce the risk of complications and ensure that the patient does not suffer a needless complication. We have successfully performed laparoscopic varix ligation in patients who previously have undergone appendectomy, hernia repair, omphalocele, and pyloromyotomy without complication [4, 6]. We currently use the "open" laparoscopic technique in varix ligation utilizing a blunt 10/11 mm cannula in all laparoscopic varix ligations.

We have not operated upon patients with recurrent varix who have undergone prior varix ligation by the Palomo approach. The laparoscopic varix ligation identifies the spermatic vessels immediately cephalad to the internal ring – the site of varix ligation in the retroperitoneal approach. These patients are best served by a different approach such as transvenous ablation of collateral venous channels missed at the initial operation [13, 27]. We have successfully performed repeat varicocelectomy in patients who have undergone failed transvenous varix ablation and inguinal varix ligation.

Patient Preparation

We discuss with each patient the possible consequences of a varicocele and the anticipated benefits of varix ablation. We also review the available approaches to varix ablation including operative and non-operative techniques mentioned above and compare the advantages and disadvantages of each (success, recurrence, recovery, cost, anesthetic) [8].

Each patient is informed of the potential risks of the procedure with special emphasis on risks which are peculiar to laparoscopy. While review of all possible risks is not practical, the patient is informed of the possibility of injury to intestine and/or blood vessels which would require immediate celiotomy and repair, thus eliminating any potential advantage of laparoscopy with respect to rapid recovery. We discuss precautions taken to avoid such mishaps including the use of the open laparoscopy and the Doppler probe. In addition, the patient is informed that the varix ligation may not be possible using the laparoscopy approach, thus necessitating a traditional operative technique. Although we have not yet failed to complete a varix ligation by the laparoscopic approach in 82 patients, we realize that extensive adhesions or other unexpected intra-peritoneal conditions (inflammation, infection, cancer) might preclude or contraindicate the laparoscopic varix ligation.

Operative Technique

Laparoscopy is typically performed under general anesthesia. The use of local anesthesia in laparoscopic varix ligation has been reported in conjunction with varix ligation where no attempt was made to preserve the testicular artery [25]. We have found that the preservation of the spermatic artery is a delicate and time consuming process which would preclude the use of local or regional anesthetic and therefore have performed laparoscopic varix ligation exclusively with general anesthesia.

Following induction of general anesthesia and endotracheal intubation, a nasogastric tube may be inserted and the gastric contents aspirated. This is especially important *if one suspects gastric distention has occurred* during induction. The skin is scrubbed and prepped with topical antiseptic solution, then draped with sterile sheets to provide access to the entire abdomen and the genitals. Although we no longer insert an indwelling bladder catheter, we pass a straight urethral catheter to drain the bladder. Skin preparation of the testes permits traction during laparoscopy facilitating identification of the spermatic vessels traversing the internal ring and thus define the necessary limits of dissection.

Pneumoperitoneum

Although we experienced no complications due to the use of the Veress needle, we sought to minimize any potential complications, especially those which would be unique to the laparoscopic approach to varix ligation (i.e., bowel or vascular injury – complications virtually impossible in other methods of varix ablation); therefore, we currently perform laparoscopic varix ligation using the "open" technique with the Hasson-type cannula.

A 2–3 cm vertical midline incision extends inferiorly from the umbilicus (the length of the incision varies proportionate to the depth of the subcutaneous fat). A 2-cm incision in the linea alba permits insertion of the 10 mm trocar while maintaining an occlusive seal with the cone-shaped sleeve. Stay sutures (2 PDS) are placed in a horizontal mattress on either side of the linea alba incision. The transversalis fascia and the peritoneum are incised under direct vision and a finger is passed into the peritoneal cavity to confirm the absence of adhesions. The shaft of the blunt-tipped Hasson trocar is positioned in the peritoneal cavity and the cone-shaped sleeve plugged into the fascial opening and secured with the previously placed stay sutures wrapped tightly around the cleat device.

The Hasson cannula is designed to fix the laparoscopic trocar to the fascia while occluding the fascial defect to prevent escape of pneumoperitoneum. Some have suggested insertion of Vaseline gauze into the wound around the cone-tip sleeve to minimize escape of CO_2. We have found that the Vaseline gauze is more likely to occlude the incision at the level of the skin rather than at the level of the fascia. Consequently, gas may still escape around the Hasson cannula but be trapped in the subcutaneous tissues resulting in subcutaneous emphysema. We prefer to tolerate the CO_2 leak as long as the insufflator can keep pace and maintain adequate intraperitoneal pressure (12–15 mmHg). If the rate of gas escape from the peritoneal cavity compromises the exposure of the operative site, then a fascial suture is placed to tighten the fascial seal around the cone-tipped sleeve.

Once the Hasson cannula is fixed to the fascia, the peritoneal cavity is insufflated with CO_2. Through the large caliber 10-mm trocar, insufflation proceeds at a rate of 6–8 liters per minute. Total insufflation time is approximately 1 minute in comparison to approximately 5 minutes through the Veress needle (at 1–2 liters per minute). Thus, the additional time required to insert the Hasson cannula is compensated by the more rapid insufflation.

Insertion of Trocars

Once the subumbilical sheath is secure, the laparoscope is inserted and the peritoneal contents are inspected. The optimal sites for insertion of the additional trocars providing access for the operative instruments are then identified. The site of varix ligation is 3–5 cm cephalad to the internal ring, a point which can be identified and located topically by transilluminating the abdominal wall from within the peritoneal cavity. A point is identified in each lower quadrant near enough to permit the instruments to reach the internal ring easily, but far enough to prevent encumbrance of the laparoscopic instruments. When the instrument sheath is too close to the operative site, the trocar sleeve will interfere with proper operation of the instruments (i.e., scissors and curved dissector unable to open). When the instrument sheath is too far away, the fulcrum created by fixation of the instrument at the site of abdominal wall penetration exaggerates the movements of the instrument tip, making separation of artery from vein more difficult. In general, the optimal port placement will be near the level of the umbilicus lateral to the rectus muscle – higher than McBurney's point as we originally recommended [4, 6]. We currently place lower quadrant trocars on each side of the umbilicus lateral to the rectus muscle and just caudad to the umbilical port (Fig. 1).

The abdominal wall is transilluminated at the intended site of trocar insertion and the silhouette of subcutaneous vessels identified. Skin incisions long enough to accommodate the instrument trocars are made – 5 mm for standard instruments and 10.5 mm for the disposable hemo-clip appliers. The trocars are inserted while monitoring the intraperitoneal space to prevent injury to the peritoneal contents. With the advent of reusable 5 mm clip appliers, we now use 5 mm trocars in each lower quadrant. Clips can be placed on either ipsilateral or contralateral spermatic veins when the trocar is positioned cephalad to the site of ligation. The trocars are secured to the abdominal wall with suture.

Instruments

Primarily, we use a curved scissors and curved dissector to accomplish most of the steps in the procedure. A 5 mm laparoscopic Doppler probe can speed identification and isolation of the spermatic artery (Meadox, Medsonics). Hemo-clip appliers (Hemoclip by USSC) ligate the veins which are then divided. With the recently introduced 5 mm reusable clip applier, we note that small clips are capable of ligating small caliber vessels but may be inadequate for ligation of multiple veins and adventitial tissues. Consequently, as suggested by Sanchez de Badajoz [24], we have incorporated the use of suture ligation by placing short (5 cm) ligatures of 2–0 silk near the operative site to be used when large or multiple veins are to be occluded.

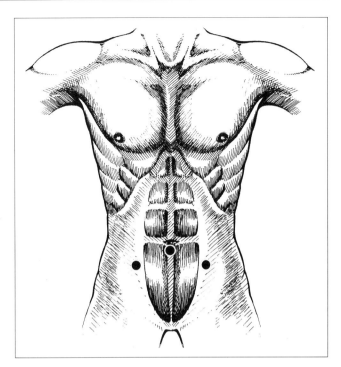

Fig. 1. Trocar placement for laparoscopic varix ligation. The laparoscope is inserted through the umbilical port, the instrument ports are positioned lateral to the rectus muscle and 2–3 cm below the umbilicus

Dissection

Once the laparoscope and instrument trocars have been established, attention is turned to the isolation and ligation of the spermatic veins. If the sigmoid colon is fixed over the spermatic veins above the internal ring, we mobilize the colon to provide the necessary exposure (Fig. 2). A 3–5 cm incision is positioned lateral to the spermatic vascular bundle (Figs. 3 and 4). The medial edge of the incision is lifted and the under-

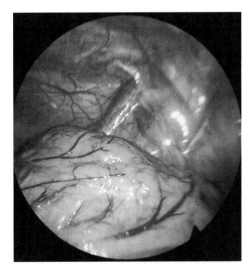

Fig. 2. In left side varicoceles, the sigmoid colon may have to be mobilized for the necessary exposure

lying spermatic vessels separated from the peritoneal flap (Figs. 5 and 6). From the midpoint of this incision, we incise the peritoneal flap medially to the edge of the iliac artery (Fig. 7). The "T" incision provides excellent exposure of the spermatic veins just cephalad to the internal ring. The surgeon may tug on the testes while observing the spermatic vascular bundle through the laparoscope, and thereby identify collateral veins adjacent to the spermatic veins which traverse the internal ring. Ligation of these vessels will reduce the incidence of subsequent persistent or recurrent varix.

The entire spermatic vascular bundle is freed from the underlying psoas muscle. In case of injury to the spermatic artery or vein, prior mobilization of the vascular packet permits quick application of hemo-clips and control of bleeding, albeit forfeiting the spermatic artery.

Following mobilization of the spermatic vessels, loose adventitial tissues are removed and the vascular bundle split into lateral and medial parts. In general, the spermatic veins number 3 to 8; the spermatic artery is located posteriorly and medially to the spermatic veins. We identify the site of the spermatic artery by careful observation, looking for evidence of pulsation in either the medial or lateral bundle. One must take care to distinguish true spermatic arterial pulsation from transmitted pulsation of the iliac artery. Our experience confirms that the use of the laparoscopic Doppler probe provides significant reduction in operative duration [20, 22]. Once the artery is located, the non-arterial tissue is clipped or ligated and divided (Fig. 8). Careful dissection of the remaining vascular packet permits separation of artery from veins which are sequentially ligated and divided until only the spermatic artery remains.

We have abandoned the use of a Nd:YAG laser contact probe (Figs. 9 and 10) [6, 7]. The discontinuation of Nd:YAG laser was in response to an intra-abdominal bleeding 21 days following surgery. At the time of celiotomy, inspection revealed the operative site covered by peritoneum with the exception of a 1 mm opening fused to the spermatic artery which was actively bleeding into the peritoneal cavity. A careful review of

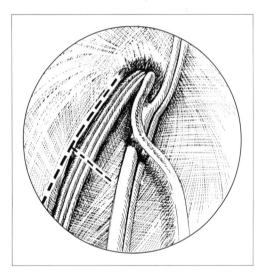
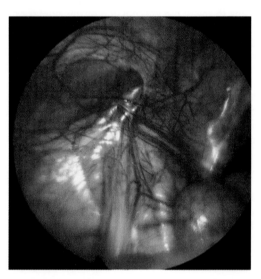

Figs. 3 and 4.   Anatomy of the spermatic vessels cephalad to the internal ring. Incision of the peritoneum is carried out in a T-shape

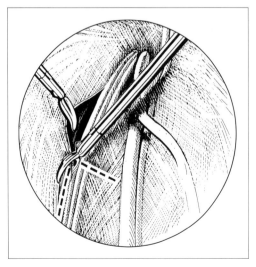
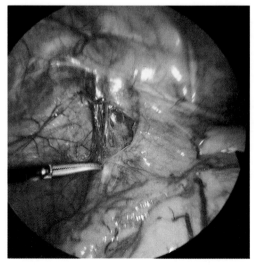

Figs. 5 and 6.   The peritoneum is lifted up with a grasper and incised with scissors over a length of 3–5 cm

video tape recorded at the original operation demonstrated free-beam injury to surrounding tissues – a defect in the "contact" probe. We concluded that the delayed presentation of the arterial wall injury is consistent with thermal damage caused by the "free-beam" energy escaping from the imperfect contact fiber tip (similar to delayed presentation of thermal injury of bowel and bladder). Consequently, we discontinued use of laser coagulation

Additional Procedures

Occasionally, patients who present for varix ligation may present with a coincident inguinal hernia. Repair of the inguinal hernia may be performed through the laparoscope using the technique described by Schultz [35]. We perform the varix ligation using the technique described above with the exception of the peritoneal incision: the incision lateral and parallel to the spermatic veins extends lateral to the internal ring and

then across the anterior abdominal wall medially to the obliterated umbilical ligament [5]. Dissection of the indirect hernia sac and floor of the inguinal canal permits exposure for prosthetic repair of the hernia defect. The indications for inguinal hernia repair are relatively vague in the absence of symptoms. In general, the presence of a clinically palpable hernia is sufficient to recommend repair especially in the young male. Other procedures which could be combined with elective varix ligation are uncommon, and we do not feel that incidental laparoscopic appendectomy is warranted.

Termination of Procedure

Once the varix ligation is complete, attention is turned to termination of the procedure. The operative site(s) is inspected with intraperitoneal pressures reduced to 8–10 mmHg pressure and active bleeding sites identified (Figs. 11 and 12). Hemostasis is secured with the use of electro-coagulation at the

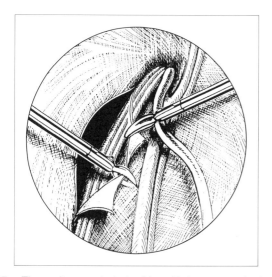

Fig. 7. The peritoneum is incised in a T-shape towards the iliac vessels

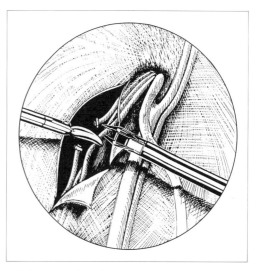

Fig. 8. 3–8 spermatic veins are clipped and transsected with scissors, taking care not to injure the artery

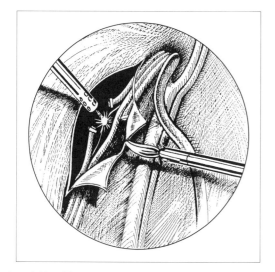
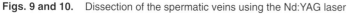

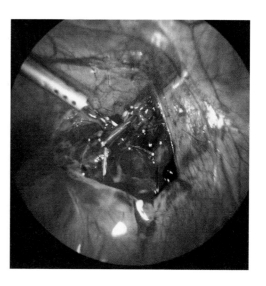

Figs. 9 and 10. Dissection of the spermatic veins using the Nd:YAG laser

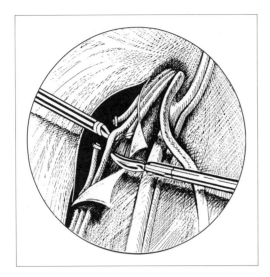

Fig. 11. Dissected spermatic artery after transsection of all the veins

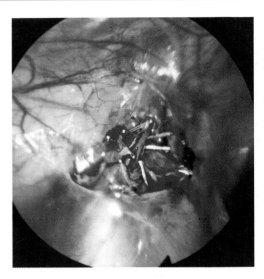

Fig. 12. The operative site is inspected for hemostasis after reducing intraabdominal pressure to 8–10 mmHg

operative site. Each trocar site is inspected to exclude any active bleeding from the anterior abdominal wall.

The patient is returned to a horizontal position and any blood or irrigant which may have collected in the pelvis is aspirated. The lower quadrant trocars are removed under direct vision and, when 10.5 mm trocars are used, the sites closed with a fascial suture of 2–0 PDS while the anterior abdominal wall remains elevated by the pneumoperitoneum. This permits placement of a secure fascial suture without the risk of injuring underlying bowel. The subumbilical port is removed last with the laparoscope inserted to prevent entrapment of small bowel which might otherwise be drawn up into the fascial defect. The peritoneal cavity is then allowed to desufflate before the fascial incision is carefully secured with the 0-PDS stay-sutures. Frequently, scrotal emphysema occurs due to extravasation of CO_2 tracking through the internal ring adjacent to the spermatic vessels. The scrotal gas is removed by careful compression of the scrotum which returns the gas to the peritoneal cavity or vents the gas through the subcutaneous tissues and out through the lower quadrant trocar sites.

Subcutaneous sutures may be placed at the discretion of the surgeon and the skin closed with either a single subcuticular stitch or skin tapes. A Tegaderm dressing is used to cover the wounds.

Results

Since June 1990, we have performed 115 laparoscopic varix ligations in 82 patients: 49 unilateral (59.8 %) and 33 bilateral (40.2 %). Patients have ranged in age from 16 to 48 years and in weight from 54 to 134 kilograms. Indications for varix ligation have included male factor infertility in 70 (85 %), adolescent testicular growth retardation in 3 (4 %), and pain in 9 (11 %). The average duration for the unilateral varix ligation is 102 minutes (range 58–199 minutes) and for the bilateral varix ligation is 156 minutes (range 105–298 minutes). We have used the Hasson cannula and the open laparoscopic technique in 48 patients with no discernible increase in operative time.

We have preserved the spermatic artery in 107 of 115 (93 %) varix ligations. We have identified and preserved duplicate spermatic arteries at the supra-inguinal level in two cases. We have used the laparoscopic Doppler probe in 41 cases. Mean duration of operation for unilateral with Doppler is 91 (±5.4) minutes and without Doppler 110 (±6.3) minutes; mean duration of bilateral varix ligation with and without Doppler are 141 (±4.8) minutes and 161 (±8.5) minutes respectively. As described by Loughlin, the use of a laparoscopic Doppler probe speeds identification of the artery and, consequently, shortens the duration of the procedure [25].

Table 1. Complications

	Number	Per Cent
Major		
Intra-abdominal Bleeding	1	1.2
Total Major	1	1.2
Minor		
Infection	1	1.2
Hydrocele	3	3.7
Pampiniform Phlebitis	2	2.4
Laryngospasm/ Pulmonary Edema	1	1.2
Total Minor	7	8.5

Complications have been rare. One major complication, a delayed postoperative bleed presumably due to thermal injury of the spermatic artery by free-beam energy from the Nd:YAG laser probe, has been described above. We have identified one wound infection confirmed by culture (per patient wound infection rate 1.2 %; per wound infection rate with three wounds per patient 0.4 %). Two wounds have exhibited inflammation presumably due to inflammatory reaction in response to absorbable suture used to approximate skin. Abdominal visceral injury has not occurred. No patient has noted testicular pain following varix ligation and we have not detected decrease in testicular size in any patient during the postoperative follow-up. Two patients (2.4 %) have, however, suffered pampiniform plexus thrombophlebitis treated with non-steroidal anti-inflammatory agents during a protracted postoperative period (14–21 days). We have identified 3 hydroceles (2.6 %) following laparoscopic varix ligation, but none has required therapy to date. One patient experienced laryngospasm following extubation; although he did not require reintubation, the extreme negative intra-thoracic pressure generated while attempting inhalation against a closed glottis resulted in pulmonary edema which resolved during an overnight in-hospital observation.

The majority of patients (80) have undergone repeat physical exam with or without color Doppler ultrasonography at six months following surgery. Four patients have subsequently undergone spermatic venogram to confirm persistent varix predicted by color Doppler (but not physical exam). Two (of 113 varicoceles evaluable at 6 month follow-up: 1.7 %) recurrent varicoceles have been identified and treated by transvenous sclerotherapy.

In principle, the laparoscopic varix ligation is an outpatient surgery. Seven of the 82 patients have been admitted for observation during recovery from anesthetic which extended beyond the hours of operation for the ambulatory surgery unit. All patients who required admission were discharged on the day following surgery. No other operative complications have been noted.

Lund recently reviewed our results in 37 patients who had completed at least 6 months follow-up and provided at least 2 semen samples for analysis. Mean sperm density has increased from 10.2 million sperm/ml to 19.7 million sperm/ml ($p = 0.001$). Motility has not changed significantly during post-therapy observation: average preoperative motility 33.5 % and average postoperative motility 36.7 %. The total motile sperm per ejaculate has increased from 13.4 million to 26.0 million ($p = 0.004$). For 64 patients who have completed a 12 month follow-up period, 30 (46.9 %) have reported pregnancy (3 patients lost to follow-up). When restricted to patients who have completed a 24 month follow-up evaluation, 50 % report pregnancy.

Recovery from laparoscopic varix ligation is rapid. Mean time to return to preoperative activity is 4.8 days and average analgesic use is 10.5 tablets of acetaminophen with codeine.

Discussion

The most obvious advantage of laparoscopic varix ligation would appear to be early return to normal activity. Very few authors report duration of convalescence using traditional techniques for operative varix ligation, although we anticipate that time to recovery will receive more attention in the future. On average, our patients return to normal preoperative activity in 4.8 days. Physical exertion is not discouraged and the resumption of strenuous activity is left to the patients' discretion. Others have noted a similarly short recovery time following laparoscopic varix ligation [1, 17]. In 10 patients, Hagood and associates note return to work or school within 48 hours. In the report by Aaberg, four patients who underwent laparoscopic varix ligation returned to regular activity the day after surgery. The early return to preoperative levels of activity following laparoscopic varix ligation is in contrast to the description by Thomas in his review of operative varix ligation: patients "who do not have physically demanding jobs generally may return to work within a few days, when they are comfort-

able. Full physical activity may be resumed 3 to 4 weeks after surgery" [37]. Using a subinguinal approach, Marmar reports that patients return to work within 48 hours, but does not specify level of activity. Enquist and associates reported no difference in return to normal activity when comparing laparoscopic to subinguinal varix ligation [10]. Despite their contention that they had achieved technical competence in laparoscopy during pelvic lymph node dissections, the major complication rate in the laparoscopy group was an unacceptable 14 % due to 2 abdominal wall injuries which required prolonged hospitalization and wound exploration. Laparoscopic techniques in general provide a speedy recovery. With the advent of minimally invasive surgical procedures, the scope of surgical outcome analysis will include the rapidity of return to the activities of daily living.

To date, few reports of laparoscopic varix ligation provide detailed follow-up for response in the infertile male [4, 6]. In our hands, laparoscopic varix repair demonstrates results comparable to those achieved with traditional approaches such as the Ivanissevitch and Palomo techniques. Patients who have completed six-month follow-up demonstrate improvement in seminal fluid characteristics as noted above. Specifically, improvement in sperm density was noted in 82 % of patients; 50 %, and 77 % of patients treated for male factor infertility achieved improved motility and motile sperm per ejaculate, respectively. This frequency of improvement is comparable to that reported by Marks and associates [23]. In a review of 15 reported series of varix ligation performed for male infertility, Pryor and Howards noted improved semen quality in 66 % of patients following varix ligation [31]. Pregnancy rates ranged from 24–53 % of couples. The preponderance of available data would suggest that varix ligation is indicated in patients who suffer male factor subfertility, although successful impregnation is not certain. In comparison to medical treatment, patients who undergo varix ligation have a significantly greater chance of conception [23, 31]. Marks and associates noted four variables which would predict a higher rate of impregnation in patients who undergo varix ablation: lack of testicular atrophy, sperm density greater than 50 million/ml, motility greater than 60 %, and FSH less than 30 ng/ml.

While all of our patients satisfied the last criteria (eugonadotrophic), only one demonstrated a sperm density greater than 50 million/ml (and motile sperm per ejaculate greater than 40 million) and one demonstrated motility greater than 60 %. Thus, further study is warranted to stratify patients according to preoperative seminal fluid analysis measurements. Given the severity of the preoperative semen analysis deficits in our patient population, one would anticipate the pregnancy rate observed.

Recurrence or persistence of varicocele is an important consideration in choice of treatment. In our series, we followed patients with physical exam and ultrasound with color Doppler. In 80 patients who have completed six-month follow-up including physical exam and ultrasound with color Doppler, we have found a persistent varix in 2 of 112 varices (1.8 %). Recurrence rates for varices treated surgically range from 0.5–20 % [12, 14, 37]. In contrast, a review of 1,894 patients treated by percutaneous ablation revealed persistence in 22 % [12].

Several disadvantages must be noted in the use of laparoscopy for treatment of varicocele. As noted above, our laparoscopic technique requires a general anesthetic while the inguinal, retroperitoneal, subinguinal, and Marmar techniques can be performed under local anesthesia with sedation. However, a survey of urologist members of the American Fertility Society in 1993 revealed that the majority utilize general anesthesia in performing varix ligation regardless of the operative technique employed. At this time, laparoscopic varix ablation appears to be a more time consuming procedure when compared to traditional approaches; consequently, the cost of the procedure may be higher when compared to the more traditional techniques.

However, to truly understand the cost of any operative procedure, one must include the cost of lost revenue (i.e., income paid to the patient during the recuperative phase). With early return to productive work, the increased charge for laparoscopic varix ligation may be offset by a decrease in lost revenue. Furthermore, the cost of the operative procedure is decreasing with experience: more rapid completion of the procedure and utilization of reusable equipment have reduced charges for the laparoscopic varix ligation by 16 % comparing the years 1990–1992 to 1992–1994 [32]. A prospective randomized study is underway which will compare laparoscopic, inguinal, and subinguinal varix ligation with attention to operative results, complications, response to treatment, convalescence, and cost.

The extended duration of the laparoscopic varix ligation must be addressed. Early in one's experience, even the rudimentary maneuvers required in laparoscopy may be difficult. Each movement requires repeated attempts to align instruments and adjust for the loss of depth perception due to monocular vision which is the current standard in laparoscopy. With practice, these surgical tasks become routine and quick. The majority of time spent in laparoscopic varix ligation is devoted to preservation of the artery. Protection of the spermatic artery requires delicate dissection of small veins (0.5 mm) which are adherent to the artery utilizing microsurgical techniques in the magnified field provided by the laparoscope. Gradually, with the addition of instruments which facilitate the identification of the artery (the laparoscopic Doppler), operating times have decreased as we climbed the learning curve. We have reports of unilateral laparoscopic varix ligation performed within 30 minutes with spermatic artery preservation in non-training situations [16, 21]. However, in a residency training program, the learning curve is sinusoidal and recurs as new, inexperienced surgeons acquire the skills in clinical laparoscopy following an introductory animal laboratory laparoscopy course. Thus, one should focus not upon the maximum time required to complete laparoscopic varix ligation in our series but rather upon the minimum time necessary- and anticipate that this time will be further reduced in the future.

Ultimately, the beneficiary of laparoscopic varix ligation is the patient. A quicker recovery and return to regular activity is a desirable goal which is difficult to quantify in monetary terms. Presumably, laparoscopic varix ligation is more expensive than alternate procedures due to general anesthesia, prolonged use of the operating room, and occasional overnight admission for anesthetic recovery. Reduction in recovery to an average of 4.8 days must be compared to the recovery in traditional procedures at approximately 10–14 days. Since third party payers do not reimburse the patient for time lost from work, a clear accounting of recovery outside the hospital is not available. We presume that employers would be in favor of reduction of paid absence during recovery since

the consequence of absent worker is: 1. worker absent but paid; 2. worker's tasks must be completed by fellow employee (presume overtime) or by temporary employee (additional salary and benefits); and 3. employee's position is left vacant for the duration of recovery. With continued improvement in laparoscopic technique, operating time will be reduced and cost of laparoscopic varix ligation will be no more than that for traditional procedures. Thus, shortened recovery may provide an over-riding difference.

The Use of the Hasson Cannula

We have used the Hasson cannula to perform "open" laparoscopy in 10 patients. This is now our routine approach to laparoscopy for varix ligation and preferred for all laparoscopic surgery (prostate, lymphadenectomy, renal). Review of the available literature suggests that the majority of injuries and complications in laparoscopy are attributable to insertion of the Veress needle or the first trocar, procedures which are performed without the benefit of intraperitoneal visualization [3, 11]. We encountered no complications related to the use of these instruments in performing laparoscopic varix ligation, and no published reports have alluded to such complications in performing laparoscopic varix ligation. However, we have received personal communication indicating that catastrophic complications have been encountered in several centers (bladder perforation, bowel perforation, vascular injury to external iliac artery and vein).

Complications of traditional techniques for laparoscopic varix ligation (inguinal, retroperitoneal) would not include such catastrophic events. Every effort must be made to reduce the potential risk to each patient subjected to surgery. In the case of laparoscopic varix ligation, the use of "open" laparoscopy is mandated. By eliminating potential complications of Veress needle and first trocar insertion, potential risk is markedly reduced and potential complications should be identical to (and no more frequent than) those encountered in the traditional operative varicocelectomy. Despite the slightly longer incision, our patients have demonstrated no increase in wound discomfort at the subumbilical site when compared to the lateral or suprapubic insertion sites. With practice, the mini-laparotomy exposure and entry into the peritoneal cavity can be performed quickly and safely.

Conclusion

With care, laparoscopic varix ligation may be performed effectively and safely, and with experience, operative times and cost will approach that of traditional operative varix ligation. The primary advantage of laparoscopic varix ligation appears to be a decrease in duration of patient morbidity following the procedure. Further study in a prospective and randomized fashion is necessary to clearly define differences in traditional operative varix ligation and laparoscopic varix ablation. At the very least, the advent of laparoscopic surgery has focused the attention of the surgical world upon the issues of patient recovery and morbidity. This does not necessarily indicate that laparoscopy is the preferred approach for all procedures, but does suggest that, if not laparoscopy, then modification of traditional surgical procedures will be demanded by the patients whom we serve.

References

1. AABERG RA, VANCAILLIE TG, SCHUESSLER WW: Laparoscopic varicocele ligation: a new technique. Fertility and Sterility 56 (4) (1991) 776–77.
2. BELMAN AB: The dilemma of the adolescent varicocele. Contemporary Urology 3 (9) (1991) 21–27.
3. BORTEN M: Laparoscopic Complications: Prevention and Management, Vol. 1. B.C. Decker Inc., Philadelphia (1986).
4. DONOVAN JF, WINFIELD HN: Laparoscopic varix ligation. J Urol 147 (1992) 77–81.
5. DONOVAN JF JR., WINFIELD HN, LUND GO: Laparoscopic hernia repair combined with urologic procedures (in preparation 1992).
6. DONOVAN JF JR.: Laparoscopic varix ligation with the Nd: YAG laser. J Endourol (1992).
7. DONOVAN JF JR.: Laparoscopic varix ligation. Atlas Urol Clin North Amer 1 (2) (1993) 15–32.
8. DONOVAN JF JR.: Legal issues in laparoscopy. Contemporary Urology 4 (6) (1992) 74–81.
9. DUBIN L, AMELAR RD: Varicocele size and results of varicocelectomy in selected subfertile men with varicocele. Fertility and Sterility 21 (8) (1970) 606–609.
10. ENQUIST E, STEIN BS, SIGMAN M: Laparoscopic versus subinguinal varicocelectomy: a comparative study. Fertility and Sterility 61 (6) (1994) 1092–1096.
11. EVANS RM, HULBERT JC, REDDY PK: Complications in laparoscopy. Seminars in Urology 10 (3) (1992) 164–168.
12. FISCH H: The surety of surgical repair of varicoceles. Contemporary Urology (1991) 68–74.
13. GILL B, KOGAN SJ, MALDONADO J, REDA E, LEVITT SB: Significance of intraoperative venographic patterns on the postoperative recurrence and surgical incision placement of pediatric varicoceles. J Urol 144 (2) (1992) 502–505.
14. GOLDSTEIN M, GILBERT BR, DICKER AP, DWOSH J, GNECCO C: Microsurgical inguinal varicocelectomy with delivery of the testis: an artery and lymphatic sparing technique. J Urol 148 (1992) 1808–1811.
15. GOLDSTEIN M: Surgery of male infertility and other scrotal disorders. In: Walsh PC et al. (eds.): Campbell's Urology, 3114–3149. W.B. Saunders Company, Philadelphia (1992).
16. GRAHAM R: Personal communication re. duration of laparoscopic varix ligation in non-training program environment (1992).
17. HAGOOD PG, MEHAN DJ, WORISCHECK JH, ANDRUS CH, PARRA RO: Laparoscopic varicocelectomy: preliminary report of a new technique. J Urol 147 (1992) 73–76.
18. HORSTMAN WG, MIDDLETON WD, MELSON GL, SIEGEL BA: Color Doppler US of the scrotum. RadioGraphics 11 (6) (1991) 941–957.
19. IVANISSEVICH O: Left varicocele due to reflux: experience with 4,470 operative cases in forty-two years. Journal of the International College of Surgeons 34 (6) (1960) 742–755.
20. JAROW J: Personal communication (1991)
21. KREDER K: Personal communication re. duration of laparoscopic varix ligation in non-training program environment (1992).
22. LOUGHLIN KR BROOKS DC: The use of a Doppler probe to facilitate laparoscopic varicocele ligation. Surgery, Gynecology, and Obstetrics 174 (1992) 326–328.
23. MARKS JL, MCMAHON R, LIPSHULTZ LI: Predictive parameters of successful varicocele repair. J Urol 136 (1986) 609–612.
24. MARMAR JL, DEBENEDICTIS TJ, PRAISS D: The management of varicoceles by microdissection of the spermatic cord at the external inguinal ring. Fertility and Sterility 43 (4) (1985) 583–588.
25. MATSUDA T, HORII Y, TAKEUCHI H, YOSHIDA O: Laparoscopic varicocelectomy (abstract). J Urol 145 (4) (1991) 325A.
26. MCCLURE RD., KHOO D., JARVI K, HRICAK H: Subclinical varicocele: the effectiveness of varicocelectomy. J Urol 145 (1991) 789–791.
27. MURRAY RR JR., MITCHELL SE, KADIR S, KAUFMAN SL, CHANG R, KINNISON ML, SMYTH JW, WHITE RI JR.: Comparison of recurrent varicocele anatomy following surgery and percutaneous balloon occlusion. J Urol 135 (1986) 286–289.
28. NAGLER HM, ZIPPE CD: Varicocele: Current concepts and treatment. In: LIPSHULTZ LI, HOWARDS SS (eds.): Infertility in the Male, 313–336, Mosby Year Book, St. Louis (1991).
29. PALOMO A: Radical cure of varicocele by a new technique: preliminary report. J Urol 61 (1949) 604.
30. PETROS JA, ANDRIOLE GL, MIDDLETON WD, PICUS DA: Correlation of testicular color Doppler ultrasonography, physical examination and venography in the detection of left varicoceles in men with infertility. J Urol 145 (1991) 785–788.
31. PRYOR JL, HOWARDS SS: Varicocele. Urologic Clinics of North America 14 (3) (1987) 499–513.
32. RASHID TM, WINFIELD HN, LUND GO, TROXEL SA, SANDLOW JI, DONOVAN JF: Comparative financial analysis of laparoscopic versus open varix ligaiton for men with clinically significant varicoceles. J Urol 151 (5) (1994) 310A.
33. SALGARELLO G, CAGOSSI M, SALGARELLO TLA, COTRONEO AR, CINQUE MD, PATANE D, FALAPPA P: Transvenous sclerotherapy of the gonadal veins for treatment of varicocele: long-term results. Journal of Vascular Diseases (1990) 427–431.
34. SANCHEZ DE BADAJOZ E: Personal communication (1994).
35. SCHULTZ L, GRABER J, PIETRAFITTA J, HICKOK D: Laser laparoscopic herniorrhaphy: a clinical trial – preliminary results. Journal of Laparoendoscopic Surgery 1 (1) (1990) 41–45.
36. SIGMAN M, HOWARDS SS: Male infertility. In: WALSH PC et al. (eds.): Campbell's Urology 661–705. W.B. Saunders Company, Philadelphia (1992).
37. THOMAS AJ JR., GEISINGER MA: Current management of varicoceles. Urologic Clinics of North America 17 (4) (1990) 893–907.
38. WALSH PC, WHITE RI JR.: Balloon occlusion of the internal spermatic vein for the treatment of varicoceles. Journal of the American Medical Association 246 (15) (1981) 1701–1702.
39. WHEATLEY JK, BERGMAN WA, GREEN B, WALTHER MM: Transvenous occlusion of clinical and subclinical varicoceles. Urology XXXVII (4) (1991) 362–365.
40. WORLD HEALTH ORGANIZATION: Comparison among different methods for the diagnosis of varicocele. Fertility and Sterility 43 (4) (1985) 575–582.

Gynecologic Surgery

Critical Comments

M. A. BRUHAT

Introduction

Since Raoul Palmer developed the marvellous diagnostic tool of gynecological laparoscopy back in 1940, this technique has gradually developed into a surgical tool and become the archetype for minimally invasive surgery.

After 25 years of practice and reflections on gynecological endoscopic surgery, I would like to make a few remarks:
- concerning the past, which may be recent, but is essentially concerned with technique
- concerning the present which is dominated by the question of economics,
- and concerning the future, in which technology will be omnipresent but will never eliminate the irreplaceable role of the surgeon.

The past essential technique

Noteworthy points about the recent past of operative laparoscopy include:
- the revolutionary aspect of this approach in which the operating field is transferred inside the peritoneal cavity
- the secondary effects which, like with any revolution, are unexpected because although the beginning may be clearly perceived, the end rarely is.

For example:

Ectopic Pregnancy for which laparoscopic treatment has become the standard for 95 % of the patients. This is crowned with success in 97 % of the thousand cases we have treated in our department since we described the technique over 20 years ago. 70 % of the patients wishing to become pregnant achieved their desire within the year. A study of 250 patients resulted in guidelines for choosing radical or conservative treatment based on the statistical weight of various factors which enable 3 groups to be defined to help with the indication for treatment.

The unexpected benefits are quite remarkable because the opportunity is provided to recognize and treat both cases in which intra-uterine pregnancy can be hoped for and those which are better referred to IVF.

Tubo-peritoneal Infertility which is approached in a radically different way today. Here too, in one and the same operation, the diagnosis of the etiology of infertility can be made, the prognosis established and the actual surgical procedure carried out: adhesiolysis without trauma for the organs and neosalpingostomy with spontaneous reversion of the tube which we have developed using the CO_2 laser.

The unexpected benefits: the absolute necessity of classifying the tubes in 4 stages according to the degree to which they are affected enables an instant decision as to the most suitable treatment and has given birth to new means of artificial fertilization such as GIFT.

Ovarian Cysts are the subject of on-going consideration in our series of 1000 cases studied over a period of 15 years,

ever since we developed the technique of laparoscopic cystectomy for macroscopic study of the cyst by extra- and intracystic examination to confirm it is benign or establish it is malignant, or, on the contrary in a very few cases, leave us waiting for the exact diagnosis.

The unexpected benefits: the search for definite arguments to confirm the benign nature by macroscopic and pathological frozen examination in all cases. This enables the ovary to be conserved without hesitation in patients desiring pregnancy: the search for pre-neoplastic ovarian dysplasia; the search for peritoneal diffusion meachnisms of malignant cells.

The recent past is more controversial

The retroperitoneal surgical techniques are an excellent example of the clinical assessments underway at present.

Laparoscopic Hysterectomy This surgical procedure, which is so highly symbolic for the gynecologist, is developing rapidly, even though it was only carried out for the first time by Harry Reich in 1989.

We consider that the operation comprises 4 phases: adnexa, uterine arteries, vaginal opening and vaginal closing, meaning that surgically we progress in the direction of increasing difficulty and at the same time towards completion of the laparoscopic procedure. The 600 hysterectomies we have carried out enable us to state today that the technique is becoming as rapid and easy as by the other classic techniques. Technology is of great help with the procedures.

The unexpected benefits concern, above all : the volume of the uterus which remains the major technical difficulty, and prompts us to search for all kinds of methods to reduce the uterus, whether surgically or medically. Combination with manoeuvres via the vaginal route sometimes makes the procedures easier and confirms the role of the vaginal route as the supreme route for gynecological surgeons.

Cancer, the inevitable symbol, which should also be able to draw some benefit from endoscopic surgery.

Lymphadenectomies
Inter iliac sub peritoneal, Daniel Dargent (1987), Inter iliac trans peritoneal, Denis Querleu (1988), latero-aortic sub mesenteric, Joël M. Childers (1992), Latero aortic, supra mesenteric and sub renal, Denis Querleu (1993), axilliary for breast cancer, François Suzanne and Arnaud Wattiez (1992) have shown themselves to be elegant techniques which are just as productive as those via a skin incision, and irreproachably radical.

The unexpected benefits are to be found in new strategies thanks to early lymphadenectomy providing accurate pathology findings. Lymphorrhoea and lymphoceles have practically disappeared. The return to normal function is extremely rapid.

Radical Hysterectomy Yes, we did indeed succumb to the temptation of testing what had become possible and carried this out for the first time in our group in 1989. Since then we have dealt with several dozen cases. To date it has proven to be feasible, and as rapid as the techniques requiring laparotomy.

The unexpected benefits: it is practically unequalled for precision and radicality for uterine cancer. There is a distinct absence of bleeding and lymphorrhea. Surgery for ovarian cancer, however, does not seem to us to be structured enough yet to be dealt with purely by laparoscopy.

Prolapse the latest frontier. Proud of being the descendants of the abdominal surgeons such as René Huguier and Georges Cerbonnet, we very quickly applied our treatments to the laparoscopic route.

Burch bladder colposuspension is a challenge which has now been met. The hundreds of cases we have dealt with and the urodynamic and ultrasonography studies demonstrate that anatomical and functional recuperation is comparable to that achieved by laparotomy or the vaginal route. Hysteropexy to the common anterior vertebral ligament or by cervicovaginal interposition of a triangle of mersylen is an efficient technique via laparotomy, as our 20 years of experience have shown. It can also be achieved by laparoscopy, as our cases demonstrate. Here too the absence of bleeding and accuracy of the procedure merit underlining.

The unexpected benefits: the advantage of revising the anatomopathology of prolapses, assisted by study of the functionality using urodynamic and morphological tests, MRI and ultrasonography. We are rediscovering which surfaces slide where and the movements of the organs relative to one other.

The present - economics and organisation

a) Economics

Health care is expensive: in France it consumed 9.8 % of G.D.P. in 1993 compared to 5.8 % in 1970.

In the USA it consumed 14.1 % of the G.D.P. in 1993 compared with 7.3 % in 1970.

If this tendency is not brought under control it may very well seriously endanger some of the basic principles of our work:
– care accessible to all the population
– top quality care provided without drawing distinctions between one patient and another
– permanent research effort.

The future of our profession is thus in question. It would seem to be necessary to use two methods of approach:
1. Greater attention needs to be paid to whether the sums spent on medical activities are justified
2. Greater involvement in the management of the quality of care provided.

The first point is highlighted by the enquiries which reveal considerable variations in medical practice.

For example, the number of Cesarean sections per 100 births in France in 1992 varied between 14.2 on average in the public sector and 16.6 in the private sector, with one of the regions reaching 22 Caesarean per 100 births. The number of hysterectomies per 100 000 women in 1998, after making allowances for age, varied between 540 in New Englang (USA) and 118 in Norway, i.e., a ratio of 4:6.

This question regarding the justification or the necessity for certain treatments prompts us to search for the best procedure to use. It should be noted that the multiplication of technologies and procedures which can be used, and which are often in competition with one other, together with the extension of treatment procedures to new fields, the multiplication of sources of information and many other factors render this type of question increasingly difficult to answer.

Certain tools which have proven their worth enable the data provided by clinical research in epidemiology and the economic dimension to be used for this analysis:
– study of costs gives information on the value of the resources mobilized,
– cost-efficiency studies when there is some means of judging the efficiency which is adequate in medical terms and has immediate significance (number of years of life gained, number of cases discovered etc.),
– the cost-usefulness studies when there are several types of results to take into account: these are then described using an overall indicator (the highly controversial OALY, for example).

Finally, concerning the question of whether treatment is appropriate, pooling and confrontation of reflections by the professional during consensus conferences, for example, or recommendations from scientific societies would seem to be efficient in the middle term.

b) Education and on-going training

The education systems are confronted with totally new problems, i.e. the increasing speed at which new techniques appear. The scientific community in its turn is confronted with the problem of managing these treatments. Basic training and on-going education are inevitably involved.

The universities must not fall behind not only in teaching the new techniques but also providing training in the intellectual tools which enable them to be acquired. They must teach people how to learn.

On-going education is going to have to take charge of teaching the more recent techniques and checking that they have been properly acquired, while respecting the irreplaceable value of the doctor's personal judgement.

33. Minimally Invasive Treatment in Gynecology and Pelviscopic Surgery

K. SEMM

Historical Review

At the beginning of the 20th century, laparoscopy quickly grew to become a routine method for diagnosis of upper abdominal complaints, particularly of the liver and spleen. The next primary technical developments were introduced by Kalk [3] and, later, Wildhirt [30]. The French physician Palmer [5] adapted the method for gynecological applications in the early 1940's and named it *celioscopy*. Further significant developments were made in Germany by Frangenheim in the late 1950's [1] and in England by Steptoe [29] and Semm in the late 1960's. Most importantly, these physicians provided the necessary impetus for the transition from diagnostic laparoscopy to pelviscopic surgery. To accomplish this feat, the surgical instruments for classical laparotomy first had to be adapted for endoscopic surgery. Moreover, it was imperative to develop new machines and instruments that made it possible to operate in the closed abdomen with the same efficiency as in the open abdomen.

In 1980, a successful pelviscopic appendectomy was the first breakthrough in general surgery [15]. This marked the beginning of the era of operative laparoscopy. However, it took

Figs. 1 and 2. Schematic representation of the differences in the surgical procedures

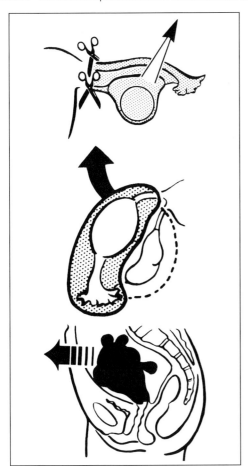

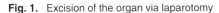

Fig. 1. Excision of the organ via laparotomy

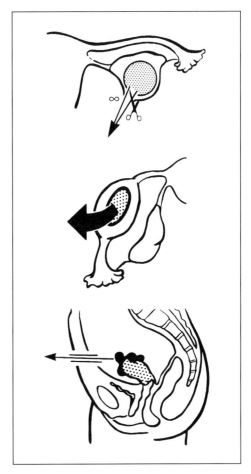

Fig. 2. Preservation of the organ via pelviscopy

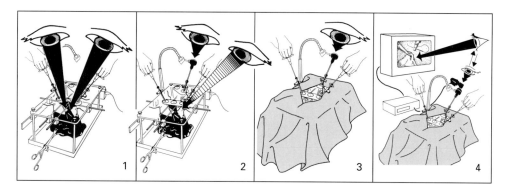

Fig. 3. Pelvi-Trainer for four-step training in pelviscopic surgical technique

almost another 10 years for the technique to gain wide acceptance in general surgery.

Rapid developments were made in the field of general surgery after laparoscopic appendectomy was adopted by Götz (1986). Cholecystectomy, herniotomy, selective vagotomy, and proctectomy were some of the main developments.

Today we generally speak of minimally invasive surgery (MIS), the main goal of which is to improve the patient's quality of life. Moreover, minimally invasive surgery places a strong emphasis on organ preservation, which was heretofore unprecedented in gynecology. In the past, the absolute goal of laparotomy was not only to cure the existing disease, but also to exclude the risk of recurrence by removing the organ in question (Fig. 1). In other words, ovarian cysts were treated via ovariectomy = castration, and tubal pregnancies were treated via tubectomy = sterilization. Due to the repeatability of minimally invasive gynecological surgeries, it is now for the first time possible to practice organ preservation in gynecology (Fig. 2).

For example, the enucleation of ovarian cysts or myomas can be carried out in such a way that the ovaries and uterus are left intact. Moreover, conservative treatment of tubal pregnancy is able to preserve fertility in over 70 % of all patients.

Tubectomy and adnexectomy were the treatments of choice for ovarian cysts until the advent of pelviscopic surgery. These procedures are performed in only a minimal number of patients today.

An estimated 50 % of all routine hysterectomies can be avoided, even in patients with uterine myomas. *Total uterine mucosa ablation* (TUMA) reduced the number of hysterectomies by more than 20 %. It seems that total hysterectomy is now outdated. There is hardly any justifiable indication for cardinal ligament dissection and culpotomy. Newer techniques such as *classical intrafascial serrated edge macro-morcellation hysterectomy* (CISH) can prevent the disastrous psychological and physical side effects which often occur following total hysterectomy.

Intrafascial hysterectomy does not disturb the topography of the pelvic floor and is thus a valuable addition to the field of operative gynecology. It can also be performed via laparotomy in patients with a large uterus or vaginally (IVH – Intrafascial Vaginal Hysterectomy). This will have two main effects on operative gynecology: In the future, the use of radical hysterectomy will be restricted to malignant tumors, and intrafascial pelviscopic hysterectomy will become the treatment of choice for benign uterine growths.

Informed Consent

Pelviscopy is performed not only for diagnostic reasons, but also for therapeutic and operative purposes. Therefore, the procedure for obtaining informed consent from the patient is similar to that of classical laparotomy, with the only difference being that one attempts to keep the surgery minimally invasive, *i.e.*, surgery is performed via pelviscopy. In any case, the surgeon must be free to make an immediate interoperative conversion to laparotomy if the situation demands such a measure. Prior informed consent of the patient is therefore essential. Only then does the endoscopic surgeon have true freedom of action. The surgeon can achieve good surgical results if he or she does not have to operate under pressure, *i.e.*, in fear that he or she may later be sued for malpractice because of the conversion from pelviscopy to laparotomy.

Physician Training for Endoscopic Surgery

Training in abdominal surgery can be acquired exclusively in open abdominal surgery via laparotomy, and the trainee must have a considerable amount of prior surgical experience. Endoscopic surgery, however, requires that the trainee first successfully switch from stereoscopic binocular operating conditions to monocular endoscopic conditions. The training period for endoscopy is therefore longer, because it is more difficult to judge the size and spatial orientation of the organs as viewed through the endoscope, and it is more difficult to guide and manipulate the surgical instruments through the restricted space of the trocar sleeves.

The trainee should first undergo four-step instruction on the training phantom to become familiar with the sequences of classical pelviscopic operations and to learn how to use the essential instruments, *e.g.*, scissors, forceps, needle, and suture material. Primary training should never be undertaken on the patient. All endoscopic operating sequences can be simulated with the Pelvi-Trainer (Fig. 3).

Four-step instruction on the Pelvi-Trainer:

Step 1: Practice in fixing membranes in position on the transparent "abdominal wall" of the Pelvi-Trainer using such dummy materials as half of a chicken or placental tissue. After inserting the instruments in the appropriate "puncture sites" at various positions on the glass abdominal wall, the trainee practices grasping with the atraumatic grasping forceps, cutting with the hook scissors, and suturing and ligation techniques. Once the trainee has gained adequate binocular spatial orientation to master the necessary intra- and extracorporal knotting techniques, he or she may proceed to Step 2.

Step 2: The trainee must now practice the surgical techniques learned in Step 1 looking through the 10-mm operating laparoscope inserted in the appropriate opening. If possible, a freshly extirpated uterus with adnexa should be used as the dummy material. The trainee practices such sequences as probing the tubes and performing ovariectomy. The endoscopic manipulations can be monitored under binocular vision, *i.e.*, by plain eyesight, until all the techniques have been mastered.

Step 3: The Pelvi-Trainer is now completely covered by a slit drape. The trainee must practice all laparoscopic sequences and techniques exclusively under endoscopic control.

Step 4: The trainee must now practice all grasping, cutting, and suturing techniques exclusively under video monitor control. This requires an even higher degree of dexterity, because the monitor completely lacks stereoscopic vision.

Anesthesiological preparation

Diagnostic and operative pelviscopy (*e.g.* tubal sterilization) can be performed under local, peridural, spinal, mask-administered, or general anesthesia. The pelviscopic surgical technique basically resembles that of the corresponding technique performed via laparotomy, and the conversion to laparotomy can be made at any time. General anesthesia via intubation is the least stressful form of anesthesia, and it is acceptable for all surgical pelviscopic operations.

Depending on the patient's condition, peridural anesthesia may be preferred in cases where other types of anesthesia carry higher risks. A gastric tube should also be inserted before the Veress needle puncture is made. This helps to prevent stomach perforation in patients who develop gastric distension due to hyperventilation after anesthesia has been initiated.

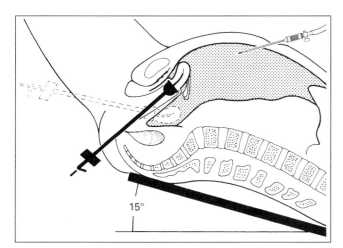

Fig. 4. 15° Trendelenburg position for creation of pneumoperitoneum

Contraindications

We distinguish between relative and absolute contraindications. The *absolute contraindications* for pelviscopy are identical to those of general surgery. The main absolute contraindications are unsuitability for anesthesia and hemorrhagic diasthesis. Large tumors (the size of a fist and larger) are one of the primary *relative contraindications,* except for patients in whom diagnostic endoscopy is performed only for histological purposes.

One or more previous abdominal surgeries via laparotomy is no longer considered to be a contraindication. However, each patient must be adequately informed of the risks and prepared for major abdominal surgery. This also applies in patients with inflammatory changes in the minor pelvis. In patients with multiple previous abdominal surgeries, the examining trocar should never be inserted blindly, but always under endoscopic control.

Preparation of the abdomen

The abdominal cavity should only be insufflated to a maximum pressure of 12 mmHg. Deep anesthesia completely relaxes the abdominal muscles, thereby enlarging the gas volume. The larger the gas volume, the simpler the operation. Preoperative intestinal lavage can greatly simplify the task of the surgeon. Orthograde intestinal lavage with 5 to 6 liters of saline solution should be performed prior to adhesiolysis – a procedure which general surgeons routinely carry out prior to intestinal surgery. The bowel is then completely empty, which minimizes the risk of contamination from bowel contents in case of accidental bowel perforation. Endoscopic intestinal suturing is a relatively simple technique.

Patient positioning

The patient is placed in a 15° Trendelenburg position with the buttocks projecting from the edge of the operating table prior to initiating pneumoperitoneum (Fig. 4). This position ensures that the greater portion of the bowel will lie in the epigastric region during insufflation. The operating table should also permit upper body elevation for appropriate repositioning of the minor pelvis in order to suction off blood or rinsing fluid in the subphrenic space. This is sometimes required in tubal pregnancy operations (Figs. 5 and 6).

Exudate can best be removed from the subdiaphragmatic space (Fig. 7), *i.e.*, between the liver and the diaphragmatic peritoneum, where no epiploic appendices or bowels, etcetera can get caught in the suction device.

Technical instrumentation for gynecological surgery

Instrumentation revolves around the tenet:

The endoscopic surgeon should strive to perform all endoscopic operations in the same manner as in open surgery.

In addition to the basic instruments for laparoscopy, the following instruments should also be on hand.

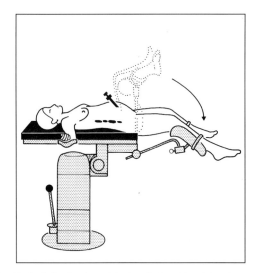

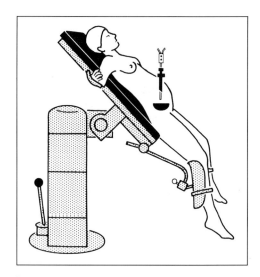

Fig. 5. Typical distribution of rinsing fluid or blood that has escaped from the minor pelvis

Fig. 6. By elevating the head as high as possible, the fluids can accumulate in the minor pelvis, where they can be removed by suction

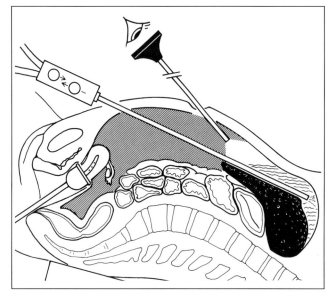

Fig. 7. Suction removal of irrigation fluid which has escaped up to subphrenic space using an extra-long bee-hive suction device

Instruments for Tubal or Transuterine Lavage

In view of the fact that sterility/infertility is one of the primary indications for pelviscopic surgery, the basic set should include an all-purpose pertubator (according to Fikentscher & Semm) and an intrauterine vacuum probe (Fig. 8). The methylene blue required for visualization of the tubes is instilled via an accessory bottle with continuous pressure (controlled by the pertubator). In the past, methylene blue was commonly injected with a syringe. However, this technique produces un-

satisfactory results and makes it more difficult to prepare the ampulla.

Instruments for Transvaginal Mobilization of the Uterus

Uterine mobilization is required to achieve an unobstructed view of the minor pelvis during surgery. The intrauterine vacuum probe can be very helpful in this regard (Fig. 8). Since most operations are performed with the uterus maximally anteverted behind the symphysis, we recommend probe fixation with weights.

Prewarming Device for Carbon Dioxide Gas

In the past few decades, carbon dioxide gas has always been insufflated into the abdomen at temperatures of approximately 18° to 20°C. Measurements in Kiel, Germany, have shown that the temperature in the abdominal cavity can thereby be reduced to as little as 28°C. Rectal temperatures of 34°C were also measured. Gas-induced hypothermia led to complaints of severe pain after the patients awoke from anesthesia.

The use of prewarmed carbon dioxide gas reduced operative shoulder pain by 50%, tachycardia was almost totally prevented, and the postoperative use of pain killers was reduced by 31% after pelviscopic and/or laparoscopic surgery. On the whole, the use of prewarmed carbon dioxide gas for creation of pneumoperitoneum substantially increased the patients' well-being, even in lengthy surgeries.

Typical Gynecologic/Endoscopic Operations

First, the importance of palpating the aorta through the umbilicus prior to making any blind puncture with the Veress needle

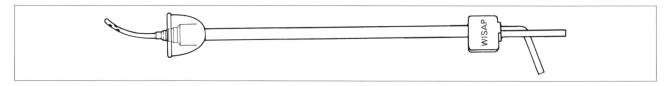

Fig. 8. SEMM intrauterine vacuum probe for atraumatic mobilization of the uterus and simultaneous insufflation of fluid or CO_2 gas

(Fig. 9) should be emphasized. Palpation makes it possible to precisely identify the location of the bifurcation site (Figs. 10–12). Once the location of the greater vessels has been identified, the Veress needle is inserted perpendicular to the abdominal wall. Careful attention to technique almost completely excludes the risk of preperitoneal emphysema and perforation or laceration of the greater vessels. The Veress needle should always be inserted perpendicular to the abdominal wall. Oblique insertion of the needle automatically turns it into a scalpel (Fig. 13).

Once optimal pneumoperitoneum is confidently confirmed by the needle test, aorta test, palpation test, click test, aspiration test, manometer test, volume test (Quadro-Test), and hissing test, the examining trocar is inserted via the **Z**-tract puncture technique under visual control.

If inspection with the subsequently inserted pelviscope confirms the preoperative diagnosis, the surgeon must decide

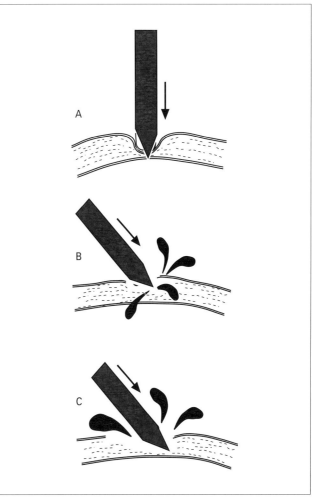

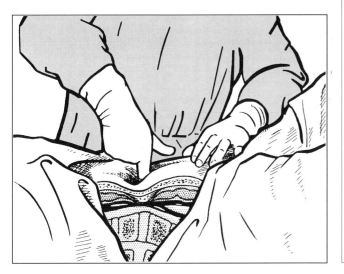

Fig. 9.   Transumbilical palpation of the aorta and bifurcation site

Fig. 13.   When held obliquely, the Veress needle is transformed into a scalpel and lacerates the vessel

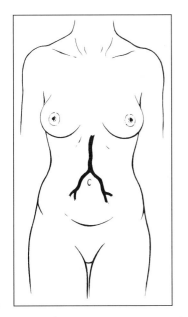

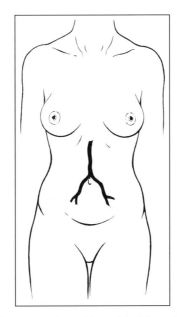

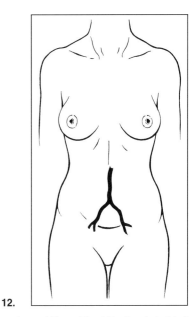

10.   11.   12.

Figs. 10–12.   Schematic representation of the possible topographic positions of the bifurcation: above the umbilicus (Fig. 10), directly behind the umbilicus (Fig. 11), and below the umbilicus (Fig. 12)

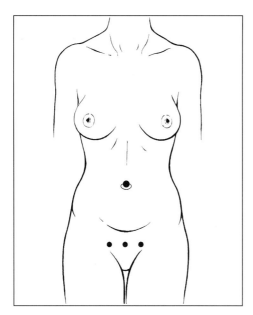

Fig. 14. Typical insertion sites for the 4 trocar sleeves: The examining trocar is inserted through a small (longitudinal) incision in the lower umbilical fossa. The remaining trocars are inserted below the pubic hairline

whether operative endoscopic correction of the condition is feasible in light of the pathological findings. Two to four secondary puncture sites are established as needed (Fig. 14). If pelviscopic surgery is to be performed, the 5-mm pelviscope is removed and exchanged for a 10-mm pelviscope after atraumatic widening of the umbilical puncture site is completed (Fig. 15).

Basic Principles

Pelviscopic surgery should be performed in basically the same manner as classical open abdominal surgery. In other words, the operator should avoid "tricks" like coagulating hemorrhages in omental tissue or leaving unsutured wounds in the ovaries, Fallopian tubes, uterus, or intestines.

Table 1 provides an "organ-oriented catalogue" of all pelviscopic surgical operations currently performed.

Plates 1 to 4 contain schematic, step-by-step diagrams of these surgical techniques, which will be described in detail in the following.

Pelviscopic Surgery of the Uterus

Because bleeding is considerably reduced in operative endoscopy as compared to surgery via laparotomy, pelviscopic surgery of the uterus can be recommended, despite the fact that the uterus contains numerous blood vessels.

Virtually bloodless enucleation of myomas can be achieved using a myoma enucleator preheated to a temperature of 120 °C in conjunction with local infiltration of vasopressin (0.05 IU/ml). The coagulated wound surface, which can be relatively large in some cases, forms a protein film that protects the area against postoperative intestinal or omental adhesion formation. In contrast, postoperative adhesion formation is virtually unavoidable in laparotomy, due to the exudation of such substances as fibrin. We distinguish between subserous myoma enucleation and intramural myoma enucleation.

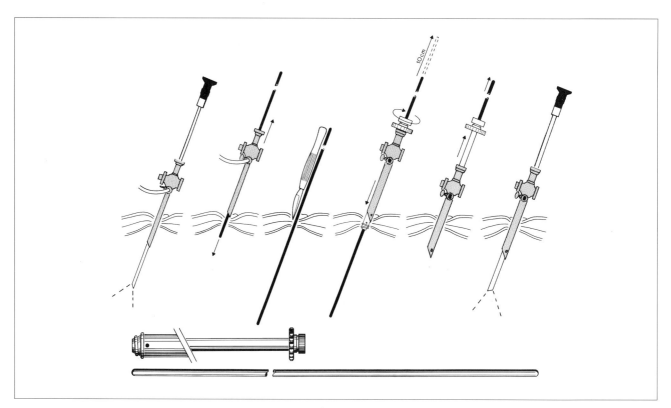

Fig. 15. Atraumatic widening of the 5-mm insertion site to accommodate a 10, 15, or 20-mm trocar sleeve using the Semm atraumatic dilatation set

Table 1. Organ-Oriented Catalogue of Pelviscopic Surgery

Uterus

1. Correction of perforation:
   due to sound, curette, etc.
   due to IUD
2. Myoma enucleation: subserous location, intramural location
3. Extrauterine fibroma enucleation
4. Myolysis (hyperthermia treatment)
5. Intrafascial hysterectomy (CISH)
6. Total uterine mucosa ablation (TUMA)

Adnexa, conservative

1. Ovariolysis
2. Ovarian biopsy
3. Ovarian cyst biopsy
4. Ovarian cyst enucleation
5. Fimbriolysis
6. Salpingolysis
7. Fimbrioplasty
8. Salpingostomy
9. End-to-end anastomosis
10. Excision of Morgagni hydatids
    pedunculated
    retroperitoneal
11. Parovarian cyst enucleation
12. Partial Oophorectomy
13. Pyo-ovarium, pyosalpinx

Adnexa, total

1. Oophorectomy
2. Tubal sterilization (interruption)
3. Tubectomy
   partial
   total
4. Adnexectomy

Extrauterine pregnancy

1. Fallopian tube
   total
   conservative
2. Ovary
3. Abdominal cavity

Endometriosis

1. Peritoneal
2. Sacrouterine ligament region
3. Ovarian
4. Uterine
5. Tubal
6. Dome of the bladder region
7. Intestinal
8. Retrocervical
9. Appendiceal region
10. Splenic region

Follicular puncture and gamete transfer

1. In vitro fertilization and embryo transfer (IVF-ET)
2. Gamete intra-Fallopian tube transfer (GIFT)
3. Intrauterine insemination (IUI)
4. Intra-peritoneal insemination (IPI)

Intraabdominal adhesiolysis

1. Hypogastrium
2. Mesogastrium
3. Epigastrium

Bowel

1. Intestinal adhesiolysis (parietal peritoneum)
2. Intestinal adhesiolysis (visceral peritoneum)
3. Intestinal/omental adhesiolysis and resection
4. Intestinal suturing

Intra-abdominal cancer diagnosis

1. Exploratory laparoscopy
2. Aspiration of ascites
3. Tumor biopsy
4. Tumor reduction
5. Tumor staging
6. Lymph node enucleation

Induction of Temporary Uterine Ischemia via Ligation

The induction of hemostasis via destructive heat is inappropriate in uterine surgeries where considerable blood loss is expected (i.e. enucleation of very large myomas). Complete uterine ischemia can be achieved by applying uterine ligatures with extracorporal knotting (Fig. 19).

Uterine Suturing After Perforation

If the uterus has been perforated by a probe, dilator, curette (Fig. 16/1), intrauterine device grasper, or other instruments, the location and position of the perforation and the presence or absence of intestinal injury is determined pelviscopically (patient history).

Uterine bleeding is stopped by means of point coagulation and infiltration with vasoconstrictor solution if necessary. The wound is then closed with an endosuture (Fig. 16/2). None of our patients developed any postoperative complications. No adhesion formation at the suture site was observed in patients who were later re-pelviscopied.

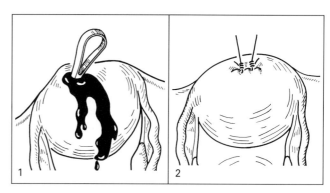

Fig. 16. Closure of a perforation wound caused by a curette in the fundus corporis uteri

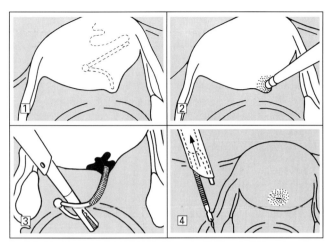

Fig. 17. Operation sequence in transuterine extraction of a "lost IUD" with subsequent hemostasis by means of point coagulation (and endosuturing with extra- or intracorporal knotting if necessary)

Transabdominal Removal of a "Lost" Intrauterine Device

Infrequently, an intrauterine device (IUD) may partially or completely transmigrate the muscle walls of the uterus. In most cases, the IUD has been incorrectly inserted. If the intramural position of the IUD has been determined by ultrasound, x-ray, and hysteroscopy, but the IUD cannot be removed transcervically, the intrauterine device is probably located in the subperitoneal region, or it may have partially perforated the fundus corporis uteri or the cervix.

Once the precise location of the IUD has been identified (Fig. 17/1), the dome of uterine tissue projecting above the IUD is first point coagulated through the 2nd and 3rd ports. A vasoconstrictor solution can also be injected into the area if necessary (Fig. 17/2). Once bloodless division of the uterine tissue and liberation of a tip of the IUD has been achieved, the IUD is removed from the uterus under traction with biopsy forceps (Fig. 17/3). Subsequent bleeding is usually minor and can be stopped by means of point coagulation.

The IUD can be removed after dilating the 5-mm puncture site to accommodate the 11-mm trocar sleeve (Fig. 17/4).

If the IUD is located in the free omentum, the region is ligated, and the IUD is bloodlessly removed *in toto* with omental tissue. The omentum must be inspected to make sure that no perforations are present. Such undetected injuries could lead to postoperative bowel prolapse with delayed subileus complaints. Any such omental perforations can be closed via endosuture.

Enucleation of Subserous Myomas

Using the myoma enucleator, virtually bloodless enucleation of pedunculated myomas can be achieved when the myoma enucleator is heated to 120 °C and guided very slowly through the myoma tissue (Plate I-1.2.1). This ensures that the divided vessels are already coagulated before they spiral back into the uterine muscle tissue due to the effects of heat.

Uterine muscle retraction or "collaboration of the uterus" is essential for achieving bloodless surgery. The residual amputation scar must be point coagulated to ensure good results. No further wound treatment is required. Healthy peritoneal tis-

sue cannot attach to the coagulated surface. Coagulated protein, *i.e.* tissue, is re-epithelialized from within via histiocyte and fibroblast migration.

In hard fibromyomas, the suprasymphyseal 5-mm puncture site should be dilated to 11–20 mm. The myoma can then be grasped with the large clawed forceps or lanced with the myoma drill, then morcellated with the S.E.M.M. Set morcellator (Fig. 18).

Pedunculated myomas can be ligated with Semm safety loop ligatures, which even permits bloodless removal of some myomas. It is very important to point coagulate the pedicle afterwards to prevent postoperative adhesion formation with the peritoneum.

In myoma enucleation, the problem is morcellation, not excision, of the myoma. The myoma can also be removed transvaginally by means of a posterior colpotomy. This "trick" was used at our hospital only in the early years of operative pelviscopy, and it has become completely obsolete since the advent of morcellation.

A colpotomy incision carries the risk of uncontrolled infection and later development of adhesions. Therefore, it is incompatible with the tenets of minimally invasive surgery.

Enucleation of Intramural Myomas

The enucleation of intramural myomas can be very helpful, particularly in infertility. A bloodless surgical technique is also decisive. Once the myoma capsule has been coagulated and infiltrated with a vasoconstrictor (Plate I-1.2.2), it is held with biopsy forceps and carefully cut with microscissors. The myoma drill is wound into the myoma fixing it and allowing the surgeon to manipulate it. Further enucleation is done with the myoma enucleator attachement of the WISAP-Endocoagulator set at 120 °C.

One detail that the surgeon should pay careful attention to is the fact that the 120 °C myoma knife should be guided *very slowly* through the tissue. This dispenses with the need for additional coagulation. Large arterioles also respond well after slow coagulation with the myoma knife.

Once the first hole has been drilled in the myoma (see Figs. 32–34) with the 10, 15, or 20 mm S.E.M.M. Set instrument (Figs. 18 and 32) the myoma is held with clawed forceps and is thoroughly enucleated. The edges of the wound are brought into apposition using endosutures with extracorporeal knotting. Two or three sutures are usually sufficient for gross wound apposition. Adhesions seldom develop at the wound

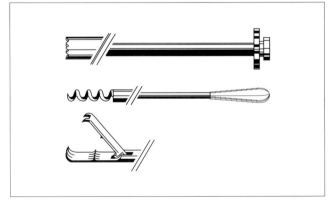

Fig. 18. Combined use of the Serrated Edge Macro-Morcellator (S.E.M.M.), the myoma drill and a large, two-pronged clawed forceps

site as endocoagulation prevents adhesion formation by production of a protective protein film. Profuse abdominal lavage must always be performed at the end of the procedure.

Myomas as large as 14 cm can be morcellated with the S.E.M.M. Set instruments.

Supravesicular myomas (Fibromas in the Dome of the Bladder) occur infrequently. They can be nonproblematically enucleated once the peritoneum has been opened. The myo-

mas can then be removed through an 11-mm trocar sleeve after they have been morcellated. For bloodless enucleation of medium-sized to large myomas, we recommend transitory ligation of the ascending branches of the uterine arteries by applying parametrial and cervical ligatures, known as the TOURNIQUET-Technique according to RUBIN (Figs. 19/1–3 and 19/6) [8]. A Robinson drain should be routinely placed during the first 24 hours after surgery.

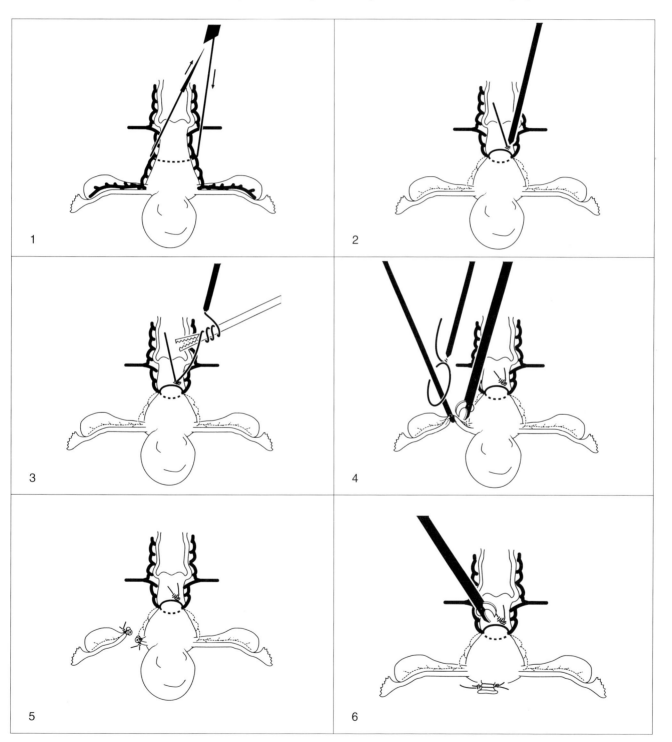

Fig. 19. Ischemia of the fundus corporis uteri is achieved by transitory ligation of the ascending branches of the uterine arteries using a Semm Security Ligature. Tourniquet Technique according to Rubin

Pelviscopic Intrafascial Hysterectomy Without Colpotomy

Total hysterectomy via the vaginal and abdominal route has been performed with colpotomy and enucleation of the extrauterine fasciae of the corpus uteri since around 1962. A new technique of pelviscopic hysterectomy makes it possible to leave the highly vascularized, extrafascial vascular trunk, the corresponding nerves, and the topography of the ureter intact, as is compatible with the tenets of minimally invasive surgery. Moreover, the method fulfills all the previous demands of total hysterectomy, including the prevention of carcinoma of the cervix stump.

We distinguish between three types of hysterectomies:

1. *Subtotal hysterectomy:* Only the body of the uterus is excised with or without adnexectomy. The cervix and the pelvic floor ligaments are left completely intact
2. *Total hysterectomy:* Excision of the entire uterus including the cervical portio with colpotomy
3. *Radical hysterectomy:* Malignant tumors

Postoperative cervix stump carcinomas were found to develop in 0.3 to 1.8 % of all patients treated with the supravaginal technique. Therefore, it has been more or less completely abandoned since around 1962.

The new technique of pelviscopic hysterectomy, called classical intrafascial serrated edged macro-morcellated hysterectomy (CISH), can be performed via laparotomy via pelviscopy, or vaginally. It provides the following advantages:

Surgical Advantages
1. Safe transvaginal excision of the cervical muscles, including the transformation zone
2. The cardinal ligaments are left intact
3. The pericervical nervous plexus is left intact, and such structures as the ureter, the uterine arteries, the bladder, and the rectum are not endangered
4. No need for colpotomy, *i.e.*, incision of the vagina
5. No need to shorten the vagina
6. No risk of abdominal infection due to contamination with vaginal bacteria
7. No need for technique-related secondary healing of the amputated vaginal canal
8. Minimal traumatization and little loss of blood
9. The ligamentous apparatus is suspended from the cervix, not the vaginal stump
10. Marks the beginning of a new era in the surgical treatment of prolapse

Medical Advantages
1. Absolute prevention of cervical stump carcinoma
2. The topography of the pelvic floor remains completely intact, because the support apparatus, *i.e.*, the cardinal ligaments, is left intact
3. Little physical stress on the patient
4. The hospitalization time is reduced from weeks to a few days
5. The recovery time is reduced from months to days
6. The sense of sexual sensations, both vaginal and cervical, remains fully intact
7. The sexual partner function in the vaginal organ remains completely intact

Psychosomatic Advantages
1. The woman's self-confidence remains intact; there is no feeling of mutilation
2. Improved quality of life, despite hysterectomy

In addition to the usual endoscopic instruments, only a needle and sutures are required for CISH. No high-frequency electrocoagulation or laser are necessary.

CISH can, of course, be modified. For example, uni- or bipolar high-frequency electrocoagulation can be used for division of the round ligaments or adnexa, and laser or suturing devices such as the *Endo GIA* can be used. However, these modifications do not change the basic principle of the technique, which is to preserve the pelvic floor and to make hysterectomy as risk-free as in 1960. Back then, subtotal hysterectomy was the technique of choice because of its high relative safety.

Operative Technique

Transvaginal Preparation

The preoperative work-up is the same as for laparotomy: Diagnosis of flora with preoperative eradication, cytology, and colposcopy if indicated. The diameter and length of the cervix are determined via transvaginal ultrasound with bimanual control, and the diameter of the calibrated uterine resection tool (CURT) is selected accordingly. Tenaculums are placed paracervically at 3 and 9 o'clock. The cervix and the uterine cavity are transvaginally probed with a bulb-headed probe. The cervical canal is dilated to Hegar 5. The CURT perforating rod is inserted up to the middle of the uterine cavity (Fig. 20) and is attached anterior to the vulva via a fixation clamp on ball forceps. This completes the transvaginal preoperative preparations.

Pelviscopic Surgery
(see Plate VA p. 388)
The initial phase of pelviscopy begins with the 8 safety tests, the creation of pneumoperitoneum, insertion of the 5-mm diagnostic pelviscope, a 360° inspection, and confirmation of the diagnosis and indication for pelviscopy. If necessary, an assistant can start transvaginal preparations at this time. The pelvis must be examined to secure an exact diagnosis of

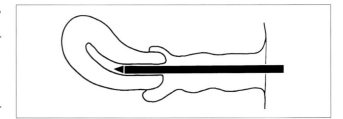

Fig. 20. Transvaginal insertion of the 50 cm perforating rod in intrafascial hysterectomy

Müller's tract and to determine the size, shape, position, and mobility of the uterus and the topography of the adnexa. The feasibility of operative transabdominal pelviscopy is then reconfirmed.

The following operational steps are performed in accordance with the concept of surgery (with or without adnexecto-

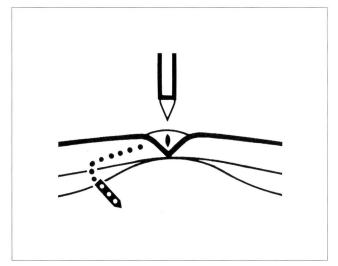

Fig. 21. Z-tract puncture when a cutting trocar is used for prevention of postoperative omental and intestinal adhesions or herniation which occurs due to injury of the umbilical fascia or linea alba

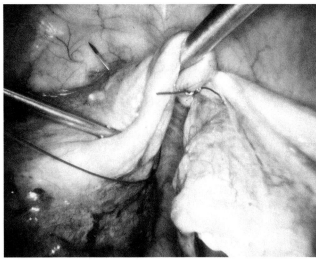

Fig. 23. The second stitch through the broad ligament is placed around the adnexal bundle proximal to the uterus

my): Two 5-mm conical point trocars, which should be placed as far apart as possible, are inserted below the pubic hairline making a Z-tract puncture (Fig. 21). The upwardly directed Z-tract puncture prevents injury to the urinary bladder (Fig. 14). A 10-mm trocar is inserted in the medial parafascial region, i.e., adjacent to the linea alba in the pubic region.

The uterus is fixed in place in a central position using the fixation instruments. After loosening the fixation screw, the fundus corporis uteri is transvaginally perforated with the perforation probe (s. Plate VA p. 388). Prior to perforation, the perforation site is clearly marked by ischemia. The fixed uterus is mobilized by means of extracorporal, i.e., transvaginal, manipulation of the perforation probe. The position, size, and mobility of the uterus is then rechecked. Classical bloodless lysis of adhesions in the region of the adnexa, uterus, or roof of the bladder is performed.

Pelviscopic Hysterectomy with Adnexectomy

The infundibular pelvic ligament in question (right or left) is put on stretch and is doubly ligated as deep as possible. The first extracorporeally prepared safety knot is tied with a surgical safety knot. An additional safety ligature is placed around the ovarian artery using a Roeder loop (see Plate VC-1 p. 388). The Fallopian tube is pushed as far downward as possible without causing bleeding. Two suture ligatures are applied through the round ligaments, which are then separated by a bloodless incision.

The same procedure is repeated on the contralateral side. The uterus is now bilaterally mobilized up to the level of the uterine arteries in the parametrial region (Plate VC-1 p. 388).

The techniques for cervical cylinder resection and uterine excision will be described later on.

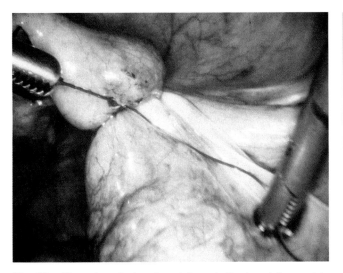

Fig. 22. The suture ligature is put through the broad ligament to achieve ligation of the round ligament, Fallopian tube, and utero-ovarian ligament. The picture shows how the second safety knot is knotted

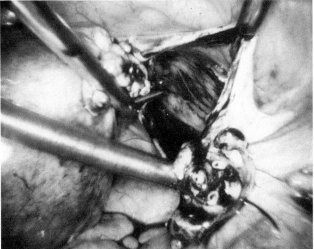

Fig. 24. The anterior and posterior leaves of the broad ligament are separated after bloodless division of the adnexal bundle

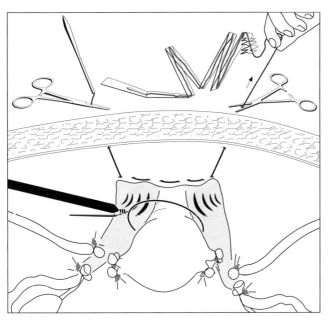

Fig. 25. Schematic representation of peritoneal suspension during classical intrafascial S.E.M.M. hysterectomy (CISH) (S.E.M.M. = **S**errated **E**dge **M**acro-**M**orcellated)

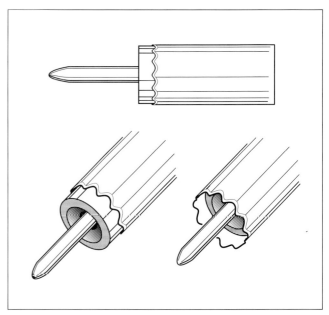

Fig. 27. The calibrated uterine resection tool (CURT) in non-cutting and cutting positions

Pelviscopic Hysterectomy without Adnexectomy

The ligamentum teres uteri and the Fallopian tube are each doubly ligated with an endosuture and extracorporeal knotting, then bloodlessly divided (see Plate VB p. 388 and Figs. 22–23). Parallel ligation of the uterine portion of the Fallopian tube and ovarian ligaments (together with the round ligament if necessary) and subsequent bloodless division between the two ligatures can also be performed (Fig. 24).

Identical ligatures are applied on the contralateral side to achieve bilateral isolation of the uterus from its adnex stumps (see Plate VC-2 p. 388). Two 10-ml doses of *POR 8 solution*

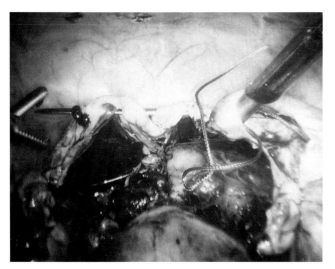

Fig. 26. Once the uterus has been isolated on both sides and the dome of the bladder has been dissected off the uterus the vesico uterine peritoneum is fixed in a ventral position posterior to the symphysis with a stay suture. A 7-cm-long needle is used to pass the suture through the vesical peritoneum

(5 IU of ornipressin dissolved in 100 ml saline solution) are injected into the cervix through the vesico-uterine peritoneum. This step can alternatively be performed during transvaginal attachment of the two portio clamps. Two additional 10-ml doses are injected subperitoneally below the roof of the bladder for aquadissection purposes (Plate VD p. 388).

The dissection off of the vesico-uterine peritoneum is generously performed to ensure that enough peritoneum is left for extraperitonealization of the stumps. The roof of the bladder is dissected with a swab from the lower portion of the corpus uteri and cervix until it lies 2 to 3 cm in the cervical region. This provides a view of the ascending branch of the uterine artery and makes it possible to identify the ureter.

Transabdominal fixation of the vesico-uterine peritoneum is performed with the CISH needle set to achieve a completely unobstructed view of the perivesical space (see Plate VD p. 388 and Figs. 25–26). Using suture material with a very high tensile strength, a safety loop is extracervically guided around the cervical tube and ascending branches of the uterine arteries. The ligature is pulled tight after the correct position of the loop around the insertions of the sacrouterine ligaments (also from posterior) has been confirmed.

The fixation clamp is removed from the perforating rod. The CURT cylinder resector is then attached (Fig. 27) and rotated transvaginally through the cervical and corpus tissue region until the rotating shaft of the CURT exits from the fundus (see Plate VD p. 388 and Fig. 28). The cylinder of tissue and the perforating rod are withdrawn transvaginally with the resector tube.

The ligature, previously set around the cervix, is pulled tight simultaneous with the collapsing of cervical fascia upon retraction of the CURT cylinder resector. The safety knot is tied to the plastic rod under strong extracorporeal traction. This totally closes off the cervix and completely interrupts the blood supply in areas above the ascending branches of the uterine arteries.

Once hemostasis has thus been achieved, the pericervical tissue tube is closed with two additional Roeder loops (triple-loop ligature according to SEMM, 1978). The uterus is then sharply dissected with hook scissors or a scalpel (see p. 388 F and Fig. 29).

Warning: Be careful not to cut the ligatures.

Modified Technique

The adnexal ligation step can be omitted to save time (Plate VB to C2 p. 388), provided that the ascending branches are ligated as described in Figures 19.1 to 19.3. The adnexal stumps are held with a large clawed forceps (preferably the CISH grasper), bloodlessly divided, and ligated with a Roeder loop.

The excised uterus is placed in the pouch of Douglas or the epigastrium. In one case of "lost uterus", laparotomy had to be performed because the uterus was hidden behind the spleen. We therefore recommend provisional fixation of the uterus to the lateral gastric wall.

The tissue stump is then point coagulated and treated with iodine solution for desinfection and prevention of abscess formation.

The round ligaments with or without adnexal stumps are attached to the lateral portion of cervical fasciae proximal to the ligature (see p. 388 G and Fig. 30). Slowly absorbable suture material should be used for optimal elevation and tightening of the pelvic floor, *i.e.*, for elimination of moderate prolapse.

The pouch of Douglas is then carefully rinsed. Once the small needle of the CISH needle set has been retracted, the suture is attached to the sacrouterine ligaments and both ends are knotted. The peritoneum then drops like a stage curtain across the adnexal stumps and completely extraperitonealizes them.

Morcellation: The 10-mm puncture site is first dilated to accommodate a 15 or 20-mm trocar, depending on the size of the uterus. The myoma is removed with the help of the S.E.M.M. Set morcellator or "tissue puncher" (Fig. 31).

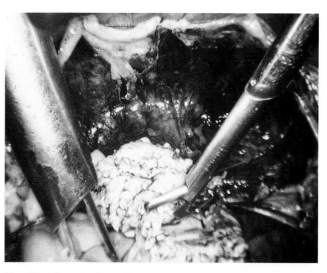

Fig. 29. Completely unobstructed view of the carefully dissected minor pelvis. The uterus is separated from the pericervical stump with the scissors

For best results, the myoma should first be drilled into with the myoma drill, then morcellated "bite-by-bite". Although long and repetitive, even large myomas can be removed in this manner. Once the myoma is manageable enough, it can be thoroughly morcellated with the help of clawed forceps.

After morcellation, the entire abdominal cavity is copiously rinsed with several liters of saline solution. Two Robinson drains are then inserted through the 5-mm ports and left in place for the next few hours for detection of potential bleeding.

The patient should be placed on a light diet for the first postoperative day and hospitalized for 2 to 4 days. The Robinson drains should be removed within 12 to 24 hours.

The CISH technique can be learned best in the frame of hysterectomy via laparotomy.

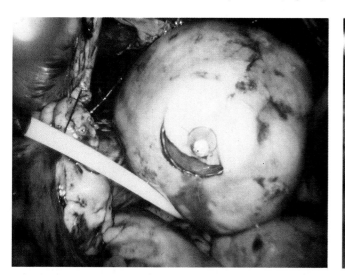

Fig. 28. After loosely applying a Roeder loop from the left, a cylinder of tissue from the cervix, cavum uteri, and fundus is resected. In this picture, the CURT is just emerging from the other side. We recommend using the Moto-Drive for cylinder resection

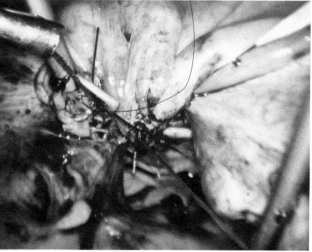

Fig. 30. After both round ligaments have been attached to the pericervical fascial stumps, the vesical peritoneum is draped like a stage curtain across the stumps and attached to the sacrouterine ligaments

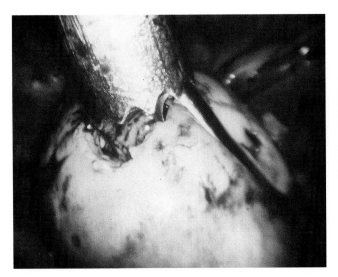

Fig. 31. Intra-abdominal morcellation of the uterine corpus

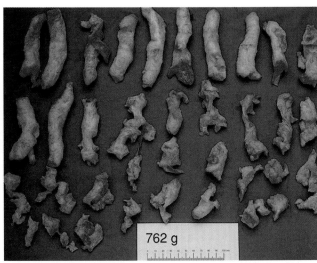

Fig. 33. Macro-morcellated tissue of myoma (762 g) (see Fig. 18)

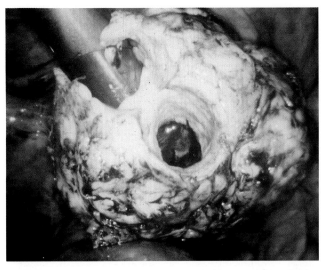

Fig. 32. Endoscopic demonstration of starting the myoma enucleation in situ: one hole has been excised and the second hole is in progress (see Fig. 18)

Longitudinal and cross-sectional specimens of the cervical conus (Plate VF p. 388) are submitted for histological diagnosis. This permits histopathological confirmation of complete removal of the cervical transfomation zone.

The defect in the cervix heals within approximately 6 weeks.

Intra-abdominal Morcellation

Intra-abdominal morcellation for reduction in size of myoma and uterine tissue following endoscopic isolation is efficiently performed using the S*E*M*M* System which consists of the Serrated Edged Macro Morcellator, the large Claw Forceps, and a Myoma Drill (see Fig. 18). The morcellator can be manually or motor powered.

The manually driven morcellator is principally recommended for reduction of the size of myoma tissue which remains in situ (Fig. 32). Once a central core has been removed from the myoma it may be easily grasped and extracted from the uterus.

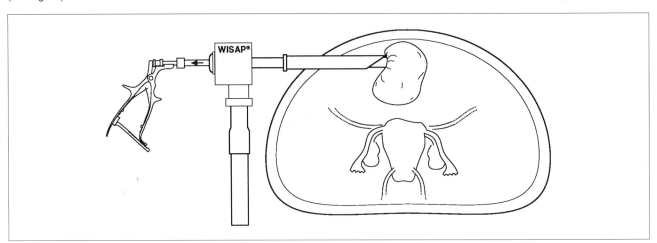

Fig. 34. Classic horizontal positioning of the Moto-Drive for morcellation using the 15 or 20 mm Ø S*E*M*M*. The Moto-Drive is only recommended for isolated tissue masses (see Fig. 18)

In cases where a large myoma has been isolated surgically, the motor driven morcellator with a diameter of 15 or 20 mm is a most useful instrument (Fig. 33).

The manually driven or Moto-Drive Morcellator offers a practicable solution to the problem of reduction of isolated intraabdominal tissue (Fig. 34). Removal by posterior colpotomy or Mini-Lap incision should thus be abandonned in favor of this technique.

Total Uterine Mucosa Ablation (TUMA)

Hysteroscopic endometrial ablation was established in the spirit of minimally invasive surgery. However, its clinical results are not very satisfactory. TUMA, a new technique of transvaginal, pelviscopically controlled cavum uteri and cervix ablation (SEMM 1992), is recommended for total excision of the uterine endometrium. TUMA combines techniques of pelviscopy, excoreation, and coagulation. We believe that TUMA is able to prevent hysterectomy in patients with certain indications.

Technique of total uterine mucosa ablation
(see Plate VI p. 389).
1. After the cervix has been dilated to Hegar 3-5, the 50 cm CURT perforating rod is inserted up to the uterine fundus
2. The corpus uteri is transformed into a straight muscle tube under pelviscopic vision. The cervix is transvaginally fixed at 3 and 9 o'clock. With the help of spacers, the perforating rod is firmly attached to two tenaculums that are firmly fixed in the cardinal ligaments at 3 and 9 o'clock
3. A safety loop to temporarily ligate the ascending branches of the uterine artery is guided underneath the tubal origin angles using two biopsy forceps
4. The safety loop is knotted twice to keep it from coming undone during cylinder resection
5. The uterine cervix and corpus muscles are infiltrated with two 10-ml injections of POR 8 solution each (0.05 IU/ml)
6. The CURT cylinder resector is inserted and the uterine mucosal tissue cylinder resected
7. After the resector tube has been removed, the ligature is cut, and a hemostaser that has been heated to 120 ° C is inserted under pelviscopic control. The tissue cylinder must be carefully inspected for possible defects (Fig. 35). The remaining endometrium is then denatured under pelviscopic/hysteroscopic control, which automatically stops any residual bleeding
8. The cylindrical defect in the uterine cavity is closed with a suture

Obliteration of the cylindrical defect and healing of the vagina should be observed within 6 weeks (vaginal ultrasound follow-up).

Intrafascial Vaginal Hysterectomy (IVH)

In light of the successful application of CISH via laparotomy and pelviscopy, and in view of its functional success with total uterine mucosa ablation, it was only logical that intrafascial vaginal hysterectomy should be attempted. This was all the more understandable, since the pelviscopic CISH technique and the laparoscopic assisted vaginal hysterectomy (LAVH) developed by REICH (1989) both require highly specialized equipment. Also, as many years of worldwide practice have shown, the two techniques are somewhat more time-consum-

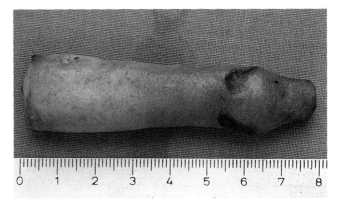

Fig. 35. Example of resected cylinder of tissue from the cervix, uterine cavity, fundus in CISH and TUMA. The tube origin angles are clearly visible

ing than laparotomy, and they are much more time-consuming than the vaginal hysterectomy technique.

Moreover, due to the removal of the cervical tissue cylinder, intrafascial vaginal hysterectomy (IVH) is technically less demanding than vaginal classical extrafascial hysterectomy with colpotomy (i.e. total hysterectomy). The reason is that forward delivery of the uterus is easier due to collapsing down of the cervix in the former technique.

The individual steps of intrafascial vaginal hysterectomy (IVH) are described in Plate VIII p. 391.

The anterior lip of the os uteri is held at the 3 and 9 o'clock positions, as is routine procedure in vaginal incisions, and the uterovesical pouch is opened (A). Each tenaculum is next positioned deep in the parametrium at 3 and 9 o'clock, and the precise length of the cavity is determined (B). Two 10-ml doses of 0.05 IU/ml POR 8 solution each are injected intracervically, and the blunt end of the CURT perforating rod is inserted into the uterine cavity (C). The CURT resector tube (15-, 20-, or 24-mm diameter) is attached, and a cylinder of cervical muscle tissue is excised (D).

The maximum cutting depth equals two-thirds of the measured probe length. This should be carefully monitored using the gauge on the CURT (calibrated guide cylinder). Manual cylinder resection is possible but, for optimum results, we recommend using the Auto-Moto-Drive, which cuts down to the millimeter with high precision. After the CURT has been removed, a claw forceps is inserted deep within the incision wound and the cervical canal. It is used to rotate the cylinder of cervical tissue, as in excision of a myoma in statu nascendi (E).

The cylinder of tissue detaches in the region of the thin-walled endometrium and can be removed from the cervix with almost no loss of blood (F).

Once two stay sutures have been placed, vaginal hysterectomy is performed using two claw hooks (cats paws) for forward delivery of the uterus (G), a technique that has been tried and proven effective for decades. The absence of the cylinder of cervical muscle tissue makes it much easier to deliver the uterus.

Pelviscopic-assisted intrafascial vaginal hysterectomy is performed when adnexectomy is indicated (SEMM 1984). The adnexa and the divided infundibulo-ovarian ligaments are drawn downwards. A Roeder loop is pulled tight around the uterine fundus. This marks the waist of the cervix and serves as a "rein" which makes it easier to ligate the ascending branches of the right and left uterine arteries with deep interrupted sutures placed below the loop.

Next, the uterus is cut supravaginally between the loops of the ligature and the rein with a scalpel (I).

The round ligaments are sewn onto the cervix stump so as to simultaneously close the abdominal excoriation wound with the same stitches (K). A running suture placed around the roof of the bladder peritoneum on the posterior wall of the cervix closes the abdominal cavity while simultaneously extraperitonealizing the stumps (L). The vaginal wound is closed with interrupted sutures. A T-drain can be placed if this is routine hospital procedure (L).

Summary: This procedure basically corresponds to classical vaginal hysterectomy with forward delivery of the uterus. However, the difference is that the vaginal mucosa is incised only from 3 to 9 o'clock, not in circular fashion. Furthermore, the cervical mucosa is excoreated using the Calibrated Uterine Resection Tool (CURT).

This intrafascial vaginal hysterectomy technique offers the same advantages as those of pelviscopic intrafascial hysterectomy without colpotomy. The technique requires neither division of the cardinal and sacrouterine ligaments, nor colpotomy, nor ligation of the uterine arteries. It does not alter the patient's sex life, and it provides ideal conditions for preservation of the pelvic floor topography.

Pelviscopic Adnex Surgery (Conservative)

Modern pelviscopic surgery is setting the pace for abdominal diagnosis of female infertility.

Endoscopic Ovariolysis and Salpingolysis

Adhesiolysis can be performed virtually anywhere in the tube or ovarian region with the help of one or two atraumatic graspers, hook scissors, and microscissors. In some cases, crocodile forceps must be used to apply heat coagulation to the vascularized area. The myoma enucleator, which reaches

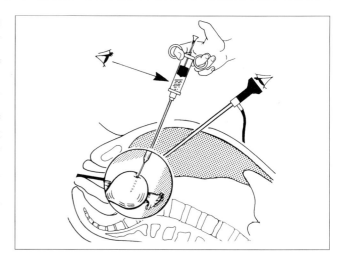

Fig. 37. Ovarian cyst biopsy with the atraumatic vacuum aspirator

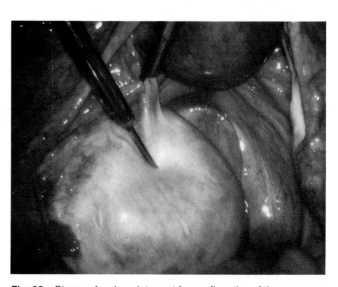

Fig. 38. Biopsy of a chocolate cyst for confirmation of the preoperative diagnosis. Subsequent rinsing of cyst contents and infiltration of vasopressin in the mesovarium using two 10-ml doses of POR 8 solution (0.05 IU/ml) (also see Fig. 63)

temperatures of 110–120 °C, is an excellent instrument for removing adhesive foci from the ovaries and tubes (see Plate II-2.5). The instrument induces protein coagulation and the subsequent formation of a protein film that helps to prevent postoperative adhesion formation.

Particularly in sharp-dissection adnexal surgery, maximum ischemia should preferably be achieved infiltrating the area with *POR 8* solution (see Fig. 63). Hemostasis can then be maintained with little or no use of destructive heat.

Pelviscopic Ovarian Biopsy

Bidentate biopsy forceps are needed for ovarian biopsy (Plate I-2.2). A tissue cylinder is resected by pushing down on the elliptical trocar sleeve. Hemostasis is achieved by point coagulation. In contrast with high-frequency electrocoagulation, the point coagulator does not cause heat destruction of healthy surrounding ovarian tissue.

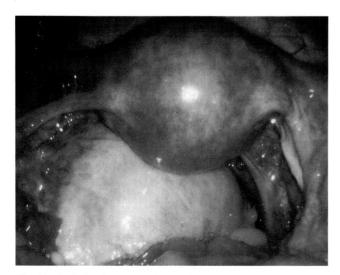

Fig. 36. Left-sided, 8-cm single-chambered chocolate cyst in situ

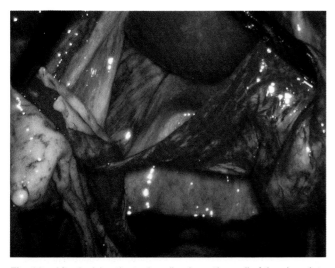

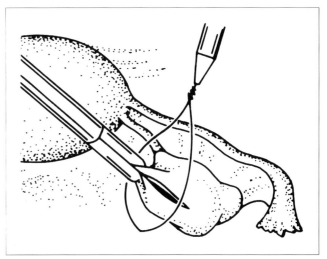

Fig. 39. After incising the tunica albuginea, the wall of the chocolate cyst is fully enucleated, in part with the curler technique

Fig. 40. The edges of the ovarian wound are appositioned with a Roeder loop

Ovarian Cyst Biopsy

In most cases, the patient is referred for ovarian biopsy with a preoperative diagnosis obtained either by bimanual examination or ultrasound. The first step in ovarian cyst biopsy is to assess the external appearance of the cyst (Fig. 36).

Next, a sample of the cyst contents is removed with a biopsy aspirator (Figs. 37–38) for macroscopic evaluation (clear, turbid, mucinous, etc.). Thorough rinsing is then performed.

The surgeon should never rely solely on the results of the histological examination, but should also open the cyst and carefully inspect its interior walls. If there is the slightest suspicion of irregularity (e.g., papilloma, solid structures), it would not be wise to continue the endoscopic procedure. Enucleation can be performed if no signs of malignancy are found.

Ovarian Cyst Enucleation and Ovarian Suture

The following technique is recommended if the results of biopsy and interior wall inspection showed beyond a doubt that the cyst is benign (94 % of all ovarian cysts are benign), and that the sac of the cyst is large enough to permit in toto excision.

POR 8 solution is injected into the mesovarium as shown in Plate I-2.4. The contents of the cysts are then removed by suction, and the cyst is rinsed repeatedly. Once refilled, 2 to 5 cm of the tunica albuginea should be point coagulated and divided.

The sac of the cyst is enucleated step by step with two biopsy forceps (Fig. 39). In most cases, it is not possible to enucleate the cyst without damaging it. Therefore, chocolate cysts or dermoids should be enucleated after thorough rinsing has been completed, as this is technically easier. Any bleeding at the base of the cyst can be stopped with the point coagulator. Finally, the edges of the wound are brought into apposition.

Two alternatives are possible:
1. Apposition of the wound edges with the help of a biopsy forceps, which is manoeuvred through a Roeder loop in such a way that the Roeder knot appositions the wound edges (Fig. 40)
2. In large gaping ovarian wounds, wound adaptation should be performed by means of **Z** endosuture placement (Figs. 41–43)

Minor bleeding can also be stopped by generous suturing of the ovarian parenchyma. In contrast to laparotomy, painstaking apposition of the wound edges is not necessary, because they quickly adapt. Postoperative adhesions almost never develop, because the peritoneum is not injured by the technique, and peristalsis is hardly affected.

At the end of any ovarian surgery, the minor pelvis must be rinsed with at least 1 to 2 liters of saline solution to achieve a completely dry area and to ensure that no residual tissue particles are left in the minor pelvis. When doing so, an atraumatic grasper must be used to hold the epiploic appendices, the bowels and the ampulla, away from the bivalent rinsing and suction tube.

A higher than average amount of transudation develops after such procedures. Therefore, a Robinson drain should be routinely inserted and left in place for 24 hours after any conservative ovarian surgery (see Fig. 55).

Endoscopic Fimbrioplasty

Endoscopic fimbrioplasty is a very promising technique for surgical correction of infertility due to tubal disease. First the obstructed end of the ampulla is dilated (with the tubal sound if necessary) as shown in Plate II-2.7. Next atraumatic holding or grasping forceps are used to carefully widen the obstructed end just large enough to accommodate the closed grasper of an atraumatic holding forceps. Patency of the ampulla can be restored with little or no loss of blood by withdrawing the open atraumatic grasper one or more times through the opening.

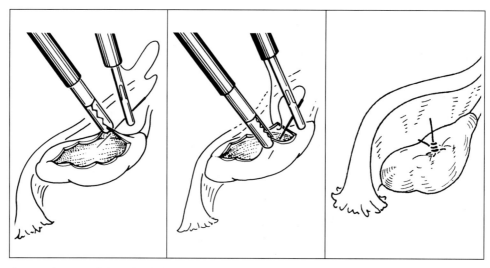

Fig. 41. Closure of an ovarian wound via endosuturing

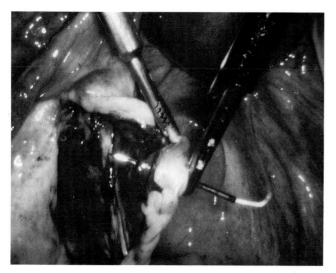

Fig. 42. The wound edges (tunica albuginea) are brought into apposition with a Z-tract endosuture and extracorporeal knotting

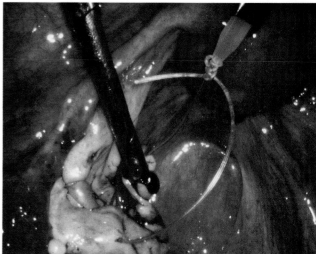

Fig. 43. Final situs after apposition of wound edges (suture material: catgut, mono- or multifil absorbable suture material of up to 6-0 can be used; needle: straight sharp needle is best, sliding needle or round needle can also be used). In principle, it is not necessary to painstakingly approximate the wound edges. However, failure to suture the wound can lead to severe adhesions

Simultaneous chromosalpingoscopy can be used to monitor the results, *i.e.*, the collapse of the dilated pre-ampullary neck of the tube and the escape of methylene blue and CO_2 gas.

Endoscopic Salpingostomy

Plate II-2.8. p. 383 gives a schematic representation of the technique of endoscopic salpingostomy. When performed with 20 fold screen magnification, the results of the technique are comparable to those of microsurgery. The first step is either coagulation of the obstructed ampulla opening or injection of a vasoconstrictor such as *POR 8* followed by classical opening of the ostium using the microscissors with subsequent eversion of the ampulla. 4-0 or 6-0 PDS microsutures with intracorporeal knotting are applied for fixation of the

everted ampulla. The results are monitored by continuous ascending chromosalpingoscopy. Isthmic salpingostomy with end-to-end anastomosis is another technique for surgical endoscopic correction of infertility due to tubal disease (Fig. 44).

Extensive adhesiolysis, salpingolysis, or ovariolysis is often initially performed in preparation for microsurgical refertilization.

Pelviscopic Excision of Parovarian Cysts

Attempts to perform pelviscopic cystectomy are justified, even in parovarian cysts that are as large as a fist. After using the point coagulator to create a coagulation streak along the peritoneum (Fig. 45.1), the tissue is divided and the cyst is enucleated *in toto* with the help of two biopsy forceps (Fig. 45.2). Usually, the results are surprisingly good. A triple-loop ligature

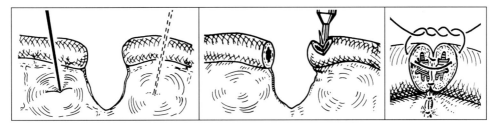

Fig. 44. Bloodless end-to-end anastomosis with micro-endosutures can be achieved after tubal sterilization if vasopressin infiltration is used (0.05 IU/ml)

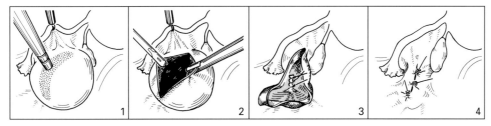

Fig. 45. Division of the broad ligament and enucleation of a parovarian cyst, followed by application of the triple-loop ligation technique and peritoneal suturing

is placed around the residual pedicle (Fig. 45.3), and a continuous Z-tract endosuture is applied to close the loose edges of the peritoneum (Fig. 45.4).

Pelviscopic Adnexal Surgery (Total)

In patients, in whom conservative ovarian surgery is not indicated because of their age we recommend the triple-loop ligature technique in ovariectomy or adnexectomy for *in toto* excision of cystic ovarian tumors.

Mobile ovaries (ovarian cysts) and ovaries that can easily be freed from adhesions are excised via the triple-loop ligature technique. The recommended procedure is as follows:

The surgeon first makes an umbilical puncture for the pelviscope and 3 punctures in the pubic hairline region (see Fig. 14), *i.e.*, two lateral punctures for the 5-mm trocar sleeves, and one puncture site midway between them for the 11- or 15-mm trocar sleeve. Following the diagram in Plate II-3.1 the ovary is grasped using a large 11-mm clawed forceps passed through a Roeder loop. The loop can be positioned behind the ovary by applying strong traction on the contralateral side with atraumatic grasping forceps. The utero-ovarian ligament and the mesovarium are ligated with the first knot.

Next, two additional loops are placed posterior to the ovary. Ideally, they should be positioned close to the first loop. Hook scissors are introduced through the port on the side where an ovary is to be resected. The ovary is then dissected with the hook scissors at a right angle to the tissue stump. A small tissue stump should be left intact; the stump should be point coagulated to prevent postoperative adhesion formation. Intensive coagulation can damage the catgut sutures and should be avoided.

If the ovary is too large to be removed *in toto* through the 11-mm trocar, it can be longitudinalized and narrowed by cutting small notches in it with the hook scissors (Fig. 46) until it is manageable enough to fit through the trocar. Alternatively, the ovary may be morcellated with the S.E.M.M. Set before it is extracted (see Fig. 18).

Next, the minor pelvis is carefully rinsed with 1 to 3 liters of saline solution until the peritoneum glistens. One should be careful not to let any rinsing solution run off into the mesogastrium or epigastrium.

The only potential complication is the risk that the three catgut loops may slip after resection of the ovary. Should this occur, the infundibulo-pelvic ligament and the utero-ovarian ligament must again be caught in a Roeder loop and ligated (Fig. 19). Bleeding from the ascending branch of the uterine artery and the ovarian artery is minor, due to the absence of vessel paralysis. Therefore, the surgeon can carefully and safely complete ligation without being pressed for time.

Pelviscopic Tubal Sterilization

Pelviscopic tubal sterilization (see Plate II-3.2 p. 383) was the main reason for the enthusiastic acceptance of pelviscopy.

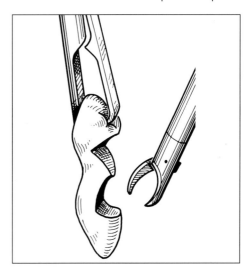

Fig. 46. Notching makes it easier to remove the ovary through the 11-mm trocar sleeve. Larger ovarian fibromas can be morcellated with the S.E.M.M. Set (see Fig. 18)

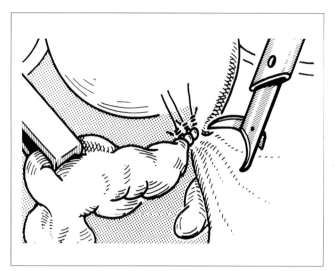

Fig. 47. Excision of a hydrosalpinx using the triple-loop ligature technique

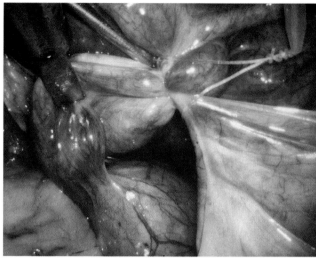

Fig. 49. Placement of the 3rd Roeder loop for right-sided adnexectomy with a parovarian cyst that is as large as a chicken egg

Tubectomy for Hydrosalpinx

Hydrosalpinx, which frequently occurs after tubal sterilization, can be safely and unproblematically excised after a triple-loop ligature has been applied (Fig. 47). The hydrosalpinx is grasped *in toto* using a clawed forceps inserted through a Roeder loop. The hydrosalpinx then usually drains. The stump is then triply ligated before resecting the tube.

Pelviscopic Adnexectomy

Pelviscopic adnexectomy with triple-loop ligature is technically less demanding than ovariectomy. This is because a larger tissue stump can be created by including the Fallopian tube in the ligature. Ovariolysis or salpingolysis is performed beforehand if indicated. The triple-loop technique proceeds as follows if the ovary and the tube are mobile.

Following the technique shown in Plate III-3.4, the tube and ovary are grasped with a large clawed forceps inserted through a Roeder loop. While exerting strong traction, the atraumatic forceps is used to push the Roeder loop far into the mesosalpinx. This ensures deep ligation of the tube, the infundibulo-pelvic ligament, and the utero-ovarian ligament (Figs. 48 and 49). If prior adhesiolysis was performed, correct position of the ureter must be reconfirmed.

Once the three Roeder loops have been properly applied, the adnexal bundle is dissected with hook scissors while applying strong traction. This should be done stepwise at a 90° angle to the tissue stump. The right adnex should never be cut from left to right, or vice versa. Careful attention to technique can prevent damage to the ligature loops and parametrial injuries.

Next, the tube is grasped with spoon forceps inserted through the 11-mm trocar sleeve. The ovary can usually be

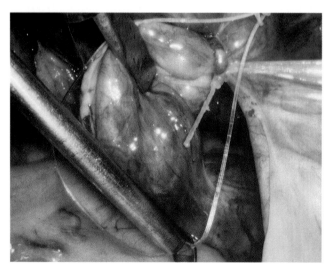

Fig. 48. Guidance of a Roeder loop for right-sided adnexectomy using the triple-loop technique. In this picture, the 2nd Roeder loop is being guided around the infundibulo-pelvic ligament, the Fallopian tube, and the ovarian ligament

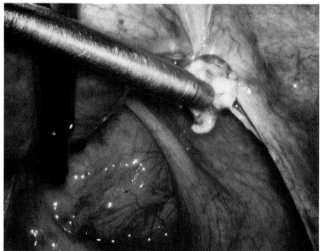

Fig. 50. Triple-loop ligation technique for adnexectomy: Once the right adnexa has been bloodlessly divided, the ligated stump is coagulated to prevent postoperative adhesion formation

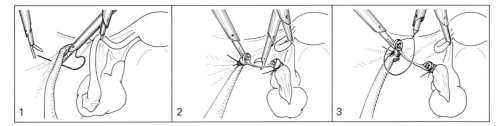

Fig. 51. Operation sequence for division of the infundibulo-pelvic ligament prior to excision of an ovarian tumor during the course of a vaginal hysterectomy

removed through the sleeve at this point. However, large ovarian fibromas must be morcellated beforehand.

As in ovariectomy, the last step is point coagulation of the tissue stump to prevent postoperative adhesion formation (Fig. 50).

If the adnexal bundle is not mobile, the infundibulo-pelvic ligament should be doubly ligated and bloodlessly divided as shown in Figure 51. This technique can also be very useful in vaginal hysterectomy in patients with large ovarian tumors (pelviscopy-assisted vaginal hysterectomy, (SEMM 1984).

Should the loops slip, the same corrective technique is performed as in ovariectomy. The loosened tissue stumps are grasped and can be ligated with individual Roeder loops or sutures (Fig. 52). This complication does not constitute an indication for laparotomy.

The adnexa can also be anteriorly and posteriorly ligated and divided, as in classical laparotomy. However, this technique is more time-consuming.

Pelviscopic Surgery in Extrauterine Pregnancy

Until recently, due to the risk of recurrence, salpingectomy was the treatment of choice for ectopic pregnancy, (see Figs. 1 and 2). In this sense, the development of new microsurgical techniques has improved the quality of life of these patients.

We distinguish between radical tubectomy (semicastration) and conservative operative treatment of tubal ectopic pregnancy. The latter technique allows the surgeon to preserve the rete ovarii. Therefore, it is the preferred method for patients of childbearing age (Fig. 53).

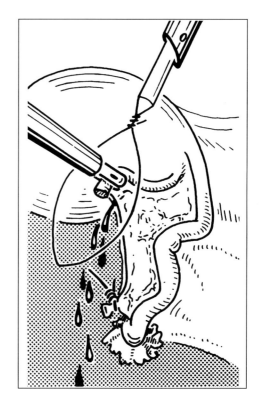

Fig. 52. If the triple-loop ligature should slip, the oozing branch of the tubal-ovarian or other vessel is ligated again with a Roeder loop (or sutures)

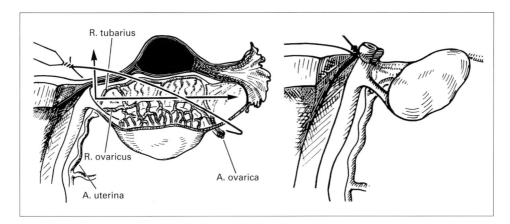

Fig. 53. Schematic representation of destruction of the rete ovarii and interruption of the ovarian blood supply at tubal dissection due to tubal ectopic pregnancy. The blood supply to the ovary is reduced by over 60 % = semi-castration

Triple-loop Tubectomy in Tubal Pregnancy

After applying the three loop ligatures (see Plate III-4.1 p. 385), the tube is sharply transected at a right angle and extracted through the 11-mm trocar with the help of large spoon forceps. The residual tissue stump is coagulated to prevent postoperative adhesion formation in the bowel or omentum.

In extrauterine ectopic pregnancies, *e.g.*, in the pouch of Douglas or intestinal region, the products of conception can be extracted under traction using the large spoon forceps and an atraumatic grasper. Infiltration with vasoconstrictor solution can also be helpful.

A pregnancy test must always be performed on days 7 and 14 after surgical excision of the ectopic pregnancy to determine whether residual chorial tissue exists.

Conservative Correction of Tubal Pregnancy

In contrast with laparotomy, this technique allows quick regeneration of the tubal fragments. Therefore, this technique of conservative surgery of the uterine Fallopian tubes gives us new medical perspectives.

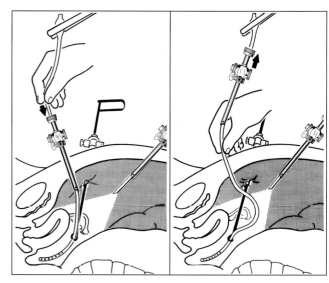

Fig. 55. Placement of a Robinson-Douglas drain through the 5-mm (or 11-mm) trocar sleeve for identification of postoperative-bleeding and drainage of rinsing fluid

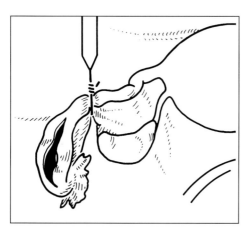

Fig. 54. Transitory or "light" ligation of the Fallopian tube in very bloody conservative surgery of a ruptured tubal pregnancy

Partial salpingectomy can also be performed via pelviscopy. This procedure is reserved for cases where subsequent end-to-end anastomosis via laparotomy is to be performed. However, most hospitals have abandoned the technique.

A vasoconstrictor solution is injected around the interstitial or medially located products of conception. It usually is not necessary to use the point coagulator to create a coagulated line in the convex antimesosalpinx. A longitudinal incision is made in the tubal wall using microscissors and biopsy forceps. The usefulness of a sagittal incision is being debated. In most cases, the products of conception are spontaneously expelled from the tube. However, a large spoon forceps can be used if necessary. The nidation cavity should always be thoroughly rinsed to prevent chorionic tissue from remaining (risk of recurrence). The serosal edges of the wound are brought into apposition using 4-0 microsutures with intracorporeal knotting. Postoperative tubal fistulae develop in 8 to 17 percent of these patients without wound suturing.

Any tubal pregnancy in the ampullary region is more likely to be a tubal abortion. In this case, three suprasymphyseal puncture sites are made (two for the 5-mm trocar, and one for the 11-mm trocar; see Fig. 14). Working through the trocars, the bowel is mobilized into the epigastric region, and the blood is thoroughly rinsed out of the pouch of Douglas. Transampullary suction removal of the chorial tissue can usually be achieved. If necessary, the chorial tissue can be dislodged with the biopsy forceps.

Minor bleeding is stopped by infiltrating vasoconstrictor solution into the mesosalpinx (see Fig. 63). Areas with spurting hemorrhages can be ligated with a Roeder loop or controlled with endosutures. If the bleeding cannot be controlled in this fashion, the ampullary end of the tube can be provisionally ligated by applying a Roeder loop under light traction (Fig. 54). An attempt to remove the loops should be made within 5 to 10 minutes, because the bleeding has usually stopped by then. This should be followed by routine placement of a Robinson drain (Fig. 55).

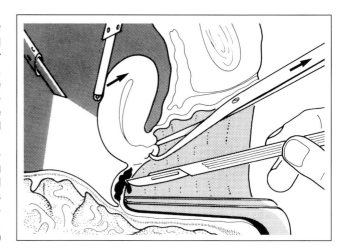

Fig. 56. Vaginal incision of retrocervical endometrial foci while simultaneously monitoring the pouch of Douglas via pelviscope or on the video monitor

The Fallopian tube usually contracts considerably during the approximately 15 to 20-minute operation. Even grossly "ragged" tubes can reconfigurate surprisingly well.

Transitory Roeder loop ligature of the adnexa is often very helpful in cases where venous bleeding from the mesosalpinx cannot be stopped (see Fig. 54). Salpingectomy with triple-loop ligature provides another surgical option which, however, is a rarely used technique. It is important to rinse the entire abdominal cavity with 2 to 3 liters of physiological saline solution in order to prevent postoperative adhesion formation and to reduce the recovery time. Seepage of blood and rinsing solution into the diaphragm can be drained by elevating the head end of the table (see Fig. 6). The accumulated fluids can then be thoroughly suctioned out of the minor pelvis or subdiaphragmatic space (see Fig. 7). This should be followed by routine placement of a Robinson drain (Fig. 55).

In tubal pregnancies where conservative treatment is not indicated, pelviscopic partial salpingectomy is performed following triple-loop ligature (see Plate III-4.1.1). The tubal incision can be made with high-frequency coagulating current or laser. However, laser and electrocoagulation do not have any technical advantages over loop ligature.

Operative Pelviscopic Treatment of Endometriosis

Endometrial foci can be heat-denatured at 100 to 120 °C. This procedure can also be applied in the roof of the bladder region, but not in the bowel region. The combined pelviscopy and vaginal incision technique enables the surgeon to safely remove retrovaginal and retrocervical endometrial foci (Fig. 56).

Virtually complete healing of endometriosis genitalis externa can be achieved using the 3-phase technique described below (SEMM 1980).

Three-phase technique:
1. Surgical pelviscopy for removal of endometrial foci
2. 3- to 4-month hormone treatment of endometriosis
3. Repelviscopy for removal of residual foci

Pelviscopic Surgery for Follicular Puncture and Gamete Transfer

From a technical point of view, it is easy to puncture a ready-to-burst follicle, especially when the necessary instrumentation is available. These patients are usually candidates for *in vitro* fertilization with subsequent return of the embryo. Extensive adhesiolysis is necessary in most cases, because these patients have usually had one or more previous abdominal surgeries. Transvaginal follicular puncture under vaginal ultrasound control is the method of choice today.

Pelviscopic Surgery for Intra-abdominal Adhesiolysis

Omental Adhesiolysis without Omental Resection

We distinguish between bloody and bloodless adhesiolysis of omental tissue. The latter technique is the method of choice. Although the former technique might appear to be quicker in the beginning, it may be slower in the long run if the source of bleeding cannot be found quickly enough to permit Roeder loop ligature.

Bloody Adhesiolysis
Avascular omental adhesions secondary to laparotomy are usually found along the midline in the region of the peritoneal suture or in the adnex region (Fig. 57). Hook scissors can be used to sharply dissect the adhesions proximal to the peritoneum (Fig. 58). If bleeding should occur, a Roeder loop introduced through the two routinely place trocars is used to ligate the oozing vessel stump (see Plate IV-7.1 p. 387, Fig. 59). Any long omental lobes that develop after resection are generously ligated and resected. Lavage with saline solution is the best way to identify p 387 bleeding (Fig. 60).

Bloodless Adhesiolysis
Following the technique for ligation of adhesions shown in Plate IV-7.2 p. 387, adhesions are sharply divided after vas-

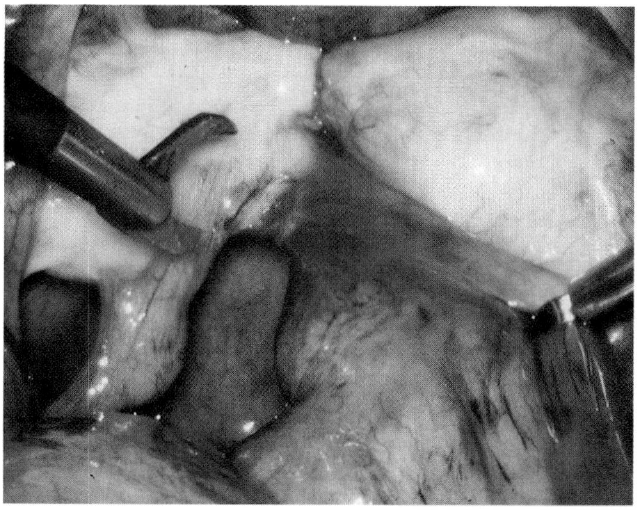

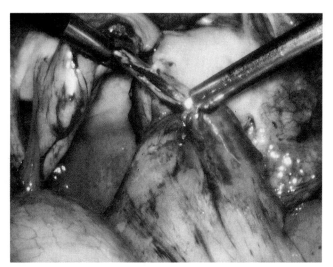

Fig. 57. Formation of ovary to ovary, sigma to ovary, and omental adhesions secondary to right-sided tubal pregnancy. The sigma is stretched between the two ovaries for sharp adhesiolysis

Fig. 58. The sigmoid colon is sharply dissected with the scissors

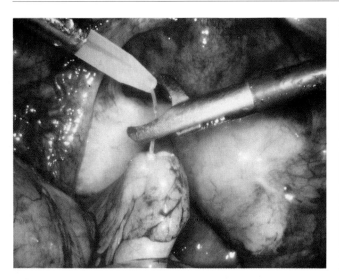

Fig. 59. Bleeding in the appendicea epiploicae was stopped with a Roeder loop

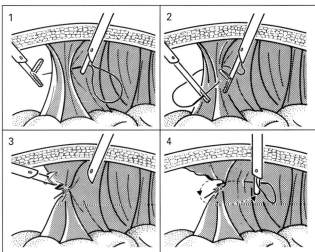

Fig. 61. Bloodless adhesiolysis by stepwise ligation of broad-based omental adhesions

cularized tissue bridges have been ligated. Endoligature without suturing is usually sufficient for this purpose. Some larger tissue bridges must be ligated in a stepwise manner; the endosuture is useful in this regard (Fig. 61). General comment: In the long run, early prophylactic hemostasis is usually less time-consuming than later hemostasis.

Vascularized tissue strands should never be overzealously resected in order to apply Roeder loop ligatures. Complications frequently develop, particularly when operating in the epigastrium, and much time is lost trying to locate oozing omental vessels – a fact which is well-known in laparotomy.

Occasionally, these two techniques are performed in preparation for later laparotomy, *e.g.*, prior to microsurgical correction of infertility due to tubal disease. Once all the adhesions have been lysed in a previous diagnostic/operative pelviscopy, one can concentrate totally on the tubes during microsurgery 1 to 2 months later. This significantly enhances the results of infertility operations.

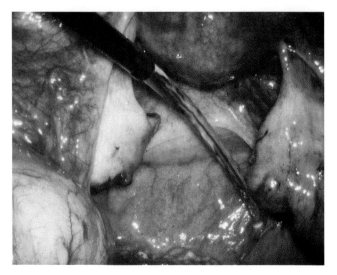

Fig. 60. Once adhesiolysis is completed, the wound area is copiously rinsed in order to identify bleeding

Pelviscopic Surgery of the Bowel

Intestinal Adhesiolysis in the Parietal Peritoneum

Omental or intestinal adhesions subsequent to gynecological surgeries usually develop parallel to the peritoneal suture. They can be pelviscopically removed with virtually no risk of recurrence. Microscissors should be used to prevent accidental and inadvertent perforation of the intestinal lumen. Serosal defects can be repaired by endosutures with either extra- or intracorporal knotting.

A perforated bowel loop can be endoscopically repaired with a single-layer suture. Peristalsis is generally restored within a few hours, as compared to the longer term intestinal paralysis normally observed after laparotomy. The wound area is thoroughly rinsed upon completion of the procedure (see Fig. 60).

Intestinal Adhesiolysis in the Visceral Peritoneum

In patients with subileus complaints due to the formation of omental bridges between loops of bowel and the epiploic appendages, the bridges are double ligated and bloodlessly divided through the middle (see Plate IV-8.2 p. 387), as in the corresponding laparotomy technique. For safety reasons, a secondary Roeder loop ligature is applied according to the bloody adhesiolysis technique (Plate IV-7.1 p. 387).

Pelviscopic Monitoring of Neovagina Surgery

In placement of an artificial vagina via the vaginal route in patients with Rokytansky-Küstner-Mayer-Hauser syndrome, it is always difficult to achieve ideal preparation of the topographic vaginal cavity up to the level of the peritoneum in the pouch of Douglas. Heretofore, a wide abdominal incision was made to ensure visualization of the abdomen. However, pelviscopic monitoring of vaginal surgery is recommended today (Fig. 62). Using the combined technique, it is possible to optimally prepare the available cavity while avoiding the risk of perforation injury.

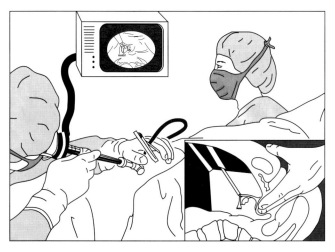

Fig. 62. An artificial vagina is prepared while simultaneously monitoring the pouch of Douglas via an accessory telescope or a television link (substitute for laparotomy)

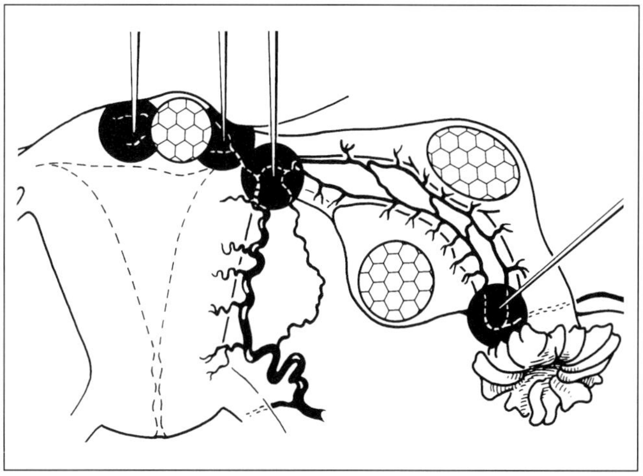

Fig. 63. Typical injection sites for 10-ml POR 8 infiltration in the main vascular supply regions of the uterus and adnexal vessels in preparation for tubal pregnancy operation or myoma enucleation. Dilution of *POR 8:* 5 IU (= 1 ml) in 100 ml NaCl solution

Intraoperative Conversion from Surgical Endoscopy to Laparotomy

Because patient preparation for surgical endoscopy is generally the same as for laparotomy, and because informed consent is obtained before starting the procedure, it is always possible to make the conversion to laparotomy at any time during surgical endoscopy. In some cases, the indication for laparotomy is dictated by the situation, *i.e.* complications. In others, laparotomy was regularly scheduled for the same session due to the preoperative diagnosis. This is the case with a tentative diagnosis of ovarian carcinoma.

Single-session surgical endoscopy with laparotomy is a borderline situation. In other words, it is generally accepted if operative pelviscopy is planned. Operative pelviscopy always comprises an attempt to avoid wide incision of the abdominal cavity. However, it should never be undertaken compulsively.

Postoperative Care

Postoperative care after endoscopic abdominal surgery is generally the same as for abdominal surgery via laparotomy. Following infertility surgery, *i.e.* refertilization surgery, hydropertubation is routinely performed on 5 consecutive postoperative days using the following solution:

1. 0.1 g hydrocortisone acetate
   4.0 g streptomycin sulfate
   0.4 g procaine hydrochloride
   enough distilled water to yield 100 ml
2. +5 mg α-chymotase to 20 ml hydrotubation solution directly prior to instillation

The procedure is painless if the flexible portio adapter is used together with the universal pertubation device designed by Fikentscher & Semm.

Because the endoscopic operation can be repeated without subjecting the patient the great physical stress, the range of indications differs from that of laparotomy. In the treatment of endometriosis genitalis, for example, we routinely perform 3-phase therapy according to SEMM (1980), which calls for routine repelviscopy after completion of hormone therapy and initial diagnostic and therapeutic pelviscopy.

The patient is usually discharged on the same day in minor pelviscopic surgery. In major operations such as hysterectomy, the hospitalization time is 1 to 3 days.

Documentation

The documentation of pelviscopic operations on film (full-format color slides) and on videotape has already been fully perfected. We will have to wait and see whether and to what extent the new charged coupled device (CCD) sensor technique will be capable of replacing photo-optical transmission systems.

Documentation will also be influenced by other rapid developments in the field of electronics in the next few years. The degree of sharpness and color fidelity of display images will continue to grow and enhance the potential for surgery under video monitor control (videoscopy). Beam-splitters are needed only in extremely difficult surgical techniques such as salpingostomy and intestinal suturing.

Errors and Complications and Their Prevention

The prerequisites for endoscopic abdominal surgery are:
1. Total mastery of the corresponding organ surgeries via laparotomy
2. Thorough training in diagnostic pelviscopy and laparoscopy
3. Adequate experience ín assisting and observing endoscopic abdominal surgeries
4. Availability of all the necessary instruments
5. Completion of four-phase Pelvi-Trainer instruction to ensure mastery of all endoscopic techniques (see Figs. 3/1– 3/4)

If these rules are observed, the technique-related operation risk can be kept extremely low. According to statistical data for the Federal Republic of Germany provided by Semm [12], Riedel and Semm [6], and Riedel et al. [7], fatalities were observed in 0.051 % of a total of 807,809 diagnostic and operative pelviscopies performed from 1945 to 1982, and in 0.024 % of 249,467 surgeries performed from 1983 to 1985.

The cause of death in the total of 15 fatalities reported in the 2nd pelviscopy survey was failure to promptly identify intestinal lesions in 9 cases, vessel injury in 3 cases, and anesthesia-related complications in 2 cases. The cause of death was not specified in one case.

The cause of death in a total of 6 fatalities reported in the 3rd pelviscopy survey (1988) was anesthesia-related complications in 2 cases, peritonitis and septic shock due to intestinal lesions in 2 cases, and vessel injury in 2 cases.

A total of 518 severe complications (requiring repelviscopy or laparotomy) were reported in the 2nd pelviscopy survey (1985). Of these complications, 36 % were due to laceration of the great vessels with the Veress needle or examining trocar, 25 % were due to inadvertent perforation of the bowel or stomach, and 14 % were due to burns in such organs as the intestine, bladder, or ureter. The rest were summarized as "other complications".

The hospitals that participated in the 3rd pelviscopy survey (1988) reported a total of 429 severe complications. Of these, 23.3 % were due to laceration of the great vessels, 38 % were due to inadvertent perforation of the bowel or stomach, and 15.2 % were due to burns in such organs as the intestine, bladder and ureter (65 % of which were attributable to high-frequency current). Such injuries as bleeding from lysed omental lobes, bleeding from divided Fallopian tubes, postpelviscopic bleeding, and anesthesia-related complications were summarized as "other complications".

Endoscopic abdominal surgery is a valuable technical addition to gynecologic surgery; it was able to prevent the use of laparotomy in around 80 % of these patients. For the patient, the technique provides considerable relief and reduction of physical operation-related stress due to the avoidance of large abdominal wall incisions. For the insurance company, the major benefit is a significant reduction in hospitalization and recovery times.

Short Description of Suturing and Knotting Techniques

Despite all the efforts to achieve hemostasis by means of tissue coagulation (*e.g.*, endocoagulation, high-frequency electrocoagulation, laser), hemostasis is still best achieved by means of optimal suturing. Also, whether in endoscopic surgery or classical surgery, optimal apposition of wound edges is best achieved by means of suturing, despite the availability of modern bonding and stapling techniques.

The most important knotting and suturing techniques are summarized in Plate VII p. 390. The Roeder knot for simple ligation of oozing vessels or omental segments is shown in Plate VII-1 p. 390. If tissue is under traction as in the CISH technique (e.g. adnex bundles, cervical fasciae stumps), the Semm safety knot should be used. The Roeder sliding knot remains absolutely intact after tying on an additional surgical knot (see Plate VII-2 p. 390 for technique).

If the tissue to be ligated cannot be drawn through a loop, i.e. an adhesional strand fixed at both ends, the suture is guided around it, and a Roeder knot with extracorporeal knotting is applied (Plate VII-3 and VII-4 p. 390). The knot can also be converted into a Semm safety knot by aftertying the knot keeping the "tail" long (Plate VII-2 p. 390). The extracorporal knot can be transformed into a "sliding knot" using a simple knot pusher (Plate VII-5 p. 390). Tissue under traction is not held very securely by the first knot. Therefore, 4 to 5 additional loops must be tied on with the help of the knot pusher.

The intracorporeal knotting technique shown in Plate VII-6 p. 390 should be used to apposition wound edges subjected to strong traction. In this technique, tight knotting is achieved by applying strong outward traction with the long end of the suture.

The knotting technique shown in Plate VII-7 p. 390 should be used when fine 4-0 to 6-0 sutures are required, *e.g.*, in surgery of the fimbria (eversion of the neck of the ampulla) or intestine. In this technique, a double surgical knot is also applied to ensure fixation of the knot (A-F). Complete security is achieved by the application an additional knot (G-I).

The emergency needle is used if bleeding from the abdominal wall occurs (Plate VII-8 p. 390). Very strong suture material that is quickly absorbed is recommended in this case.

Use of Laser

The dangers associated with high-frequency current, *i.e.* its uncontrollability, led to the introduction of endocoagulation. In endocoagulation, hemostasis is achieved at temperatures of around 100 °C. Thanks to miniaturization, it is possible to use the laser beam in surgical endoscopy for bloodless division of tissue not supplied by greater vessels. The available technology to date includes the CO_2 laser, the Nd:YAG laser, the argon laser, and the KTP laser, to name a few. These lasers are valuable additions to operative pelviscopic instrumentation.

In principle, the use of lasers often facilitates the operation. However, the laser has no other specific advantages. On the contrary, the rate of postoperative adhesion formation is much higher with lasers than with high-frequency electrocoagulation or endocoagulation.

References

1. FRANGENHEIM H: Die Bedeutung der Laparoskopie für die gynäkologische Diagnostik. Fortschr Med 76 (1958) 451.
2. HASSON HM: Clinical application of the wing sound device. Obstet. Gynec 43 (1974) 498-506.
3. KALK H: Erfahrungen mit der Laparoskopie. Z Klin Med 111 (1929) 303-348.
4. KÖNIG UD: Technik der offenen Pelviskopie: eine neue Methode für bessere Sicherheit in der Laparoskopie. Fortschr Med 97 (1979) 1850-1953.
5. PALMER R: La coelioscopie gynécologique. Rapport du Professeur Mocquot. Acad de Chir 72 (1946) 363-368.
6. RIEDEL HH, SEMM K: Die deutsche Pelviskopiestatistik der Jahre 1978-1982. Geburtsh Frauenheilk 39 (1985) 537-544.
7. RIEDEL HH et al.: Die Häufigkeitsverteilung verschiedener pelviskopischer (laparoskopischer) Operationsverfahren und deren Komplikationsraten. Geburtsh Frauenheilk 48 (1988) 791-799.
8. RUBIN JC: Technical principles in myomectomy with special references to hemostais. J Mt. Sinai Hosp. 17 (1951) 565.
9. SEMM K: Zur Technik der Eileiterdurchblasung. Z Geburts Gynäk 162 (1964) 48-53

10. SEMM K: Die gezielte und dosierbare Wärmekoagulation der gutartigen Portio-Veränderung. Geburtsh Frauenheilk 25 (1965) 795-802.
11. SEMM K: Pelviskopie und Hysteroskopie: Farbatlas und Lehrbuch. Schattauer, Stuttgart (1976).
12. SEMM K: Statistischer Überblick über die Bauchspiegelung in der Frauenheilkunde bis 1977 in der Bundesrepublik Deutschland. Geburtsh Frauenheilk 39 (1979) 537-544.
13. SEMM K: Die Automatisierung des Pneumoperitoneums für die endoskopische Abdominalchirurgie. Arch Gynaek 232 (1980) 738-739.
14. SEMM K (ed): Pelviskopie, Hysteroskopie und Fetoskopie. Stuttgart, Schattauer (1980).
15. SEMM K: Die operative Pelviskopie. In: Schwalm H, Döderlein G, Wulf K-H (eds): Klinik der Frauenheilkunde und Geburtshilfe. Bd 1,3 Ergänzung. Urban & Schwarzenberg, München Wien Baltimore (1983) 353-424.
16. SEMM K: Die endoskopische Appendektomie. Gynäkol Praxis 7 (1983) 131-140.
17. SEMM K: Operationslehre für endoskopische Abdominalchirurgie – operative Pelviskopie, operative Laparoskopie. Schattauer, Stuttgart (1984).
18. SEMM K: Differentialdiagnose der Endometriose 2 (1985) 21-37.
19. SEMM K: Endometriose. In: Schneider HPC, Lauritzen CH, Niemann H (eds): Grundlagen und Klinik der menschlichen Fortpflanzung. De Gruyter, Berlin (1986) 1009-1057.
20. SEMM K: Pelvi-Trainer, ein Übungsgerät für die operative Pelviskopie zum Erlernen endoskopischer Ligatur und Nahttechnik. Geburtsh Frauenheilk 46 (1986) 60-62.
21. SEMM K: Drainage der Bauchhöhle nach operativer Pelviskopie. Böhringer, Ingelheim (1988).
22. SEMM K: Sichtkontrollierte Peritoneumperforation zur operativen Pelviskopie. Geburtsh Frauenheilk 48 (1989) 381-468.
23. SEMM K (ed): Pelviskopie: ein operative Leitfaden. 2. Aufl. Kiel (1991).
24. SEMM K: Morzellieren und Nähen per pelviskopiam – kein Problem mehr. Geburtsh Frauenheilk 51 (1991) 843-846.
25. SEMM K: Das Pneumoperitoneum: Fehler und Gefahren. Laparo-Endosk Chir 1 (1992) 1-20.
26. SEMM K: Hysterektomie per laparotomiam oder per pelviskopiam. Geburtsh Frauenheilk 51 (1992) 996-1003.
27. SEMM K: Total Uterus Mucosa Ablatio (TUMA) – C*U*R*T anstelle Endometrium-Ablation. Das geheizte Pneumoperitoneum. Thieme, Stuttgart (1992).
28. SEMM K, METTLER L: Local infiltration of Ornithine 8-Vasopression (POR 8) as a Vasconstrictive Agent in Surgical Pelviscopy (applied to myoma enucleation, salpingotomy in cases of tubal pregnancy and peripheral salpingostomy. Endoscopy 20 (1988) 298-304.
29. STEPTOE PC: Laparoscopy in Gynaecology. Livingstone, Edinburgh (1964).
30. WILDHIRT E: Mediastinalemphysem bei Laparoskopie und zur Luftembolie bei Laparoskopien. Münch Med Wschr 98 (1956) 48-58.
31. WILDHIRT E, KALK H: Lehrbuch und Atlas der Laparoskopie und Leberpunktion. Thieme, Stuttgart (1965).

References for IVH

1. FREUND WA: Bemerkungen zu meiner Methode der Uterus-Exstirpation. Ztbl 2 (1978) 497-500.
2. REICH H, DECAPIRO J, McGLYNN F: Laparoscopic Hysterectomy. J Gynecol. Surg. 5 (1989) 213.
3. SEMM K: Intrafasziale vaginale Hysterektomie (IVH) mit oder ohne pelviskopischer Assistenz. Geburtsh. Fraueneheilk. 53 (1993) 873-878.

1.2.1 Enucleation of subserous myomas

1.2.1
Schematic representation of the enucleation of subserous or partially subserous myomas

1.2.2 Enucleation of intramural myomas

1.2.2
Enucleation of intramural myomas with subsequent capsule suturing

1.4 Hysterectomy without colpotomy

1.4
Intrafascial hysterectomy (CISH): After classical ligation of the adnexal bundle (with or without adnexectomy), a cylinder of tissue in the cervix and uterine cavity up to the uterine fundus is resected. The uterus is triply ligated with Semm safety loops and divided. The cervical stump is recoagulated and the tissue stumps are extraperitonealized

2.1 Ovariolysis

2.1
Ovariolysis with scissors or laser

2.2 Ovarian biopsy

2.2
Ovarian biopsy with double-pronged biopsy forceps and cylinder resection using the elliptical trocar sleeve. Hemostasis is achieved by point coagulating the tissue at 120 ° C.

2.4 Ovarian cyst enucleation and ovarian suture

2.4
The ovarian cyst is enucleated following infiltration with POR 8 solution. The edges of the tunica albuginea are brought into apposition by an endoscopic suture (extracorporeal knotting)

Plate I
Organ-Oriented Catalogue of Pelviscopic Surgery

1.2.1 Enucleation of subserous myomas

1.2.2 Enucleation of intramural myomas

1.4 Hysterectomy without colpotomy

2.1 Ovariolysis   2.2 Ovarian biopsy

2.4 Ovarian cyst enucleation and ovarian suture

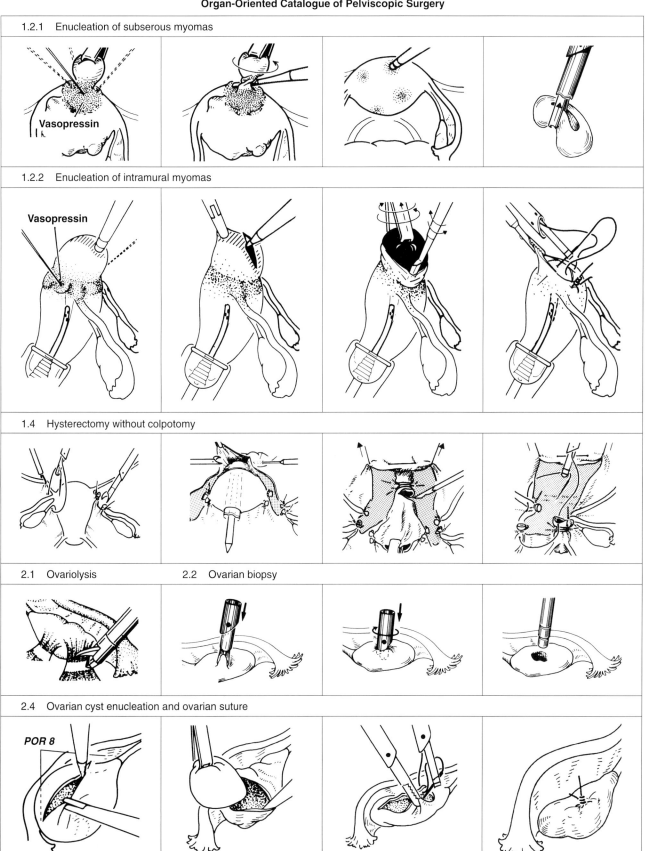

2.5 Fimbriolysis	2.6 Salpingolysis
2.5 Fimbriolysis with myoma enucleator preheated to 110 ° C and crocodile forceps, or sharp dissection with micro-scissors or laser	2.6 Salpingolysis with microscissors

2.7   Fimbrioplasty
2.7 Blunt fimbrioplasty with the help of atraumatic grasping forceps

2.8   Salpingostomy
2.8 Salpingostomy with or without endocoagulator after POR 8 injection with subsequent microsuture and endocorporeal knotting

3.1   Oophorectomy with triple-loop ligature
3.1 Oophorectomy (triple-loop ligature according to SEMM) and morcellation with S.E.M.M. Set if indicated

3.2   Tubal sterilization with endocoagulation and sharp dissection
3.2 Tubal sterilization with sharp dissection of the Fallopian tubes after achieving hemostasis with the crocodile forceps at 120 ° C

Plate II
Organ-Oriented Catalogue of Pelviscopic Surgery

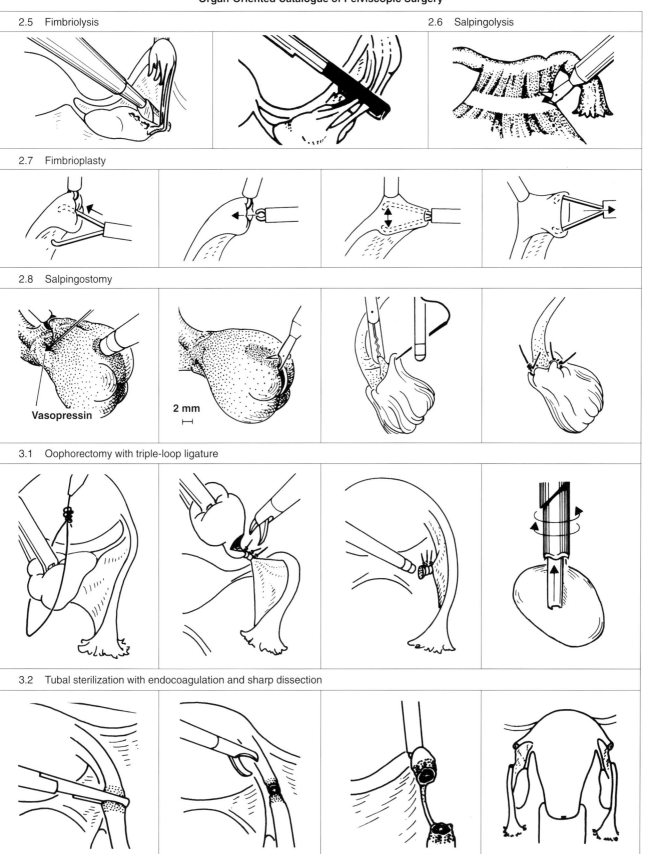

2.5 Fimbriolysis

2.6 Salpingolysis

2.7 Fimbrioplasty

2.8 Salpingostomy

Vasopressin

2 mm

3.1 Oophorectomy with triple-loop ligature

3.2 Tubal sterilization with endocoagulation and sharp dissection

3.4   Adnexectomy with triple-loop ligation technique

3.4
Adnexectomy (triple-loop ligature according to SEMM) and subsequent coagulation of the tissue stumps with the point coagulator pre-heated to 120 ° C for prevention of postoperative adhesion formation

4.1.1   Tubectomy with triple-loop ligation technique for tubal pregnancy or hydrosalpinx

4.1.1
Radical treatment of tubal pregnancy; tubectomy (with triple-loop ligature) with or without excision of tubal origin

4.1.2   Conservative treatment of tubal pregnancy

4.1.2
Conservative, i.e. tube-preserving, therapy of tubal pregnancy with POR 8 infiltration and microsutures with endocorporal knotting for apposition of serosal wound edges

Coagulation of endometrial foci in the

5.1 Peritoneum	5.2 Sacrouterine lig.	5.3 Ovary	5.7 Dome of the bladder
5.1 Point coagulation of endometrial foci with peritoneal suturing for apposition of wound edges if necessary	5.2 Coagulation of endom etrial foci in the region of the sacrouterine ligament with enucleation of nodules if indicated	5.3 Removal of retro-ovarian foci	5.7 Point coagulation of foci on the dome of the bladder (Endocoagulator)

Plate III
Organ-Oriented Catalogue of Pelviscopic Surgery

3.4   Adnexectomy with triple-loop ligation technique

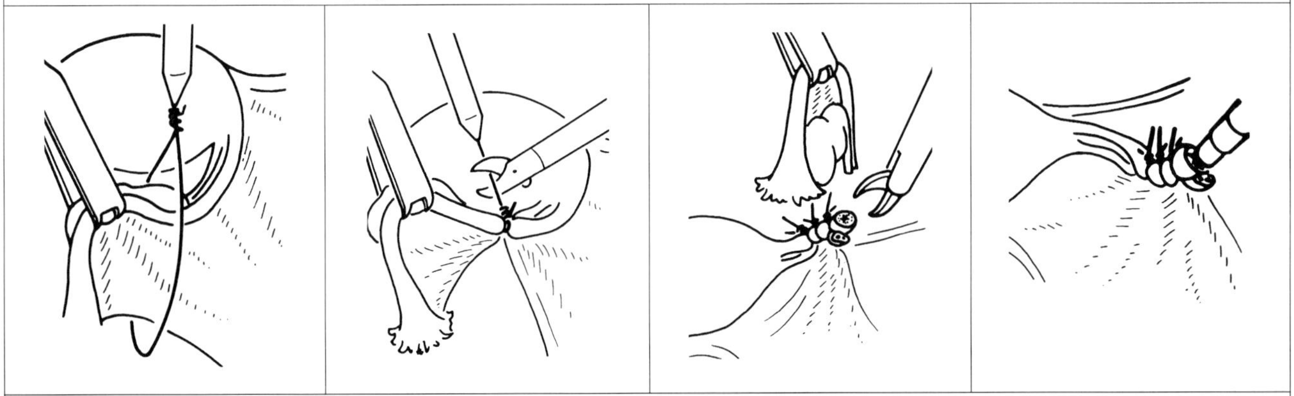

4.1.1   Tubectomy with triple-loop ligation technique for tubal pregnancy or hydrosalpinx

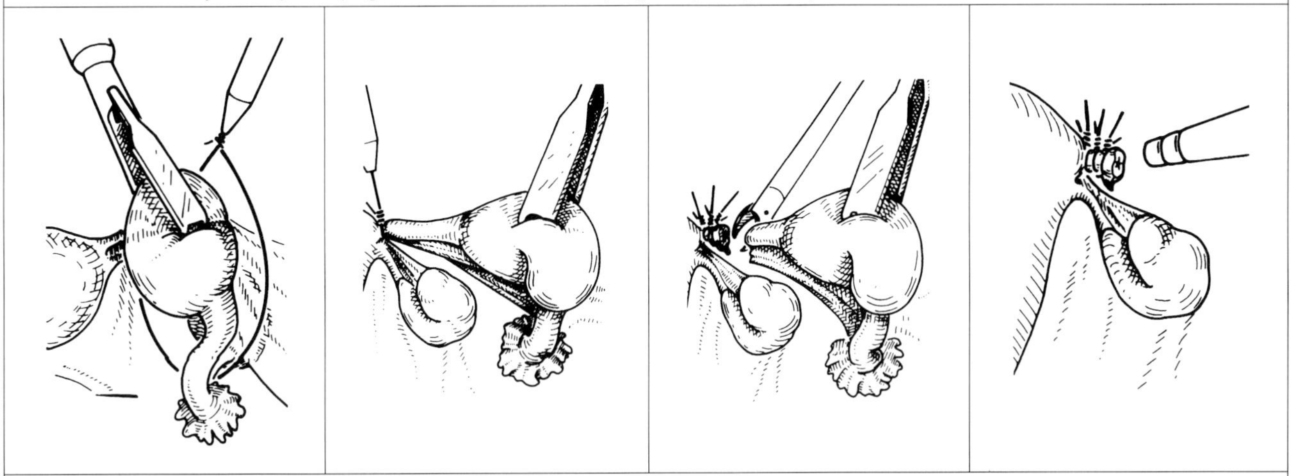

4.1.2   Conservative treatment of tubal pregnancy

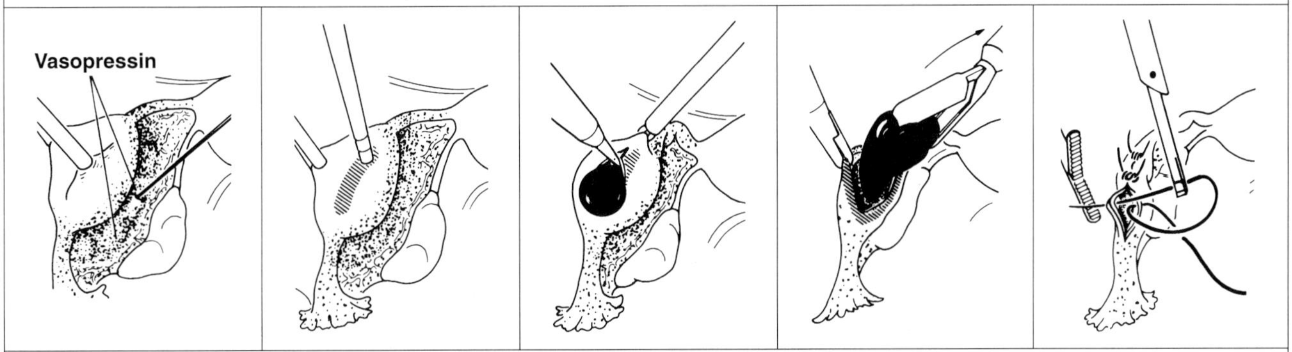

Vasopressin

Coagulation of endometrial foci in the

5.1 Peritoneum   5.2 Sacrouterine lig.   5.3 Ovary   5.7 Dome of the bladder

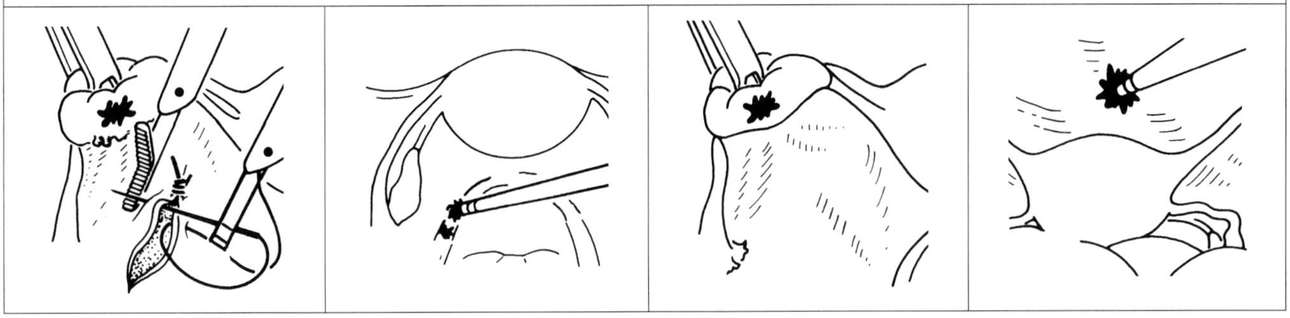

7.1   Bloody adhesiolysis

7.1
Bloody adhesiolysis: Sharp dissection of adhesions followed by Roeder loop ligature for hemostasis

7.2   Bloodless adhesiolysis

7.2
Bloodless adhesiolysis: Ligation and subsequent dissection of highly vascularized adhesions

8.1   Intestinal adhesiolysis and suturing

8.1
Dissection of adherent bowel and parietal peritoneum followed by serosal microsuturing or transverse intestinal closure in 1 to 2 layers

8.2   Intestinal adhesiolysis, omental resection

8.2
Dissection of highly vascularized intestinal adhesions via double endoligature with extracorporeal knotting

Plate IV
Organ-Oriented Catalogue of Pelviscopic Surgery

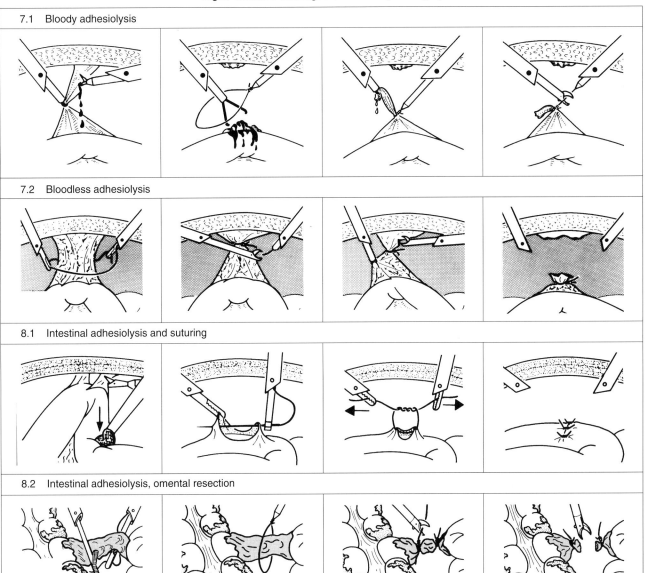

7.1 Bloody adhesiolysis

7.2 Bloodless adhesiolysis

8.1 Intestinal adhesiolysis and suturing

8.2 Intestinal adhesiolysis, omental resection

Plate V
Classical Intrafascial Serrated Edge Macro-Morcellated (S.E.M.M.) Hysterectomy (CISH) with the Classical Uterine Resection Tool (CURT)

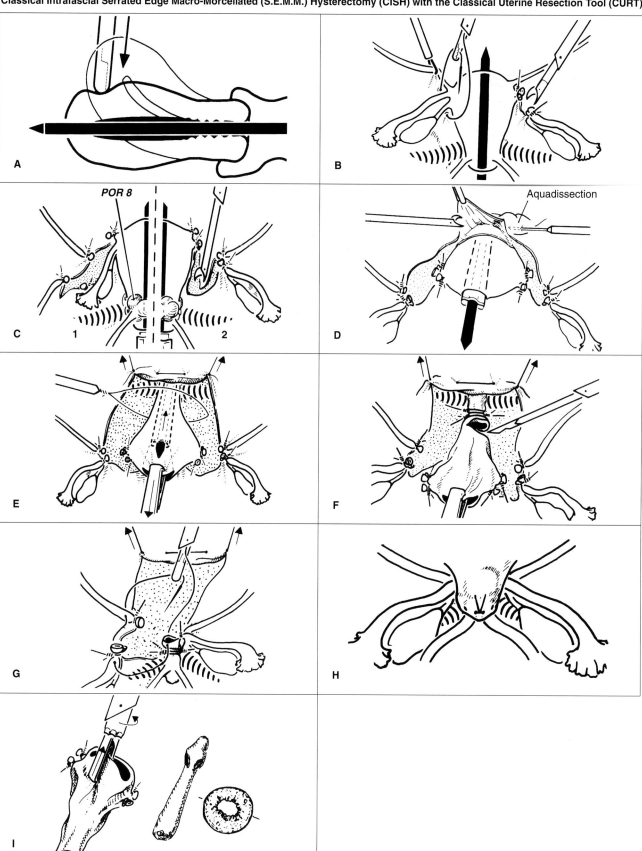

Plate VI
Total Uterine Mucosa Ablation (TUMA)

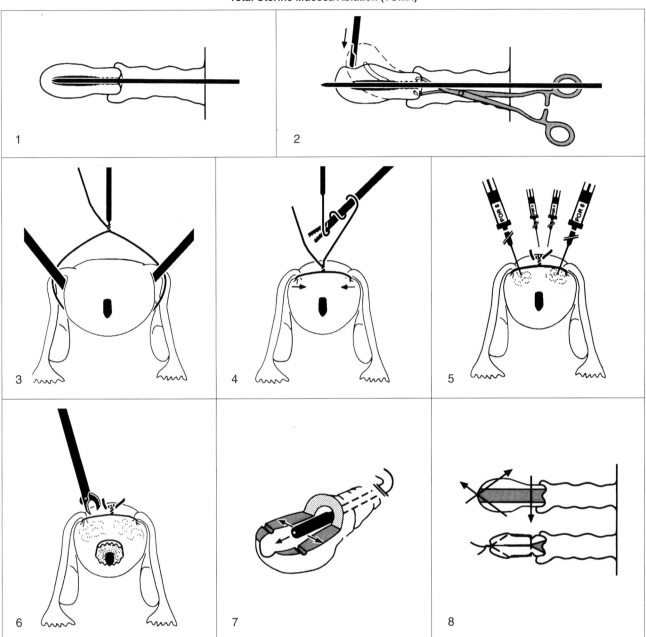

Plate VII
Endoscopic Knotting Techniques

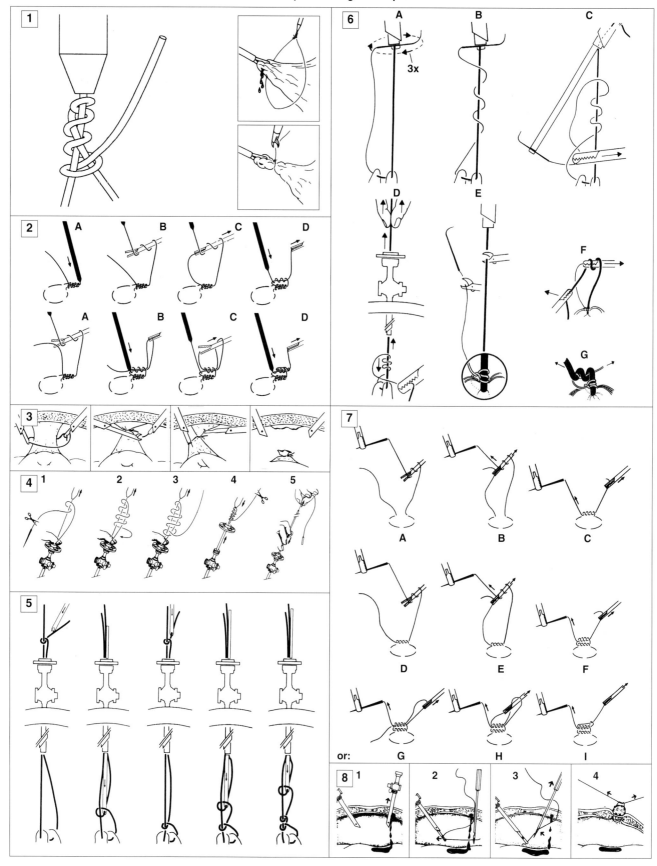

Plate VIII
Steps of Intrafascial Vaginal Hysterectomy (IVH)

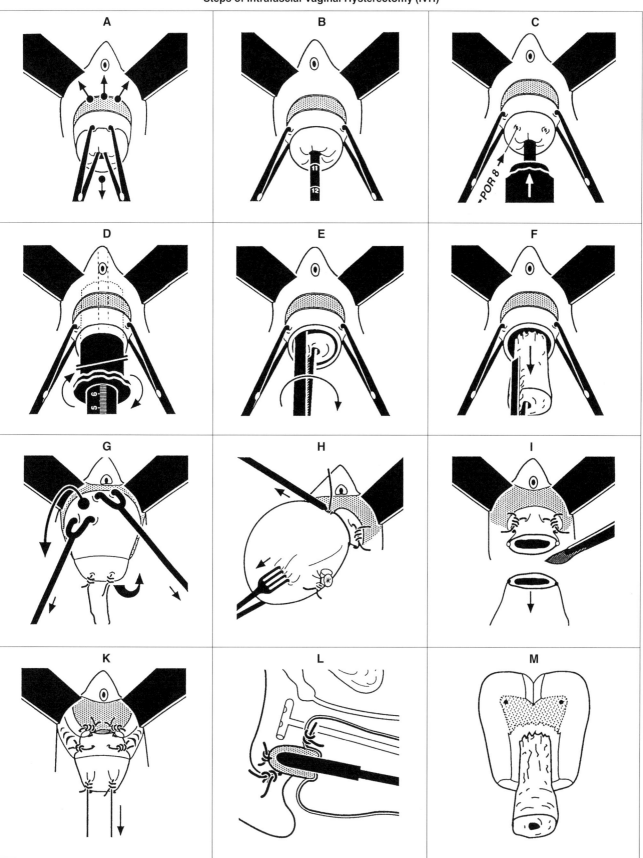

Index

A

abdomen
-, acute 215-217
Abdominal Cavity Expander (ACE) 21
abscess 144, 207
-, periappendiceal 203
-, pericolic 216
achalasia 109
-, esophageal 85
achlorhydria 116
acidosis 231
acid secretion
-, basal 92
-, pentagastrin stimulated 92
adenocarcinoma *see* carcinoma
adenoma
-, tubular 173
-, tubulovillous 173
adenomatous polyposis
-, familial 152, 163, 166
adhesiolysis 165, 304, 331, 355, 368, 370, 375
-, bloodless 375f
-, bloody 375
adhesion 109, 114, 143, 152, 215f, 263, 268, 304f, 334, 340
-, intestinal 13
-, intra-abdominal 50
-, (to the) liver bed 52
-, omental 13
-, pleural 275, 282
-, prophylaxis 239
adnexectomy 371-373
adrenalectomy 144, 301, 335
-, transperitoneal 323
adrenal gland 301
air leak 293
analgetics 234
anastomosis 144, 151
-, colo-anal 181
-, double-stapled 161, 163, 165f
-, end-to-end 157, 161, 165
-, extracorporeal 156f
-, gastrojejunal 124
-, hand-sutured 123, 127, 163
- -, gastroenterostomy 123
- -, gastrojejunostomy 123
-, ileorectal 166

-, intra-abdominal 37f
-, intracorporeal 154, 157
-, side-to-side 157
-, stapled 122, 124, 127, 191
-, transanal hand-sewn 191
-, triple-stapling 163, 181
-, vesicourethral 312
anastomotic leak 124, 128, 151, 157, 163
anemia
-, hemolytic 209
anesthesia
-, local 220
aneurysma 237
angiography
-, mesenteric 143
-, radionuclide 339
angioinfarction 301
angioma 237
Angle of His 97
animal experiments 191
anorchidism 242
-, congenital 242
antibiotic(s) 41, 49, 153, 204, 264
-, bowel preparation 174
-, prophylaxis 41f, 120, 123, 198
- -, choice of 41
antrectomy 91f, 102
aortic bifurcation 16
aperistalsis
-, (of) esophagus 109
appendectomy 7, 42, 152, 203-208, 216, 235, 238, 353
appendiceal stump
-, everted 206
-, inverted 206
-, leak 207
appendicitis 152
-, acute 203f, 216
appendix
-, abscess 144, 207
- -, periappendiceal 203
-, pelvic 205
-, perforated 205
-, retrocecal 205
ascites 216
aspiration 231
atelectasis 115